Hematologic Cancers: Essentials in Oncology

Hematologic Cancers: Essentials in Oncology

Edited by Wesley Ortiz

hayle medical

New York

Hayle Medical,
750 Third Avenue, 9th Floor,
New York, NY 10017, USA

Visit us on the World Wide Web at:
www.haylemedical.com

ISBN: 978-1-63241-850-0

Cataloging-in-Publication Data

Hematologic cancers : essentials in oncology / edited by Wesley Ortiz.
p. cm.
Includes bibliographical references and index.
ISBN 978-1-63241-850-0
1. Hematological oncology. 2. Lymphoproliferative disorders. 3. Blood--Cancer.
4. Oncology. I. Ortiz, Wesley.

RC280.H47 H46 2020
616.994 18--dc21

Table of Contents

Preface IX

Chapter 1 **Inhibition of MDM2 by Nilotinib Contributes to Cytotoxicity in Both Philadelphia-Positive and Negative Acute Lymphoblastic Leukemia** 1
Hailong Zhang, Lubing Gu, Tao Liu, Kuang-Yueh Chiang and Muxiang Zhou

Chapter 2 **Multi-Agent Chemotherapy Overcomes Glucocorticoid Resistance Conferred by a *BIM* Deletion Polymorphism in Pediatric Acute Lymphoblastic Leukemia** 9
Sheila Xinxuan Soh, Joshua Yew Suang Lim, John W. J. Huang, Nan Jiang, Allen Eng Juh Yeoh and S. Tiong Ong

Chapter 3 **The Progeroid Phenotype of Ku80 Deficiency is Dominant over DNA-PK$_{CS}$ Deficiency** 21
Erwin Reiling, Martijn E. T. Dollé, Sameh A.Youssef, Moonsook Lee, Bhawani Nagarajah, Marianne Roodbergen, Piet de With, Alain de Bruin, Jan H. Hoeijmakers, Jan Vijg, Harry van Steeg and Paul Hasty

Chapter 4 **Comparison between Karyotyping-FISH-Reverse Transcription PCR and RNA- Sequencing-Fusion Gene Identification Programs in the Detection of *KAT6A-CREBBP* in Acute Myeloid Leukemia** 30
Ioannis Panagopoulos, Synne Torkildsen, Ludmila Gorunova, Anne Tierens, Geir E. Tjønnfjord and Sverre Heim

Chapter 5 **Inhibition of the MDM2 E3 Ligase Induces Apoptosis and Autophagy in Wild-Type and Mutant p53 Models of Multiple Myeloma and Acts Synergistically with ABT-737** 37
Dongmin Gu, Shuhong Wang, Isere Kuiatse, Hua Wang, Jin He, Yun Dai, Richard J. Jones, Chad C. Bjorklund, Jing Yang, Steven Grant and Robert Z. Orlowski

Chapter 6 **Risk of Multiple Myeloma in Rheumatoid Arthritis** 49
Kaini Shen, Gufeng Xu, Qing Wu, Daobin Zhou and Jian Li

Chapter 7 **MYC Expression in Concert with BCL2 and BCL6 Expression Predicts Outcome in Chinese Patients with Diffuse Large B-Cell Lymphoma, not Otherwise Specified** 57
Li-Xu Yan, Yan-Hui Liu, Dong-Lan Luo, Fen Zhang, Yu Cheng, Xin-Lan Luo, Jie Xu, Jie Cheng and Heng-Guo Zhuang

Chapter 8 **The Deficiency of Tumor Suppressor *Prep1* Accelerates the Onset of *Meis1- Hoxa9* Leukemogenesis** 73
Leila Dardaei, Livia Modica, Giorgio Iotti and Francesco Blasi

Chapter 9 **A Gene Panel, Including *LRP12*, is Frequently Hypermethylated in Major Types of B-Cell Lymphoma** 80
Nicole Bethge, Hilde Honne, Kim Andresen, Vera Hilden, Gunhild Trøen, Knut Liestøl, Harald Holte, Jan Delabie, Guro E. Lind and Erlend B. Smeland

Chapter 10 **Serum Levels of Interleukin-9 Correlate with Negative Prognostic Factors in Extranodal NK/T-Cell Lymphoma** 88
Jing Zhang, Wei-da Wang, Qi-rong Geng, Liang Wang, Xiao-qin Chen, Cheng-cheng Liu and Yue Lv

Chapter 11 **The use of Novel Drugs can Effectively Improve Response, Delay Relapse and Enhance Overall Survival in Multiple Myeloma Patients with Renal Impairment** 98
Katarina Uttervall, Adil D. Duru, Johan Lund, Johan Liwing, Gösta Gahrton, Erik Holmberg, Johan Aschan, Evren Alici and Hareth Nahi

Chapter 12 **Effects of ^{28}Si Ions, ^{56}Fe Ions and Protons on the Induction of Murine Acute Myeloid Leukemia and Hepatocellular Carcinoma** 108
Michael M. Weil, F. Andrew Ray, Paula C. Genik, Yongjia Yu, Maureen McCarthy, Christina M. Fallgren and Robert L. Ullrich

Chapter 13 **Loss of Function of TET2 Cooperates with Constitutively Active KIT in Murine and Human Models of Mastocytosis** 116
Serena De Vita, Rebekka K.Schneider, Michael Garcia, Jenna Wood, Mathilde Gavillet, Benjamin L.Ebert, Alexander Gerbaulet, Axel Roers, Ross L. Levine, Ann Mullally and David A. Williams

Chapter 14 **Serum Thymidine Kinase Activity: Analytical Performance, Age-Related Reference Ranges and Validation in Chronic Lymphocytic Leukemia** 129
Eszter Szánthó, Harjit Pal Bhattoa, Mária Csobán, Péter Antal-Szalmás, Anikó Újfalusi, János Kappelmayer and Zsuzsanna Hevessy

Chapter 15 **FTY720 Induces Apoptosis of M2 Subtype Acute Myeloid Leukemia Cells by Targeting Sphingolipid Metabolism and Increasing Endogenous Ceramide Levels** 136
Limin Chen, Liu-Fei Luo, Junyan Lu, Lianchun Li, Yuan-Fang Liu, Jiang Wang, Hong Liu, Heng Song, Hualiang Jiang, Sai-Juan Chen, Cheng Luo and Keqin Kathy Li

Chapter 16 **Phenotypic, Genomic and Functional Characterization Reveals no Differences between CD138^{++} and CD138^{low} Subpopulations in Multiple Myeloma Cell Lines** 149
Teresa Paíno, María E.Sarasquete, Bruno Paiva, Patryk Krzeminski, Laura San-Segundo, Luis A. Corchete, Alba Redondo, Mercedes Garayoa, Ramón García-Sanz, Norma C. Gutiérrez, Enrique M. Ocio and Jesús F. San-Miguel

Chapter 17 **Dissecting the Regulatory Microenvironment of a Large Animal Model of Non-Hodgkin Lymphoma: Evidence of a Negative Prognostic Impact of FOXP3^{+} T Cells in Canine B Cell Lymphoma** 161
Dammy Pinheiro, Yu-Mei Chang, Hannah Bryant, Balazs Szladovits, Tim Dalessandri, Lucy J. Davison, Elizabeth Yallop, Emily Mills, Chiara Leo, Ana Lara, Anneliese Stell, Gerry Polton and Oliver A. Garden

Chapter 18 **NSFC Health Research Funding and Burden of Disease** 176
Gelin Xu, Zhizhong Zhang, Qiushi Lv, Yun Li, Ruidong Ye, Yunyun Xiong, Yongjun Jiang and Xinfeng Liu

Chapter 19 **Cellular Intrinsic Mechanism Affecting the Outcome of AML Treated with Ara-C in a Syngeneic Mouse Model** 186
Wenjun Zhao, Lirong Wei, Dongming Tan, Guangsong Su, Yanwen Zheng, Chao He, Zhengwei J Mao, Timothy P. Singleton and Bin Yin

Chapter 20 **The *NPM1* Mutation Type has no Impact on Survival in Cytogenetically Normal AML** 197
Friederike Pastore, Philipp A. Greif, Stephanie Schneider, Bianka Ksienzyk, Gudrun Mellert, Evelyn Zellmeier, Jan Braess, Cristina M. Sauerland, Achim Heinecke, Utz Krug, Wolfgang E. Berdel, Thomas Buechner, Bernhard Woermann, Wolfgang Hiddemann and Karsten Spiekermann

Chapter 21 **Establishment of a Humanized APL Model via the Transplantation of *PML-RARA*-Transduced Human Common Myeloid Progenitors into Immunodeficient Mice** 203
Hiromichi Matsushita, Takashi Yahata, Yin Sheng, Yoshihiko Nakamura, Yukari Muguruma, Hideyuki Matsuzawa, Masayuki Tanaka, Hideki Hayashi, Tadayuki Sato, Anar Damdinsuren, Makoto Onizuka, Mamoru Ito, Hayato Miyachi, Pier Paolo Pandolfi and Kiyoshi Ando

Permissions

List of Contributors

Index

Preface

Hematologic cancers are the malignancies of the hematopoietic and lymphoid tissues that affect the blood, lymph, bone marrow and lymphatic system. These derive from two blood lineages- lymphoid and myeloid cell lines. Lymphomas, myeloma and lymphocytic leukemias are lymphoid line malignancies, while myelodysplastic syndromes, myeloproliferative diseases, and acute and chronic myelogenous leukemia are myeloid in origin. A blood film and a complete blood count are essential for the diagnosis of a blood cancer. A bone marrow biopsy is usually needed for the analysis of these disorders. These cancers are targeted through symptomatic treatment or more aggressively with immunotherapy, chemotherapy, radiotherapy and a bone marrow transplant. In case of a successful treatment, patients are followed up at regular intervals to detect recurrences and secondary malignancies. This book provides comprehensive insights into the field of oncology. It unfolds the innovative aspects of hematologic cancers, which will be crucial for the progress of this field in the future. It will help the readers in keeping pace with the rapid changes in this field.

The information shared in this book is based on empirical researches made by veterans in this field of study. The elaborative information provided in this book will help the readers further their scope of knowledge leading to advancements in this field.

Finally, I would like to thank my fellow researchers who gave constructive feedback and my family members who supported me at every step of my research.

Editor

1

Inhibition of MDM2 by Nilotinib Contributes to Cytotoxicity in both Philadelphia-Positive and Negative Acute Lymphoblastic Leukemia

Hailong Zhang[9], **Lubing Gu**[9], **Tao Liu, Kuang-Yueh Chiang, Muxiang Zhou***

Department of Pediatrics and Aflac Cancer and Blood Disorders Center, Emory University School of Medicine, Atlanta, Georgia, United States of America

Abstract

Nilotinib is a selective BCR-ABL tyrosine kinase inhibitor related to imatinib that is more potent than imatinib. Nilotinib is widely used to treat chronic myelogenous leukemia (CML) and Philadelphia-positive (Ph+) acute lymphoblastic leukemia (ALL). The present study identifies Mouse double minute 2 homolog (MDM2) as a target of nilotinib. In studying ALL cell lines, we found that the expression of MDM2 in both Philadelphia positive (Ph+) and Philadelphia negative (Ph-) ALL cells was remarkably inhibited by nilotinib, in a dose- and time-dependent manner. Further studies demonstrated that nilotinib inhibited MDM2 at the post-translational level by inducing MDM2 self-ubiquitination and degradation. Nilotinib-mediated MDM2 downregulation did not result in accumulation and activation of p53. Inhibition of MDM2 in nilotinib-treated ALL cells led to downregulation of the anti-apoptotic protein X-linked inhibitor of apoptosis protein (XIAP), a translational target of MDM2, resulting in activation of caspases. Inhibition of XIAP following nilotinib-mediated downregulation of MDM2 resulted in apoptosis of MDM2-expressing ALL; however, similar nilotinib treatment induced stronger apoptosis in Ph+/MDM2+ ALL than in Ph-/MDM2+ or Ph+/MDM2- ALL. The ALL cells that were Ph-/MDM2- were totally resistant to nilotinib. These results suggested that nilotinib can inhibit MDM2 and induce a p53-independent apoptosis pathway by downregulating XIAP; thus, nilotinib can treat not only Ph+, but also Ph- ALL patients whose cancer cells overexpress MDM2.

Editor: Andrei L. Gartel, University of Illinois at Chicago, United States of America

Funding: This work was supported by the National Institutes of Health (R01 CA123490 and R01CA143107 to MZ) and CURE (to MZ and LG). The funders had no role in study design, data collection and analysis, decision to publish, or preparation of the manuscript.

Competing Interests: The authors have declared that no competing interests exist.

* Email: mzhou@emory.edu

[9] These authors contributed equally to this work.

Introduction

The tyrosine kinase inhibitors (TKIs) such as imatinib, dasatinib and nilitinib were designed and developed for the treatment of chronic myelogenous leukemia (CML) and certain acute lymphoblastic leukemia (ALL), based on the knowledge that the protein kinase ABL is constitutively activated in patients with these disease. It is known that the constitutive activation of ABL observed in CML and ALL patients is due to a t(9;21) chromosome translocation (Ph), in which the BCR protein becomes fused to ABL, to generate the BCR-ABL oncoprotein that drives both transformation and leukemogenesis [1]. This Philadelphia or Ph chromosome is found in almost all patients with CML and in 25-30% patients with ALL, where it produces a 210-KD and a 190-KD form of the BCR-ABL protein, respectively, in CML and ALL [2,3]. BCR-ABL then activates a large number of signaling pathways in the cells [4,5]; however, many of these pathways are thought to act in a redundant fashion as only a few signaling components such as PI3K/AKT, NF-KB and STAT are reported to be critical for BCR-ABL-mediated oncogenic transformation and leukemogenesis [5–7].

Inhibition of the BCR-ABL tyrosine kinase activity by imatinib, the first generation of specific BCR-ABL inhibitors, results in durable cytogenetic and molecular remissions in the majority of CML and Ph+ ALL; however, not all patients benefit from treatment, due to drug resistance and intolerance [8,9]. This led to the development of second-generation TKIs, such as nilotinib, which is more potent than imatinib and is currently approved for the treatment of newly diagnosed, imatinib-resistant or imatinib-intolerant CML and Ph+ ALL [10]. Although very successful hematologic and cytogenetic responses are obtained in nilotinib-treated patients, in recent years there have been cases with resistance to nilotinib [11,12]. On the other hand, imatinib and nilotinib are also reported to induce apoptosis in BCR-ABL– cells of lymphoid origin [13] and are used for treatment of other types of cancer, such as advanced gastrointestinal stromal tumors [14]. The fact that some BCR-ABL+ cases are not sensitive to imatinib nor nilotinib and that some BCR-ABL– cancer cells are still killed by imatinib or nilotinib suggests the existence of additional pathways regulated by BCR-ABL in leukemia cell growth, and multiple mechanisms of action of imatinib and nilotinib in inducing cancer cell apoptosis. For example, it is reported that several cell survival and anti-apoptotic proteins such as BCL-X, survivin and histone deacetylases are downregulated by imatinib and nilotinib, which contribute to their cytotoxic and apoptotic activities [15–17].

MDM2, an oncoprotein, is also a regulatory target of BCR-ABL. BCR-ABL activates MDM2 mRNA translation [18] and the existence of MDM2 is required for the survival effects of BCR-ABL in hematopoietic cells [19]. In addition, c-ABL phosphorylates MDM2, facilitating formation of the MDM2-MDM4 complex, and MDM2 becomes stabilized in the MDM2-MDM4 complexes [20,21]. The main oncogenic function of MDM2 is to inhibit the tumor suppressor p53 [22,23]; thus, p53 function becomes inactivated in MDM2-overexpressing cells, resulting in cancer cell growth. MDM2 also plays p53-independent roles in oncogenesis. Increasing evidence suggests that even in p53-deficient cancer patients, MDM2 overexpression is still involved in cancer promotion and progression, as well as resistance to treatment [24]. This is because, in addition to interacting with and regulating p53, MDM2 interacts with other molecules involved in oncogenesis. We recently reported that binding of the C-terminal RING domain of the MDM2 protein to XIAP mRNA regulates translation of this apoptosis regulator, which allows for development of resistance to anticancer treatment [25]. Overexpression of MDM2 due to genomic amplification occurs in a variety of human cancers [26]. High levels of MDM2 expression can still be observed even in malignancies without MDM2 gene amplification, as occurs in leukemia [27]. Although no detailed studies on MDM2 expression in CML have been reported, it is known that overexpression of MDM2 is observed in 20 to 30% of patients with ALL [28-30] and is found to be associated with early treatment failure and a poor prognosis [31–34].

Because MDM2 is positively regulated by c-ABL and BCR-ABL, we evaluated whether inhibition of the ABL activity by nilotinib had effects on MDM2 expression. We found that nilotinib strongly inhibited MDM2 expression and induced apoptosis of both BCR-ABL positive and negative ALL cells. Herein, we delineate the mechanism by which nilotinib inhibits MDM2 expression and the mechanistic steps involved in MDM2 downregulation that induce ALL cell apoptosis.

Materials and Methods

Cells and reagents

This study used six established cell lines derived from children with ALL. Four of these cell lines (EU-1, EU-5, EU-6 and EU-9) were established at Emory University by Dr. Muxiang Zhou, and two (UOC-B1 and SUP-B15) were established at University of Chicago by Dr. Stephen D. Smith. All cell lines were authenticated and their phenotypes, including the status of p53 and BCR-ABL as well as MDM2 expression levels, were characterized by Drs. Zhou and Smith in prior publications [28,35]. All cell lines grew in standard culture medium (RPMI 1640 containing 10% FBS, 2 mM L-glutamine, 50 U penicillin and 50 µg/ml streptomycin), at 37°C in 5% CO_2. The nilotinib (>98% pure) used was purchased from Caymanchem (Ann Arbor, MI, USA), and stock solution was prepared at a concentration of 10 mM, in deionized water. The treatment of cells was by exposure to 0.25–5 µM of nilotinib, for the time periods given. Antibody to Bcr-Abl (Ab-3) was purchased from Calbiochem. We also purchased antibody to MDM2 (SMP14) from Sigma, antibody to p53 (DO-1) from Santa Cruz, antibodies to p21 (12D1) and PARP (7D3-6) from Cell Signaling, and antibody to XIAP (2F1) from Abcam. The concentrations of all antibodies were used according to the manufacturers' instructions. The caspase-3 and caspase-9 ELISA kits were purchased from Enzo.

Plasmid, siRNA and transfection

The XIAP expression plasmid pCDNA3-6myc-XIAP was provided by Dr. L. Yang (Emory University). For XIAP gene transfection, SUP-B15 cells in exponential growth were transfected with pCDNA3-6myc-XIAP plasmid and vehicle control plasmid by electroporation at 300 V, 950 µF using a Gene Pulser II System (Bio-Rad, Hercules, CA). The p53 siRNA and control siRNA were purchased from Santa Cruz. Transfection of these siRNAs was performed using the HiPerFect transfection reagent (Qiagen), following the manufacturer's manual.

Immunoprecipitation (IP) and western blot assay

Cells were lysed in a buffer composed of 50 mM Tris-HCl, pH 7.6, 150 mM NaCl, 1% Nonidet P-40, 10 mM sodium phosphate, 10 mM NaF, 1 mM sodium orthovanadate, 2 mM phenylmethylsulfonyl fluoride (PMSF), 10 µg/ml aprotinin, 10 µg/ml leupeptin and 10 µg/ml pepstatin. After centrifugation, the clarified cell lysate was incubated with 15 µl Protein G plus/ Protein A-agarose and 1 µg of antibodies, overnight at 4°C. Cell lysates or immunoprecipitates were resolved by sodium dodecyl sulfate - polyacrylamide gel electrophoresis (SDS-PAGE). Following transfer of the gel contents to a nitrocellulose filter, the filter was blocked for 1 h at room temperature, with buffer containing 20 mM Tris-HCl (pH 7.5), 500 mM NaCl and 5% non-fat milk; then incubated with specific antibodies for 3 h at room temperature, washed, and incubated with a HRP-labeled secondary antibody for 1 h. Finally, the blots were developed using a chemiluminescent detection system (ECL, Amersham Life Science, Buckinghamshire, England).

Reverse transcription (RT)-PCR

The total RNA was extracted with the RNeasy Mini Kit (Qiagen, Hilden, Germany). For testing MDM2 mRNA expression, First-strand cDNA synthesis was performed with mixture of random nonamers and oligo-dT as primers (Qiagen). Amplification of MDM2 was performed with a 7500 Real-Time RT-PCR System (Applied Biosystems, Foster City, CA), using QuantiFast SYBR Green RT-PCR kit (Qiagen) according to the manufacturer's instructions. The MDM2 primers and the house-keeper gene GAPDH and Actin were purchased from Qiagen (sequences of the primers not provided).

Pulse-chase assay

The protein turnover was assessed by a standard protein-synthesis inhibitor cycloheximide (CHX) assay. Briefly, cells were treated with 50 µg/ml CHX for different times before lysis, in the presence or absence of nilotinib. Western blot analysis of the products revealed concurrent expression levels of MDM2.

Polysome preparation and analysis

Polysome profiling was carried out essentially as described previously [25]. Briefly, SUP-B13 cells, with or without exposure to nilotinib, were incubated with 100 µg/ml CHX for 15 min to arrest polyribosome migration. Cells were then lysed to isolate cytoplasmic RNA in a buffer containing 20 mM Tris-HCl at pH 8.0, 100 mM NaCl, 5 mM $MgCl_2$, 0.5% Triton X-100, 500 U/ml RNAsin, and a cocktail of protease inhibitors, followed by fractionation on 15–45% (w/v) sucrose gradient. The gradient was centrifuged in a SW41Ti rotor at 39,000 rpm for 1 hr. Fractions were collected from each gradient tube by up-ward replacement with monitored absorption at OD_{254} by using a fractionator (Brandel, Inc). The RNA in each fraction was extracted and subjected to quantitative PCR as described above.

WST assay

The cytotoxic effect of triptolide on ALL cells was determined using the water-soluble tetrazolium salt (WST) assay. Briefly, cells cultured in 96-well microtiter plates were given different concentrations of triptolide, for a 20-h period. Following this, WST (25 µg/well) was added and incubation continued for an additional 4 h before the optical density (OD) of the wells was read with a microplate reader (set at a test wavelength of 450 nm and a reference wavelength of 620 nm). Appropriate controls lacking cells were included, to determine background absorbance.

Flow cytometry

Flow cytometry was performed to analyze the cell cycle position and degree of apoptosis induced by nilotinib. For the cell-cycle analysis, cells were collected, rinsed twice with phosphate buffered saline (PBS), fixed in 70% ethanol for 1 h at 4°C, washed twice in PBS and re-suspended in 0.5 ml PBS containing 20 µg/ml of propidium iodide (PI) and 20 µg/ml of RNase A. Following incubation at 4°C for at least 30 min, the samples were analyzed using a FACScan (Becton Dickinson) with WinList software (Verity Software House, Inc.).

For the quantitative detection of apoptotic cells, flow cytometry of annexin-V stained cells was performed. Briefly, cells with or without nilotinib treatment were washed once with PBS and stained with Annexin-V and PI, according to the manufacturer's instructions, prior to flow analysis.

Statistical analysis

All comparative data was statistically analyzed using Statistical Package for the Social Sciences (SPSS) software. The differential significance was determined via Student's *t*-test and presented the data as the mean ± SD. The statistically significant difference was considered at $p<0.05$.

Results

Nilotinib inhibits MDM2 expression in ALL

To investigate whether nilotinib can inhibit MDM2, we tested a group of ALL cell lines (three were BCR-ABL+ and three were BCR-ABL-) that were known to express different levels of MDM2 (Fig. 1) and have various p53 status (EU-1, UOC-B1 and SUP-B13: wild-type (wt)-p53; EU-6: mutant p53; EU-5 and EU-9: p53-null) [28]. First, we found that there seemed to be no correlation between BCR-ABL expression and the MDM2 protein levels in ALL. As seen in Fig. 1A, overexpression of MDM2 and lack of MDM2 expression were detected in both BCR-ABL positive and negative ALL. Also, the BCR-ABL+ cell lines either had wt, mutant or had a null p53 phenotype, whereas high-level MDM2 expression was always associated with an enhanced expression of MDM4 and with a wt-p53 phenotype. All six cell lines studied expressed similar levels of XIAP. Treatment with nilotinib potently downregulated MDM2 expression in two MDM2-overexpressing ALL cell lines (Fig. 1B). The protein levels of either BCR-ABL or ABL appeared not to be changed by nilotinib. Also, MDM4 expression was not significantly affected by nilotinib treatment. Nilotinib inhibited the expression of XIAP in the two MDM2-overexpressing cell lines, but not in the MDM2-negative line, suggesting that inhibition of XIAP by nilotinib is MDM2-dependent. Nilotinib inhibited MDM2 and XIAP expression in a dose-dependent manner, spanning 0.5–5 µM (Fig. 1C). Inhibition of MDM2 and XIAP by nilotinib occurred at about 2–4 h after treatment and was followed by steady-state downregulation (Fig. 1D).

Nilotinib downregulates MDM2 at the post-translational level

We wished to investigate further how MDM2 is regulated by nilotinib. First, we performed quantitative RT-PCR for the expression of MDM2 mRNA in nilotinib-treated SUP-B15 cells. We found that nilotinib did not inhibit MDM2 mRNA expression (Fig. 2A), as compared with a previously identified MDM2 inhibitor triptolide, which downregulates MDM2 through inhibition of mRNA expression [36]. Nilotinib also did not inhibit MDM2 mRNA expression in the BCR-ABL– line, EU-1 (data not shown). Because a previous study demonstrates that BCR-ABL increases MDM2 mRNA translation [18], we investigated whether presumable inhibition of BCR-ABL by nilotinib in SUP-B15 cells could result in a decrease of MDM2 mRNA translation. In our experimental mode and setting, we did not detect an effect of nilotinib on MDM2 mRNA translation, because we detected no effect of nilotinib on the polyribosome profile of MDM2 (Fig. 2B). Furthermore, we measured the turnover of MDM2 after nilotinib treatment by pulse-chase assay. The half-life of MDM2 in untreated cells was larger than 90 min, whereas treatment with nilotinib decreased the MDM2 half-life to <60 min (Fig. 2C), indicating that nilotinib treatment induced MDM2 protein degradation. Nilotinib did not significantly alter the half-life of MDM4. The nilotinib-induced degradation of MDM2 was blocked by the proteasome inhibitor MG132 (Fig. 2D). As also seen in this figure, downregulation of XIAP was not inhibited by MG132, indicating that nilotinib-mediated inhibition of XIAP did not occur at the post-translational level.

Previous studies show that MDM2 protein degradation is regulated by an autolytic mechanism, through ubiquitination, and that MDM2 becomes unstable when it is dissociated from the MDM2-MDM4 complex [21]. Also, previous studies demonstrate that phosphorylation of MDM2 by c-BAL facilitates MDM2-MDM4 complex formation [20]. Thus, we tested whether nilotinib, which inhibits BCR-ABL and c-ABL, is able to block the MDM2-MDM4 interaction and induce MDM2 ubiquitination. As expected, co-IP/western blot assay results showed that the MDM2-MDM4 complexes were disrupted by nilotinib treatment (Fig. 2E), resulting in ubiquitination of MDM2 in both BCR-ABL positive and negative cells (Fig. 2F).

The effects of nilotinib on p53 and XIAP functions

Because MDM2 is an inhibitor of p53, we investigated the consequences of nilotinib-mediated downregulation of MDM2 on p53 expression. As is seen in Fig. 3A, the protein levels of p53 were not significantly changed by nilotinib in two wt-p53 cell lines with BCR-ABL (SUP-B15) or without BCR-ABL (EU-1) expression. Consistent with having no change in p53 expression, there was neither detectable alteration of p21 protein levels (Fig. 3A) nor G1 cell-cycle arrest (Fig. 3B) in these nilotinib-treated ALL cells. These results suggest that neither p53 accumulation nor activation occur following nilotinib-mediated-downregulation of MDM2. However, we detected a significant cleavage of the death substrate PARP in both cell lines after nilotinib treatment (Fig. 3A). Because PARP cleavage is always a result of activation of caspases such as caspase-9 and -3, we looked for activation of these caspases in nilotinib-treated cells: caspase-9 and -3 were indeed activated in both BCR-ABL positive and negative ALL cells (Fig. 3C and Fig. 3D), suggesting that the function of XIAP is inhibited by nilotinib, because XIAP specifically inhibits both these caspases [37,38]. In comparing the activation levels of caspase-9 and -3 induced by nilotinib between BCR-ABL positive and negative ALL, we did not detect any significant differences, as $p>0.5$ (Fig. 3C and D).

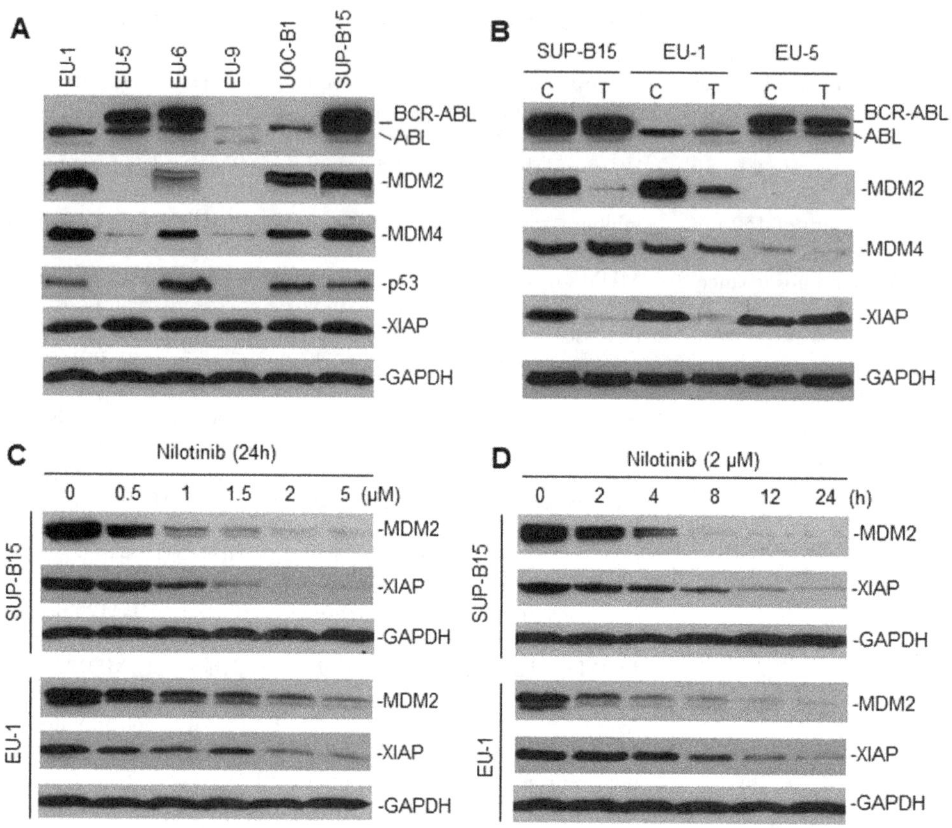

Figure 1. Downregulation of MDM2 by nilotinib in ALL. A, western blot assay for the expression of BCR-ABL, MDM2, p53 and XIAP in six cultured ALL cell lines. The p53 status of these lines (EU-1, UOC-B1 and Sup-B15: wt-p53; EU-6: mutant-p53; EU-5 and EU-9: p53-null) was previously characterized [28]. **B**, changes of the expression levels of MDM2 and XIAP by nilotinib treatment. Representative cell lines, as indicated, were treated (T) with 2 μM nilotinib for 24 h. Untreated cells served as a control (C). The expression of proteins was detected by western blot, as indicated. **C** and **D**, western blot assays showed the dose-response and time-course of MDM2 and XIAP inhibition by nilotinib, in both BCR-ABL positive (SUP-B15) and negative (EU-1) ALL cell lines.

Nilotinib induced different degrees of apoptosis in ALL with distinct BCR-ABL and MDM2 expression

To investigate where nilotinib-mediated downregulation of MDM2 contributes to nilotinib's cytotoxic and apoptotic activities, we evaluated and compared the cytotoxic and apoptotic effects of nilotinib on ALL cells with different BCR-ABL and MDM2 expression status. We found that the degree of cytotoxicity and apoptosis induced by nilotinib in BCR-ABL+ cells was related to their expression levels of MDM2. WST cytotoxic assay results showed that nilotinib exhibited very strong cytotoxic effects on the BCR-ABL+ ALL cell line SUP-B15, which overexpresses MDM2 (Fig. 4A); while EU-6 cells with lower expression of MDM2 had relatively low sensitivity to nilotinib ($p<0.05$); and EU-5 cells with no expression of MDM2 had much lower sensitivity ($p<0.01$), when compared with SUP-B15. Even in the BCR-ABL– ALL cells, the cytotoxic effects of nilotinib were associated with the expression of MDM2, so the EU-9 BCR-ABL– ALL cells with no MDM2 expression were totally resistant to nilotinib. We also tested for induction of apoptosis by nilotinib in the 6 cell lines, by annexin-V and PI staining and flow cytometry. In consistency with the results of the WST assay, nilotinib induced very strong apoptosis in SUP-B15 (BCR-ABL+, MDM2 overexpressing) and less apoptosis in those cell lines that were either BCR-ABL+ with no and low levels of MDM2 expression, or BCR-ABL– cell lines with MDM2 overexpression. We detected no apoptotic effect for nilotinib-treated EU-9, a BCR-ABL– and MDM2– cell line (Fig. 4B).

We presented the data in Fig. 3A and 3B showing that neither p53 expression nor p53 function was altered by nilotinib, suggesting that the nilotinib-induced cytotoxicity and apoptosis are p53-independent. To confirm this, we performed an experiment using p53 siRNA to knock down p53 in SUP-B15 and treated these cells with nilotinib. Inhibition of p53 did not significantly alter the sensitivity of SUP-B15 to nilotinib (Fig. 4C). In contrast, our data in Fig. 1 and 3 apparently indicated a subsequent inhibition of XIAP expression and function following nilotinib-mediated downregulation of MDM2. We transfected a XIAP expression plasmid into SUP-B15 cells, and then treated the cells with nilotinib. Because the expression of the transfected XIAP was not driven by the XIAP Internal ribosome entry site (IRES), downregulation of MDM2 did not inhibit its expression. Cell death triggered by nilotinib was significantly attenuated by the enforced overexpression of ectopic XIAP (Fig. 4D), which suggests that inhibition of XIAP indeed confers, at least in part, to apoptosis induced by nilotinib.

Discussion

Although the use of second-generation TKIs such as nilotinib to treat imatinib-resistant Ph+ ALL significantly improved the clinical outcome, there still existed cases that failed to respond to

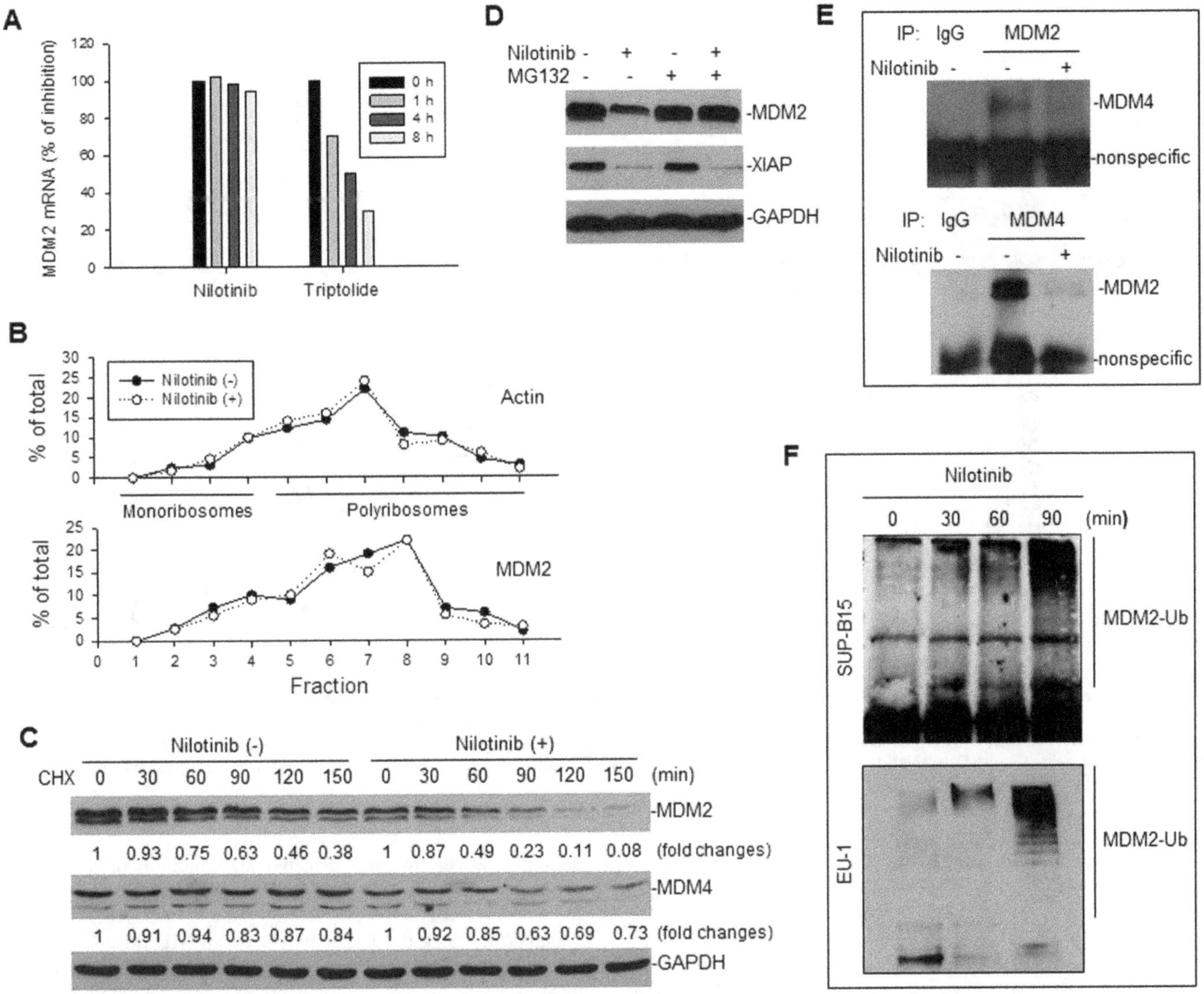

Figure 2. Evaluation of the mechanism by which nilotinib inhibits MDM2. A, RT-PCR for MDM2 mRNA expression in SUP-B15 cells, treated with 2 µM nilotinib and 0.2 µM triptolide (as a control) for the different times, as indicated. **B**, SUP-B15 cells were treated with or without 2 µM nilotinib for 4 h; then their cytoplasmic lysates were fractionated on a sucrose gradient. RNA was extracted from each of the fractions and subjected to quantitative RT-PCR for analysis of the distribution of MDM2 and actin mRNAs. Data represent the percentage of the total amount of corresponding mRNA in each fraction. **C**, CHX pulse-chase assay for detection of MDM2 turnover in SUP-B15 cells treated with or without 2 µM nilotinib for 4 h. Numerical labels under each protein band represent protein expression levels after normalization for GAPDH, compared with the untreated (0) samples (defined as 1 unit). **D**, SUP-B15 cells with or without nilotinib exposure were treated with 10 µM MG32 for 4 h and then the expression of proteins as indicated was assessed by Western blot. **E**, co-IP and western blot assay to detect the effect of nilotinib on the interaction between MDM2 and MDM4. Cell lysates from SUP-B15 treated with or without nilotinib were immunoprecipitated with the indicated antibodies. Normal mouse IgG served as a control. Proteins in immune complexes were separated on denaturing gels, transferred to filters, and then detected by western blotting with antibodies, as indicated. Antibodies for western blotting were from different species than those used in the IP. **F**, IP-western blot assay for detection of MDM2 ubiquitination after nilotinib treatment. SUP-B15 cells were treated with 2 µM nilotinib for the indicated length of time. Cellular lysates were immunoprecipitated with anti-MDM2 antibody, and then the MDM2 ubiquitination (MDM2-Ub) was detected by Western blot using anti-ubiquitin antibody.

nilotinib. In a clinical trial of 126 patients treated with nilotinib after imatinib failure, the complete hematologic and major cytogenetic responses reported are only 33% and 50%, respectively, in Ph+ ALL [39]. This suggests that additional mechanisms exist in Ph+ ALL for resistance to nilotinib. For example, the *Ikaros* gene is identified as frequently deleted in Ph+ ALL, which is associated with resistance to TKIs [40,41]. In the present study, we demonstrated that the expression level of MDM2 in ALL seems to be associated with the sensitivity of the cells to nilotinib. The ALL cell lines having both MDM2 overexpression and BCR-ABL expression were found to be very sensitive to nilotinib, whereas BCR-ABL-expressing ALL lines with no or low levels of MDM2 expression were less sensitive to nilotinib. We discovered that nilotinib specifically and strongly induced degradation of MDM2, through disruption of the interaction between MDM2 and MDM4; however, downregulation of MDM2 in nilotinib-treated cells did not result in activation of p53. Instead, we observed a reduction of XIAP expression and activation of

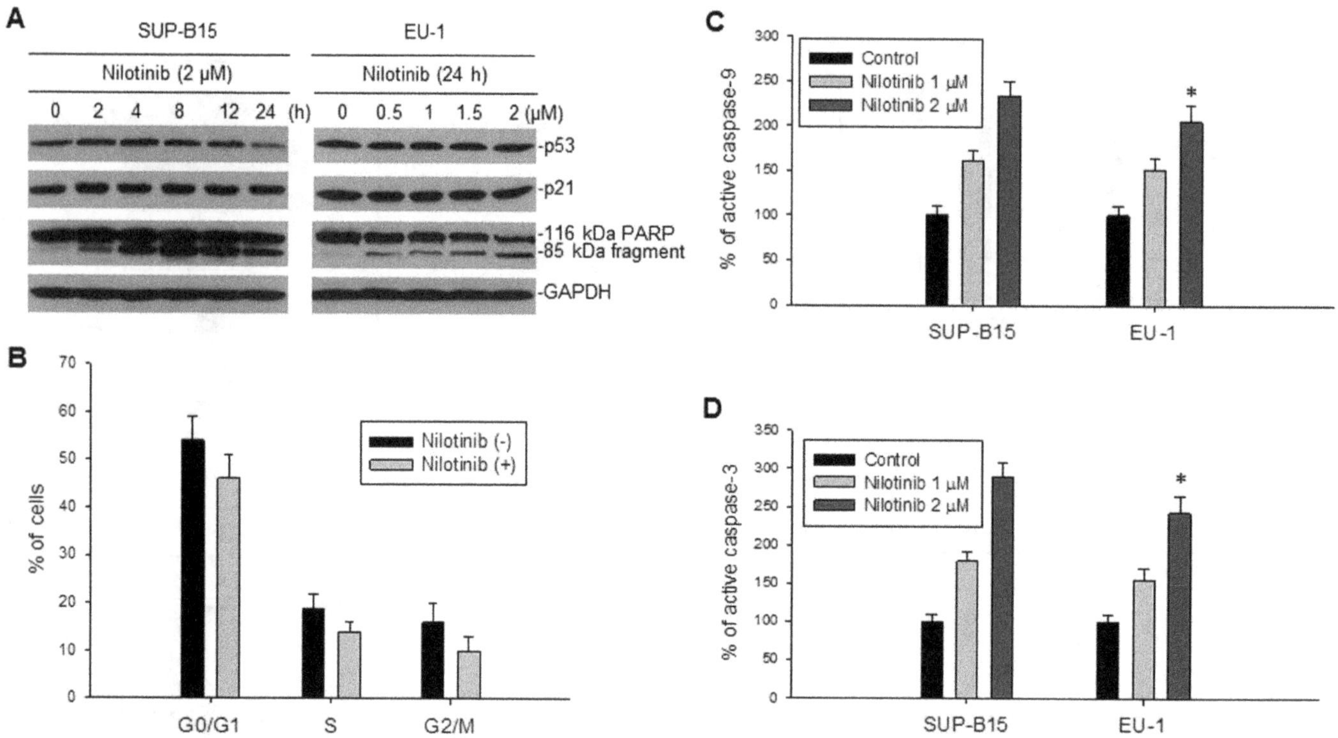

Figure 3. The effect of nilotinib-mediated downregulation of MDM2 and XIAP on activation of p53 and caspases. A, SUP-B15 (BCR-ABL+) and EU-1 (BCR-ABL–) were treated with 2 μM nilotinib for different times and different doses for 24 h, respectively. The expression of p53, p21 and PARP was detected by western blotting. **B**, cell-cycle analysis in SUP-B15 cells performed 4 h post-treatment with 2 μM nilotinib, as compared with untreated cells. **C** and **D**, activation of caspase-9 (C) and -3 (D) in nilotinib-treated SUP-B15 and EU-1 cells was detected by enzyme-linked immunosorbent assay (ELISA), *p>0.05.

caspase-3 and -9, following MDM2 inhibition in these nilotinib-treated cells, leading to their apoptosis.

The expression of MDM2 is regulated mainly at the post-translational level, through a self-ubiquitination mechanism, although previous studies report that MDM2 is transcriptionally activated by p53 [42] and translationally induced by BCR-ABL [18]. In the set of ALL cell lines that we studied, there was an association of MDM2 overexpression with wt-p53, while we detected no correlation with regard to the levels of MDM2 with BCR-ABL expression. Treatment of these cell lines with nilotinib detected neither reductions of p53 nor decreases in BCR-ABL and ABL expression. However, nilotinib remarkably inhibited MDM2 expression in all the MDM2-expressing cell lines, including the BCR-ABL positive and negative lines. We performed RT-PCR and polysome profiling assays, finding that nilotinib-mediated downregulation of MDM2 did not occur at the transcriptional nor translational levels. We observed that the half-life of the MDM2 protein was significantly reduced in nilotinib-treated cells. Further studies showed that the MDM2 and MDM4 complexes were separated by nilotinib; thus, increased ubiqitination of MDM2 was detected in these nilotinib-treated cells.

A well-characterized finding is that c-ABL phosphorylates MDM2, which facilitates the formation of the MDM2-MDM4 complex [20], where MDM2 becomes stabilized [21]. Our results indicating that nilotinib, the ABL inhibitor, disrupted the MDM2-MDM4 interaction and induced MDM2 degradation, seems a validation of the previous observation. It is easy to understand that the constitutive activation of ABL in BCR-ABL+ ALL is inhibited by nilotinib, which leads to the dissociation of MDM2 from the MDM2-MDM4 complex, resulting in ubiquitination and degradation; however, we also detected an inhibition of MDM2 by nilotinib in the BCR-ABL– ALL. This suggested that inhibition of the normal c-ABL activity by nilotinib in any BCR-ABL– cells was adequate to block the interaction between MDM2 and MDM4, resulting in MDM2 degradation. The degradation of MDM2 is most likely the mechanism for nilotinib to induce the apoptosis of BCR-ABL– cells.

The expression level of MDM2 seemed to play a partial role in induction of apoptosis by nilotinib. For example, the BCR-ABL– cell lines EU-1 and UOC-B1, which express high levels of MDM2, were sensitive to nilotinib; whereas the EU-9 cell line lacking both BCR-ABL and MDM2 expression was not killed by nilotinib. Most normal cells/tissues express no or very low levels of MDM2, which is probably the reason for nilotinib to be developed as a drug for clinical use.

Previous studies also demonstrate that c-ABL is a positive regulator of p53 [43], interacting with p53, which can activate its downstream target p21 [44]. Treatment of CML with imatinib impairs p53 accumulation and function [45]. Similarly, we did not detect an induction of p53 after downregulation of its inhibitor MDM2 in the nilotinib-treated cell lines, both BCR-ABL positive and negative. This could be explained by considering that the induction of p53 and its target p21, due to inhibition of MDM2, is diminished or abrogated by the direct inhibitory effect nilotinib has on p53 and p21, through its inhibition of BCR-ABL or c-ABL. Thus, neither p53 activation nor inhibition was detected in the nilotinib-treated cells.

MDM2 also regulates cancer cell growth and resistance to apoptosis in a p53-independent manner. For example, MDM2 is a positive regulator of the anti-apoptotic factor XIAP, binding the

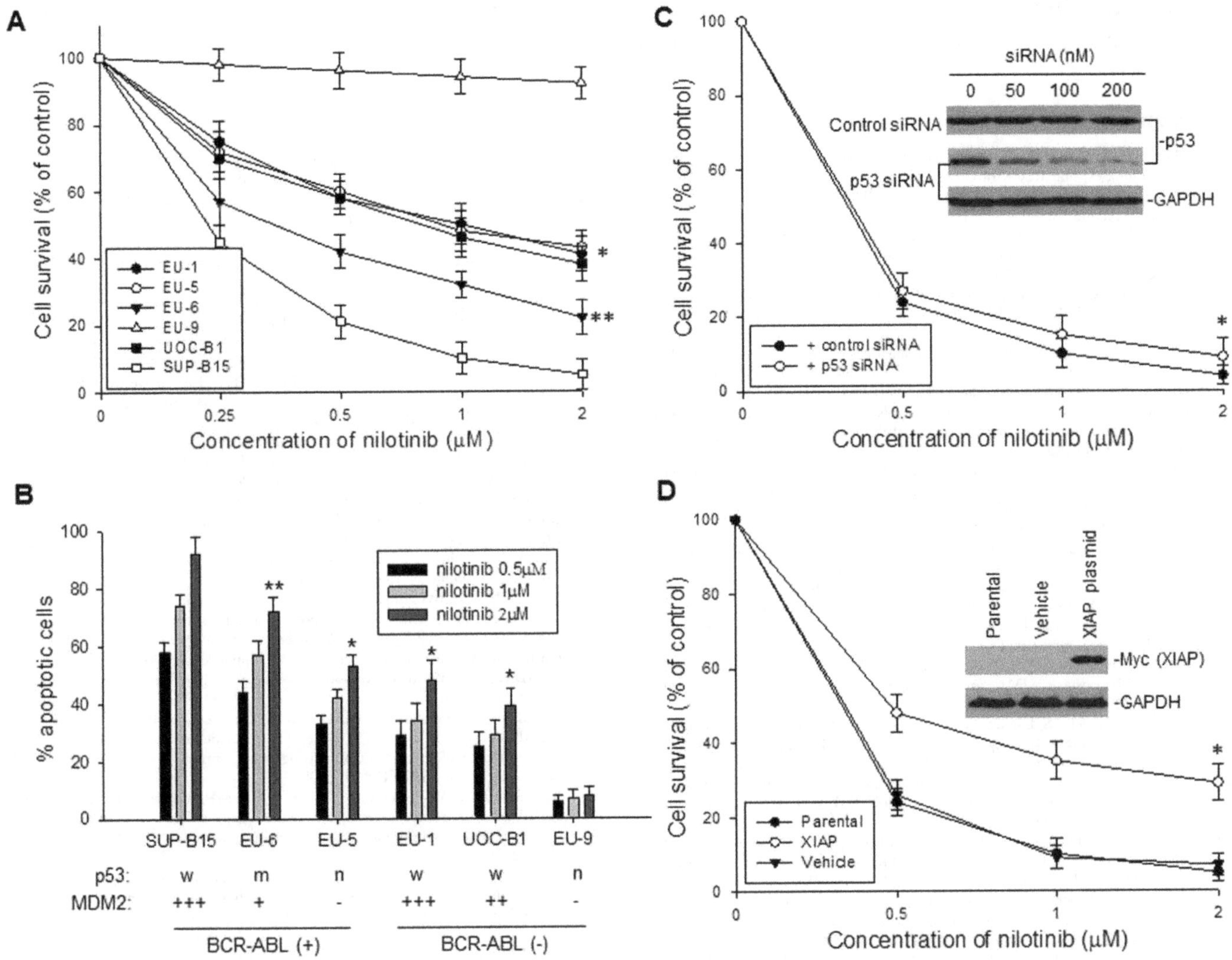

Figure 4. Cytotoxic and apoptotic effects of nilotinib on ALL cells. A, dose-dependent cytotoxic response to nilotinib in the six ALL cell lines, as tested for Fig. 1A. The viability of cells incubated with different concentrations of nilotinib for 24 h was determined by WST assay. Data from three independent experiments is represented by the mean percentage ± SD of surviving cells, as compared to the untreated controls. *$p<0.01$; **$p<0.05$ (as compared with SUP-B15) **B**, dose-response of apoptosis of the six cell lines treated with the nilotinib doses indicated for 24 h, as quatitatively detected by flow cytometry. *$p<0.01$; **$p<0.05$ (as compared with SUP-B15). **C**, the effect of p53 knockdown on sensitivity of BCR-ABL+ cells to nilotinib. SUP-B15 cells, transfected with 200 nM of either p53 siRNA or control siRNA, were treated with different dose of nilotinib for 24 h, and cell viability was detected by WST assay, *$p>0.5$. The expression of p53 in SUP-B15 cells transfected with p53 siRNA was determined by Western blot assay (*insert*). **D**, the effect of enforced overexpression of XIAP on sensitivity of ALL cells to nilotinib. SUP-B15 cells, transfected with pCDNA3-6myc-XIAP plasmid and vehicle control, were treated with different dose of nilotinib for 24 h, and cell viability was detected by WST assay, *$p<0.05$. Western blot showing the expression of ectopic XIAP (as detected by Myc antibody) in SUP-B15 cells (*insert*).

XIAP IRES to induce XIAP mRNA translation, which results in resistance of cancer cells to radio-chemotherapy [25]. Inhibition of MDM2 by specific siRNA or specific inhibitors, such as triptolide, is always followed by a downregulation of XIAP [25,36]. In the present study, we also found a concomitant downregulation of XIAP and activation of caspase-9 and caspase-3, following nilotinib-mediated inhibition of MDM2. Based on our results, we now believe that the potent apoptosis induced by nilotinib in BCR-ABL+ and MDM2-overexpressing ALL cells are partially attributable to the downregulation of XIAP. In contrast, lack of XIAP downregulation in BCR-ABL+ cells due to loss of their MDM2 expression, which usually occurs in p53-deficient cancer cells such as the EU-5 cell line, could be one of the mechanisms for these cells' resistance to nilotinib.

The significance of the present study is our finding that nilotinib can inhibit MDM2 expression in BCR-ABL– ALL cells. Overexpression of MDM2 is detected in about 20-30% of ALL and is associated with refractory disease. Although nilotinib is unable to induce the activation of p53 in the MDM2-overexpressing ALL, it can induce the downregulation of the anti-apoptotic protein XIAP, following its inhibition of MDM2. Thus, we believe nilotinib should be an interesting candidate drug for therapy against high-risk, refractory ALL, including in Ph– patients whose leukemic cells overexpress MDM2.

Author Contributions

Conceived and designed the experiments: HZ LG MZ. Performed the experiments: HZ LG TL. Analyzed the data: HZ MZ KYC. Contributed reagents/materials/analysis tools: KYC. Wrote the paper: MZ.

References

1. Hantschel O, Superti-Furga G (2004) Regulation of the c-Abl and Bcr-Abl tyrosine kinases. Nat Rev Mol Cell Biol 5: 33–44.
2. Deininger MW, Goldman JM, Melo JV (2000) The molecular biology of chronic myeloid leukemia. Blood 96: 3343–3356.
3. Lee HJ, Thompson JE, Wang ES, Wetzler M (2011) Philadelphia chromosome-positive acute lymphoblastic leukemia: current treatment and future perspectives. Cancer 117: 1583–1594.
4. Hazlehurst LA, Bewry NN, Nair RR, Pinilla-Ibarz J (2009) Signaling networks associated with BCR-ABL-dependent transformation. Cancer Control 16: 100–107.
5. Skorski T, Bellacosa A, Nieborowska-Skorska M, Majewski M, Martinez R, et al. (1997) Transformation of hematopoietic cells by BCR/ABL requires activation of a PI-3k/Akt-dependent pathway. EMBO J 16: 6151–6161.
6. Nawata R, Yujiri T, Nakamura Y, Ariyoshi K, Takahashi T, et al. (2003) MEK kinase 1 mediates the antiapoptotic effect of the Bcr-Abl oncogene through NF-kappaB activation. Oncogene 22: 7774–7780.
7. Klejman A, Schreiner SJ, Nieborowska-Skorska M, Slupianek A, Wilson M, et al. (2002) The Src family kinase Hck couples BCR/ABL to STAT5 activation in myeloid leukemia cells. EMBO J 21: 5766–5774.
8. Kantarjian H, Sawyers C, Hochhaus A, Guilhot F, Schiffer C, et al. (2002) Hematologic and cytogenetic responses to imatinib mesylate in chronic myelogenous leukemia. N Engl J Med 346: 645–652.
9. Talpaz M, Silver RT, Druker BJ, Goldman JM, Gambacorti-Passerini C, et al. (2002) Imatinib induces durable hematologic and cytogenetic responses in patients with accelerated phase chronic myeloid leukemia: results of a phase 2 study. Blood 99: 1928–1937.
10. Kantarjian H, Giles F, Wunderle L, Bhalla K, O'Brien S, et al. (2006) Nilotinib in imatinib-resistant CML and Philadelphia chromosome-positive ALL. N Engl J Med 354: 2542–2551.
11. Mahon FX, Hayette S, Lagarde V, Belloc F, Turcq B, et al. (2008) Evidence that resistance to nilotinib may be due to BCR-ABL, Pgp, or Src kinase overexpression. Cancer Res 68: 9809–9816.
12. Camgoz A, Gencer EB, Ural AU, Baran Y (2013) Mechanisms responsible for nilotinib resistance in human chronic myeloid leukemia cells and reversal of resistance. Leuk Lymphoma 54: 1279–1287.
13. Chow KU, Nowak D, Trepohl B, Hochmuth S, Schneider B, et al. (2007) The tyrosine kinase inhibitor AMN107 (Nilotinib) exhibits off-target effects in lymphoblastic cell lines. Leuk Lymphoma 48: 1379–1388.
14. Montemurro M, Schoffski P, Reichardt P, Gelderblom H, Schutte J, et al. (2009) Nilotinib in the treatment of advanced gastrointestinal stromal tumours resistant to both imatinib and sunitinib. Eur J Cancer 45: 2293–2297.
15. Oetzel C, Jonuleit T, Gotz A, van der Kuip H, Michels H, et al. (2000) The tyrosine kinase inhibitor CGP 57148 (ST1 571) induces apoptosis in BCR-ABL-positive cells by down-regulating BCL-X. Clin Cancer Res 6: 1958–1968.
16. Carter BZ, Mak DH, Schober WD, Cabreira-Hansen M, Beran M, et al. (2006) Regulation of survivin expression through Bcr-Abl/MAPK cascade: targeting survivin overcomes imatinib resistance and increases imatinib sensitivity in imatinib-responsive CML cells. Blood 107: 1555–1563.
17. Shaker ME, Ghani A, Shiha GE, Ibrahim TM, Mehal WZ (2013) Nilotinib induces apoptosis and autophagic cell death of activated hepatic stellate cells via inhibition of histone deacetylases. Biochim Biophys Acta 1833: 1992–2003.
18. Trotta R, Vignudelli T, Candini O, Intine RV, Pecorari L, et al. (2003) BCR/ABL activates mdm2 mRNA translation via the La antigen. Cancer Cell 3: 145–160.
19. Goetz AW, van der Kuip H, Maya R, Oren M, Aulitzky WE (2001) Requirement for Mdm2 in the survival effects of Bcr-Abl and interleukin 3 in hematopoietic cells. Cancer Res 61: 7635–7641.
20. Waning DL, Lehman JA, Batuello CN, Mayo LD (2011) c-Abl phosphorylation of Mdm2 facilitates Mdm2-Mdmx complex formation. J Biol Chem 286: 216–222.
21. Sharp DA, Kratowicz SA, Sank MJ, George DL (1999) Stabilization of the MDM2 oncoprotein by interaction with the structurally related MDMX protein. J Biol Chem 274: 38189–38196.
22. Momand J, Zambetti GP, Olson DC, George D, Levine AJ (1992) The mdm-2 oncogene product forms a complex with the p53 protein and inhibits p53-mediated transactivation. Cell 69: 1237–1245.
23. Honda R, Tanaka H, Yasuda H (1997) Oncoprotein MDM2 is a ubiquitin ligase E3 for tumor suppressor p53. FEBS Lett 420: 25–27.
24. Zhang Z, Zhang R (2005) p53-independent activities of MDM2 and their relevance to cancer therapy. Curr Cancer Drug Targets 5: 9–20.
25. Gu L, Zhu N, Zhang H, Durden DL, Feng Y, et al. (2009) Regulation of XIAP translation and induction by MDM2 following irradiation. Cancer Cell 15: 363–375.
26. Momand J, Jung D, Wilczynski S, Niland J (1998) The MDM2 gene amplification database. Nucleic Acids Res 26: 3453–3459.
27. Bueso-Ramos CE, Yang Y, deLeon E, McCown P, Stass SA, et al. (1993) The human MDM-2 oncogene is overexpressed in leukemias. Blood 82: 2617–2623.
28. Zhou M, Yeager AM, Smith SD, Findley HW (1995) Overexpression of the MDM2 gene by childhood acute lymphoblastic leukemia cells expressing the wild-type p53 gene. Blood 85: 1608–1614.
29. Gustafsson B, Stal O, Gustafsson B (1998) Overexpression of MDM2 in acute childhood lymphoblastic leukemia. Pediatr Hematol Oncol 15: 519–526.
30. Zhou M, Gu L, Abshire TC, Homans A, Billett AL, et al. (2000) Incidence and prognostic significance of MDM2 oncoprotein overexpression in relapsed childhood acute lymphoblastic leukemia. Leukemia 14: 61–67.
31. Marks DI, Kurz BW, Link MP, Ng E, Shuster JJ, et al. (1996) High incidence of potential p53 inactivation in poor outcome childhood acute lymphoblastic leukemia at diagnosis. Blood 87: 1155–1161.
32. Marks DI, Kurz BW, Link MP, Ng E, Shuster JJ, et al. (1997) Altered expression of p53 and mdm-2 proteins at diagnosis is associated with early treatment failure in childhood acute lymphoblastic leukemia. J Clin Oncol 15: 1158–1162.
33. Gustafsson B, Christenson B, Hjalmar V, Winiarski J (2000) Cellular expression of MDM2 and p53 in childhood leukemias with poor prognosis. Med Pediatr Oncol 34: 117–124.
34. Gustafsson B, Axelsson B, Gustafsson B, Christensson B, Winiarski J (2001) MDM2 and p53 in childhood acute lymphoblastic leukemia: higher expression in childhood leukemias with poor prognosis compared to long-term survivors. Pediatr Hematol Oncol 18: 497–508.
35. Naumovski L, Morgan R, Hecht F, Link MP, Glader BE, et al. (1988) Philadelphia chromosome-positive acute lymphoblastic leukemia cell lines without classical breakpoint cluster region rearrangement. Cancer Res 48: 2876–2879.
36. Huang M, Zhang H, Liu T, Tian D, Gu L, et al. (2013) Triptolide inhibits MDM2 and induces apoptosis in acute lymphoblastic leukemia cells through a p53-independent pathway. Mol Cancer Ther 12: 184–194.
37. Shiozaki EN, Chai J, Rigotti DJ, Riedl SJ, Li P, et al. (2003) Mechanism of XIAP-mediated inhibition of caspase-9. Mol Cell 11: 519–527.
38. Riedl SJ, Renatus M, Schwarzenbacher R, Zhou Q, Sun C, et al. (2001) Structural basis for the inhibition of caspase-3 by XIAP. Cell 104: 791–800.
39. Fava C, Kantarjian HM, Jabbour E, O'Brien S, Jain N, et al. (2009) Failure to achieve a complete hematologic response at the time of a major cytogenetic response with second-generation tyrosine kinase inhibitors is associated with a poor prognosis among patients with chronic myeloid leukemia in accelerated or blast phase. Blood 113: 5058–5063.
40. Mullighan CG, Miller CB, Radtke I, Phillips LA, Dalton J, et al. (2008) BCR-ABL1 lymphoblastic leukaemia is characterized by the deletion of Ikaros. Nature 453: 110–114.
41. Iacobucci I, Lonetti A, Messa F, Cilloni D, Arruga F, et al. (2008) Expression of spliced oncogenic Ikaros isoforms in Philadelphia-positive acute lymphoblastic leukemia patients treated with tyrosine kinase inhibitors: implications for a new mechanism of resistance. Blood 112: 3847–3855.
42. Juven T, Barak Y, Zauberman A, George DL, Oren M (1993) Wild type p53 can mediate sequence-specific transactivation of an internal promoter within the mdm2 gene. Oncogene 8: 3411–3416.
43. Levav-Cohen Y, Goldberg Z, Zuckerman V, Grossman T, Haupt S, et al. (2005) C-Abl as a modulator of p53. Biochem Biophys Res Commun 331: 737–749.
44. Jing Y, Wang M, Tang W, Qi T, Gu C, et al. (2007) c-Abl tyrosine kinase activates p21 transcription via interaction with p53. J Biochem 141: 621–626.
45. Goldberg Z, Levav Y, Krichevsky S, Fibach E, Haupt Y (2004) Treatment of chronic myeloid leukemia cells with imatinib (STI571) impairs p53 accumulation in response to DNA damage. Cell Cycle 3: 1188–1195.

2

Multi-Agent Chemotherapy Overcomes Glucocorticoid Resistance Conferred by a *BIM* Deletion Polymorphism in Pediatric Acute Lymphoblastic Leukemia

Sheila Xinxuan Soh[1], Joshua Yew Suang Lim[2], John W. J. Huang[1], Nan Jiang[2], Allen Eng Juh Yeoh[2,3,4,5], S. Tiong Ong[1,6,7,8]*

1 Cancer and Stem Cell Biology Program, Duke-NUS Graduate Medical School, Singapore, Singapore, **2** Department of Paediatrics, Yong Loo Lin School of Medicine, National University of Singapore, Singapore, Singapore, **3** National University Cancer Institute, National University Health System, Singapore, Singapore, **4** Viva-University Children's Cancer Centre, University Children's Medical Institute, National University Health System, Singapore, Singapore, **5** Cancer Science Institute, National University of Singapore, Singapore, Singapore, **6** Department of Haematology, Singapore General Hospital, Singapore, Singapore, **7** Department of Medical Oncology, National Cancer Centre, Singapore, Singapore, **8** Division of Medical Oncology, Duke University Medical Center, Durham, North Carolina, United States of America

Abstract

A broad range of anti-cancer agents, including glucocorticoids (GCs) and tyrosine kinase inhibitors (TKIs), kill cells by upregulating the pro-apoptotic BCL2 family member, BIM. A common germline deletion in the *BIM* gene was recently shown to favor the production of non-apoptotic BIM isoforms, and to predict inferior responses in TKI-treated chronic myeloid leukemia (CML) and EGFR-driven lung cancer patients. Given that both *in vitro* and *in vivo* GC resistance are predictive of adverse outcomes in acute lymphoblastic leukemia (ALL), we hypothesized that this polymorphism would mediate GC resistance, and serve as a biomarker of poor response in ALL. Accordingly, we used zinc finger nucleases to generate ALL cell lines with the *BIM* deletion, and confirmed the ability of the deletion to mediate GC resistance *in vitro*. In contrast to CML and lung cancer, the *BIM* deletion did not predict for poorer clinical outcome in a retrospective analysis of 411 pediatric ALL patients who were uniformly treated with GCs and chemotherapy. Underlying the lack of prognostic significance, we found that the chemotherapy agents used in our cohort (vincristine, L-asparaginase, and methotrexate) were each able to induce ALL cell death in a BIM-independent fashion, and resensitize *BIM* deletion-containing cells to GCs. Together, our work demonstrates how effective therapy can overcome intrinsic resistance in ALL patients, and suggests the potential of using combinations of drugs that work via divergent mechanisms of cell killing to surmount *BIM* deletion-mediated drug resistance in other cancers.

Editor: Linda Bendall, University of Sydney, Australia

Funding: STO was supported by the Leukemia & Lymphoma Society Translational Research Program Grant (R913-302-026-597) www.lls.org. AEY was supported by the Singapore National Medical Research Council (NMRC/0582/2001, NMRC/CSA/003/2008). www.nmrc.gov.sg, and by A*STAR (SCS-POU98, NMRC/CSI/004/2005). www.a-star.edu.sg, and by Children's Cancer Foundation, Singapore. www.ccf.org.sg, and by VIVA Foundation for Children with Cancer, Singapore. www.viva.sg. The funders had no role in study design, data collection and analysis, decision to publish, or preparation of the manuscript.

Competing Interests: The authors have declared that no competing interests exist.

* Email: sintiong.ong@duke-nus.edu.sg

Introduction

Genome-wide profiling studies of acute lymphoblastic leukemia (ALL) have revealed it to be a highly heterogeneous disease [1]. In spite of this, the majority of ALL subtypes are treated with a remission-induction protocol that invariably consists of a glucocorticoid, vincristine and at least one other chemotherapy agent (L-asparaginase, an anthracycline, or both) [2]. Unfortunately, 15-20% of patients continue to relapse, and outcome remains poor for these individuals [3]. Consequently, there have been ongoing efforts to identify genetic factors that could account for this response heterogeneity and serve as prognostic markers for risk stratification or novel druggable targets in order to improve patient outcomes [4–6].

At the same time, recent reviews have underscored the notion that response heterogeneity can arise from not only somatic mutations but also germline polymorphisms [7,8]. A number of examples of the latter have been described, including genetic variants that influence the pharmacokinetic and pharmacodynamic phenotype of the host, as well as those affecting the underlying biology of the leukemic cell and thereby cell intrinsic drug resistance/sensitivity [9–15]. Notably, however, studies correlating genetic variants with clinical phenotypes have been largely based on genetic epidemiology data and lack experimental validation at a mechanistic level. Such mechanistic studies have been hampered in part by the difficulty and cost of generating isogenic cell lines that either possess or lack a mutation of interest. More recently, a variety of methods that enable genome engineering to faithfully recapitulate mutations of interest have been developed and these will aid the functional validation of these variants *in vitro* [16].

Using such an approach, we recently validated the functional consequences of a germline deletion in the *BIM* gene in chronic myeloid leukemia (CML) [17]. Unlike in ALL, a single causative lesion, the 9;22 translocation, is known to be present in >95% of chronic myeloid leukemia (CML) cases [18]. Despite the targeted nature of tyrosine kinase inhibitors (TKIs), response heterogeneity is also a significant challenge in CML [19]. From a group of TKI-resistant CML patients, we identified a 2.9 kb intronic deletion in the *BIM* gene, and later verified it to be a polymorphism found in 12.3% of East Asians [17]. *BIM* encodes a potent pro-apoptotic BH3-only protein that is required for specific anti-cancer therapies to induce apoptotic cell death [20–25]. When we introduced the deletion into a CML cell line using zinc finger nuclease-based technology, the polymorphism was sufficient to cause intrinsic resistance to tyrosine kinase inhibitors. Mechanistically, we showed that the *BIM* deletion biases splicing toward BIM isoforms that lack the BH3 domain encoded in exon 4, resulting in the expression of BIM isoforms incapable of inducing apoptosis. Consistent with the *in vitro* data, both CML and EGFR-driven lung cancer patients carrying the polymorphism experienced inferior responses to treatment with tyrosine kinase inhibitors.

Since BIM is required for GC-induced apoptosis in lymphoid lineage cells, including ALL cells [26–32], and both *in vitro* and *in vivo* GC response has been shown to predict favorable treatment outcome in ALL [33–37], we wondered if the polymorphism could contribute to response heterogeneity in ALL patients. If this were the case, we expect that pharmacological restoration of BIM function using drugs such as BH3 mimetics would enable us to improve response in patients with the polymorphism [17,25]. Furthermore, because multi-agent chemotherapy is essential to the long-term control of pediatric ALL, the clinical model of ALL could allow us to determine the interaction between a single germline variant and combination therapy.

Accordingly, we used zinc finger nucleases to generate *de novo* ALL cell lines with the *BIM* deletion polymorphism in both heterozygous and homozygous configurations. Using these lines, we found that the *BIM* deletion polymorphism was sufficient to confer GC resistance *in vitro*. However, analysis of a pediatric ALL cohort uniformly treated with GCs and chemotherapy [38] revealed that patients with the *BIM* deletion did not experience inferior response rates nor poorer clinical outcomes. Mechanistically, we determined that GC resistance conferred by the *BIM* polymorphism could be overcome with the addition of chemotherapeutic agents used in standard ALL protocols, and which likely act via a BIM-independent mechanism to cause cell death. Together, our data demonstrate that, whilst the *BIM* deletion is sufficient to confer resistance to GCs, the negative impact of polymorphic variants on single agent therapy can be overcome with multi-agent chemotherapy that kill cancer cells via divergent mechanisms. These results highlight the challenge of identifying genetic markers predictive of clinical outcome in populations treated with multi-agent therapy, the utility of genome editing technologies in the study of polymorphic variants, as well as the importance of using drug combinations that kill cancer cells via non-overlapping mechanisms.

Methods

Cell lines and culture conditions

CCRF-CEM was purchased from the American Type Culture Collection (Manassas, VA, USA). Cells were maintained in RPMI-1640 media (Nacalai Tesque, Japan) supplemented with 20% FBS, penicillin/streptomycin and L-glutamine (all from Thermo Scientific, Rockford, IL, USA). Dexamethasone (Rotexmedica, Germany), methotrexate (ABIC Ltd, Israel), vincristine (Korea United Pharm Inc, Korea) and L-asparaginase (Kyowa Hakko Kirin, Japan) were used at the dosages and times indicated in the figure legends. All experiments using cell lines were performed at least 3 times.

Creation of genome-edited lines

The zinc finger nucleases (ZFNs) targeting the *BIM* gene were custom-made (Sigma-Aldrich, St Louis, MO, USA) and the repair template was generated as described in a previous paper [17]. Plasmids encoding the repair template and ZFNs were transfected into CCRF-CEM cells using the Neon system (Invitrogen, Carlsbad, CA, USA). Clones were isolated by dilution cloning and screened for presence of the deletion using the following primers: Forward (5′-GGCCTTCAACCACTATCTCAGTG-CAATGG-3′) and Reverse (5′- GGTTTCAGAGACA-GAGCTGGGACTCC-3′). qPCR to determine exon 3 to exon 4 ratio was performed as previously described [17].

MTS assays

Cells were seeded at a density of 4×10^4 per well in a 96-well plate and incubated with the indicated drugs. In each experiment, every treatment condition was repeated in triplicate wells. After 48 h, CellTiter AQueous One Solution Cell Proliferation reagent (Promega, Fitchburg, WI, USA) was added to each well and incubated for 2 h before an absorbance reading at 490 nm was taken.

Immunoblotting

Cells were washed once in PBS and lysed in RIPA lysis buffer (Millipore, Billerica, MA, USA) containing proteinase inhibitor (Roche, Indianapolis, IN, USA). Protein concentrations were assayed using the Quick Start Bradford protein assay kit (Bio-Rad) and bovine serum albumin as a standard. The following antibodies were used at these concentrations: phospho-glucocorticoid receptor (S211) (Cell Signaling Technology, Danvers, MA, USA #4161, 1:1 000), glucocorticoid receptor (BD Transduction Laboratories, San Jose, CA, USA, 1:2 000), β-actin (Sigma-Aldrich, 1:10 000), PARP (Cell Signaling Technology #9542, 1:2 000), caspase 3 (Cell Signaling Technology #9663, 1:500) and BIM (Cell Signaling Technology #2819, 1:1 000). HRP-conjugated secondary antibodies against mouse or rabbit IgG (Santa Cruz Biotechnology, Santa Cruz, CA, USA) were used at 1:10 000. Western Lightning ECL reagent (PerkinElmer, Waltham, MA, USA) was used to visualize the protein bands. Any adjustments to contrast and intensity were applied uniformly to the images.

Patient recruitment

411 patients with newly-diagnosed ALL from the Malaysia-Singapore (Ma-Spore) acute lymphoblastic leukemia (ALL) 2003 study [38] were included on the basis of DNA availability. Written informed consent was obtained from the parents or the legal guardians of the patients. The study was approved by the National Healthcare Group Domain Specific Review Board (NHG DSRB). Since the *BIM* deletion is germline in nature, and will be present in both normal and leukemic samples, we were able to employ both remission (n = 362) and diagnostic (n = 49) samples for genotyping for this study. Patient risk stratification, details of the treatment protocol, minimal residual disease monitoring and molecular subgrouping were described previously [38].

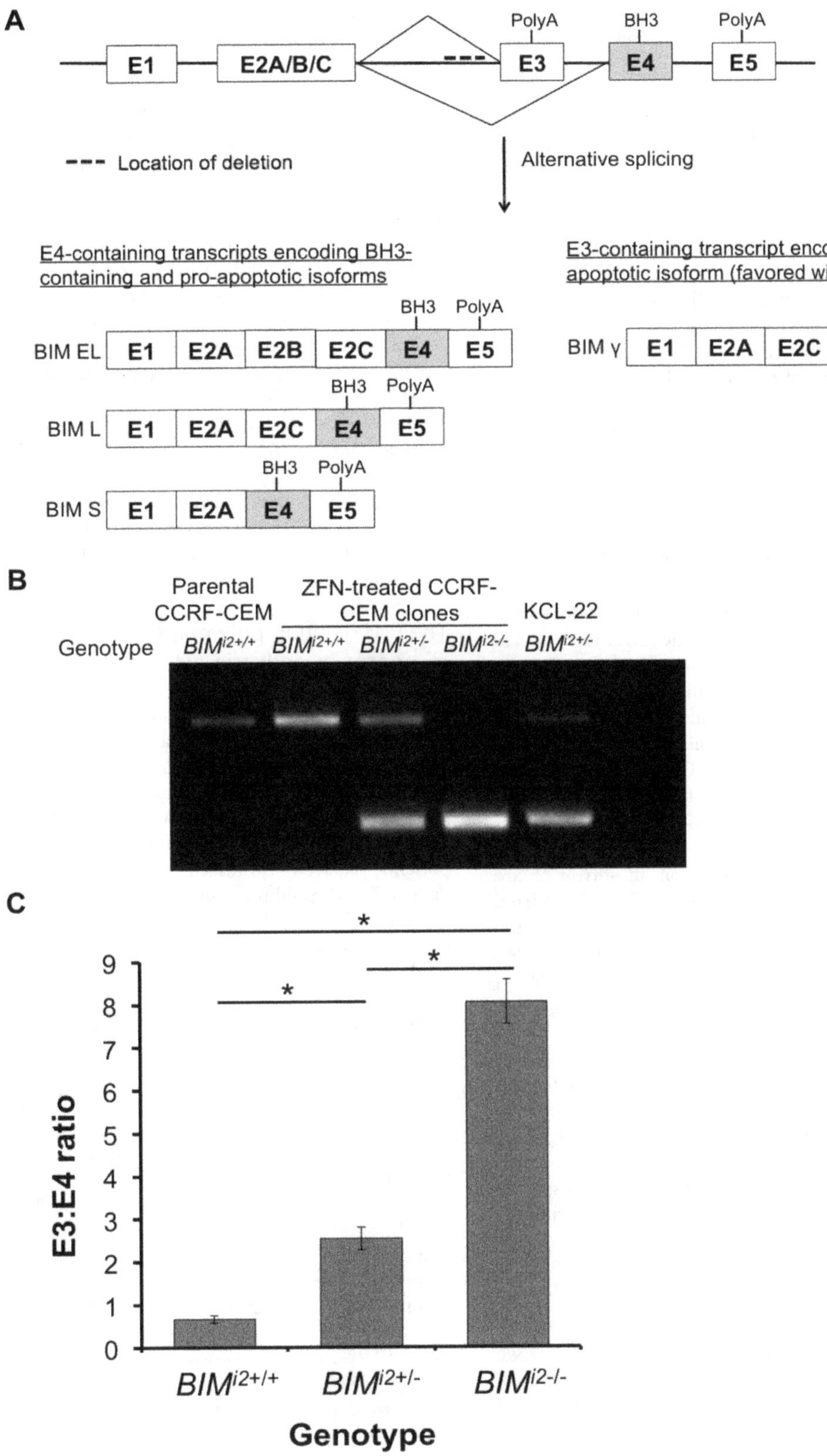

Figure 1. Generation of isogenic CCRF-CEM cell lines with the *BIM* deletion polymorphism. (**A**) Structure of the *BIM* gene and major splice isoforms. The *BIM* deletion polymorphism lies within intron 2 and upstream of exon 3, as indicated by the dashed line. Exon 4 contains the crucial BH3 domain required for apoptosis. Exon 3 (E3) and 4 (E4) are spliced in a mutually exclusive fashion, leading to the generation of either E4-containing isoforms with the BH3 domain (BIM EL, BIM L and BIM S) or E3-containing isoforms without the BH3 domain (BIM γ). When present, the deletion biases splicing towards E3-containing non-apoptotic isoforms. (**B**) Agarose gel of the products from a PCR reaction to detect the polymorphism in zinc finger nuclease (ZFN)-treated CCRF-CEM subclones, with the lower band indicating the presence of the deletion. Parental CCRF-CEM and KCL-22 cells (a CML cell line known to be heterozygous for the *BIM* deletion polymorphism) were included as controls. (**C**) The ratio of exon 3 to exon 4-

containing transcripts (E3:E4) in CCRF-CEM $BIM^{i2+/+}$, $BIM^{i2+/-}$ and $BIM^{i2-/-}$ clones as measured by qPCR. Error bars indicate mean ± SEM (n = 3). A student's t-test was performed for pairwise comparisons of E3:E4 ratio between genotypes. * indicates a significant difference with $P<0.05$.

Statistical analyses

Statistical analysis was performed using SPSS software (version 16.0 for Windows; IBM Corporation, Armonk, NY, USA). Comparisons between groups were examined by Fisher's exact test for categorical variables. A statistically significant difference was defined as a P value of <0.05. Survival curves were evaluated using Kaplan–Meier analysis. Event-free survival (EFS) was defined as the time from diagnosis to first recurrence of the disease, including induction failure, or death. Induction failure was defined as failure to achieve complete remission and considered as an event at one day after date of diagnosis. Overall survival (OS) was defined as the time from diagnosis to death. Patients who were alive and had no progression of disease or relapse were censored at the time of their last follow-up.

Results

De novo generation of ALL cell lines bearing the *BIM* deletion polymorphism

To determine if the *BIM* deletion polymorphism is sufficient to confer GC resistance to ALL cells, we used zinc finger nucleases to derive *de novo* ALL cell lines bearing the deletion. Because human cell lines vary in their amenability to transfection and genome editing by zinc fingers (personal communication, TK Ko and unpublished observations), we tested the ability of our approach to edit 3 different GC-sensitive ALL cell lines (CCRF-CEM, RS4;11, and PALL-2) [39–41] that did not have the polymorphism. Of these lines, we were only able to successfully generate clones containing the deletion in CCRF-CEM cells. The structure of the *BIM* gene and the location of the deletion in intron 2 are illustrated in Figure 1A. Using PCR primers that flank the deleted region, we identified subclones that either did not have the deletion (denoted $BIM^{i2+/+}$) or were heterozygous (denoted $BIM^{i2+/-}$) or homozygous (denoted $BIM^{i2-/-}$) for the deletion polymorphism (Figure 1B). The deleted region contains splicing elements that either promote the production of functional, exon 4-containing isoforms or suppress the production of non-apoptotic, exon 3-containing isoforms [42]. Consequently, when deleted, an increase in exon 3 to exon 4-containing transcripts is expected. To confirm that the deletion produced the expected changes in the splicing of *BIM*, we measured the ratio of exon 3- to exon 4-containing transcripts in clones of each genotype by exon-specific RT-PCR, and found that it was increased in a polymorphism-dosage-dependent manner (Figure 1C).

The *BIM* deletion polymorphism is sufficient to confer GC resistance in ALL cells

To determine if the deletion conferred resistance to GCs, we compared the effect of treating clones of each genotype with a range of dexamethasone concentrations. First, we quantified cell viability using the MTS assay and found that across the range tested, the deletion-containing clones exhibited increased cell viability in a polymorphism dosage-dependent manner (Figure 2A). Following this, we assessed the extent of apoptosis using the induction of cleaved poly ADP-ribose polymerase (PARP), as well as the level of cleaved caspase 3, using immunoblots performed on lysates of cells treated as in Figure 2A. We also probed for BIM using an antibody that only detects the pro-apoptotic E4-containing isoforms (BIM EL, L, and S). As a marker of glucocorticoid receptor (GR) activation, we probed for phospho-GR (S211). As predicted, when compared to wildtype clones, upregulation of E4-containing BIM isoforms was impaired in a polymorphism dosage-dependent manner. Furthermore, apoptosis was attenuated in clones with the deletion, as evidenced by an increase in cleaved PARP, as well as cleaved caspase 3 (Figure 2B). Importantly, this occurred in spite of equivalent GR phosphorylation and auto-induction upon GC treatment across the genotypes (Figure 2C). These results indicate that GC resistance in the deletion-containing clones takes place downstream of the GR, and is consistent with our hypothesis that GC resistance results from impaired expression of BH3-containing BIM isoforms. Taken together, our data demonstrate that the presence of the *BIM* deletion polymorphism is sufficient to confer GC resistance in ALL cells.

Because prior work has shown that *in vitro* GC responses *per se* is an important prognostic factor in childhood ALL [33,34], we predicted that patients with the *BIM* deletion polymorphism would have inferior outcomes compared to those without.

The *BIM* deletion polymorphism does not predict inferior responses in pediatric ALL

To test our prediction that the *BIM* deletion polymorphism confers a poorer clinical outcome in pediatric ALL, we conducted a retrospective analysis correlating treatment outcome with the presence of the polymorphism in a group of uniformly-treated pediatric patients from the Malaysia-Singapore (Ma-Spore) ALL 2003 multicenter study. The Ma-Spore ALL 2003 protocol was based on a modified Berlin-Frankfurt-Münster regimen, where all patients received intrathecal methotrexate together with seven days of oral prednisolone at the point of diagnosis. Patients subsequently completed the rest of their induction regimen based on a common backbone of vincristine, L-asparaginase, and methotrexate, followed by risk-adapted consolidation and maintenance therapy as directed by their MRD status at day 33. Importantly, the design of this study allowed us to determine if the *BIM* deletion predicts for inferior clinical outcomes at three distinct assessment points: initial GC response (defined as absolute blast count ≥1000/μl at day 8), day 33 MRD following multi-agent induction chemotherapy, as well as overall survival (OS) and event-free survival (EFS) after consolidation and maintenance therapy.

Sufficient DNA from 411 individuals (out of a total of 556) from the Ma-Spore study was available for analysis for the *BIM* deletion polymorphism. Importantly, there was no difference in treatment outcome between this subgroup of 411 patients compared to the 556 patients in the full study (5-year EFS 82.0% vs 80.6%). Using this sample set, we determined the incidence of the *BIM* deletion to be 12.2%, which is consistent with the ethnic make up of the Ma-Spore cohort, as well as the incidence of the polymorphism in the normal population (Table 1, [17]). We also found that the *BIM* deletion polymorphism did not segregate according to any patient demographic except for Chinese ethnicity, which is as expected, or adverse prognostic indicators such as genetic subtype (Table 1).

We next determined if the *BIM* deletion predicted for inferior outcomes at each of the three response assessment points described above. Here, and to our surprise, we found that there was no significant difference between patients with or without the deletion for GC response at day 8 ($P = 0.804$), MRD response at day 33

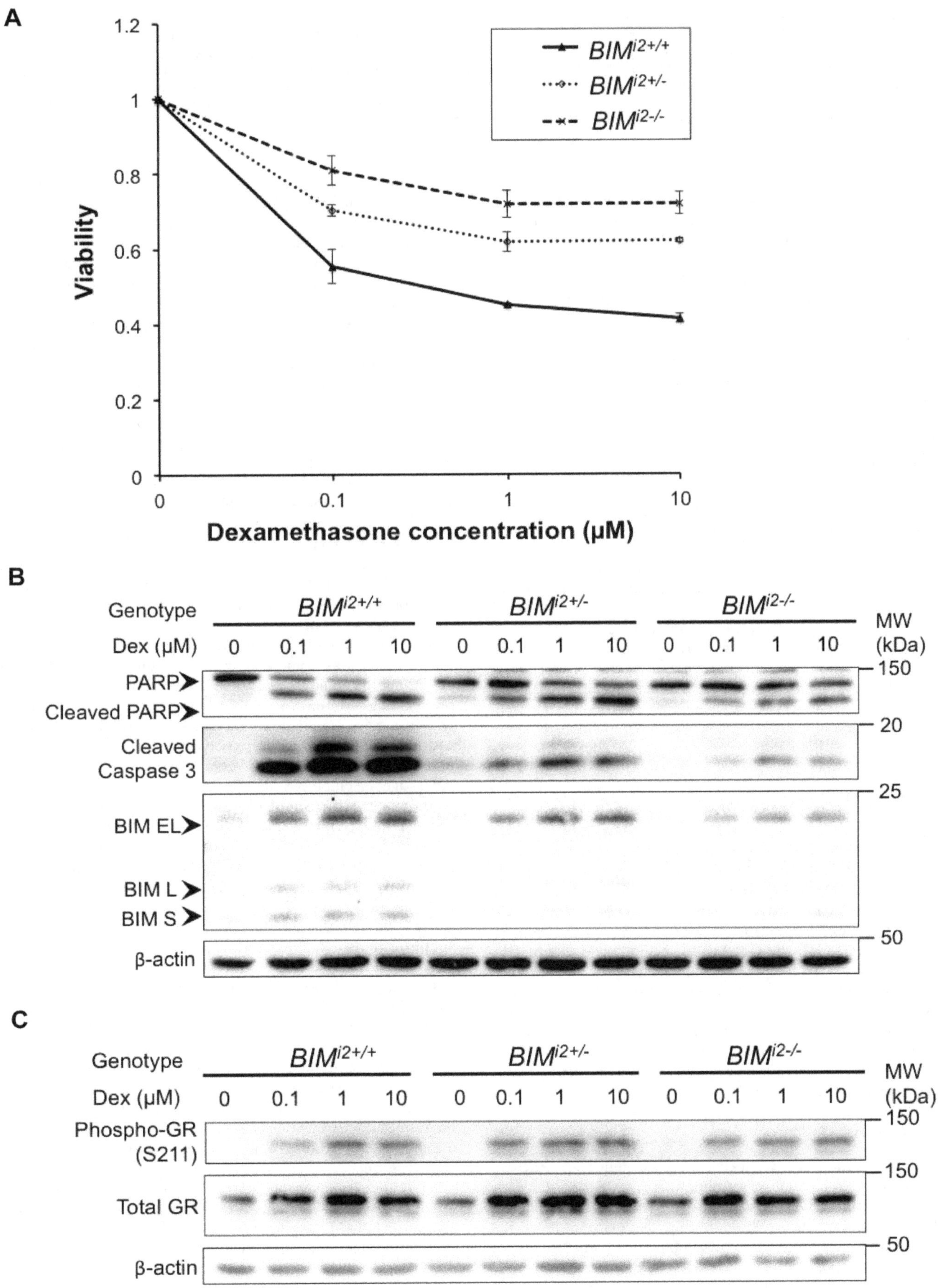
A
Viability
Dexamethasone concentration (μM)
BIMi2+/+
BIMi2+/-
BIMi2-/-
B
Genotype
Dex (μM)
PARP
Cleaved PARP
Cleaved Caspase 3
BIM EL
BIM L
BIM S
β-actin
MW (kDa)
C
Phospho-GR (S211)
Total GR

Figure 2. The *BIM* deletion confers dexamethasone resistance in CCRF-CEM cells. (**A**) Cell viability following exposure of CCRF-CEM subclones to increasing concentrations of dexamethasone. Viability was measured by MTS assay at 48 h. Error bars indicate mean ± SEM (n = 3) of 3 independent replicates. (**B**) Western blot of cell lysates from CCRF-CEM $BIM^{i2+/+}$, $BIM^{i2+/-}$ and $BIM^{i2-/-}$ clones following treatment with increasing doses of dexamethasone for 48 h. The induction of cleaved PARP and cleaved caspase 3 were used as readouts for apoptosis. An antibody that recognizes pro-apoptotic exon-4 containing BIM isoforms (BIM EL, L and S) was used to show the extent of BIM upregulation following GC exposure. β-actin was used as a loading control. (**C**) Western blot showing phosphorylation of the glucocorticoid receptor (Phospho-GR S211) in CCRF-CEM $BIM^{i2+/+}$, $BIM^{i2+/-}$ and $BIM^{i2-/-}$ clones upon treatment with dexamethasone.

($P = 0.970$), nor EFS ($P = 0.427$) or overall OS ($P = 0.646$) (Table 1, Figures 3A and 3B). Additionally, subgroup analysis by genetic subtype, race and risk category at diagnosis did not uncover any associations between the *BIM* deletion polymorphism and treatment outcome (data not shown). Together, these results demonstrate that the *BIM* deletion polymorphism does not predict for inferior outcomes following the administration of a modern GC-containing three-drug remission-induction regimen. Our clinical observations led us to propose that at least one or more of the chemotherapy agents employed during induction is able to overcome GC resistance conferred by the *BIM* deletion polymorphism.

Chemotherapy overcomes GC resistance conferred by the *BIM* deletion polymorphism

To determine if any of the chemotherapy agents used in the induction regimen was able to overcome *BIM* deletion-mediated GC resistance, we treated the *BIM* deletion-containing clones with methotrexate, vincristine, and L-asparaginase individually, and in combination with dexamethasone. Cells were then assessed for activation of apoptotic cell death, BIM protein induction, and cell viability.

First, using immunoblot, we found that each of the three chemotherapy agents was individually able to induce equivalent levels of apoptotic cell death (as measured by the production of cleaved PARP and caspase 3) in the absence and presence of the *BIM* deletion (Figures 4A–C, compare lanes 3, 7 and 11). Importantly, we also observed that chemotherapy-induced apoptosis occurred without significant induction of any of the three BIM isoforms (BIM EL, L, and S) reported to be important for GC-induced apoptosis [31]. These results demonstrate that methotrexate, vincristine, and L-asparaginase are each able to induce ALL cell death in a BIM-independent manner, and that this occurred regardless of the *BIM* deletion status of the cell line.

Next, we found that when dexamethasone was combined with methotrexate, vincristine or L-asparaginase, there was a consistent increase in the level of activated PARP and caspase 3 compared to GC alone (Figures 4A–C, lanes 4, 8 and 12). Similarly, when cell viability was assayed, the addition of methotrexate (Figure 5A), vincristine (Figure 5B), or L-asparaginase (Figure 5C) to dexamethasone augmented cell death in deletion-containing clones. Taken together, our *in vitro* data suggest that the ability of the *BIM* deletion polymorphism to confer GC resistance can be overcome by the co-administration of several of the cytotoxic components of the Ma-Spore regimen, including methotrexate, vincristine, and L-asparaginase.

Discussion

In the current work, we used a genome-editing approach to demonstrate that a common germline variant in the *BIM* gene is sufficient to confer GC resistance in ALL cell lines. Mechanistically, we confirm that cells harboring the deletion favor the splicing and expression of non-apoptotic isoforms of BIM, impairing the apoptotic response to GC exposure, and thereby promoting ALL cell survival. However, using a cohort of 411 uniformly-treated ALL patients, we also find that the deletion does not predict inferior responses to GC-containing multi-agent chemotherapy, and that this is associated with the ability of chemotherapy to induce BIM-independent cell death.

By generating CCRF-CEM subclones that were either wildtype, heterozygous or homozygous for the *BIM* polymorphism, we were able to demonstrate that the *BIM* deletion polymorphism is able to confer GC resistance in a T-ALL cell line. In these clones, the expected changes in splicing to favor the E3-containing, non-apoptotic splice variants were recapitulated in a polymorphism dose-dependent manner. We then showed that both upregulation of the E4-containing *BIM* isoforms and apoptosis upon GC treatment were impaired in the deletion-containing clones. Overall, our results are consistent with prior work demonstrating a critical role for BIM induction in GC-induced ALL cell death, particularly the EL, L, and S isoforms which harbor the E4- and BH3-containing isoforms capable of activating apoptosis [27,31]. One limitation of our *in vitro* studies is the use of a single cell line, CCRF-CEM, which is a T-ALL line. Although we were unable to generate deletion-containing lines of other lineages, we expect that introduction of the deletion, which phenocopies a BIM knock-down of BIM, will likely confer glucocorticoid resistance in other ALL cell lines [27,31,32].

The inability of the *BIM* deletion to segregate poor versus good risk patients was somewhat surprising given previous reports describing the ability of *in vitro* as well as clinical GC responses to predict long-term outcomes in pediatric ALL [33–37]. Importantly, because we were able to generate isogenic cell lines with and without the *BIM* deletion, we could explore the mechanisms underlying our clinical observations. Here, we found that three other agents employed in the Ma-Spore ALL 2003 regimen, methotrexate, vincristine, and L-asparaginase, are each individually able to overcome *BIM* deletion-associated GC resistance. Our *in vitro* results also indicate that each of these drugs activate apoptotic cell death in a largely BIM-independent manner, and that this is likely to underlie their clinical efficacy in overcoming *BIM* deletion-mediated GC resistance. While the precise mechanisms by which methotrexate and L-asparaginase induce apoptosis remain ill-defined [43], it is interesting to note that the mechanism of vincristine-induced apoptosis has recently been described [44]. Here [44], and consistent with our observations, vincristine-induced apoptosis was shown to occur via the depletion of the pro-survival protein MCL1, a factor that has itself been shown to mediate GC resistance in ALL [45].

It is also important to highlight that *in vitro* resistance to GC, which has been shown to correlate with clinical responses [33,34], may not necessarily readout for GC resistance *per se*. This is because such assays will also read out for more general mechanisms of resistance that would be expected to mediate cross-resistance among different drug classes, a conclusion that other studies have suggested [46,47]. More recent work has also implicated other germline *BIM* variants in mediating drug resistance [48,49]. Importantly, and reminiscent of our data, we note that it was the combination of a functional SNP in *BIM* with a SNP in the *MCL1* promoter (associated with increased *MCL1* expression) that best predicted OS in pediatric ALL [49,50].

Table 1. Biological and clinical features of patients from the Ma-Spore ALL 2003 trial genotyped for the *BIM* polymorphism.

Characteristics	Wildtype (n = 361)		*BIM* polymorphism present (n = 50)		*P* value
	No.	%	No.	%	
Age at diagnosis					1.000
<1 or >10	71	19.7	10	20	
1–10	290	80.3	40	80	
Sex					0.094
Male	213	59	23	46	
Female	148	41	27	54	
Molecular subtype^					0.127
ETV6-RUNX1	68	19	7	14.3	
TCF-PBX1	17	4.7	7	14.3	
BCR-ABL1	16	4.5	1	2	
MLL rearrangements	9	2.5	3	6.1	
Hyperdiploidy	65	18.2	12	24.5	
Hypodiploidy	4	1.1	0	0	
T-ALL	30	8.4	3	6.1	
Others	149	41.6	16	32.7	
NCI Risk					0.642
High	138	38.2	17	34	
Low	223	61.8	33	66	
Day 8 Prednisolone Response^					0.804
Good	320	88.9	44	91.7	
Poor	40	11.1	4	8.3	
Day 33 PCR MRD^					0.970
<0.01%	146	43.6	19	46.3	
0.01–1%	155	46.4	18	43.9	
≥1%	34	10	4	9.8	
PCR MRD Risk^					0.966
Standard	134	38.4	17	37	
Intermediate	194	55.6	27	58.7	
High	21	6	2	4.3	
Ma-Spore Risk^					0.463
Standard	109	30.2	14	28	
Intermediate	177	49	29	58	
High	75	20.8	7	14	
Ma-Spore Outcome					0.608
CCR	295	81.7	42	84	
Induction Failure	16	4.4	1	2	
Relapse	21	5.8	1	2	
Death	17	4.7	3	6	
Abandonment	12	3.3	3	6	
Race					<0.001
Chinese	156	43.2	35	70	
Malay	147	40.7	14	28	
Indian & Others	58	16.1	1	2	

Incidence of the *BIM* polymorphism is 50 out of 411 patients, or 12.2%. Abbreviations: Ma-Spore, Malaysia- Singapore; MRD, minimal residual disease; NCI, National Cancer Institute; PCR, polymerase chain reaction; CCR, continuous complete remission.
^indicates that data was unavailable for some patients.

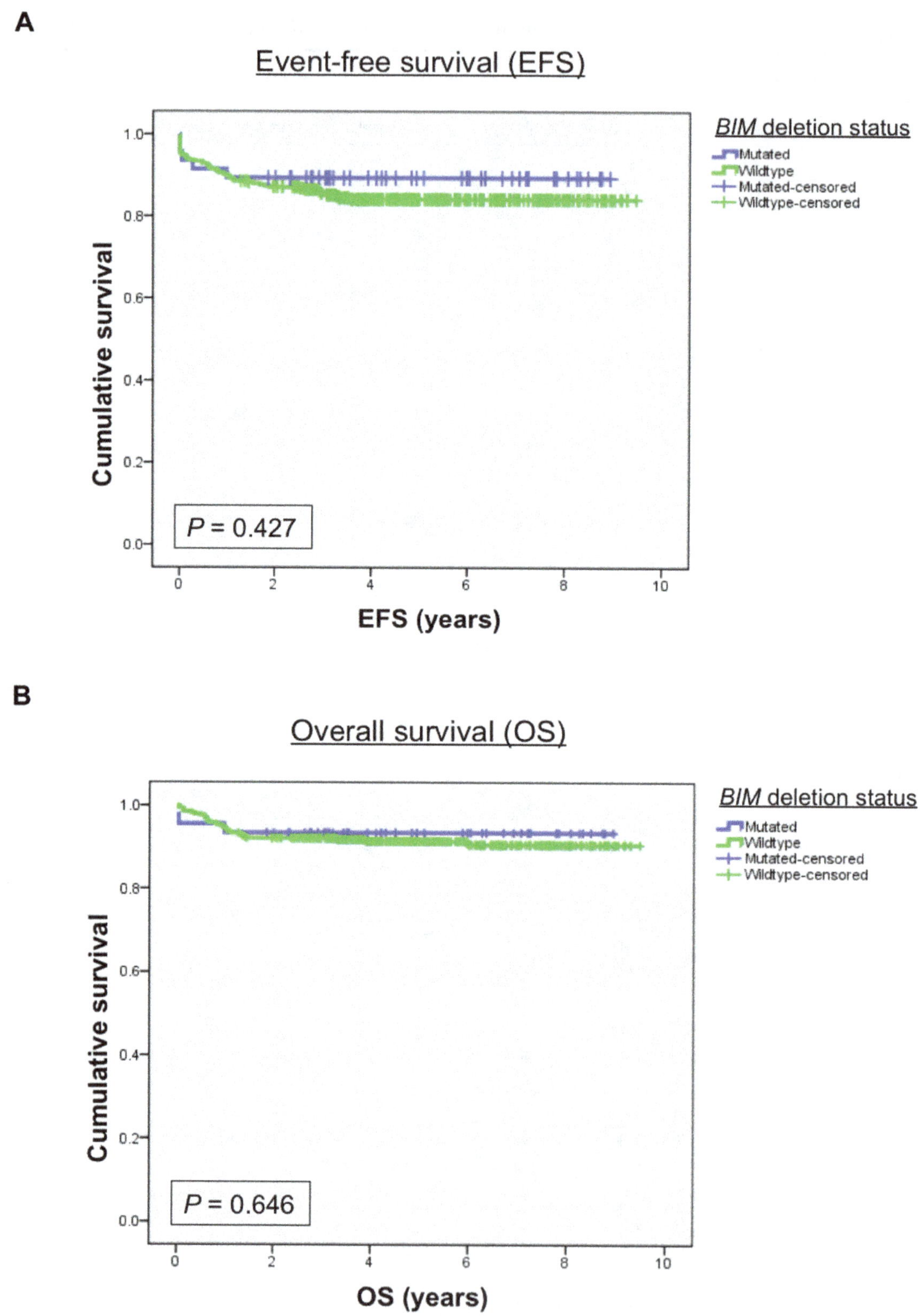

Figure 3. Retrospective analysis of the Ma-Spore ALL 2003 cohort according to the presence or absence of the *BIM* deletion polymorphism. Kaplan-Meier curves comparing event-free survival (**A**) or overall survival (**B**) in patients with or without the *BIM* deletion polymorphism are shown.

Together, our observations are consistent with a "BCL-2 rheostat" model where the cellular apoptotic threshold is set by the balance of pro-apoptotic BCL-2 family members such as BIM and anti-apoptotic members like MCL1 [27]. This model would predict

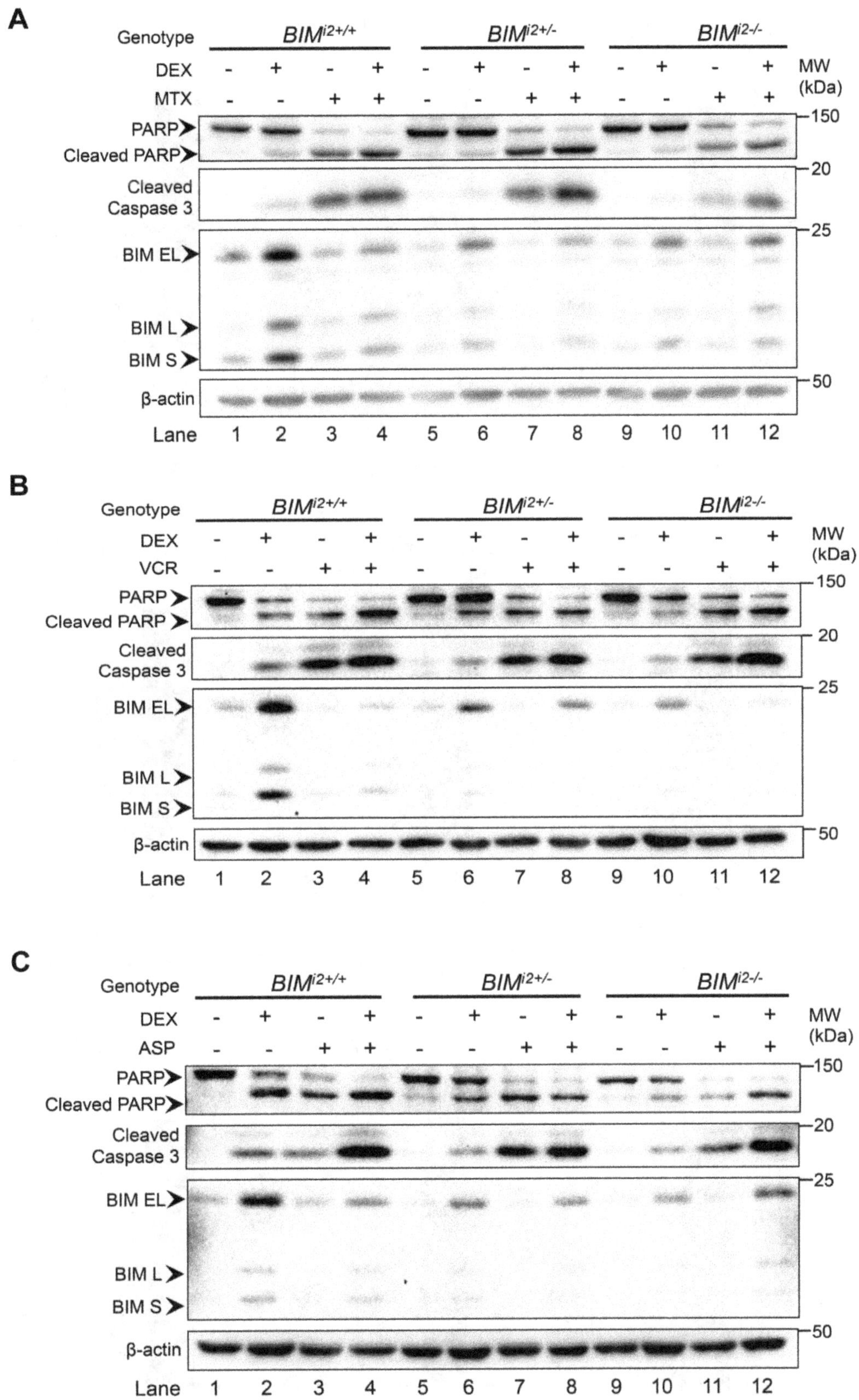

Figure 4. Methotrexate, vincristine, and L-asparaginase activate apoptosis in a BIM-independent manner, and overcome *BIM* deletion-mediated GC resistance. CCRF-CEM clones were treated with dexamethasone (DEX) (0.1 μM) with or without (**A**) methotrexate (MTX) (1 μM), (**B**) vincristine (VCR) (2 ng/ml), or (C) L-asparaginase (ASP) (0.5 IU/ml) for 48 h. Following incubation, cell lysates were obtained and analyzed for cleaved PARP and caspase 3, as well as BIM induction. β-actin was used as a loading control.

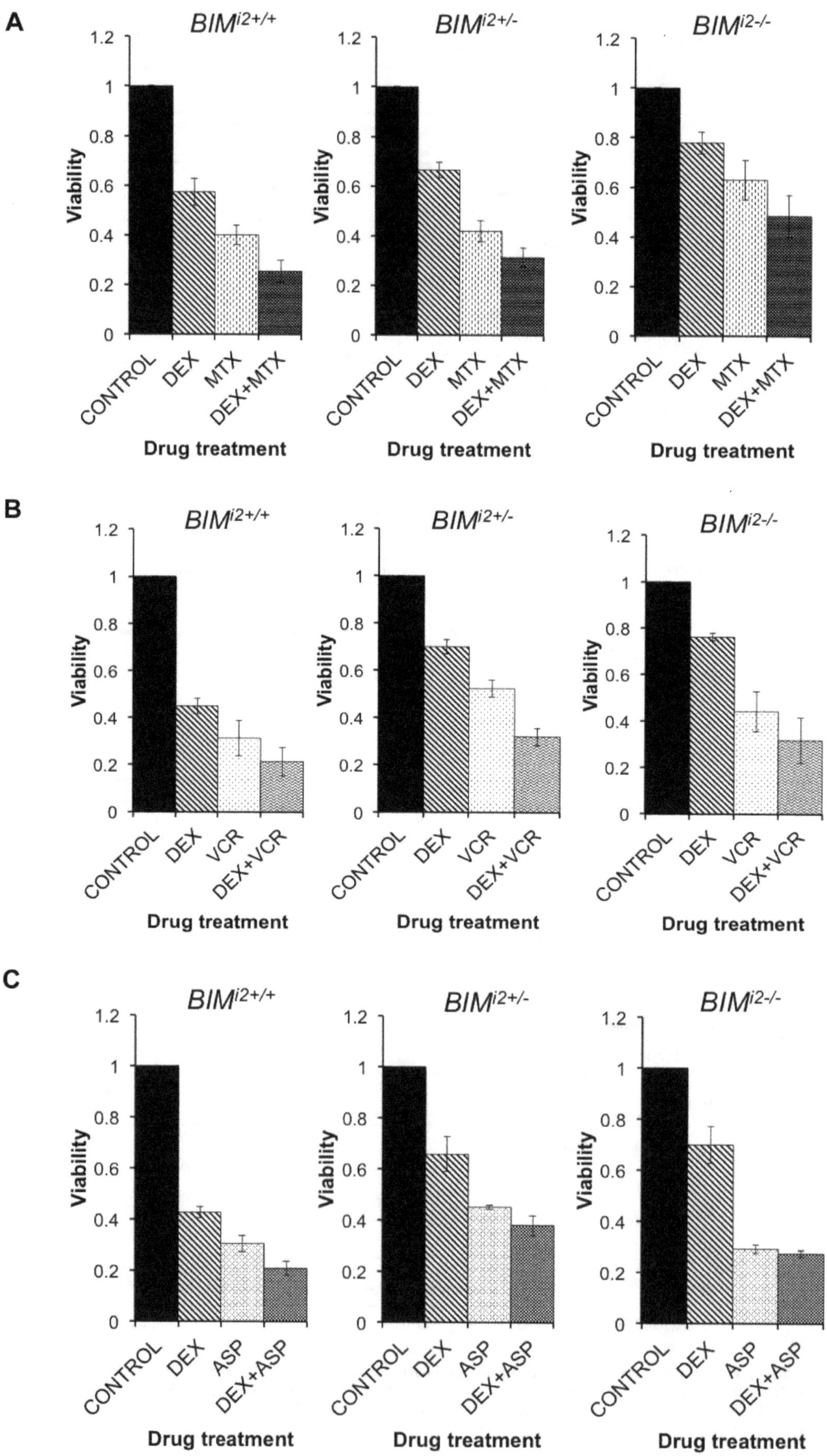
A
BIMi2+/+
BIMi2+/-
BIMi2-/-
Viability
0
0.2
0.4
0.6
0.8
1
1.2
CONTROL
DEX
MTX
DEX+MTX
Drug treatment
B
BIMi2+/+
BIMi2+/-
BIMi2-/-
Viability
CONTROL
DEX
VCR
DEX+VCR
Drug treatment
C
BIMi2+/+
BIMi2+/-
BIMi2-/-
Viability
CONTROL
DEX
ASP
DEX+ASP
Drug treatment

Figure 5. The addition of methotrexate, vincristine or L-asparaginase resensitizes *BIM* deletion-containing CCRF-CEM clones to dexamethasone. Cell viability was measured by MTS assay after (**A**) methotrexate (MTX) (1 μM), (**B**) vincristine (VCR) (2 ng/ml), or (**C**) L-asparaginase (ASP) (0.5 IU/ml) was used singly or in combination with dexamethasone (DEX) (0.1 μM) for 48 h. Values obtained for treated cells were normalized to the untreated control for the same genotype. Error bars indicate SEM (n =) of 3 independent replicates.

that genetic variants affecting BCL2 family members may only be clinically important when two or more act in concert to alter the apoptotic threshold.

While there is increasing evidence that germline polymorphisms contribute to clinical heterogeneity in ALL [13–15], it is likely that only those variants capable of conferring alterations in biological behavior and/or multi-drug resistance will be associated with clinically meaningful endpoints. Thus, as we have demonstrated with the *BIM* deletion, polymorphisms that confer single-drug resistance in the setting of modern multi-agent ALL therapy are less likely to be of clinical importance. Indeed, variants that have been shown to predict poor response are enriched for genes expected to confer a multi-drug resistance phenotype, and include those that influence systemic drug clearance and intracellular drug concentrations [9,12].

Finally, our observations also highlight the ability of at least three cytotoxic agents to induce apoptosis independently of BIM, and suggest that the success of modern day ALL regimens is due to the ability of individual agents to kill leukemia cells via targeting different components of the "BCL-2 rheostat". Indeed, this general lesson may be applied to cancers where we have found that the *BIM* deletion does play a part in clinical drug resistance [17], and supports the use of judiciously chosen combination therapies to overcome *BIM* deletion-mediated drug resistance in these patients.

Acknowledgments

The authors thank the collaborators and patients in the Ma-Spore ALL 2003 study, as well as TK Ko for advice on genome editing and SK Kham for technical assistance.

Author Contributions

Conceived and designed the experiments: STO AEJY. Performed the experiments: SXS JYL JWJH. Analyzed the data: SXS JYL NJ STO AEJY. Contributed to the writing of the manuscript: SXS STO.

References

1. Mullighan CG (2012) The molecular genetic makeup of acute lymphoblastic leukemia. Hematology Am Soc Hematol Educ Program 2012: 389–396.
2. Pui CH, Evans WE (2006) Treatment of acute lymphoblastic leukemia. N Engl J Med 354: 166–178.
3. Locatelli F, Schrappe M, Bernardo ME, Rutella S (2012) How I treat relapsed childhood acute lymphoblastic leukemia. Blood 120: 2807–2816.
4. Yeoh EJ, Ross ME, Shurtleff SA, Williams WK, Patel D, et al. (2002) Classification, subtype discovery, and prediction of outcome in pediatric acute lymphoblastic leukemia by gene expression profiling. Cancer Cell 1: 133–143.
5. Martinelli G, Iacobucci I, Storlazzi CT, Vignetti M, Paoloni F, et al. (2009) IKZF1 (Ikaros) deletions in BCR-ABL1-positive acute lymphoblastic leukemia are associated with short disease-free survival and high rate of cumulative incidence of relapse: a GIMEMA AL WP report. J Clin Oncol 27: 5202–5207.
6. Roberts KG, Morin RD, Zhang J, Hirst M, Zhao Y, et al. (2012) Genetic alterations activating kinase and cytokine receptor signaling in high-risk acute lymphoblastic leukemia. Cancer Cell 22: 153–166.
7. McLeod HL (2013) Cancer pharmacogenomics: early promise, but concerted effort needed. Science 339: 1563–1566.
8. Coate L, Cuffe S, Horgan A, Hung RJ, Christiani D, et al. (2010) Germline genetic variation, cancer outcome, and pharmacogenetics. J Clin Oncol 28: 4029–4037.
9. Radtke S, Zolk O, Renner B, Paulides M, Zimmermann M, et al. (2013) Germline genetic variations in methotrexate candidate genes are associated with pharmacokinetics, toxicity, and outcome in childhood acute lymphoblastic leukemia. Blood 121: 5145–5153.
10. Xu H, Cheng C, Devidas M, Pei D, Fan Y, et al. (2012) ARID5B genetic polymorphisms contribute to racial disparities in the incidence and treatment outcome of childhood acute lymphoblastic leukemia. J Clin Oncol 30: 751–757.
11. Trevino LR, Shimasaki N, Yang W, Panetta JC, Cheng C, et al. (2009) Germline genetic variation in an organic anion transporter polypeptide associated with methotrexate pharmacokinetics and clinical effects. J Clin Oncol 27: 5972–5978.
12. Rocha JC, Cheng C, Liu W, Kishi S, Das S, et al. (2005) Pharmacogenetics of outcome in children with acute lymphoblastic leukemia. Blood 105: 4752–4758.
13. Perez-Andreu V, Roberts KG, Harvey RC, Yang W, Cheng C, et al. (2013) Inherited GATA3 variants are associated with Ph-like childhood acute lymphoblastic leukemia and risk of relapse. Nat Genet 45: 1494–1498.
14. Yang JJ, Cheng C, Devidas M, Cao X, Campana D, et al. (2012) Genome-wide association study identifies germline polymorphisms associated with relapse of childhood acute lymphoblastic leukemia. Blood 120: 4197–4204.
15. Yang JJ, Cheng C, Yang W, Pei D, Cao X, et al. (2009) Genome-wide interrogation of germline genetic variation associated with treatment response in childhood acute lymphoblastic leukemia. JAMA 301: 393–403.
16. Gaj T, Gersbach CA, Barbas CF 3rd (2013) ZFN, TALEN, and CRISPR/Cas-based methods for genome engineering. Trends Biotechnol 31: 397–405.
17. Ng KP, Hillmer AM, Chuah CT, Juan WC, Ko TK, et al. (2012) A common BIM deletion polymorphism mediates intrinsic resistance and inferior responses to tyrosine kinase inhibitors in cancer. Nat Med 18: 521–528.
18. Morel F, Ka C, Le Bris MJ, Herry A, Morice P, et al. (2003) Deletion of the 5′ABL region in Philadelphia chromosome positive chronic myeloid leukemia: frequency, origin and prognosis. Leuk Lymphoma 44: 1333–1338.
19. Jabbour E, Cortes JE, Kantarjian HM (2009) Suboptimal response to or failure of imatinib treatment for chronic myeloid leukemia: what is the optimal strategy? Mayo Clin Proc 84: 161–169.
20. Aichberger KJ, Mayerhofer M, Krauth MT, Vales A, Kondo R, et al. (2005) Low-level expression of proapoptotic Bcl-2-interacting mediator in leukemic cells in patients with chronic myeloid leukemia: role of BCR/ABL, characterization of underlying signaling pathways, and reexpression by novel pharmacologic compounds. Cancer Res 65: 9436–9444.
21. Bouillet P, Metcalf D, Huang DC, Tarlinton DM, Kay TW, et al. (1999) Proapoptotic Bcl-2 relative Bim required for certain apoptotic responses, leukocyte homeostasis, and to preclude autoimmunity. Science 286: 1735–1738.
22. Cragg MS, Kuroda J, Puthalakath H, Huang DC, Strasser A (2007) Gefitinib-induced killing of NSCLC cell lines expressing mutant EGFR requires BIM and can be enhanced by BH3 mimetics. PLoS Med 4: 1681–1689; discussion 1690.
23. Gong Y, Somwar R, Politi K, Balak M, Chmielecki J, et al. (2007) Induction of BIM is essential for apoptosis triggered by EGFR kinase inhibitors in mutant EGFR-dependent lung adenocarcinomas. PLoS Med 4: e294.
24. Kuribara R, Honda H, Matsui H, Shinjyo T, Inukai T, et al. (2004) Roles of Bim in apoptosis of normal and Bcr-Abl-expressing hematopoietic progenitors. Mol Cell Biol 24: 6172–6183.
25. Kuroda J, Puthalakath H, Cragg MS, Kelly PN, Bouillet P, et al. (2006) Bim and Bad mediate imatinib-induced killing of Bcr/Abl+ leukemic cells, and resistance due to their loss is overcome by a BH3 mimetic. Proc Natl Acad Sci U S A 103: 14907–14912.
26. Erlacher M, Michalak EM, Kelly PN, Labi V, Niederegger H, et al. (2005) BH3-only proteins Puma and Bim are rate-limiting for gamma-radiation- and glucocorticoid-induced apoptosis of lymphoid cells in vivo. Blood 106: 4131–4138.
27. Ploner C, Rainer J, Niederegger H, Eduardoff M, Villunger A, et al. (2008) The BCL2 rheostat in glucocorticoid-induced apoptosis of acute lymphoblastic leukemia. Leukemia 22: 370–377.
28. Wang Z, Malone MH, He H, McColl KS, Distelhorst CW (2003) Microarray analysis uncovers the induction of the proapoptotic BH3-only protein Bim in multiple models of glucocorticoid-induced apoptosis. J Biol Chem 278: 23861–23867.
29. Schmidt S, Rainer J, Riml S, Ploner C, Jesacher S, et al. (2006) Identification of glucocorticoid-response genes in children with acute lymphoblastic leukemia. Blood 107: 2061–2069.
30. Bachmann PS, Piazza RG, Janes ME, Wong NC, Davies C, et al. (2010) Epigenetic silencing of BIM in glucocorticoid poor-responsive pediatric acute lymphoblastic leukemia, and its reversal by histone deacetylase inhibition. Blood 116: 3013–3022.
31. Abrams MT, Robertson NM, Yoon K, Wickstrom E (2004) Inhibition of glucocorticoid-induced apoptosis by targeting the major splice variants of BIM mRNA with small interfering RNA and short hairpin RNA. J Biol Chem 279: 55809–55817.

32. Jiang N, Koh GS, Lim JY, Kham SK, Ariffin H, et al. (2011) BIM is a prognostic biomarker for early prednisolone response in pediatric acute lymphoblastic leukemia. Exp Hematol 39: 321–329.
33. Kaspers GJ, Pieters R, Van Zantwijk CH, Van Wering ER, Van Der Does-Van Den Berg A, et al. (1998) Prednisolone resistance in childhood acute lymphoblastic leukemia: vitro-vivo correlations and cross-resistance to other drugs. Blood 92: 259–266.
34. Den Boer ML, Harms DO, Pieters R, Kazemier KM, Gobel U, et al. (2003) Patient stratification based on prednisolone-vincristine-asparaginase resistance profiles in children with acute lymphoblastic leukemia. J Clin Oncol 21: 3262–3268.
35. Lauten M, Moricke A, Beier R, Zimmermann M, Stanulla M, et al. (2012) Prediction of outcome by early bone marrow response in childhood acute lymphoblastic leukemia treated in the ALL-BFM 95 trial: differential effects in precursor B-cell and T-cell leukemia. Haematologica 97: 1048–1056.
36. Dordelmann M, Reiter A, Borkhardt A, Ludwig WD, Gotz N, et al. (1999) Prednisone response is the strongest predictor of treatment outcome in infant acute lymphoblastic leukemia. Blood 94: 1209–1217.
37. Schrappe M, Arico M, Harbott J, Biondi A, Zimmermann M, et al. (1998) Philadelphia chromosome-positive (Ph+) childhood acute lymphoblastic leukemia: good initial steroid response allows early prediction of a favorable treatment outcome. Blood 92: 2730–2741.
38. Yeoh AE, Ariffin H, Chai EL, Kwok CS, Chan YH, et al. (2012) Minimal residual disease-guided treatment deintensification for children with acute lymphoblastic leukemia: results from the Malaysia-Singapore acute lymphoblastic leukemia 2003 study. J Clin Oncol 30: 2384–2392.
39. Foley GE, Lazarus H, Farber S, Uzman BG, Boone BA, et al. (1965) Continuous Culture of Human Lymphoblasts from Peripheral Blood of a Child with Acute Leukemia. Cancer 18: 522–529.
40. Stong RC, Korsmeyer SJ, Parkin JL, Arthur DC, Kersey JH (1985) Human acute leukemia cell line with the t(4;11) chromosomal rearrangement exhibits B lineage and monocytic characteristics. Blood 65: 21–31.
41. Miyagi T, Ohyashiki J, Yamato K, Koeffler HP, Miyoshi I (1993) Phenotypic and molecular analysis of Ph1-chromosome-positive acute lymphoblastic leukemia cell lines. Int J Cancer 53: 457–462.
42. Juan WC, Roca X, Ong ST (2014) Identification of cis-Acting Elements and Splicing Factors Involved in the Regulation of BIM Pre-mRNA Splicing. PLoS One 9: e95210.
43. DeVita VT Jr, Lawrence TS, Rosenberg SA (2008) DeVita, Hellman, and Rosenberg's Cancer: Principles & Practice of Oncology. Philadelphia, PA, USA: Wolters Kluwer/Lippincott Williams & Wilkins. pp 427, 451, 490.
44. Wertz IE, Kusam S, Lam C, Okamoto T, Sandoval W, et al. (2011) Sensitivity to antitubulin chemotherapeutics is regulated by MCL1 and FBW7. Nature 471: 110–114.
45. Wei G, Twomey D, Lamb J, Schlis K, Agarwal J, et al. (2006) Gene expression-based chemical genomics identifies rapamycin as a modulator of MCL1 and glucocorticoid resistance. Cancer Cell 10: 331–342.
46. Pieters R, Kaspers GJ, van Wering ER, Huismans DR, Loonen AH, et al. (1993) Cellular drug resistance profiles that might explain the prognostic value of immunophenotype and age in childhood acute lymphoblastic leukemia. Leukemia 7: 392–397.
47. Kaspers GJ, Pieters R, Van Zantwijk CH, Van Wering ER, Veerman AJ (1995) Clinical and cell biological features related to cellular drug resistance of childhood acute lymphoblastic leukemia cells. Leuk Lymphoma 19: 407–416.
48. Augis V, Airiau K, Josselin M, Turcq B, Mahon FX, et al. (2013) A Single Nucleotide Polymorphism in cBIM Is Associated with a Slower Achievement of Major Molecular Response in Chronic Myeloid Leukaemia Treated with Imatinib. PLoS One 8: e78582.
49. Gagne V, Rousseau J, Labuda M, Sharif-Askari B, Brukner I, et al. (2013) Bim polymorphisms: influence on function and response to treatment in children with acute lymphoblastic leukemia. Clin Cancer Res 19(18): 5240–5249.
50. Sanchez R, St-Cyr J, Lalonde ME, Healy J, Richer C, et al. (2013) Impact of promoter polymorphisms in key regulators of the intrinsic apoptosis pathway in childhood acute lymphoblastic leukemia outcome. Haematologica. doi: 10.3324/haematol.2013.085340.

3

The Progeroid Phenotype of Ku80 Deficiency is Dominant over DNA-PK$_{CS}$ Deficiency

Erwin Reiling[1,2], Martijn E. T. Dollé[1], Sameh A. Youssef[3], Moonsook Lee[4], Bhawani Nagarajah[1], Marianne Roodbergen[1], Piet de With[1], Alain de Bruin[3], Jan H. Hoeijmakers[2], Jan Vijg[4], Harry van Steeg[1,5], Paul Hasty[6]*

1 National Institute for Public Health and the Environment, Bilthoven, The Netherlands, **2** Department of Cell Biology and Genetics, Center for Biomedical Genetics, Erasmus MC, Rotterdam, The Netherlands, **3** Faculty of Veterinary Medicine, Department of Pathobiology, Utrecht University, Utrecht, The Netherlands, **4** Department of Genetics, Albert Einstein College of Medicine, Bronx, New York, United States of America, **5** Department of Toxicogenetics, Leiden University Medical Center, Leiden, The Netherlands, **6** Department of Molecular Medicine and Institute of Biotechnology, Barshop Institute for Longevity and Aging Studies, Cancer Therapy and Research Center, University of Texas Health Science Center at San Antonio, San Antonio, Texas, United States of America

Abstract

Ku80 and DNA-PK$_{CS}$ are both involved in the repair of double strand DNA breaks via the nonhomologous end joining (NHEJ) pathway. While *ku80*$^{-/-}$ mice exhibit a severely reduced lifespan and size, this phenotype is less pronounced in *dna-pk$_{cs}$*$^{-/-}$ mice. However, these observations are based on independent studies with varying genetic backgrounds. Here, we generated *ku80*$^{-/-}$, *dna-pk$_{cs}$*$^{-/-}$ and double knock out mice in a C57Bl6/J*FVB F1 hybrid background and compared their lifespan, end of life pathology and mutation frequency in liver and spleen using a lacZ reporter. Our data confirm that inactivation of Ku80 and DNA-PK$_{CS}$ causes reduced lifespan and bodyweights, which is most severe in *ku80*$^{-/-}$ mice. All mutant mice exhibited a strong increase in lymphoma incidence as well as other aging-related pathology (skin epidermal and adnexal atrophy, trabecular bone reduction, kidney tubular anisokaryosis, and cortical and medullar atrophy) and severe lymphoid depletion. LacZ mutation frequency analysis did not show strong differences in mutation frequencies between knock out and wild type mice. The *ku80*$^{-/-}$ mice had the most severe phenotype and the Ku80-mutation was dominant over the DNA-PK$_{CS}$-mutation. Presumably, the more severe degenerative effect of Ku80 inactivation on lifespan compared to DNA-PK$_{CS}$ inactivation is caused by additional functions of Ku80 or activity of free Ku70 since both Ku80 and DNA-PK$_{CS}$ are essential for NHEJ.

Editor: Robert W. Sobol, University of Pittsburgh, United States of America

Funding: This work was supported by a National Institutes of Health grant (P01 AG17242). The funders had no role in study design, data collection and analysis, decision to publish, or preparation of the manuscript.

Competing Interests: The authors have declared that no competing interests exist.

* E-mail: hastye@uthscsa.edu

Introduction

DNA damage is known to be involved in tumorigenesis and aging. There are multiple DNA repair pathways that specialize in repairing a specific DNA lesion. One such pathway is nonhomologous end joining (NHEJ), which plays an import role in the repair of double strand breaks (DSBs). Ku80 and DNA-PK$_{CS}$ are both components of the NHEJ pathway. Ku80 forms a heterodimer with Ku70, known as Ku, which binds to DNA ends at a DSB [1]. DNA-dependent protein kinase (DNA-PK) is a holo enzyme formed by a complex between Ku and DNA-depended protein kinase catalytic subunit (DNA-PK$_{CS}$). DNA-PK$_{CS}$, together with Artemis, Xrcc4-DNA ligase and Xrcc4-like factor, process DNA overhangs and ligation [2–4].

Cells with deletion of any of these NHEJ components show severe combined immunodeficiency (SCID) due to defects in assembling variable (diverse) joining (V(D)J) segments of antigens, genetic instability and hypersensitivity to DSB inducing agents [5–9]. However, there is some phenotypic variation. For instance, deletion of Ku70 and Ku80 results in reduced size, severely decreased lifespan, neuronal apoptosis and accelerated aging. Strikingly, in previous experiments using mixed backgrounds, these mice seem to be protected against tumor development, although they show a low level of thymic lymphomas [10,11]. In contrast, such a phenotype is less pronounced in DNA-PK$_{CS}$ knock out mice. Compared to the *ku70*$^{-/-}$ and *ku80*$^{-/-}$ mice, the early aging phenotype for the *dna-pk$_{cs}$*$^{-/-}$ mice is less severe and best observed with shortened telomeres [12–14]. Yet, these studies were performed in different genetic backgrounds in different labs. Therefore, phenotypic differences could be the result of inconsistent genetic backgrounds and environments. On the other hand, some phenotype differences can be explained by additional functions of the deleted NHEJ components or that a non-deleted NHEJ component is deleterious in absence of the deleted protein. Such deleterious effects have been observed previously [15,16]. For instance, DNA ligase IV deficiency is lethal in presence of Ku80 but lethality is rescued by deletion of Ku80 [16]. Furthermore, the prenatal lethal phenotype of Xrcc4 deficient mice is partly rescued by p53 knock out [15], that negates neuronal apoptosis.

Here, we generated cohorts of *ku80*$^{-/-}$, *dna-pk$_{cs}$*$^{-/-}$, double knockout and wild type mice in an identical genetic background and compared lifespan, development of body weight, end-of-life pathology and accumulation of genetic insults (LacZ mutant frequencies in liver and spleen). We find that *ku80*$^{-/-}$ mice exhibit a more sever phenotype than *dna-pk*$_{cs}$$^{-/-}$ mice while the double mutant mice are as severe as the *ku80*$^{-/-}$ mice. These observations suggest that Ku80 has additional functions that do not require DNA-PK$_{CS}$ or that free Ku70 has a deleterious affect in the absence of Ku80. Both possibilities are in line with our previous reports that show Ku70 and Ku80 have functions independent of the Ku heterodimer [17].

Results

Previous reports suggest that *ku80*$^{-/-}$ mutant mice exhibit a more severe phenotype than *dna-pk*$_{CS}$$^{-/-}$ mice. This was not predicted since both Ku80 and DNA-PK$_{CS}$ are essential for NHEJ. Thus, the phenotypic differences could be due to divergent function or divergent genetic background and environment. Alternatively, one of the components could be toxic in the absence of the deleted protein. To better understand the reason for these different phenotypes we generated *ku80*$^{-/-}$ and *dna-pk*$_{cs}$$^{-/-}$ and double mutant cohorts in the same genetic background using double heterozygous breeders (*ku80*$^{+/-}$ *dna-pk*$_{CS}$$^{+/-}$) as shown in figure 1. The breeding pairs were composed of C57Bl6/J-pUR288 males and FVB females so the cohorts were F1 brothers and sisters raised in the same cages. Thus, all cohorts are controlled for genetic background and environment so any phenotypic difference between the *ku80*$^{-/-}$ and *dna-pk*$_{cs}$$^{-/-}$ cohorts must be due to divergent function. The double mutant mice will also help determine if one component assumes a toxic activity after the other is deleted.

During the longevity study, all mice were weighed every two weeks. As can be seen in figure 2, all mutant mice were smaller compared to wild type mice. *ku80*$^{-/-}$ and double knock out mice weighted between 10 and 20 grams, while *dna-pk*$_{cs}$$^{-/-}$ mice weighted between 15 and 35 grams and were therefore considerably heavier than *ku80*$^{-/-}$ and double knock out mice. Due to differences in body size, organ weights differed significantly between the different genotypes (Figure S1). However, after correction for bodyweight, most organ weights were comparable. The exception is the testis, which was significantly heavier in *dna-pk*$_{cs}$$^{-/-}$ mice compared to the other knock out mice. Marginal significant differences were observed for males in relative organ weight for kidney, liver, spleen and heart. The wild type cohort was terminated after the final mutant mouse died since their life span appeared much longer; therefore, no end of life organ weight data were collected for this cohort. Thus, deletion of either Ku80 or DNA-PK$_{CS}$ reduced body weight with Ku80-deletion being more severe and dominant to DNA-PK$_{CS}$ -deletion.

All mutant mice displayed a severely reduced lifespan compared to wild type mice (Fig. 3). Previously, we showed that *dna-pk*$_{cs}$$^{-/-}$ mice were loner-lived than *ku80*$^{-/-}$ mice for both males and females ($p = 0.01$ and $p = 8.7*10^{-6}$ respectively) [17]. Here we also show that the double knock out mice had the same short life span as *ku80*$^{-/-}$ mice (Fig. 3). Thus, deletion of either Ku80 or DNA-PK$_{CS}$ reduced life span with Ku80-deletion being more severe and dominant to DNA-PK$_{CS}$ -deletion.

We screened for aging pathology in a selected set of animals (n = 4–5). Results are shown in table 1. Evidence of aging was found in the kidney. Mild increased renal tubular anisokaryosis was observed in all knock out models. Moderate to severe renal tubulonephrosis was present in all mutant cohorts compared to wild type animals. Analysis of skin revealed moderate to severe epidermal and adnexal atrophy. Dermis and epidermis thickness was reduced in all mutant mice. Finally, all mutant mice showed mild to moderate reduction in trabecular bone thickness, which is indicative of osteopenia. There were no differences between genotypes in anisokaryosis or lipofuscin accumulation in liver, which was previously observed in aged wild type mice [18]. Thus, deletion of either Ku80 or DNA-PK$_{CS}$ caused an early onset of many but not all aging characteristics previously reported for wild type mice.

Mutant cohorts showed a high tumor incidence at the time of death compared to age-matched controls (table 2). Most tumors were observed in the thymus followed by liver tumors. Pathological examination showed that tumors were almost exclusively

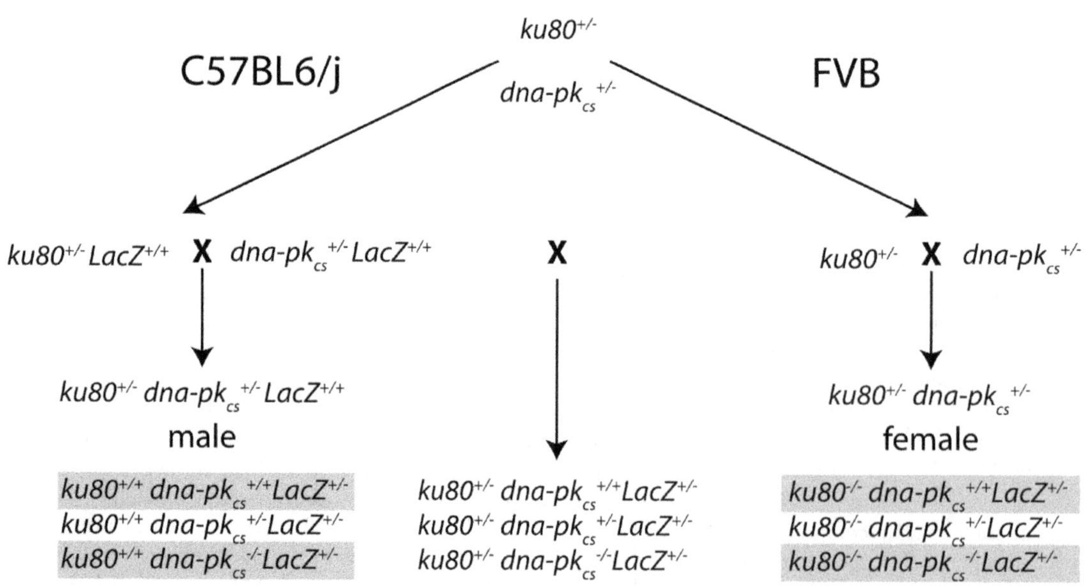

Figure 1. Breeding strategy to generate the knockout cohorts. *Ku80*$^{+/-}$ and *dna-pk*$_{cs}$$^{+/-}$ animals are backcrossed for multiple generations to C57Bl6/J-pUR288 (left of dashed line) and FVB (right of dashed line) background. Double heterozygous knock out C57BL6/J male mice are crossed with double heterozygous knock out FVB female mice. Using this strategy all four desired cohorts are generated as F1 hybrids (grey boxes).

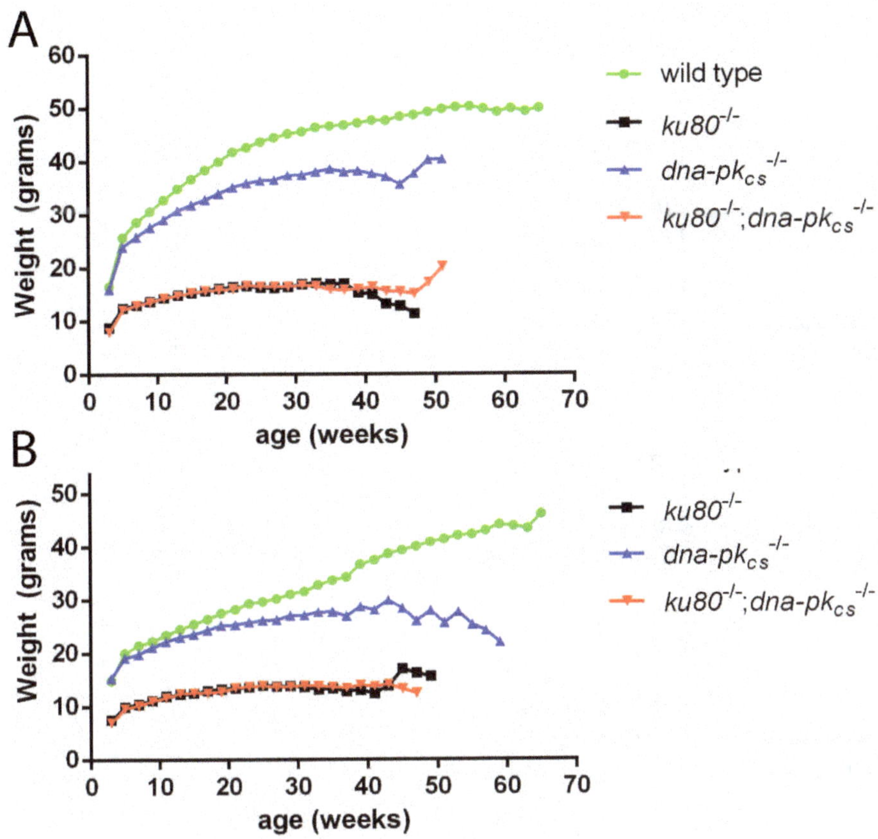

Figure 2. Mean body weights. (A) Males. (B) Females.

lymphomas. CD3 staining showed lymphomas to be of t-cell origin (three mice analyzed for each genotype). There were also rare hepatic adenomas (n = 6), a hepatic carcinoma (n = 1) and a bronchiolo-alveolar carcinoma (n = 1), which might be caused by the C57Bl6/J background according to the Mouse Tumor Database (http://tumor.informatics.jax.org/mtbwi/index.do). Lymphomas were also present in other organs than thymus with a high frequency in liver, kidney, spleen and lymph nodes. Lymphoid tissues of mutant animals, not affected by lymphomas, showed severe lymphoid depletion (table 1) as expected due to the failure to complete V(D)J recombination. This was observed in spleen and mesenterial lymph nodes and was severe in most mutant animals, with exception of female *dna-pk*$_{cs}$$^{-/-}$ mice, which showed a mild to moderate lymphoid depletion in mesenterial lymph nodes. Animals affected by lymphoid depletion also showed an increased myeloid/erythroid ratio. Although tumor incidence was slightly higher in *ku80*$^{-/-}$ mice compared to *dna-pk*$_{cs}$$^{-/-}$ and the highest in double knock out mice, this did not reach statistical significance. No synergistic effects of DNA-PK$_{CS}$ deletion in addition to Ku80 deletion were found nor did deletion of one protein ameliorate the phenotype for deletion of the other protein.

Since Ku80 and DNA-PK$_{CS}$ are DNA damage repair proteins, it would be expected that deletion of these proteins affect mutant frequency. In order to test the LacZ mutant frequencies in liver and spleen, 5 *ku80*$^{-/-}$, *dna-pk*$_{cs}$$^{-/-}$ and double knock males were killed at 38.7, 41.3 and 33.7 weeks, which corresponds approximately with their median lifespan (figure 3). Because the wild type cohort was not maintained beyond median age, we selected the 5 oldest wild type males available at the same observation time (mean age is 37.3 weeks). No significant differences in mutant frequency were observed between genotypes in both liver as spleen (figure 4). We did observe a trend towards increased mutant frequency in double knock out compared to wild type mice in spleen, but this did not reach statistical significance ($p = 0.07$).

Discussion

Previously, it was reported that Ku80 inactivation resulted in reduced cancer and accelerated aging [12,14,19] while a similar but less pronounced phenotype was observed with DNA-PK$_{CS}$ inactivation [12–14]. This phenotypic variance is unexpected since both Ku80 and DNA-PK$_{CS}$ are essential for NHEJ. Therefore, these different phenotypes could be due to differences in genetic background and/or environment. However, our experiment presented here does not support either possibility since we controlled for both genetic background and environment but still observed a disparity in phenotypes. Alternatively, *ku80*$^{-/-}$ mice could exhibit a more severe phenotype than *dna-pk*$_{CS}$$^{-/-}$ mice, if DNA-PK$_{CS}$ is toxic in the absence of Ku80. There is president for this possibility since Ku80-deletion rescued embryonic lethality for *DNA ligase IV*-null mice showing that Ku80 was toxic in the absence of DNA ligase IV. However, deleting DNA-PK$_{CS}$ did not ameliorate the Ku80-mutant phenotype. Instead the double-mutant mice exhibited the same severe phenotype as the Ku80-mutant mice. Therefore, our experiment suggests that Ku80 has extra-NHEJ function or that free Ku70 has a toxic activity in the absence of Ku80.

Our previously published data supports both possibilities. First we found that Ku80 has extra-NHEJ activity in mice by comparing p53-mutant mice deleted for Ku80 or Ku70 or both

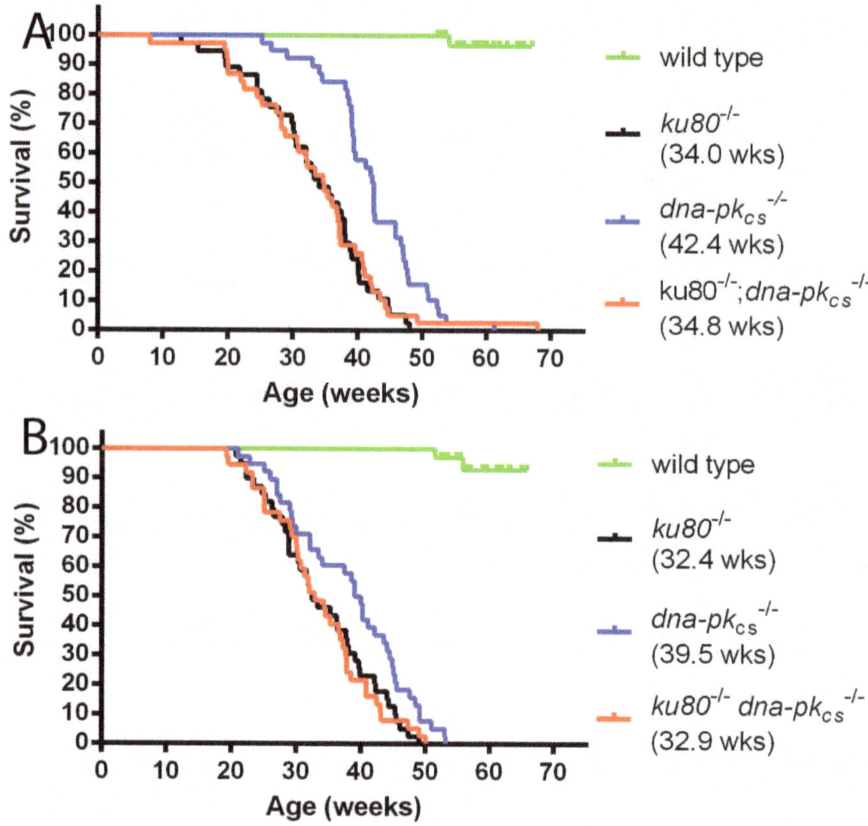

Figure 3. Survival curves. Median survivals are shown in the figure legends in parentheses. *dna-pk*$_{cs}$$^{-/-}$ mice live significantly longer compared to *ku80*$^{-/-}$ mice in both male ($p=0.01$) and females ($p=8.7*10^{-6}$) mice. Survival of double knock out mice is identical to *ku80*$^{-/-}$. (A) Males. (B) Females.

[20]. For this experiment, we found that *ku70*$^{-/-}$ *p53*$^{-/-}$ mice lived longer than *ku80*$^{-/-}$ *p53*$^{-/-}$ mice. This life span extension required Ku80 since the triple-mutant mice had the same life span as the *ku80*$^{-/-}$ *p53*$^{-/-}$ mice. The *ku70*$^{-/-}$ *p53*$^{-/-}$ mice lived longer because they had a lower incidence of pro-B cell lymphoma that was restored with deletion of Ku80. Therefore, these experiments suggest that Ku80 has extra-NHEJ activity. In addition, we showed that free Ku70 and free Ku80 bind to apurinic/apyrimidinic (AP) sites and that free Ku70 inhibits AP endonuclease 1 [17]. Another group also showed that Ku and DNA-PK$_{CS}$ inhibited AP site cleavage by APE1 [21]. Thus, Ku80 and Ku70 have activity that is separable from the Ku heterodimer and NHEJ that could exacerbate the Ku80-mutant phenotype and account for the phenotypic disparity between deleting Ku80 and DNA-PK$_{CS}$.

Ku80 as well as DNA-PK$_{CS}$ inactivation accelerated aging. These characteristics included skin atrophy, femur osteopenia, renal tubular anisokaryosis and cortical and medullar atrophy. Accelerated aging was observed previously in Ku80 and DNA-PK$_{CS}$ negative mice in different genetic backgrounds and environments suggesting that early aging is not sensitive to genetic and environmental changes [10,22] [19].

Deletion of either Ku80 or DNA-PK$_{CS}$ also increased cancer risk. Pathological examination revealed that tumors were predominantly lymphomas. Most lymphomas were observed in the thymus. Lymphomas in non-lymphoid tissues (e.g. liver and lung) are presumably metastases.

By contrast to this report, our prior reports show that *ku80*$^{-/-}$ and *ku70*$^{-/-}$ mice exhibited low levels of cancer [10,11]. Furthermore, deleting Ku80 in a familial adenomatous polyposis mouse model (APC^{MIN}) reduced intestinal tumors and increased life span [23]. We proposed that Ku80-deletion reduced cancer levels due to constitutive activation of the p53 DNA damage response and possibly other responses [24]. In support, deleting p53 greatly enhanced pro-B cell lymphomas and medulloblastoma in *ku80*$^{-/-}$ and *ku70*$^{-/-}$ mice [20,25,26]. Thus, difference in cancer incidences between our prior reports and this report suggest genetic background influence cancer incidence in the *ku80*$^{-/-}$ mice. This is possible since the former reports described mice derived from a 129*C57Bl6/J hybrid background while the current report describes mice derived from a C57Bl6/J*FVB F1 hybrid background.

Furthermore, we observed an increased myeloid/erythroid ratio that suggests true myeloid hyperplasia. However, complete blood counts are needed to confirm this. By contrast, we observed severe lymphoid depletion in all knock out cohorts. Lymphoid depletion is a known phenotype in SCID mice, which have a defective V(D)J recombination [27,28]. Since *ku80*$^{-/-}$ and *dna-pk*$_{cs}$$^{-/-}$ are SCID [9,22], it is not surprising that lymphoid depletion was found in the knock out cohorts. Therefore, this element of the phenotype is not age-related. The increased myeloid/erythroid ratio could be the result of a compensatory response to this lymphoid depletion, triggering myeloid hyperplasia and lymphoma development.

Since Ku80 and DNA-PK$_{CS}$ mutant mice have a defective DSB repair system, one expects accumulation of DNA damage. However, LacZ mutant frequency analysis could not confirm the previously observed increased mutant frequency in spleen [29]. Although our data do show a weak trend into the same direction,

Table 1. Histopathology non-neoplastic lesions.

Lesion	Median pathology score (min – max)							
	ku80$^{-/-}$		*dna-pk*$_{cs}^{-/-}$		*k-/-;d-/-*		**Wild type**	
	Male (41w)	**Female (42w)**	**Male (45w)**	**Female (45w)**	**Male (42w)**	**Female (40w)**	**Male (37w)**	**Female (40w)**
Liver anisokaryosis	2 (1-3)	1.5 (1-3)	3 (1-3)	2* (2-3)	2 (2-3)	2.5 (1-3)	1 (1-2)	1 (1-2)
Liver lipofuscin	1 (1-1)	1 (1-1)	1 (1-1)	1 (1-2)	1 (1-1)	1 (1-1)	1 (1-1)	1 (1-1)
Renal tubular anisokaryosis	2 (1-3)	2 (1-3)*	2 (1-3)	2 (2-3)	3* (2-3)	2 (1-3)	1 (1-2)	1 (1-1)
Renal tubulonephrosis	3*** (1-3)	3*** (2-4)	3*** (1-3)	4*** (2-4)	2*** (1-3)	3*** (1-3)	0 (0-0)	0 (0-0)
Epidermal atrophy	2** (1-3)	2* (1-3)	3** (2-4)	3* (2-3)	3** (1-4)	3* (2-3)	0 (0-0)	0 (0-0)
Adnexal atrophy	1** (1-2)	1* (0-1)	2.5** (1-4)	3** (1-3)	2* (0-4)	2** (1-3)	0 (0-0)	0 (0-0)
Lymphoid depletion spleen	4* (3-4)	4* (3-5)	3* (3-3)	3* (3-3)	4* (3-5)	3** (2-4)	0 (0-0)	0 (0-0)
Lymphoid depletion mes ln	4* (4-5)	3.5** (2-5)	2* (1-2)	1* (1-2)	4** (4-4)	4** (4-4)	0 (0-0)	0 (0-0)
Tissue thickness in μm (St. dev.)								
Dermis and epidermis	253.8* (56.9)	151.3* (11.7)	222.0** (38.3)	172.8 (58.7)	252.0* (99.0)	159.0 (86.3)	374.3 (50.6)	247.3 (43.4)
Trabecular bone	130.8* (36.7)	131.0* (38.2)	124.5* (18.8)	139.8* (25.5)	138.4 (43.1)	118.8** (10.6)	184.0 (19.4)	185.3 (22.4)

4–5 animals examined per group. All selected mutant mice are at end of life, wild type mice are aged matched to mutant mice.
Mean age in weeks is shown (w).
mes ln: mesenterial lymph node.
k-/-;d-/-: *ku80*$^{-/-}$; *dna-pk*$_{cs}^{-/-}$.
St. Dev.: Standard deviation.
p-values based on comparison with wild type animals.
* $p<0.05$.
** $p<0.01$.
*** $p<0.001$.

Table 2. Histopathology neoplastic lesions.

Organ	Tumor	$ku80^{-/-}$		$dna\text{-}pk_{cs}^{-/-}$		*k-/-;d-/-*	
		Male (n = 25)	**Female (n = 15)**	**Male (n = 27)**	**Female (n = 10)**	**Male (n = 24)**	**Female (n = 21)**
Liver	lymphoma	9	5	4	7	5	2
	adenoma	1	1			3	1
	carcinoma					1	
Lung	lymphoma	1					
	carcinoma		1				
Pancreas	lymphoma					1	
Kidney	lymphoma	5	2	3	6	4	5
Thymus	lymphoma*	23	14	21	9	19	15
ovary/uterus	lymphoma		1		2		
Spleen	lymphoma	4		2	3	3	
mes. lm. nd.	lymphoma	3	2	5	5	3	
ax. lm. nd.	lymphoma	3	3	5	5	5	
Skin	lymphoma				1		
Testis	lymphoma	1					
bone marrow**	lymphoma	2	1	2	2	1	1
pituitary gland	lymphoma				1		
Tumor incidence (%)		67	39	55	24	75	51

Mentioned n-numbers are tumor bearing animals available for microscopical examination.
k-/-;d-/-: ku80-/-; $dna\text{-}pk_{cs}^{-/-}$.
mes. lm. nd.: mesenterial lymph node.
ax. lm. nd.: axillary lymph node.
*~5 thymus tumor preparations were microscopically examined per group and found to be all lymphomas. All other macroscopic neoplastic lesions observed in thymus are assumed to be lymphomas as well.
** analyzed in femur.
Tumor incidence based on all animals from longevity cohort, including those not microscopically examined.

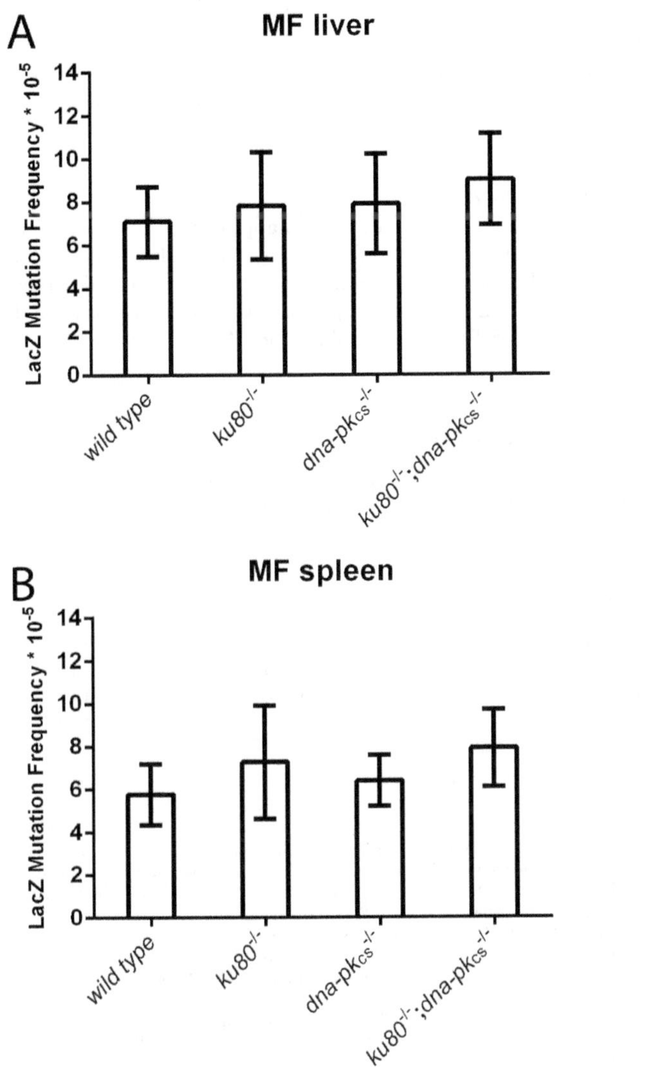

Figure 4. LacZ mutant frequency. Error bars represent standard deviation. (A) Mutant frequency in liver. (B) Mutant frequency in spleen.

variation is too large and effect sizes too small to achieve statistical significance. Previously we had to separate the small mutations from the big mutations before a difference could be seen since the former was reduced while the latter was increased.

In conclusion, we have shown that deletion of the NHEJ components Ku80 and DNA-PK_{CS} in a C57Bl6/J*FVB F1 hybrid background resulted in a accelerated aging phenotype and a strongly increased incidence of lymphomas and that simultaneous deletion does not further enhance these characteristics. Yet, Ku80-deletion was more severe than DNA-PK_{CS} –deletion. This observation is consistent with the possibility that Ku80 has an extra-NHEJ function or that free Ku70 is toxic in the absence of Ku80.

Materials and Methods

Ethics Statement

All animal work was approved by the ethics committee of the National Institutes for Public Health and the Environment (RIVM), Antonie van Leeuwenhoeklaan, Bilthoven, The Netherlands, IACUC protocol #:99047x.

Mice breeding

Ku80 null mice are not viable in a pure C57BL6/J background [30]. Therefore, we generated F1 hybrid animals with a C57Bl6/J*FVB background. This resulted in viable offspring and prevented C57BL6/J related ulcerative dermatitis [31]. $ku80^{-/-}$ mice [9] and $dna\text{-}pk_{cs}^{-/-}$ mice [32] were imported in our SPF facility, rederived and back crossed to C57Bl6/JIco (Charles River, France) and FVB/NHanHsd (Harlan, Germany) using a speed congenics approach [33]. Knock out mice in C57Bl6/JIco background were maintained by backcrossing with C57Bl6/J-pUR288 (LacZ locus integrated at chromosome 13 [34]) generating heterozygous knock out animals which are homozygous for pUR288. Knock out mice on FVB background were maintained by backcrossing with pure FVB wild type animals. Cohorts with single and double knock out animals were generated using double heterozygous knock out breeders ($ku80^{+/-}$; $dna\text{-}pk_{cs}^{+/-}$). All male breeders were on C57Bl6/J-pUR288 and all female breeders on FVB background. Using this breeding strategy, all genotypes could be generated from the same breeding colony and all experimental mice were C57Bl6/J*FVB F1 hybrids carrying one LacZ allele. The breeding scheme is depicted in figure 1.

This study was carried out in strict accordance with institutional guidelines and regulations. All animal work was approved by the ethics committee of the National Institutes for Public Health and the Environment (RIVM), Antonie van Leeuwenhoeklaan, Bilthoven, The Netherlands, IACUC protocol #:99047x. These were survival studies; therefore, mice were monitored every day without intervention. Moribund mice were sacrificed with ketamine/xylazine anesthesia followed by cervical dislocation and all efforts were made to minimize suffering and discomfort. Criteria for moribund were >15% weight loss within 2 weeks, not responsive to touch, prominent appearance of ribs, spine and hips, hunch body position, matted fur, or a visible tumor.

Study setup

Each cohort consisted of 45 males and 45 females. All animals were maintained under specific pathogen free conditions and were fed ad libitum using CRM pelleted maintenance diet (Special Diet Services, UK). A 12 hr/12 hr dark/light cycle was maintained and temperature was 20°C. Animals were maintained until death or moribund. Moribund animals were euthanized by exsanguinations and major organs were isolated and partly stored in formaldehyde and partly snap frozen in liquid nitrogen. Results from $ku80^{-/-}$ and $dna\text{-}pk_{cs}^{-/-}$ longevity cohorts were also used in a study comparing Ku70 and Ku80 function [17]. In addition, 5 male animals of all genotypes were euthanized at approximately median lifespan for LacZ mutant frequency analysis.

Pathology

Pathology lesions in mutant animals were compared with those in age matched wild type littermates. Representative sections from the liver, kidney, thymus, spleen, axillary and mesenteric lymph nodes, femur, vertebra, uterus, ovaries, testes, and accessory male genital glands were processed (n = 4–5 per genotype), stained with Hematoxylin and Eosin, and microscopically examined for the presence of histopathologic lesions. All tumors macroscopically identified during necropsy were also prepared for histopathologic examination Severity score of all recorded lesions was semi-quantitatively assessed. Scores were given as absent (0), subtle (1), mild (2), moderate (3), severe (4), and massive (5) for each criteria. Digital images from the femur cortical bone at mid-shaft area, and skin were taken for morphometric analysis using Labsense image analysis software (Olympus). The thickness of femur cortical bone thickness, and skin thickness (dermis and epidermis with exclusion of subcutaneous fat) were measured using arbitrary line option.

CD3 staining

After deparaffinization, rehydration and citrate buffer pretreatment, sections were incubated with rabbit polyclonal antibody to the human CD3 molecule (DAKO Corporation- Code-Nr. A 0452), diluted 1:250 in 10% normal goat serum, for 30 minutes at room temperature. The remainder of the procedure was accomplished according to the manufacturer's instructions. Normal goat serum was substituted for the primary antibody as a negative control. Mouse lymphoid tissue was used as a positive control.

LacZ mutant frequency analysis

LacZ mutant frequency was assessed in liver and spleen using the pUR288(lacZ) reporter. This assay has been described previously [34]. In short, total DNA was extracted from liver and spleen using a phenol/chloroform/iso-amyl alcohol extraction (25:24:1) and digested with the endonuclease HindIII in the presence of magnetic beads, coated with lacI-lacZ fusion protein. After digestion, magnetic beads were washed and DNA fragments eluted using isopropyl-L-thio-B-D-galactopyranoside. DNA fragments were circularized with T4 DNA ligase and transformed into *E. Coli* (ΔlacZ, galE-) bacteria. Of the transformed bacteria, one thousandth was plated on x-gal plates and the remainder on selective p-gal plates. The mutant frequency was defined as the amount of colonies on the selective plate divided by the amount of colonies on the X-gal plate multiplied by 1000 (dilution factor).

Statistical analysis

Survival curves were analyzed using a log rank test (Graphpad Prism 5.04, GraphPad Software Inc, La Jolla, CA, USA). Pathological scores were compared using a two-tailed Mann-Whitney U test and mutant frequencies were compared using a T-Test (IBM SPSS Statistics 19, SPSS Inc - IBM, New York, USA).

Acknowledgments

We thank Dr. G.E.Taccioli for providing DNA-PK_{CS} knock out mice and S. Imholz and A. Verhoef for technical support.

Author Contributions

Conceived and designed the experiments: ER METD JHH JV HVS PH. Performed the experiments: ER SAY ML BN MR PDW ADB. Analyzed the data: ER METD JHH JV HVS PH. Wrote the paper: ER PH.

References

1. Liang F, Romanienko PJ, Weaver DT, Jeggo PA, Jasin M (1996) Chromosomal double-strand break repair in Ku80-deficient cells. Proc Natl Acad Sci U S A 93: 8929–8933.
2. Ahnesorg P, Smith P, Jackson SP (2006) XLF Interacts with the XRCC4-DNA Ligase IV Complex to Promote DNA Nonhomologous End-Joining. Cell 124: 301–313.
3. Grawunder U, Wilm M, Wu X, Kulesza P, Wilson TE, et al. (1997) Activity of DNA ligase IV stimulated by complex formation with XRCC4 protein in mammalian cells. Nature 388: 492–495.
4. Ma Y, Pannicke U, Schwarz K, Lieber MR (2002) Hairpin opening and overhang processing by an Artemis/DNA-dependent protein kinase complex in nonhomologous end joining and V(D)J recombination. Cell 108: 781–794.
5. Biedermann KA, Sun JR, Giaccia AJ, Tosto LM, Brown JM (1991) scid mutation in mice confers hypersensitivity to ionizing radiation and a deficiency in DNA double-strand break repair. Proc Natl Acad Sci U S A 88: 1394–1397.
6. Fulop GM, Phillips RA (1990) The scid mutation in mice causes a general defect in DNA repair. Nature 347: 479–482.
7. Gu Y, Jin S, Gao Y, Weaver DT, Alt FW (1997) Ku70-deficient embryonic stem cells have increased ionizing radiosensitivity, defective DNA end-binding activity, and inability to support V(D)J recombination. Proc Natl Acad Sci U S A 94: 8076–8081.
8. Taccioli GE, Gottlieb TM, Blunt T, Priestley A, Demengeot J, et al. (1994) Ku80: product of the XRCC5 gene and its role in DNA repair and V(D)J recombination. Science 265: 1442–1445.
9. Zhu C, Bogue MA, Lim DS, Hasty P, Roth DB (1996) Ku86-deficient mice exhibit severe combined immunodeficiency and defective processing of V(D)J recombination intermediates. Cell 86: 379–389.
10. Li H, Vogel H, Holcomb VB, Gu Y, Hasty P (2007) Deletion of Ku70, Ku80, or both causes early aging without substantially increased cancer. Mol Cell Biol 27: 8205–8214.
11. Vogel H, Lim DS, Karsenty G, Finegold M, Hasty P (1999) Deletion of Ku86 causes early onset of senescence in mice. Proc Natl Acad Sci U S A 96: 10770–10775.
12. Espejel S, Martin M, Klatt P, Martin-Caballero J, Flores JM, et al. (2004) Shorter telomeres, accelerated ageing and increased lymphoma in DNA-PKcs-deficient mice. EMBO Rep 5: 503–509.
13. Gu Y, Sekiguchi J, Gao Y, Dikkes P, Frank K, et al. (2000) Defective embryonic neurogenesis in Ku-deficient but not DNA-dependent protein kinase catalytic subunit-deficient mice. Proc Natl Acad Sci U S A 97: 2668–2673.
14. Gao Y, Chaudhuri J, Zhu C, Davidson L, Weaver DT, et al. (1998) A targeted DNA-PKcs-null mutation reveals DNA-PK-independent functions for KU in V(D)J recombination. Immunity 9: 367–376.
15. Frank KM, Sharpless NE, Gao Y, Sekiguchi JM, Ferguson DO, et al. (2000) DNA ligase IV deficiency in mice leads to defective neurogenesis and embryonic lethality via the p53 pathway. Mol Cell 5: 993–1002.
16. Karanjawala ZE, Adachi N, Irvine RA, Oh EK, Shibata D, et al. (2002) The embryonic lethality in DNA ligase IV-deficient mice is rescued by deletion of Ku: implications for unifying the heterogeneous phenotypes of NHEJ mutants. DNA Repair (Amst) 1: 1017–1026.
17. Choi YJ, Li H, Son MY, Wang XH, Fornsaglio JL, et al. (2014) Deletion of Individual Ku Subunits in Mice Causes an NHEJ-Independent Phenotype Potentially by Altering Apurinic/Apyrimidinic Site Repair. PLoS ONE 9: e86358.
18. Dolle ME, Kuiper RV, Roodbergen M, Robinson J, de Vlugt S, et al. (2011) Broad segmental progeroid changes in short-lived Ercc1(-/Delta7) mice. Pathobiol Aging Age Relat Dis 1.
19. Espejel S, Klatt P, Menissier-de Murcia J, Martin-Caballero J, Flores JM, et al. (2004) Impact of telomerase ablation on organismal viability, aging, and tumorigenesis in mice lacking the DNA repair proteins PARP-1, Ku86, or DNA-PKcs. J Cell Biol 167: 627–638.
20. Li H, Choi YJ, Hanes MA, Marple T, Vogel H, et al. (2009) Deleting Ku70 is milder than deleting Ku80 in p53-mutant mice and cells. Oncogene 28: 1875–1878.
21. Ilina ES, Lavrik OI, Khodyreva SN (2008) Ku antigen interacts with abasic sites. Biochim Biophys Acta 1784: 1777–1785.
22. Holcomb VB, Vogel H, Hasty P (2007) Deletion of Ku80 causes early aging independent of chronic inflammation and Rag-1-induced DSBs. Mech Ageing Dev 128: 601–608.
23. Holcomb VB, Rodier F, Choi Y, Busuttil RA, Vogel H, et al. (2008) Ku80 deletion suppresses spontaneous tumors and induces a p53-mediated DNA damage response. Cancer Res 68: 9497–9502.
24. Hasty P (2008) Is NHEJ a tumor suppressor or an aging suppressor? Cell Cycle 7: 1139–1145.
25. Lim DS, Vogel H, Willerford DM, Sands AT, Platt KA, et al. (2000) Analysis of ku80-mutant mice and cells with deficient levels of p53. Mol Cell Biol 20: 3772–3780.
26. Holcomb VB, Vogel H, Marple T, Kornegay RW, Hasty P (2006) Ku80 and p53 suppress medulloblastoma that arise independent of Rag-1-induced DSBs. Oncogene 25: 7159–7165.
27. Shinkai Y, Rathbun G, Lam KP, Oltz EM, Stewart V, et al. (1992) RAG-2-deficient mice lack mature lymphocytes owing to inability to initiate V(D)J rearrangement. Cell 68: 855–867.
28. Mombaerts P, Iacomini J, Johnson RS, Herrup K, Tonegawa S, et al. (1992) RAG-1-deficient mice have no mature B and T lymphocytes. Cell 68: 869–877.
29. Busuttil RA, Munoz DP, Garcia AM, Rodier F, Kim WH, et al. (2008) Effect of Ku80 deficiency on mutation frequencies and spectra at a LacZ reporter locus in mouse tissues and cells. PLoS ONE 3: e3458.
30. Reliene R, Goad ME, Schiestl RH (2006) Developmental cell death in the liver and newborn lethality of Ku86 deficient mice suppressed by antioxidant N-acetyl-cysteine. DNA Repair (Amst).

31. Sundberg JP, Rozell B, Everts H (2011) Association between hair-induced oronasal inflammation and ulcerative dermatitis in C57BL/6 mice. Comp Med 61: 204–205; author reply 205.
32. Taccioli GE, Amatucci AG, Beamish HJ, Gell D, Xiang XH, et al. (1998) Targeted disruption of the catalytic subunit of the DNA-PK gene in mice confers severe combined immunodeficiency and radiosensitivity. Immunity 9: 355–366.
33. Wakeland E, Morel L, Achey K, Yui M, Longmate J (1997) Speed congenics: a classic technique in the fast lane (relatively speaking). Immunol Today 18: 472–477.
34. Dolle ME, Martus HJ, Gossen JA, Boerrigter ME, Vijg J (1996) Evaluation of a plasmid-based transgenic mouse model for detecting in vivo mutations. Mutagenesis 11: 111–118.

4

Comparison between Karyotyping-FISH-Reverse Transcription PCR and RNA- Sequencing-Fusion Gene Identification Programs in the Detection of *KAT6A-CREBBP* in Acute Myeloid Leukemia

Ioannis Panagopoulos[1,2]*, Synne Torkildsen[1,2,3], Ludmila Gorunova[1,2], Anne Tierens[4], Geir E. Tjønnfjord[3,5], Sverre Heim[1,2,5]

1 Section for Cancer Cytogenetics, Institute for Cancer Genetics and Informatics, The Norwegian Radium Hospital, Oslo University Hospital, Oslo, Norway, **2** Centre for Cancer Biomedicine, Faculty of Medicine, University of Oslo, Oslo, Norway, **3** Department of Hematology, Oslo University Hospital, Oslo, Norway, **4** Department of Pathology, The Norwegian Radium Hospital, Oslo University Hospital, Oslo, Norway, **5** Faculty of Medicine, University of Oslo, Oslo, Norway

Abstract

An acute myeloid leukemia was suspected of having a t(8;16)(p11;p13) resulting in a *KAT6A-CREBBP* fusion because the bone marrow was packed with monoblasts showing marked erythrophagocytosis. The diagnostic karyotype was 46,XY,add(1)(p13),t(8;21)(p11;q22),der(16)t(1;16)(p13;p13)[9]/46,XY[1]; thus, no direct confirmation of the suspicion could be given although both 8p11 and 16p13 seemed to be rearranged. The leukemic cells were examined in two ways to find out whether a cryptic *KAT6A-CREBBP* was present. The first was the "conventional" approach: G-banding was followed by fluorescence in situ hybridization (FISH) and reverse transcription PCR (RT-PCR). The second was RNA-Seq followed by data analysis using FusionMap and FusionFinder programs with special emphasis on candidates located in the 1p13, 8p11, 16p13, and 21q22 breakpoints. FISH analysis indicated the presence of a *KAT6A/CREBBP* chimera. RT-PCR followed by Sanger sequencing of the amplified product showed that a chimeric *KAT6A-CREBBP* transcript was present in the patients bone marrow. Surprisingly, however, *KATA6A-CREBBP* was not among the 874 and 35 fusion transcripts identified by the FusionMap and FusionFinder programs, respectively, although 11 sequences of the raw RNA-sequencing data were *KATA6A-CREBBP* fragments. This illustrates that although many fusion transcripts can be found by RNA-Seq combined with FusionMap and FusionFinder, the pathogenetically essential fusion is not always picked up by the bioinformatic algorithms behind these programs. The present study not only illustrates potential pitfalls of current data analysis programs of whole transcriptome sequences which make them less useful as stand-alone techniques, but also that leukemia diagnosis still relies on integration of clinical, hematologic, and genetic disease features of which the former two by no means have become superfluous.

Editor: Francesco Bertolini, European Institute of Oncology, Italy

Funding: This work was supported by grants from the Norwegian Cancer Society. The funders had no role in study design, data collection and analysis, decision to publish, or preparation of the manuscript.

Competing Interests: The authors have declared that no competing interests exist.

* E-mail: ioannis.panagopoulos@rr-research.no

Introduction

The chromosome aberration t(8;16)(p11;p13) was first described in 1983 in an infant in whom the leukemic cells displayed prominent hemophagocytosis [1]. The recurrence of t(8;16)(p11;p13) in acute myeloid leukemia (AML) was independently established in 1987 by three groups. Bernstein et al [2] reported two infants with AML carrying the t(8;16)(p11;p13). Heim at al [3] described three cases of AML, two teenagers and one infant, with the t(8;16) as the sole chromosome abnormality. Lai et al [4] reported three more cases of t(8;16)-positive AML with additional structural chromosome aberrations present in two of them. Monocytic differentiation and phagocytosis were distinctive features of all the patients [2,3,4]. In the Mitelman Database of Chromosome Aberration and Gene Fusions in Cancer, there are now 116 cases of AML carrying the t(8;16)(p11;p13) chromosome abnormality (http://cgap.nci.nih.gov/Chromosomes/Mitelman, database last updated on August 14, 2013).

AML with t(8;16)(p11;p13) is now recognized as a distinct disease entity characterized by monocytic differentiation of the leukemic cells and marked erythrophagocytosis [5,6], frequent skin involvement, and a tendency to develop diffuse intravascular coagulation. It often occurs at a young age and the response to treatment is poor resulting in short survival [5,7].

The translocation t(8;16)(p11;p13) disrupts *KAT6A* (also known as *MOZ* and *MYST3*) on 8p11 and *CREBBP* (also named *CBP*) on 16p13 resulting in a fusion of the two genes [8,9]. Although genomic rearrangements of *KAT6A* and *CREBBP* were repeatedly detected using fluorescence in situ hybridization (FISH) and Southern blot methodologies [8,9,10], attempts to amplify and further analyze chimeric *KAT6A-CREBBP* and *CREBBP-KAT6A* transcripts using reverse transcriptase-PCR (RT-PCR) analysis were long unsuccessful [8,9,10]. Various explanations such as low expression and/or instability of the chimeric transcripts were proposed [9]. Nevertheless, an RT-PCR strategy was developed to detect the *KAT6A-CREBBP* as well as *CREBBP-KAT6A* fusions [11] and two types of *KAT6A-CREBBP* fusion transcripts were identified: Type 1 was an in-frame transcript between codon 1117 of *KAT6A* and codon 29 of *CREBBP*, while type 2 was an out-of-frame transcript between exon codon 1117 of *KAT6A* and codon 267 of *CREBBP*. Subsequent studies confirmed the presence of *KAT6A-CREBBP* and *CREBBP-KAT6A* fusions, and it was shown that type 1 was the most frequent *KAT6A-CREBBP* fusion transcript [12,13,14]. Moreover, new *KAT6A-CREBBP* fusion transcript variants were described [15,16] and real time PCR methodology (RT-PCR) was developed to monitor minimal residual disease status throughout the entire course of the treatment [17].

Recently, RNA-sequencing (RNA-seq, also known as whole transcriptome sequencing) was shown to be an efficient tool in the detection of fusion genes in cancer [18] and has created euphoria among those working with cancer fusion genes. The methodology is in principle simple: extracted RNA from cancer cells is massively sequenced, and then the raw data are analyzed with one or more programs specifically dedicated to the task of detecting fusion transcripts such as FusionMap and FusionFinder [19,20]. However, it suffers from the shortcoming of identifying as "fusion genes" also many technical and perhaps also clinical "false positives," thus making the assessment of which fusions are important and which are noise extremely difficult. We and others have used combinations of cytogenetics and RNA-seq to detect the "primary" fusion genes of neoplasms carrying only one or a few chromosomal rearrangements. This approach was used to identify the *WWTR1-CAMTA1* and *YWHAE-FAM22A/B* chimeric genes in epithelioid hemangioendothelioma and high-grade endometrial stromal sarcomas, respectively [21,22], *ZC3H7-BCOR* in endometrial stromal sarcomas [23], *IRF2BP2-CDX1* in a mesenchymal chondrosarcoma [24], and *EWSR1-YY1* in a subset of mesotheliomas [25]. In hematologic malignancies, an *NFIA-CBFA2T3* (*NFIA* is located in 1p31) chimeric transcript was found in an acute erythroid leukemia with the translocation t(1;16)(p31;q24) [26], the *ZMYND8-RELA* fusion was detected in a congenital acute erythroid leukemia carrying a t(11;20)(p11;q13) translocation [27], and a cryptic *FUS/ERG* fusion gene was found in an acute myeloid leukemia with a rather complex karyotype [28].

We here describe a case of AML in which two translocations corresponding to a der(16)t(1;16)(p13;p13) and a t(8;21)(p11;q22) were found in the bone marrow cells. The patient had morphological features that invoked the suspicion of a t(8;16)(p11;p13) with *KAT6A-CREBBP* fusion in spite of the fact that the breakpoints suggested various other candidate genes. We therefore studied the patient's leukemic cells in two different ways looking for *KAT6A-CREBBP*: "conventionally" by karyotyping followed by FISH followed by RT-PCR, and in the modern manner using RNA-seq and programs specific for fusion genes.

Materials and Methods

Ethics Statement

The study was approved by the Regional Committee for Medical Research Ethics (Regional komité for medisinsk forskningsetikk Sør-Øst, Norge, http://helseforskning.etikkom.no). Written informed consent was obtained from the patient prior to his death. The ethics committee approval included a review of the consent procedure and all patient information has been anonymized and de-identified.

Case history

A 30 years old male was transferred to our institution with a preliminary diagnosis of acute myeloid leukemia. He presented with fever and lower back pain radiating to the left lower limb. The clinical examination was unremarkable except for the presence of gingival petecchiae. Gingival hyperplasia was not noted. Blood analysis revealed a severe thrombocytopenia and an elevated CRP and LDH, but all other parameters were normal. Magnetic resonance investigation (MRI) of the columna demonstrated a paramedian prolapse between the L5/S1 vertebrae. A chest radiography showed bilateral infiltrations in the lower pulmonary lobes. Examination of a bone marrow aspirate showed that normal hematopoiesis was replaced by intermediate to large monoblasts, often with prominent vacuolization and ingested red blood cells (Figure 1). Immunophenotypic analysis confirmed the monocytic origin of the blasts that were positive for HLA-DR antigens, CD15, CD13, CD33, and cyMPO. Molecular genetic analysis was negative for *RUNX1-RUNX1T1* and *CBFB-MYH11* fusion transcripts as well as *FLT3* and *NPM1* mutations. The patient received induction therapy for AML with daunorubicin 90 mg/m2 day 1–3 and cytarabin 200 mg/m2 day 1–7 after which he went into morphologic remission. He then received two cycles of consolidation with high dose cytarabin (3 g/m2×2 per day, day 1, 3 and 5). One month later, however, he relapsed. He now received reinduction treatment with M5A5E5 (Amsakrin 150 mg/m2 day 1–3, Cytarabin 200 mg/m2/24 hours and Etoposide 110 mg/m2 daily for 5 days). Although morphologic remission was obtained, complete hematological recovery was not achieved 2 months after re-induction treatment.The consolidation treatment M3A5E3 was therefore given with an intent to proceed to allogenic stem cell transplantation, but the patient died 3 weeks later because of liver failure and an acute abdomen caused by ischemic infarcts of the intestine and liver.

G-banding and FISH

Bone marrow cells were cytogenetically investigated by standard methods. Chromosome preparations were made from metaphase

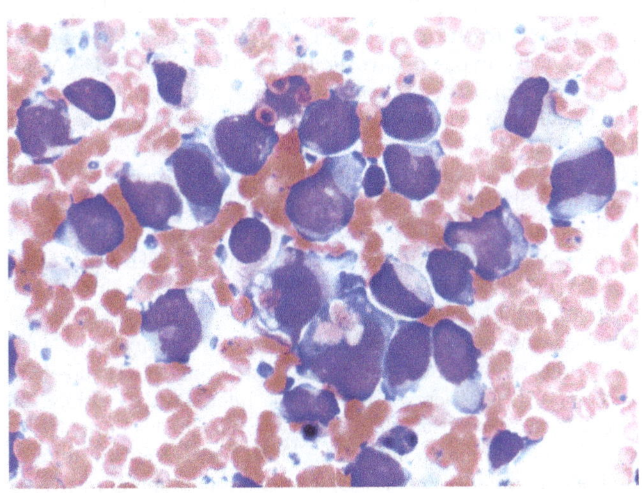

Figure 1. Bone marrow smear showing intermediate to large blasts with finely dispersed chromatin with variably abundant cytoplasm, vacuolization and phagocytosis of red blood cells (Wright-Giemsa 400 x).

cells of a 24-hours culture, G-banded using Leishman stain, and karyotyped according to ISCN 2009 guidelines [29]. FISH analysis was performed on metaphase plates.

BAC clones were retrieved from the Human genome high-resolution BAC re-arrayed clone set (the "32k set"; BACPAC Resources, http://bacpac.chori.org/pHumanMinSet.htm). The "32k set" is mapped on the UCSC Genome browser on Human May 2004 (NCBI/hg17) assembly. Mapping data for the 32k human rearray are available in an interactive web format (http://bacpac.chori.org/pHumanMinSet.htm, from the genomic rearrays page) and are obtained by activation of the ucsc browser track for the hg17 UCSC assembly from the "32k set" homepage (http://bacpac.chori.org/genomicRearrays.php). The BAC clones were selected according to physical and genetic mapping data on chromosomes 8 and 16 (see below) as reported on the Human Genome Browser at the University of California, Santa Cruz website (May 2004, http://genome.ucsc.edu/). In addition, FISH mapping of the clones on normal controls was performed to confirm their chromosomal location. The clones used were RP11-619A23 (chr16:3660077-3854572) and RP11-95J11 (chr16:3800375-3965511) mapping to 16p13.3 and which both contain the entire *CREBBP* gene (red), and RP11-642I24 (chr8:41795493-41975651) and RP11-589C21 (chr8:41992859-42155379) mapping to 8p11.21 for *KAT6A* (green). DNA was extracted and probes were labelled and hybridized according to Abbott Molecular recommendations (http://www.abbottmolecular.com/home.html). Chromosome preparations were counterstained with 0.2 μg/ml DAPI and overlaid with a 24×50 mm^2 coverslip. Fluorescent signals were captured and analyzed using the CytoVision system (Applied Imaging, Newcastle, UK).

RT-PCR analyses

Total RNA was extracted from the patients bone marrow at the time of diagnosis using Trizol reagent according to the manufacturer's instructions (Invitrogen, Life Technologies, Oslo, Norway) and used for both RT-PCR and RNA-Seq analyses. For RT-PCR, one μg of total RNA was reverse-transcribed in a 20 μL reaction volume using iScript Advanced cDNA Synthesis Kit for RT-qPCR according to the manufacturer's instructions (Bio-Rad Laboratories, Oslo, Norway). The cDNA was diluted to 30 ng equivalent of RNA/μL and 2 μL were used as templates in subsequent PCR assays. The 25 μL PCR volume contained 12.5 μL Premix Ex Taq DNA Polymerase Hot Start Version (Takara Bio Europe/SAS, Saint-Germain-en-Laye, France), 2 μL of diluted cDNA, and 0.2 μM of each of the primers, the forward MOZ-3558F (5′-GAG GCC AAT GCC AAG ATT AGA AC-3′) and the reverse primer CBP-431R (5′-GTT GAT ACT AGA GCC GCT GCC TC-3′). The PCR was run on a C-1000 Thermal cycler (Bio-Rad Laboratories) with an initial denaturation at 94°C for 30 sec, followed by 35 cycles of 7 sec at 98°C, 30 sec at 55°C and 1 min at 72°C, and a final extension for 5 min at 72°C. Four μL of the PCR products were stained with GelRed (Biotium, VWR International, Oslo, Norway), analyzed by electrophoresis through 1.0% agarose gel, and photographed. The remaining PCR products were purified using the NucleoSpin Gel and PCR Clean-up kit (Macherey-Nagel, VWR International, Oslo, Norway) and sequenced at GATC Biotech (Germany, http://www.gatc-biotech.com/en/home.html). The BLAST software (http://blast.ncbi.nlm.nih.gov/Blast.cgi) was used for computer analysis of sequence data.

RNA-sequencing (RNA-Seq)

Three μg of the total RNA extracted from the patients bone marrow at the time of diagnosis and used for RT-PCR analysis were sent for high-throughput paired-end RNA-sequencing at the Genomics Core Facility, The Norwegian Radium Hospital (http://genomics.no/oslo/). The Illumina software pipeline was used to process image data into raw sequencing data and only sequence reads marked as "passed filtering" were used in the downstream data analysis. A total of 53 million reads were obtained. The FASTQC software was used for quality control of the raw sequence data (http://www.bioinformatics.babraham.ac.uk/projects/fastqc/). Two softwares were used for the discovery of fusion transcripts: FusionMap [30] (release date 2012-04-16) together with the pre-built Human B37 and RefGene from the FusionMap website (http://www.omicsoft.com/fusionmap/) and FusionFinder [31]. In addition, the "grep" command (http://en.wikipedia.org/wiki/Grep) was used to search the fastq files of the sequence data (http://en.wikipedia.org/wiki/FASTQ_format).

Results

G-banding and FISH

G-banding analysis yielded the diagnostic karyotype. 46,XY,add(1)(p13),t(8;21)(p11;q22),der(16)t(1;16)(p13;p13)[9]/46,XY[1] (Figure 2A). Four months after diagnosis the bone marrow karyotype was: 47,Y,t(X;17)(p10;q10),der(1)(1qter->1q12::1p22->1q12::5q15->5qter),add(1)(p13),inv(2)(p21q13),der(5)t(1;5)(p22;q15), t(12;18)(q15;q21),+8,t(8;21)(p11;q22), del(13)(q21q31),der(16)t(1;16)(p13;p13)[5]/46,XY[11]. In addition to the primary t(1;16) and t(8;21) translocations, clearly many secondary aberrations had also accrued indicating clonal evolution.

Co-hybridization FISH analysis with the probes RP11-619A23/RP11-95J11 (red, for *CREBBP*) and RP11-642I24/RP11-589C21 (green, for *KAT6A*) revealed a fusion signal of the *KAT6A* and *CREBBP* BACs on the derivative chromosome 8, indicating the presence of a *KAT6A/CREBBP* chimera (Figure 2B). No corresponding fusion signal was found on the der(16)t(1;16) suggesting that the translocation was accompanied by a deletion of the reciprocal *CREBBP/KAT6A* (Figure 2B).

RT-PCR

PCR with the MOZ3558F and CBP431R primer combination amplified a 352 bp fragment from the patients cDNA (Figure 2C). To verify the presence of a *KAT6A-CREBBP* chimeric transcript, the fragment was analyzed by direct sequencing which showed the presence in the patients bone marrow of a type 1 *KAT6A-CREBBP* chimeric transcript, i.e., the nt 3764 of mRNA of *KAT6A* (accession number NM_006766.3) was fused in-frame with the nt 290 of mRNA of *CREBBP* (accession number NM_004380.2) (Figure 2D).

RNA-Seq

Using FusionMap on the raw sequencing data obtained from the Genomics Core Facility, 874 fusion transcripts were found (Table S1). The *KAT6A-CREBBP* fusion transcript was not among them (Table S1). Instead, three other *KAT6A* (referred to as *MYST3* in the FusionMap output) fusions were found: *DTX3L-MYST3* ranking 91, *MYST3-SLK* ranking 193, and *MYST-DNAJC14* ranking 606. Based on the map information on the genes, these fusions would have corresponded to the translocations t(3;8)(q21;p11), t(8;10)(p11;q24), and t(8;12)(p11;q13), respectively, none of which was seen by karyotyping. One *CREBP* fusion transcript was found, *CREBBP-TTC28* which was ranked 401 in the list of fusion transcripts (Table S1). The transcript would have corresponded to a t(16;22)(p13;q12) which was not found by G-

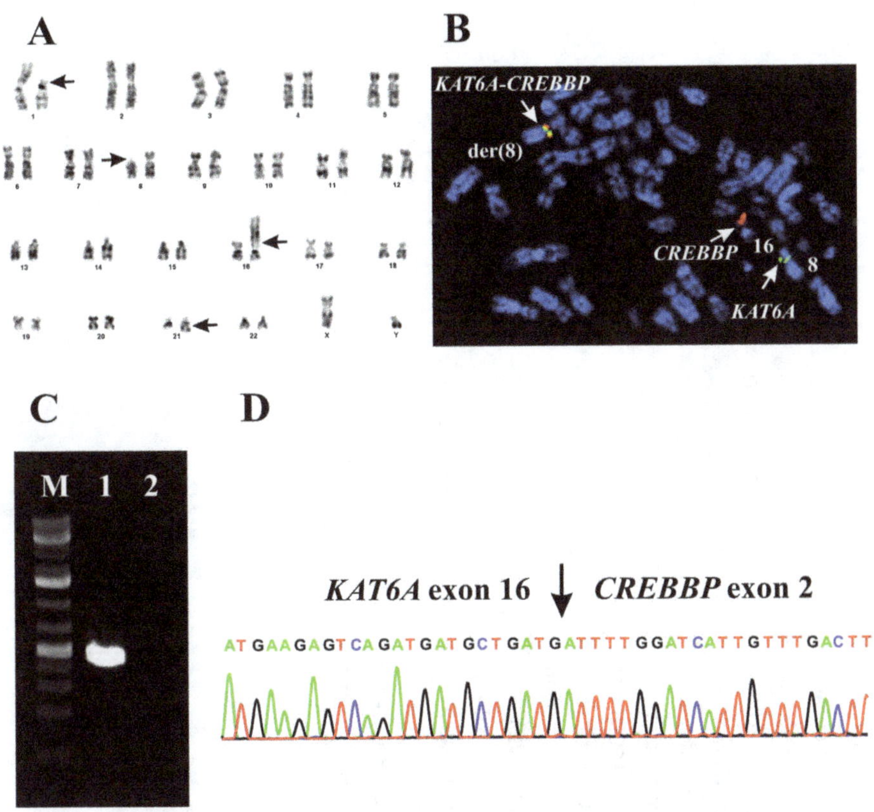

Figure 2. Cytogenetic, FISH and RT-PCR analyses. A) Karyotype at diagnosis showing the chromosome aberrations add(1)(p13), t(8;21)(p11;q22), and der(16)t(1;16)(p13;p13); breakpoint positions are indicated by arrows. B) Co-hybridization FISH analysis with the probes RP11-619A23/RP11-95J11 (red, for *CREBBP*) and RP11-642I24/RP11-589C21 (green, for *KAT6A*). A fusion signal of the *KAT6A* and *CREBBP* BACs is detected on the derivative chromosome 8, indicating the presence of a *KAT6A/CREBBP* chimera. C) Amplification of a 352 bp cDNA fragment using the primers MOZ-3558F and CBP-431R (lane 1); M, 1 Kb DNA ladder (GeneRuler, Fermentas); Lane 2, Blank, no RNA in cDNA synthesis. D) Partial sequence chromatogram of the 352 bp cDNA fragment showing that exon 16 of *KAT6A* is fused to exon 2 of *CREBBP*.

banding. The FusionFinder program detected 35 fusion transcripts none of which was *KAT6A-CREBBP* (Table S2).

Sequences which contained the first 20 nt of exon 2 of *CREBBP* (ATTTTGGATCATTGTTTGAC; nt 290–319 in sequence with accession number NM_004380.2) were retrieved from the raw sequencing data using the "grep" command. A total of 26 sequences were found (Table 1): 11 of them were *KAT6A-CREBBP* fusions, 15 sequences were exons 1–2 of *CREBBP*, and one was a genomic sequence from the chromosome band 16p13 containing the exon 2 of *CREBBP*. Similar to the results obtained by RT-PCR/Sanger sequencing, all 11 retrieved sequences showed fusion of 3764 nt of mRNA from *KAT6A* (accession number NM_006766.3) with nt 290 of mRNA from *CREBBP* (accession number NM_004380.2) (Table 1).

Discussion

The present case of AML had hematologic features highly suggestive of AML with t(8;16)(p11;p13) and a *KAT6A-CREBBP* fusion gene. The leukemic karyotype at diagnosis had two chromosome translocations, a der(16)t(1;16)(p13;p13) and a t(8;21)(p11;q22), indicating the possible generation of *KAT6A-CREBBP* via a cryptic aberration since both chromosome bands 8p11, which contains the *KAT6A* gene, and 16p13, where *CREBBP* maps, were seen rearranged. However, all the chromosome breakpoints in this particular karyotype contain also other genes known to be involved in leukemogenesis. *RBM15* in 1p13 is fused to *MKL1* in AML with t(1;22)(p13;q13) [32,33]. Likewise, chromosome band 16p13 contains, apart from *CREBBP*, also the *CBFB* gene which is fused to *MYH11* in the subset of AML with inv(16)(p13q22) [34] as well as *GLIS2* which is a partner in the fusion *CBFA2T3-GLIS2* generated by inv(16)(p13q24) [35]. On 8p11, apart from *KAT6A*, *FGFR1* is rearranged in fusions with several partner genes in the "8p11 myeloproliferative syndrome" [36,37]. For example, the fusion genes *ZNF198-FGFR1*, *CEP110-FGFR1*, *FOP-FGFR1*, and *BCR-FGFR1* result from the t(8;13)(p11;q12), t(8;9)(p11;q33), t(6;8)(q27;p11), and t(8;22)(p11q22) chromosome translocations, respectively [36,37]. On 21q22, *RUNX1* and *ERG* are fused to *RUNX1T1* and *FUS* generating the *RUNX1-RUNX1T1* and *FUS-ERG* fusion genes in AMLs carrying t(8;21)(p11;q22) and t(16;21)(p11;q22), respectively. In addition, both t(1;16)(p13;p13) and t(8;21)(p11;q22) could conceivably have generated novel leukemogenic fusion genes. Screening with FISH for all possibly rearranged genes associated with the present abnormal karyotype would have been a very laborious and time-consuming procedure. We therefore decided to perform two parallel investigations on the patients bone marrow. Based on the clinical and hematologic hunch that a *KAT6A-CREBBP* fusion was likely, we took the "conventional" approach - karyotyping and FISH followed by RT-PCR - to search for this known leukemogenic gene. In addition, we also performed RNA-Seq to search for this and other possible fusions concentrating exclusively on those fusion transcripts that had something to do with the chromosomal breakpoints. The FISH analysis showed a

Table 1. The 26 retrieved sequences from the raw sequencing data which contained the first 20 nt, ATTTTGGATCATTGTTTGAC (in bold) of *CREBBP*.

RETRIEVED SEQUENCES	*KAT6A* (NM_006766.3)	*CREBBP* (NM_004380.2)
CCCAAAAGAGCCAAACTCAGCTCGCCCGGTTTCTCGGCGAATGACAGCACAG**ATTTTGGATCATTGTTTGAC**TTGGAAAATGATCTTCCTGATGAGCTGAT		238–338 (exon 1–2)
CGGCGAATGACAGCACAG**ATTTTGGATCATTGTTTGAC**TTGGAAAATGATCTTCCTGATGAGCTGATACCCAATGGAGGAGAATTAGGCCTTTTAAACAGT		272–372 (exon 1–2)
*AAGAAGAAGATGAAGAGTCAGATGATGCTGATG***ATTTTGGATCATTGTTTGAC**TTGGAAAATGATCTTCCTGATGAGCTGATACCCAATGGAGGAGAATTA	3732–3764 (exon 16)	290–357 (exon 2)
ACTTGCTGGACGGACCGCCCAACCCCAAAAGAGCCAAACTCAGCTCGCCCGGTTTCTCGGCGAATGACAGCACAG**ATTTTGGATCATTGTTTGAC**TTGGAA		215–315 (exon 1–2)
*ATGCTGATG***ATTTTGGATCATTGTTTGAC**TTGGAAAATGATCTTCCTGATGAGCTGATACCCAATGGAGGAGAATTAAGATCGGAAGAGCGTCGTGTAGGG	3756–3764 (exon 16)	290–357 (exon 2)
*GTCAGATGATGCTGATG***ATTTTGGATCATTGTTTGAC**TTGGAAAATGATCTTCCTGATGAGCTGATACCCAATGGAGGAGAATTAGGCCTTTTAAACAGTG	3748–3764 (exon 16)	290–373 (exon 2)
*AAGAGTCAGATGATGCTGATG***ATTTTGGATCATTGTTTGAC**TTGGAAAATGATCTTCCTGATGAGCTGATACCCAATGGAGGAGAATTAGGCCTTTTAAAC	3744–3764 (exon 16)	290–369 (exon 2)
*AGAGTCAGATGATGCTGATG***ATTTTGGATCATTGTTTGAC**TTGGAAAATGATCTTCCTGATGAGCTGATACCCAATGGAGGAGAATTAGGCCTTTTAAACA	3745–3764 (exon 16)	290–370 (exon 2)
AGAACTTGCTGGACGGACCGCCCAACCCCAAAAGAGCCAAACTCAGCTCGCCCGGTTTCTCGGCGAATGACAGCACAG**ATTTTGGATCATTGTTTGAC**TTG		212–312 (exon 1–2)
GACAGCACAG**ATTTTGGATCATTGTTTGAC**TTGGAAAATGATCTTCCTGATGAGCTGATACCCAATGGAGGAGAATTAGGCCTTTTAAACAGTGGGAACCT		280–380 (exon 1–2)
AACTCAGCTCGCCCGGTTTCTCGGCGAATGACAGCACAG**ATTTTGGATCATTGTTTGAC**TTGGAAAATGATCTTCCTGATGAGCTGATACCCAATGTAGGA		251–351 (exon 1–2)
CTGGACGGACCGCCCAACCCCAAAAGAGCCAAACTCAGCTCGCCCGGTTTCTCGGCGAATGACAGCACAG**ATTTTGGATCATTGTTTGAC**TTGGAAAATGA		220–320 (exon 1–2)
AGCCAAACTCAGCTCGCCCGGTTTCTCGGCGAATGACAGCACAG**ATTTTGGATCATTGTTTGAC**TTGGAAAATGATCTTCCTGATGAGCTGATACCAGATC		246–341 (exon 1–2)
*GAAGATGAAGAGTCAGATGATGCTGATG***ATTTTGGATCATTGTTTGAC**TTGGAAAATGATCTTCCTGATGAGCTGATACCCAATGGAGGGCAGATCGGAAG	3737–3764 (exon 16)	290–350 (exon 2)
GCCAAACTCAGCTCGCCCGGTTTCTCGGCGAATGACAGCACAG**ATTTTGGATCATTGTTTGAC**TTGGAAAATGATCTTCCTGATGAGCTGATACCCAATGG		247–347 (exon 1–2)
*CTCAGGTGTCAGTCCTCTTCTAAGAGGAAGTCTAAAGATGAAGAAGAAGATGAAGAGTCAGATGATGCTGATG***ATTTTGGATCATTGTTTGAC**TTGGAAAA	3692–3764 (exon 16)	290–317 (exon 2)
CTTGCTGGACGGACCGCCCAACCCCAAAAGAGCCAAACTCAGCTCGCCCGGTTTCTCGGCGAATGACAGCACAG**ATTTTGGATCATTGTTTGAC**TTGGAAA		216–316 (exon 1–2)
AAAGAGCCAAACTCAGCTCGCCCGGTTTCTCGGCGAATGACAGCACAG**ATTTTGGATCATTGTTTGAC**TTGGAAAATGATCTTCCTGATGAGCTGATACCC		242–342 (exon 1–2)
*CAGTCCTCTTCTAAGAGGAAGTCTAAAGATGAAGAAGAAGATGAAGAGTCAGATGATGCTGATG***ATTTTGGATCATTGTTTGAC**TTGGAAAATGATCTTCC	3701–3764 (exon 16)	290–326 (exon 2)
GCCAAACTCAGCTCGCCCGGTTTCTCGGCGAATGACAGCACAG**ATTTTGGATCATTGTTTGAC**TTGGAAAATGATCTTCCTGATGAGCTGATACCCAATGG		247–347 (exon 1–2)
AAAAGAGCCAAACTCAGCTCGCCCGGTTTCTCGGCGAATGACAGCACAG**ATTTTGGATCATTGTTTGAC**TTGGAAAATGATCTTCCTGATGAGCTGATACC		241–341 (exon 1–2)
GCCAAACTCAGCTCGCCCGGTTTCTCGGCGAATGACAGCACAG**ATTTTGGATCATTGTTTGAC**TTGGAAAATGATCTTCCTGATGAGCTGATACCCAGATC		247–343 (exon 1–2)
*GATGTACTCAGGTGTCAGTCCTCTTCTAAGAGGAAGTCTAAAGATGAAGAAGAAGATGAAGAGTCAGATGATGCTGATG***ATTTTGGATCATTGTTTGAC**TT	3686–3764 (exon 16)	290–311 (exon 2)
*ATGATGCTGATG***ATTTTGGATCATTGTTTGAC**TTGGAAAATGATCTTCCTGATGAGCTGATACCCAATGGAGGAGAATTAGGAGATCGGAAGAGCGTCGTG	3753–3764 (exon 16)	290–359 (exon 2)
GTAAAGGTTGCTTAGTTTCTCATTTCCATTTCTGTTTAATTTCTAG**ATTTTGGATCATTGTTTGAC**TTGGAAAATGATCTTCCTGATGAGCTGATACCCAA		290–344 (exon 2)
*GATGATGCTGATG***ATTTTGGATCATTGTTTGAC**TTGGAAAATGATCTTCCTGATGAGCTGATACCCAATGGAGGAGAATTAGGCCTTTTAAACAGTGGGAA	3752–3764 (exon 16)	290–377 (exon 2)

KAT6A sequences are in italics.

fusion signal for *KAT6A*- and *CREBBP*- specific probes on the derivative chromosome 8, indicating the presence here of a *KAT6A/CREBBP* chimera (Figure 2B). RT-PCR analysis followed by Sanger sequencing confirmed the presence of type 1 fusion *KAT6A/CREBBP* transcript [15] (Figures 2C and 2D). The transcript retains the part of the *KAT6A* gene encoding the C4HC3 and C2HC zinc fingers, two nuclear localization signals, the HAT domain, the MYST domain, and a portion of the acidic domain, whereas the retained part of *CREBBP* encodes a domain which binds to nuclear receptor RARA, the CREB-binding domain, the three cystein/histidine rich regions, the bromodomain, and the glutamine-rich domains [11].

Surprisingly, of the 874 fusion transcripts identified by the FusionMap program [30], none was the biologically important *KAT6A-CREBBP*, nor was *KAT6A-CREBBP* featured in the list of 35 fusion genes obtained using FusionFinder [31]. Moreover, none of the two programs offered other putative fusion genes generated by the translocations der(16)t(1;16)(p13;p13) and t(8;21)(p11;q22). To find out whether the raw sequencing data contained sequences which encompassed the junction between *KAT6A* and *CREBBP*, we retrieved sequences containing the first 20 nt of exon 2 of *CREBBP* from the raw sequencing data. The rationale behind this was that exon 2 is fused to *KAT6A* (Figures 2C and 2D). Thus, the retrieved sequences should contain both *KAT6A-CREBBP* fusion transcript and wild type *KAT6A-CREBBP* transcript. Indeed, among the altogether 26 retrieved sequences, 11 were *KAT6A-CREBBP* fusions whereas 15 sequences were exons 1-2 of *CREBBP* (Table 1).

Both FusionMap and FusionFinder are among the most commonly used programs to detect fusion genes from RNA-Seq [19] and their sensitivity and specificity have been evaluated [19,30,31,38]. We, too, have in previous studies analyzed RNA-Seq data using the FusionMap program finding that it identified fusion genes that corresponded well with the available cytogenetic information and that were biologically significant [23,24,25,26,27,28]. The present study, on the other hand, shows that although the same approach detected hundreds (FusionMap) or tens (FusionFinder) of fusion genes, the programs failed to detect the biologically important *KAT6A-CREBBP* fusion gene although it was manually retrievable from the raw sequencing data.

The case illustrates that RNA-Seq with use of the FusionMap or FusionFinder programs may not be reliable as a stand-alone technique in the investigation of, at least, leukemias. Not only are there far too many false positives offered as fusion genes by this approach, but it may also fail to detect the truly important fusion gene; in the present case neither specificity nor sensitivity was satisfactory. Additional information about clinical, morphological, and cytogenetic features should be taken into account when searching for the crucial fusion genes in hematologic malignancies.

Acknowledgments

The authors thank Jim Thorsen for help with bioinformatics and Anne Mette Eibak and Hege Brandt Gehrken for their technical help.

Author Contributions

Conceived and designed the experiments: IP. Performed the experiments: IP LG. Analyzed the data: IP LG. Contributed reagents/materials/analysis tools: ST GET AT SH. Wrote the paper: IP SH. Pathological examination: AT. Medical information on the patient: ST GET.

References

1. Schouten TJ, Hustinx TW, Scheres JM, Holland R, de Vaan GA (1983) Malignant histiocytosis. Clinical and cytogenetic studies in a newborn and a child. Cancer 52: 1229–1236.
2. Bernstein R, Pinto MR, Spector I, Macdougall LG (1987) A unique 8;16 translocation in two infants with poorly differentiated monoblastic leukemia. Cancer Genet Cytogenet 24: 213–220.
3. Heim S, Avanzi GC, Billstrom R, Kristoffersson U, Mandahl N, et al. (1987) A new specific chromosomal rearrangement, t(8;16) (p11;p13), in acute monocytic leukaemia. Br J Haematol 66: 323–326.
4. Lai JL, Zandecki M, Jouet JP, Savary JB, Lambiliotte A, et al. (1987) Three cases of translocation (8;16)(p11;p13) observed in acute myelomonocytic leukemia: a new specific subgroup? Cancer Genet Cytogenet 27: 101–109.
5. Haferlach T, Kohlmann A, Klein HU, Ruckert C, Dugas M, et al. (2009) AML with translocation t(8;16)(p11;p13) demonstrates unique cytomorphological, cytogenetic, molecular and prognostic features. Leukemia 23: 934–943.
6. Hanslip JI, Swansbury GJ, Pinkerton R, Catovsky D (1992) The translocation t(8;16)(p11;p13) defines an AML subtype with distinct cytology and clinical features Leuk Lymphoma 6: 479–486.
7. Brown T, Swansbury J, Taj MM (2012) Prognosis of patients with t(8;16)(p11;p13) acute myeloid leukemia. Leuk Lymphoma 53: 338–341.
8. Borrow J, Stanton VP Jr, Andresen JM, Becher R, Behm FG, et al. (1996) The translocation t(8;16)(p11;p13) of acute myeloid leukaemia fuses a putative acetyltransferase to the CREB-binding protein. Nat Genet 14: 33–41.
9. Giles RH, Dauwerse JG, Higgins C, Petrij F, Wessels JW, et al. (1997) Detection of CBP rearrangements in acute myelogenous leukemia with t(8;16). Leukemia 11: 2087–2096.
10. Chaffanet M, Mozziconacci MJ, Fernandez F, Sainty D, Lafage-Pochitaloff M, et al. (1999) A case of inv(8)(p11q24) associated with acute myeloid leukemia involves the MOZ and CBP genes in a masked t(8;16). Genes Chromosomes Cancer 26: 161–165.
11. Panagopoulos I, Isaksson M, Lindvall C, Bjorkholm M, Ahlgren T, et al. (2000) RT-PCR analysis of the MOZ-CBP and CBP-MOZ chimeric transcripts in acute myeloid leukemias with t(8;16)(p11;p13). Genes Chromosomes Cancer 28: 415–424.
12. Rozman M, Camos M, Colomer D, Villamor N, Esteve J, et al. (2004) Type I MOZ/CBP (MYST3/CREBBP) is the most common chimeric transcript in acute myeloid leukemia with t(8;16)(p11;p13) translocation. Genes Chromosomes Cancer 40: 140–145.
13. Schmidt HH, Strehl S, Thaler D, Strunk D, Sill H, et al. (2004) RT-PCR and FISH analysis of acute myeloid leukemia with t(8;16)(p11;p13) and chimeric MOZ and CBP transcripts: breakpoint cluster region and clinical implications. Leukemia 18: 1115–1121.
14. Gervais C, Murati A, Helias C, Struski S, Eischen A, et al. (2008) Acute myeloid leukaemia with 8p11 (MYST3) rearrangement: an integrated cytologic, cytogenetic and molecular study by the groupe francophone de cytogenetique hematologique. Leukemia 22: 1567–1575.
15. Panagopoulos I, Fioretos T, Isaksson M, Mitelman F, Johansson B, et al. (2002) RT-PCR analysis of acute myeloid leukemia with t(8;16)(p11;p13): identification of a novel MOZ/CBP transcript and absence of CBP/MOZ expression. Genes Chromosomes Cancer 35: 372–374.
16. Terui K, Sato T, Sasaki S, Kudo K, Kamio T, et al. (2008) Two novel variants of MOZ-CBP fusion transcripts in spontaneously remitted infant leukemia with t(1;16;8)(p13;p13;p11), a new variant of t(8;16)(p11;p13). Haematologica 93: 1591–1593.
17. Fujiki A, Imamura T, Furutani A, Hatano W, Asai D, et al. (2012) Quantitative RT-PCR analysis of the MOZ-CBP fusion transcript in therapy-related acute myeloid leukemia with t(8;16)(p11;p13). J Pediatr Hematol Oncol 34: 402–405.
18. Maher CA, Kumar-Sinha C, Cao X, Kalyana-Sundaram S, Han B, et al. (2009) Transcriptome sequencing to detect gene fusions in cancer. Nature 458: 97–101.
19. Carrara M, Beccuti M, Lazzarato F, Cavallo F, Cordero F, et al. (2013) State-of-the-art fusion-finder algorithms sensitivity and specificity. Biomed Res Int 2013: 340620.
20. Wang Q, Xia J, Jia P, Pao W, Zhao Z (2012) Application of next generation sequencing to human gene fusion detection: computational tools, features and perspectives. Brief Bioinform 14(4): 506–519.
21. Tanas MR, Sboner A, Oliveira AM, Erickson-Johnson MR, Hespelt J, et al. (2011) Identification of a disease-defining gene fusion in epithelioid hemangioendothelioma. Sci Transl Med 3: 98ra82.

22. Lee CH, Ou WB, Marino-Enriquez A, Zhu M, Mayeda M, et al. (2012) 14-3-3 fusion oncogenes in high-grade endometrial stromal sarcoma. Proc Natl Acad Sci U S A 109: 929–934.
23. Panagopoulos I, Thorsen J, Gorunova L, Haugom L, Bjerkehagen B, et al. (2013) Fusion of the ZC3H7B and BCOR genes in endometrial stromal sarcomas carrying an X;22-translocation. Genes Chromosomes Cancer 52: 610–618.
24. Nyquist KB, Panagopoulos I, Thorsen J, Haugom L, Gorunova L, et al. (2012) Whole-Transcriptome Sequencing Identifies Novel IRF2BP2-CDX1 Fusion Gene Brought about by Translocation t(1;5)(q42;q32) in Mesenchymal Chondrosarcoma. PLoS One 7: e49705.
25. Panagopoulos I, Thorsen J, Gorunova L, Micci F, Haugom L, et al. (2013) RNA sequencing identifies fusion of the EWSR1 and YY1 genes in mesothelioma with t(14;22)(q32;q12). Genes Chromosomes Cancer 52: 733–740.
26. Micci F, Thorsen J, Panagopoulos I, Nyquist KB, Zeller B, et al. (2013) High-throughput sequencing identifies an NFIA/CBFA2T3 fusion gene in acute erythroid leukemia with t(1;16)(p31;q24). Leukemia 27: 980–982.
27. Panagopoulos I, Micci F, Thorsen J, Haugom L, Buechner J, et al. (2013) Fusion of ZMYND8 and RELA genes in acute erythroid leukemia. PLoS One 8: e63663.
28. Panagopoulos I, Gorunova L, Zeller B, Tierens A, Heim S (2013) Cryptic FUS-ERG fusion identified by RNA-sequencing in childhood acute myeloid leukemia. Oncol Rep 30: 2587–2592.
29. Schaffer LG, Slovak ML, Campbell LJ (2009) ISCN 2009: an International System for Human Cytogenetic Nomenclature. Basel: Karger.
30. Ge H, Liu K, Juan T, Fang F, Newman M, et al. (2011) FusionMap: detecting fusion genes from next-generation sequencing data at base-pair resolution. Bioinformatics 27: 1922–1928.
31. Francis RW, Thompson-Wicking K, Carter KW, Anderson D, Kees UR, et al. (2012) FusionFinder: a software tool to identify expressed gene fusion candidates from RNA-Seq data. PLoS One 7: e39987.
32. Mercher T, Coniat MB, Monni R, Mauchauffe M, Nguyen Khac F, et al. (2001) Involvement of a human gene related to the Drosophila spen gene in the recurrent t(1;22) translocation of acute megakaryocytic leukemia. Proc Natl Acad Sci U S A 98: 5776–5779.
33. Ma Z, Morris SW, Valentine V, Li M, Herbrick JA, et al. (2001) Fusion of two novel genes, RBM15 and MKL1, in the t(1;22)(p13;q13) of acute megakaryoblastic leukemia. Nat Genet 28: 220–221.
34. Liu P, Tarle SA, Hajra A, Claxton DF, Marlton P, et al. (1993) Fusion between transcription factor CBF beta/PEBP2 beta and a myosin heavy chain in acute myeloid leukemia. Science 261: 1041–1044.
35. Gruber TA, Larson Gedman A, Zhang J, Koss CS, Marada S, et al. (2012) An Inv(16)(p13.3q24.3)-encoded CBFA2T3-GLIS2 fusion protein defines an aggressive subtype of pediatric acute megakaryoblastic leukemia. Cancer Cell 22: 683–697.
36. Jackson CC, Medeiros LJ, Miranda RN (2010) 8p11 myeloproliferative syndrome: a review. Hum Pathol 41: 461–476.
37. Macdonald D, Reiter A, Cross NC (2002) The 8p11 myeloproliferative syndrome: a distinct clinical entity caused by constitutive activation of FGFR1. Acta Haematol 107: 101–107.
38. Carrara M, Beccuti M, Cavallo F, Donatelli S, Lazzarato F, et al. (2013) State of art fusion-finder algorithms are suitable to detect transcription-induced chimeras in normal tissues? BMC Bioinformatics 14 Suppl 7: S2.

5

Inhibition of the MDM2 E3 Ligase Induces Apoptosis and Autophagy in Wild-Type and Mutant p53 Models of Multiple Myeloma, and Acts Synergistically with ABT-737

Dongmin Gu[1,◔], Shuhong Wang[2,◔], Isere Kuiatse[1], Hua Wang[1], Jin He[1], Yun Dai[3], Richard J. Jones[1], Chad C. Bjorklund[1], Jing Yang[1], Steven Grant[3], Robert Z. Orlowski[1,4*]

1 Department of Lymphoma/Myeloma, The University of Texas MD Anderson Cancer Center, Houston, Texas, United States of America, **2** Department of Hematology, Chinese PLA General Hospital, Beijing, China, **3** Department of Medicine, Virginia Commonwealth University, Richmond, Virginia, United States of America, **4** Department of Experimental Therapeutics, The University of Texas MD Anderson Cancer Center, Houston, Texas, United States of America

Abstract

Intracellular proteolytic pathways have been validated as rational targets in multiple myeloma with the approval of two proteasome inhibitors in this disease, and with the finding that immunomodulatory agents work through an E3 ubiquitin ligase containing Cereblon. Another E3 ligase that could be a rational target is the murine double minute (MDM) 2 protein, which plays a role in p53 turnover. A novel inhibitor of this complex, MI-63, was found to induce apoptosis in p53 wild-type myeloma models in association with activation of a p53-mediated cell death program. MI-63 overcame adhesion-mediated drug resistance, showed anti-tumor activity *in vivo*, enhanced the activity of bortezomib and lenalidomide, and also overcame lenalidomide resistance. In mutant p53 models, inhibition of MDM2 with MI-63 also activated apoptosis, albeit at higher concentrations, and this was associated with activation of autophagy. When MI-63 was combined with the BH3 mimetic ABT-737, enhanced activity was seen in both wild-type and mutant p53 models. Finally, this regimen showed efficacy against primary plasma cells from patients with newly diagnosed and relapsed/refractory myeloma. These findings support the translation of novel MDM2 inhibitors both alone, and in combination with other novel agents, to the clinic for patients with multiple myeloma.

Editor: Carl G. Maki, Rush University Medical Center, United States of America

Funding: This study was supported by The MD Anderson Cancer Center SPORE in Multiple Myeloma (P50 CA142509). R.Z.O. is supported by the Florence Maude Thomas Cancer Research Professorship, and the Brock Family Myeloma Research Fund. The MD Anderson Flow Cytometry and Cellular Imaging Core Facility, the RPPA Core Facility, and the Characterized Cell Line Core Facility are supported by the Cancer Center Support Grant (CA16672). The funders had no role in study design, data collection and analysis, decision to publish, or preparation of the manuscript.

Competing Interests: Ascenta Therapeutics provided the MDM-2 inhibitor used in these studies. There are no further patents, products in development or marketed products to declare.

* Email: rorlowsk@mdanderson.org

◔ These authors contributed equally to this work.

Introduction

Multiple myeloma is a malignant plasma cell dyscrasia characterized clinically in patients with symptomatic disease by anemia, hypercalcemia, renal insufficiency, or bony lesions [1,2], and is the second most commonly diagnosed hematologic malignancy [3]. Novel drug classes such as proteasome inhibitors and immunomodulatory agents have had a significant impact upon the natural history of this disease, with some studies suggesting a doubling in the median overall survival [4,5,6,7,8,9]. Bortezomib and carfilzomib are the currently approved proteasome inhibitors for multiple myeloma, and exert their effects by blocking the turnover of poly-ubiquitinated proteins through the proteasome, which is the final effector of the ubiquitin-proteasome pathway [10,11,12]. Downstream effects of proteasome inhibition include activation of the endoplasmic reticulum stress response, inhibition of adherence and survival signaling through nuclear factor kappa B [10,11,12], and induction of a pro-apoptotic program, including through p53 [13,14,15,16,17]. Interestingly, recent studies of the immunomodulatory agents thalidomide, lenalidomide, and pomalidomide have indicated that they work in part through an effect on an E3 ubiquitin ligase that incorporates the immunomodulatory drug binding protein Cereblon [18,19]. This influences substrate specificity of the ligase for targets such as the Ikaros and Aiolos transcription factors [20,21], whose degradation results in anti-proliferative plasma cell effects and T cell stimulation.

Another E3 ubiquitin ligase that may be a rational target for multiple myeloma therapy is murine double minute (MDM) 2, a pleiotropic protein best known for facilitating the p53 ubiquitination required for its proteasome-mediated turnover [22]. Regulation of p53 function also occurs by binding of MDM2 to p53 amino acids 15–29, preventing p53 interactions with transcriptional machinery, forming a negative feedback loop limiting p53 accumulation and function [22]. MDM2 may be over-expressed in some cases of multiple myeloma [23,24] through mechanisms such as gene amplification or chromosomal trisomy [24]. In addition, epigenetic suppression of the promoter for the micro RNA 194-2-192 cluster may also enhance MDM2 expression [25]. This over-expression has been shown to result in enhanced cell cycle progression, proliferation, and survival of myeloma cells, in part through down-regulation of the cyclin-dependent kinase inhibitor p21 [26]. Since p21 accumulation is a part of the mechanism of action for both proteasome inhibitors [14] and immunomodulatory agents [19,27], these findings together support the possibility that approaches targeting MDM2 could be attractive options for myeloma patients.

Small molecule inhibitors of the MDM2/p53 interaction have been identified, such as the Nutlins [28], which were the first generation of agents directly targeting this pathway, and bind in MDM2's p53 binding pocket in the N-terminal region to induce p53 accumulation. These have helped in elucidating the biology of MDM2 and p53, such as by allowing identification of new MDM2 targets [29], and have shown pre-clinical activity against myeloma *in vitro* [30,31,32]. However, the low potency of these first generation agents has limited their potential clinical applicability. We therefore sought to determine if one of the second-generation MDM2 inhibitors [33], MI-63 [34,35], could be active against myeloma, and if it could fit into our armamentarium in combination with other currently approved and novel agents against this disease. In this study, we present data which indicate that MI-63 has potent activity against myeloma using both *in vitro* and *in vivo* models. Also, studies in mutant p53 models show evidence of activity, and indicate activation of autophagy. Finally, MI-63 can overcome lenalidomide resistance, can be combined with other currently approved agents, such as bortezomib or lenalidomide, and also with novel drugs including the BH3 mimetic ABT-737, to enhance activity against both myeloma cell lines and primary samples. Together, the data support the translation of approaches targeting the interaction between MDM2 and p53 to the clinic for patients with relapsed and/or refractory myeloma.

Materials and Methods

Reagents

MI-63 and MI-219 were provided by Sanofi (Bridgewater, NJ), while ABT-737, bortezomib, and lenalidomide were purchased from Selleck Chemicals (Houston, TX).

Chloroquine and 3-methyladenine were purchased from Sigma-Aldrich (St. Louis, MO).

Tissue culture and patient samples

Myeloma cell lines were purchased either from the German Collection of Microorganisms and Cell Cultures (Braunschweig, Germany), or the American Type Culture Collection (Manassas, VA), and validated by the MD Anderson Characterized Cell Line Core Facility. Primary samples were from patients who had provided written informed consent in compliance with the Declaration of Helsinki according to an MD Anderson Institutional Review Board 5 approved protocol (LAB11-0321). $CD138^+$ or $^-$ cells were isolated from these fresh bone marrow aspirates with the CD138 Positive Plasma Cell Isolation Kit (Miltenyi Biotec; Auburn, CA). Cells were cultured in RPMI 1640 medium with 2 mM L-glutamine (Invitrogen; Carlsbad, CA) supplemented with 10% fetal bovine serum (Sigma-Aldrich), 100 U/mL penicillin (Invitrogen) and 100 μg/ml streptomycin (Invitrogen). HS-5 stromal cells from the American Type Culture Collection were cultured in Dulbecco's modified Eagle's medium containing fetal bovine serum and penicillin and streptomycin as above.

Cell viability assays

Cell viability was determined using the tetrazolium reagent WST-1 (Roche Applied Science; Indianapolis, IN) according to the manufacturer's instructions and as previously described [36]. Viability curves were fitted in GraphPad Prism version 6 (La Jolla, CA) and median inhibitory concentrations (IC_{50}) were calculated using log (inhibitor) vs. response – variable slope (four parameters).

shRNA gene knockdown

Lentiviral constructs containing non-targeting shRNA sequences, or shRNAs designed to suppress expression of MDM2, p53, autophagy (ATG)-related protein 5 (ATG5) and Beclin-1 were purchased from Sigma-Aldrich. Viral particles were generated from 293T cells following standard protocols, and myeloma cells were infected and selected with the use of polybrene and puromycin, as detailed previously [37].

Reverse transcription and quantitative PCR

Total RNA was extracted using Trizol (Invitrogen), and cDNA was synthesized with High-Capacity cDNA Reverse Transcription Kits (Applied Biosystems; Grand Island, NY) as previously described [38]. TaqMan Gene Expression Master Mix and probes were purchased from Applied Biosystems and used to perform quantitative PCR (qPCR) reactions on an Applied Biosystems StepOnePlus Real-Time PCR system. Expression of glyceraldehyde 3-phosphate dehydrogenase (GAPDH) was used as an internal control.

Proteomic assays

Western blotting and immunoprecipitation of protein extracts was performed using standard procedures [39]. Antibodies which were used included: anti-p53 (DO-1) and Bax (6A7)(Santa Cruz Biotechnology; Santa Cruz, CA); anti-MDM2 (Ab-1) and -Bak (Ab-1)(Calbiochem; San Diego, CA); anti-Caspase-3 (5A1E), -9 (D2D4), -poly ADP ribose polymerase (PARP)(D64E10), -p53 upregulated modulator of apoptosis (PUMA)(D30C10), -Microtubule-associated protein 1 light chain 3 (LC3)(D3U4C & D11), -Cytochrome C (136F3), -Beclin-1 (#3738) and -ATG5 (#2630)(Cell Signaling Technology; Danvers, MA); and anti-Actin (A2066)(Sigma-Aldrich). Densitometry was performed using ImageJ software version 1.46 (National Institute of Health; Bethesda, MD). Mitochondrial isolation prior to Western blotting was performed where indicated using the Mitochondria Isolation Kit (Thermo Scientific; Rockford, IL). Reverse phase protein array (RPPA) analyses were performed by the MD Anderson Cancer Center RPPA/Functional Proteomics Core Facility.

Cell cycle analysis and apoptosis

Cell cycle analysis was performed by staining with propidium iodide (Sigma-Aldrich), and then analyzing cells by flow cytometry as described previously [40]. Annexin V staining was used to detect apoptosis by flow cytometry using the manufacturer's instructions (Invitrogen).

Drug synergy calculations and statistical analyses

Data were analyzed using CalcuSyn software (Biosoft; Cambridge, United Kingdom), and combination indices (CI) were calculated to determine if synergistic interactions were being observed. Statistical analyses were performed with unpaired t tests in GraphPad, and p-values less than 0.05 were judged to be significant.

Xenograft model

Experiments were performed in accordance with procedures and protocols approved by the MD Anderson Cancer Center Animal Care and Use Committee using xenografts developed as detailed previously [36,41]. In brief, 10^7 MM1.S cells were inoculated subcutaneously in 6-week-old nonobese diabetic severe combined immunodeficiency (NOD/SCID) gamma mice (The Jackson Laboratory; Bar Harbor, ME) to establish tumors. Vehicle (10% polyethylene glycol, 3% Cremophor EL in phosphate buffered saline) or MI-219 (100 mg/kg) was injected intraperitoneally three times a week. Tumor diameters were measured with a digital caliper, and tumor volume was calculated by the formula: volume = $(\text{width})^2 \times \text{length}/2$.

Results

MDM2 inhibition with MI-63 is cytotoxic to wild-type p53 myeloma cells

Nutlin-based inhibitors of MDM2 have been found to have activity predominantly against wild-type (wt) p53 myeloma models. To evaluate the activity of MI-63, we exposed a panel of wt p53 myeloma cell lines (MM1.S, H929, MOLP-8) to this agent, and measured viability with a tetrazolium reagent. All of these cell lines were found to be very sensitive to low drug levels over the course of a 48-hour exposure (Figure 1A), with a median inhibitory concentration (IC_{50}) in the low single μM range or less (MM1.S: 0.6 μM; H929: 0.4 μM; MOLP-8: 1.5 μM). In order to verify that MI-63 was indeed inhibiting the interaction between MDM2 and p53, we subjected extracts of MM1.S cells to immunoprecipitation with an anti-MDM2 antibody, and then analyzed these by Western blotting. Compared to vehicle-treated controls, the level of p53 immunoprecipitated in association with MDM2 was reduced after these cells were treated with MI-63 (Figure 1B). In comparison, MI-63 did not alter the interaction with MDM4, which associates with MDM2 through the RING finger domain (Figure S1) [42]. We then prepared MM1.S cells in which p53 expression had been stably suppressed at the mRNA (Figure S2A) and protein levels (Figure S2B) using a Lentiviral-delivered small hairpin (sh) RNA construct. MI-63 retained activity against MM1.S cells harboring a non-targeting shRNA construct (Figure 1C), but this was substantially blunted in the cells with decreased p53 content (control shRNA IC_{50}: 2.2 μM; p53 shRNA IC_{50}: 5.2 μM), consistent with a strong impact of p53 status. Finally, since microenvironmental effects, such as expression of interleukin (IL)-6, may modulate the expression of p53 [43], we evaluated the activity of MI-63 on myeloma cells in the presence of HS-5 human stromal cells. When MM1.S cells were co-cultured with stromal cells, the IC_{50} of MI-63 was not significantly altered (MM1.S+HS-5 IC_{50}: 1.9 μM; MM1.S IC_{50}: 3.4 μM) (Figure 1D), and similar data were obtained in MOLP-8 cells (control shRNA IC_{50}: 3.5 μM; p53 shRNA IC_{50}: 3.5 μM; Figure S3). Next, we generated a xenograft model using NOD/SCID mice and MM1.S myeloma cells. Compared to vehicle-treated mice, which experienced a substantial increase in their tumor burden over the period of the experiment, treatment with the *in vivo* analogue of MI-63, MI-219, induced a significant tumor growth delay (Figure 1E).

Molecular mechanisms of MI-63 action

Inhibition of MDM2 should result in accumulation of p53 protein with downstream activation of a p53-mediated cell death program, and we therefore examined these myeloma cell lines for evidence of this mechanism. Using qPCR, we found a significant increase of transcript levels for p53 up-regulated modulator of apoptosis (PUMA), Bcl-2 associated protein x (BAX), Noxa, p21, and MDM2 (Figure 2A). Many of these findings were then confirmed by RPPA, a high-throughput antibody-based technique developed for functional proteomics studies to evaluate protein activity in signaling networks. Results from MM1.S and MOLP-8 cells indicated an up-regulation of pro-apoptotic Bax, cell cycle regulators p21 and p27, and cleaved/active caspases-3 and -7, highlighting the activation of type I programmed cell death (Figure S4). Consistent in part with the induction of cyclin-dependent kinase inhibitors p21, p27, and with programmed cell death, cell cycle profiling showed an increased content of cells at G_0/G_1 after exposure to MI-63 (Figure 2B). Activation of apoptosis was confirmed using flow cytometry after Annexin V staining for cell surface phosphatidylserine levels, which were strongly enhanced by MDM2 inhibition (Figure 2C). Finally, at the protein level, MI-63 induced accumulation of p53, MDM2, and PUMA, and induced release of cytochrome c from mitochondria into the cytosol, resulting in activation of caspase-9 and the downstream effector caspase-3 (Figure 2D).

Inhibition of MDM2 is also active against mutant p53 myeloma

The majority of newly-diagnosed patients with myeloma are felt to have wt p53, but the incidence of deletion at the 17p locus by fluorescence *in situ* hybridization ranges from 7%–11% [44,45], and later increases to ~22% in the relapsed and/or refractory setting [46]. We therefore sought to determine if MDM2 inhibitors could retain some activity in mutant (mut) p53 models using a different cell line panel (ANBL-6, KAS-6/1, RPMI 8226, U266, and OPM-2). While single μM concentrations were, in part as expected, largely ineffective, a dose-dependent decrease in viability was nonetheless seen in these mutant cells at higher concentrations (Figure 3A), with an IC_{50} in the range of 20–40 μM (ANBL-6: 30.1 μM; KAS-6/1: 36 μM; RPMI 8226: 27.9 μM; U266: 27.9 μM; OPM-2: 20.4 μM). Cell cycle analysis showed that RPMI 8226 and U266 cells exposed to MI-63 did accumulate at G_0/G_1 (Figure 3B). Furthermore, this was associated with induction of apoptosis as measured both by Annexin V staining (Figure 3C), and by activation of caspases-9 and -3, as well as cleavage of PARP (Figure 3D). This occurred without any impact on the expression levels of p53, or on downstream targets of wt p53, such as PUMA (Figure 3D), as would be expected in a mut p53 background. Given the high MI-63 concentrations required to induce cell death, we considered the possibility that this could be occurring through an off-target effect. U266 cells were therefore prepared that expressed either a non-targeting shRNA, or one of two different shRNAs that suppressed MDM2 (Figure S5). When these were exposed to MI-63, the two clones in which MDM2 was reduced showed a lower IC_{50} and therefore greater sensitivity compared to the controls (control shRNA IC_{50}: 36.3 μM; MDM2 shRNA clone 3380 IC_{50}: 24.7 μM; MDM2 shRNA clone 3376 IC_{50}: 23.8 μM; Figure 3E). This finding is consistent with a continued role for MDM2 in the mechanism of action of MI-63 in these models, since decreased expression of MDM2 led to a need for less drug to elicit the same phenotype, whereas if MI-63 were active through a different target, MDM2 knockdown would not have changed the IC_{50}.

MDM2 inhibitors induce autophagy in mut p53 myeloma models

While RPPA studies in wt p53 cells showed induction of type I apoptosis, RPMI 8226 and KAS6/1 cells exposed to MI-63 showed induction of several targets involved in autophagy, including AMP-activated protein kinase, and p70 S6 and S6 kinase (Figure S6 and results not shown). Moreover, by Western blotting, we did detect enhanced conversion of microtubule-associated protein (MAP)-1 light chain 3 (LC3) form I to form II

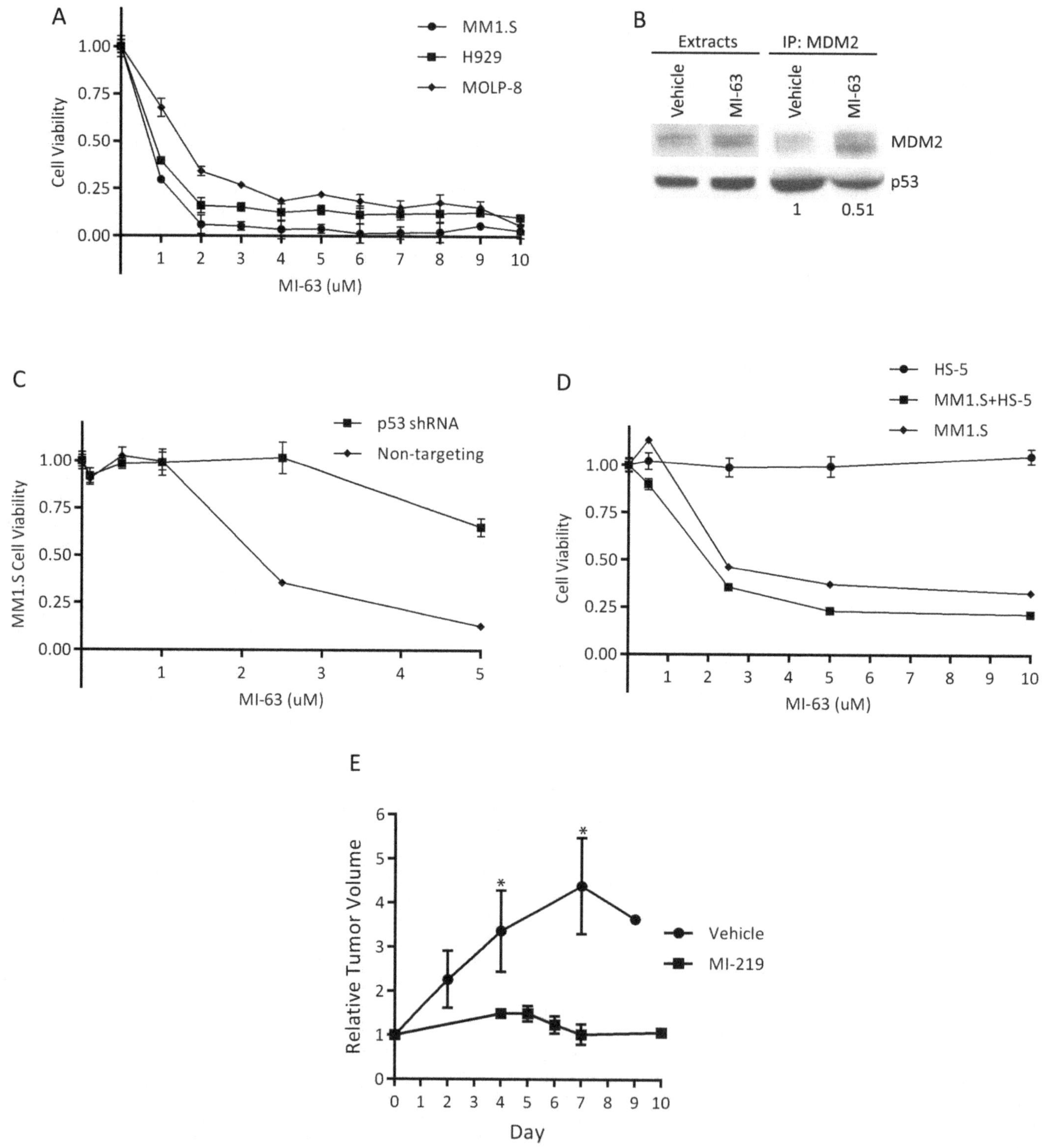

Figure 1. MI-63 is cytotoxic to wild-type p53 myeloma cells. A. Cell viability assays were performed in wild-type p53 myeloma cell lines exposed to the indicated concentrations of MI-63 for 48 hours using a tetrazolium reagent. Error bars represent standard errors of the mean from three or more replicates, and all experiments in this and later figures were repeated three times, with one representative figure shown. **B.** Whole cell extracts were prepared from MM1.S cells treated with vehicle or MI-63, and then subjected to immunoprecipitation with an antibody to MDM2. The precipitates were then probed by Western blotting using specific antibodies to MDM2 or p53, and densitometry was performed using Image J software. **C.** MM1.S cells stably infected with a Lentiviral vector expressing either a control, non-targeted shRNA or an shRNA directed at p53 were exposed to MI-63 as above, and viability was measured using the WST-1 reagent. **D.** Human stromal HS-5 cells or MM1.S myeloma cells were propagated in culture either alone, or co-cultured at a ratio of 20:1, and viability was measured in the presence of MI-63. **E.** A murine xenograft myeloma model was developed in NOD/SCID mice, and when tumor volume reached 100 mm^3, mice were treated intraperitoneally with 100 mg/kg MI-219 or vehicle, and tumor volume was monitored three times a week. Vehicle-treated mice experienced a substantial increase in the tumor burden, while MI-219 induced a significant tumor growth delay, (*$p<0.05$).

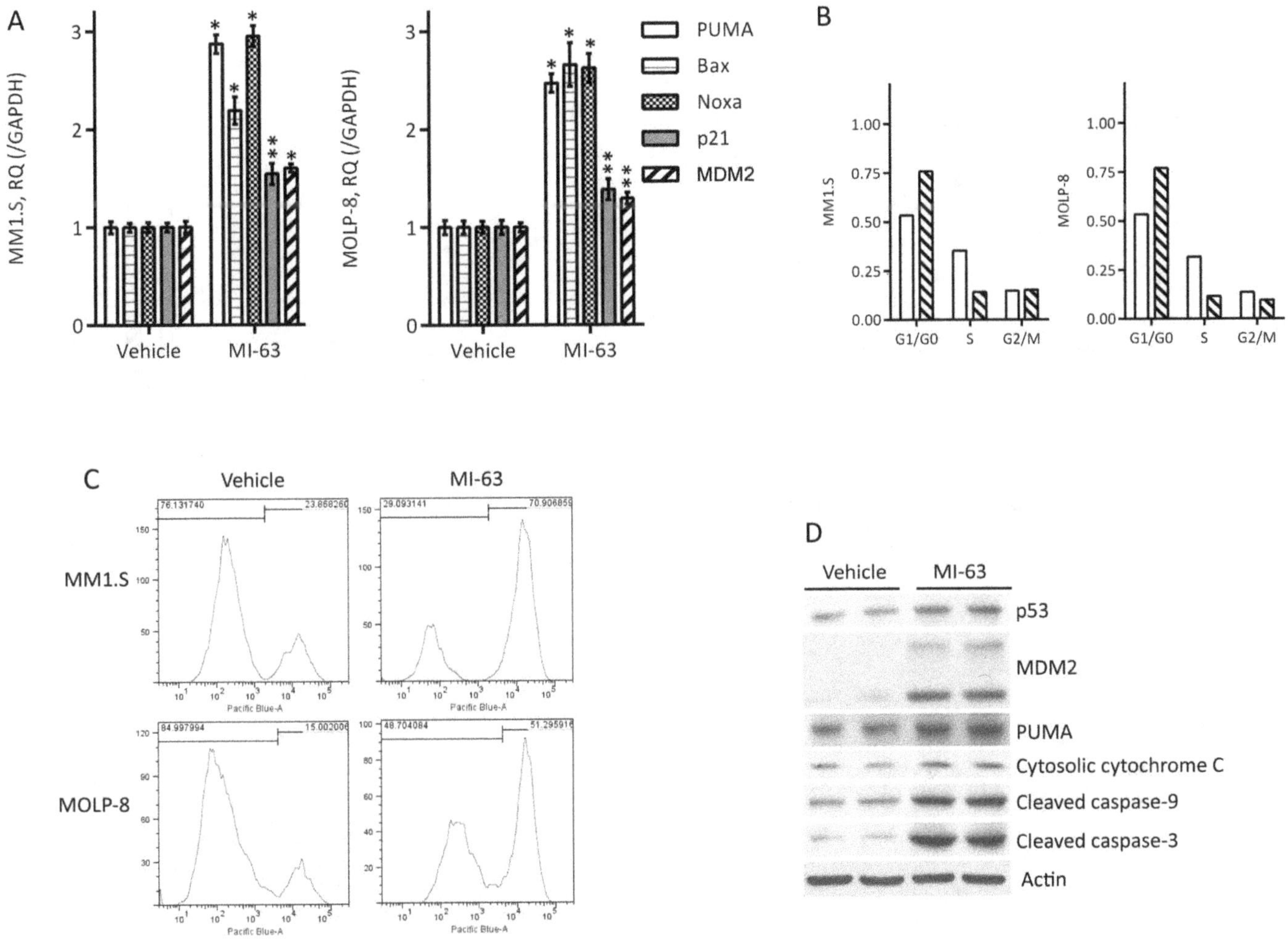

Figure 2. Molecular mechanisms underlying the action of MI-63. A. Quantitative PCR was performed of selected p53 transcriptional targets in wild-type cell lines after exposure to MI-63 at the IC_{50} for 48 hours. Values were normalized to GAPDH as a control (*p<0.005; **p<0.05). **B.** The indicated cell lines were treated with MI-63 at its IC_{50} for 48 hours, and cell cycle analysis was performed after propidium iodide staining. **C.** Activation of apoptosis was evaluated after Annexin V staining by flow cytometry in MM1.S and MOLP-8 cells treated with MI-63 for 48 hours. **D.** Western blotting of cells treated for 48 hours with MI-63 at the IC_{50} was performed to detect changes in key downstream targets, with Actin as the loading control.

(Figure 3D) after treatment with MI-63, which has been associated with autophagy. To obtain additional support for the possibility that autophagy was being induced, we stained cells with acridine orange, a hydrophobic dye that accumulates in acidic vesicles such as lysosomes and autophagic vacuoles. Compared to wt p53 MM1.S and MOLP-8 cells exposed to MI-63, which showed a slight increase in staining (Figure 4A), mut p53 RPMI 8226 and U266 cells showed a strong increase in acridine orange staining. The autophagic cell death program involves input from a number of genes, including ATG3 and 5, and we therefore performed qPCR to evaluate their expression. In wt p53 MM1.S and MOLP-8 cells exposed to MI-63, expression of ATG3 or 5 was unaltered (Figure 4B), but both were increased in mut p53 RPMI 8226 and U266 cells. Since autophagy may under some conditions promote cell survival, we evaluated the impact of MI-63 in the presence of chloroquine (ChQ), which raises lysosomal pH and inhibits autophagosome and lysosome fusion, or with 3-methyladenine (3-MA), an inhibitor of autophagic sequestration. In the context of wt p53, titrated ChQ slightly enhanced the cytotoxicity of MI-63, while 3-MA had no effect (Figure 4C). When mut p53 cells were studied, however, ChQ somewhat protected RPMI 8226 cells from MI-63, and 3-MA did so in both RPMI 8226 and U266 cells. Because these pharmacologic inhibitors can under some circumstances promote autophagy [47], we prepared RPMI 8226 cells harboring an shRNA to ATG5 (Figure S7A), and found that the IC_{50} to MI-63 was increased from 26.2 µM to 37.8 µM when ATG5 expression was suppressed (Figure 4D). Also, when the autophagy regulator Beclin-1 was suppressed (Figure S7B), the IC_{50} to MI-63 was again increased from 28.3 µM to 40.9 µM (Figure 4E). Finally, we evaluated the molecular effects of pharmacologic inhibitors of autophagy on apoptosis, and found that co-incubation of MI-63 with either ChQ or 3-MA reduced LC3 processing (Figure 4F), as expected, and also reduced the levels of activated caspase-3. Together, these findings show that MI-63 induces autophagy in mut p53 myeloma models, and suggests that there is cross-talk between autophagy and apoptosis in these plasma cells.

MI-63 acts synergistically with other agents

Novel therapeutics for myeloma typically find their greatest efficacy in combination with standard, already approved agents, and we therefore sought to determine if MI-63 could show

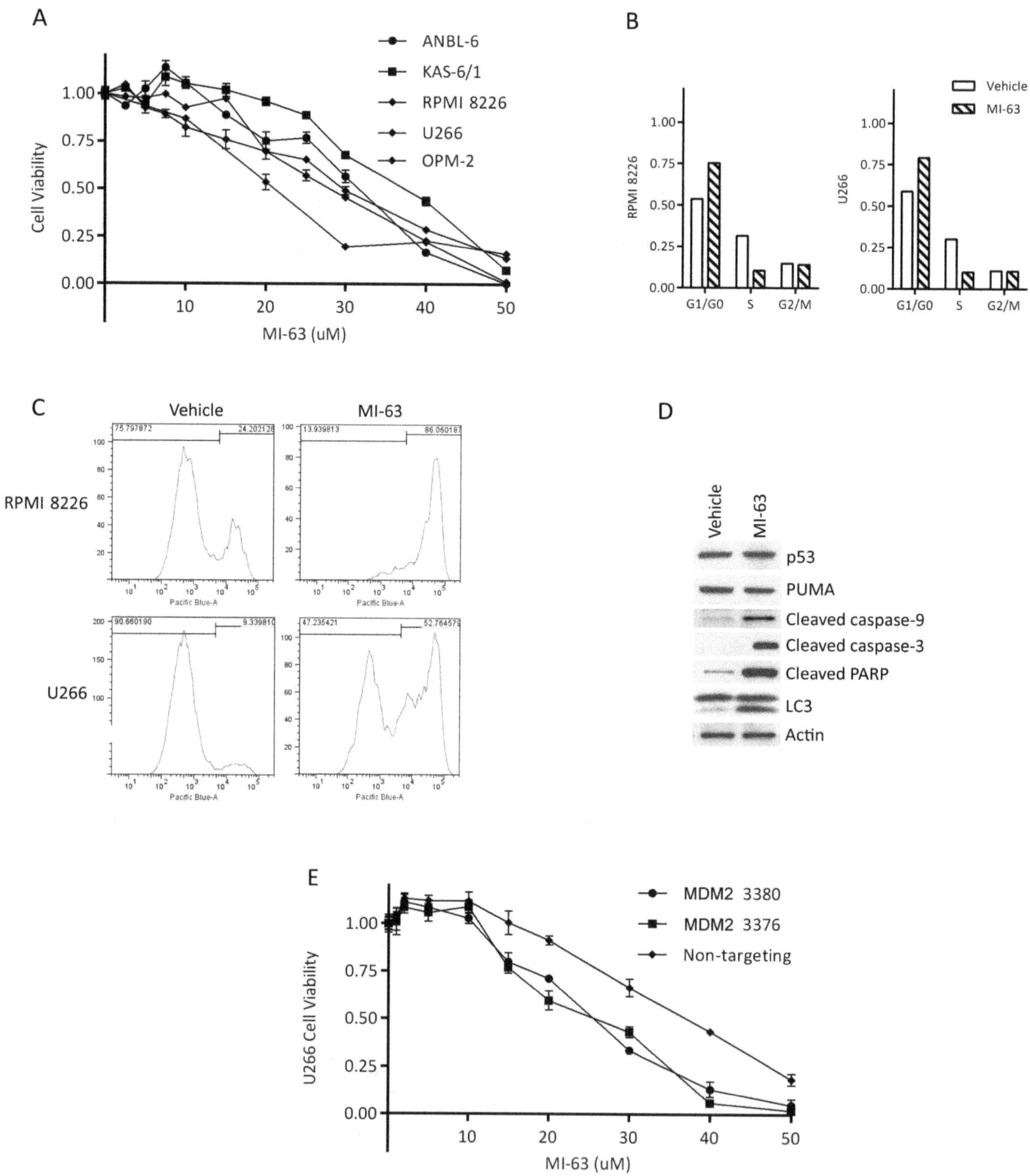

Figure 3. MI-63 is also active against mutant p53 myeloma cell lines. A. Cell viability assays were performed in a panel of mutant p53 myeloma cell lines, including ANBL-6, KAS-6/1, RPMI 8226, U266, and OPM-2 cells after exposure to MI-63 for 48 hours. **B.** Analysis of cell cycle distribution was performed in RPMI 8226 and U266 cells exposed to MI-63. **C.** Induction of apoptosis was evaluated by Annexin V staining and flow cytometry in RPMI 8226 and U266 cells treated with MI-63 at its IC_{50} for 48 hours. **D.** Extracts of RPMI 8226 cells treated with MI-63 were subjected to Western blotting to detect key intermediates in apoptosis and autophagy. **E.** The impact of MDM2 suppression on the efficacy of MI-63 was studied in U266 cells harboring either a control shRNA, or one of two different constructs that suppressed expression of MDM2.

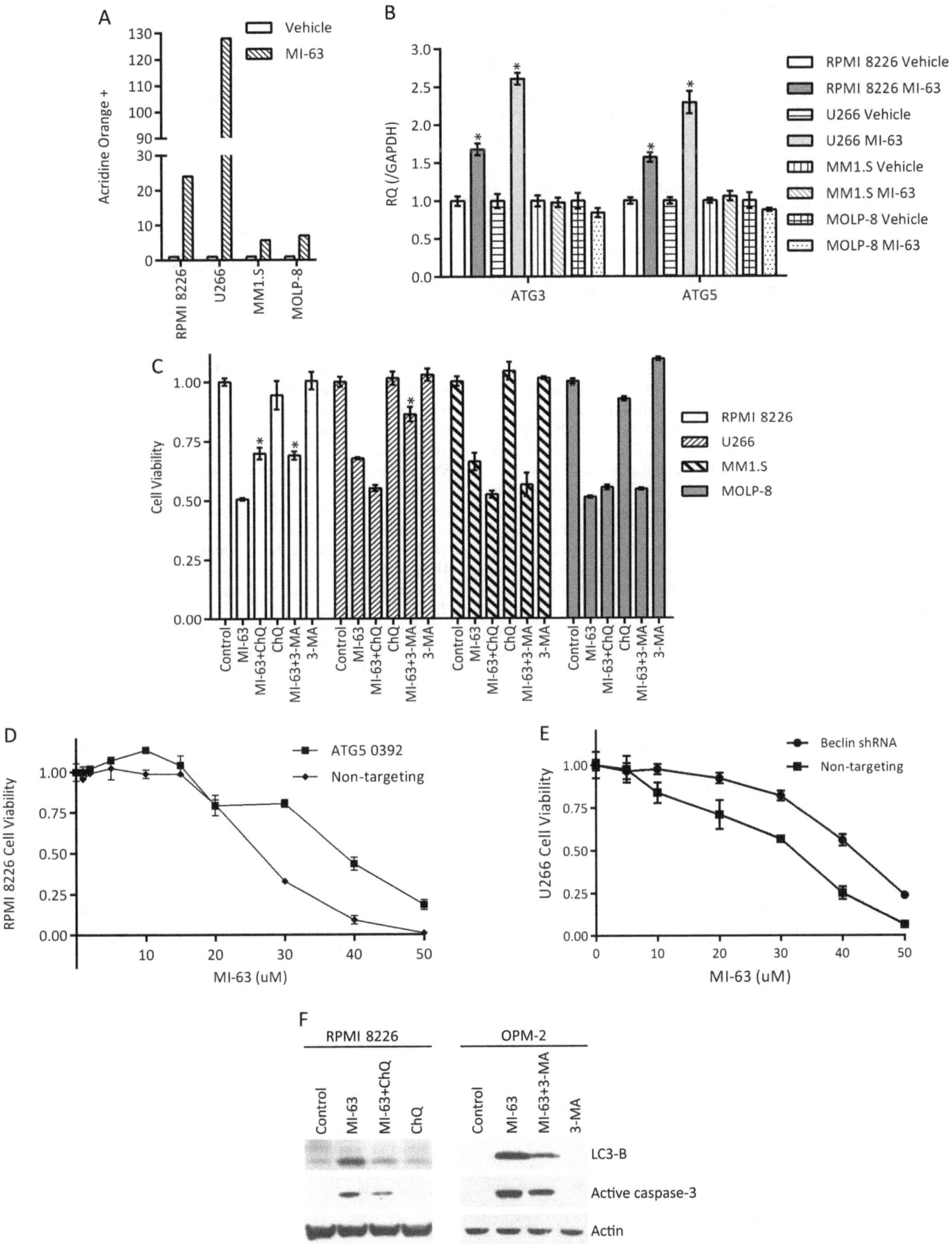
A
Vehicle
MI-63
Acridine Orange +
RPMI 8226
U266
MM1.S
MOLP-8
B
RQ (/GAPDH)
ATG3
ATG5
RPMI 8226 Vehicle
RPMI 8226 MI-63
U266 Vehicle
U266 MI-63
MM1.S Vehicle
MM1.S MI-63
MOLP-8 Vehicle
MOLP-8 MI-63
C
Cell Viability
RPMI 8226
U266
MM1.S
MOLP-8
Control
MI-63
MI-63+ChQ
ChQ
MI-63+3-MA
3-MA
D
RPMI 8226 Cell Viability
ATG5 0392
Non-targeting
MI-63 (uM)
E
U266 Cell Viability
Beclin shRNA
Non-targeting
MI-63 (uM)
F
RPMI 8226
OPM-2
Control
MI-63
MI-63+ChQ
ChQ
MI-63+3-MA
3-MA
LC3-B
Active caspase-3
Actin

Figure 4. MI-63 induces autophagy in mutant p53 myeloma models. A. Acridine orange staining and flow cytometry were used to study the appearance of acidic vacuoles in mutant p53 RPMI 8226 and U266 cells, and wild-type p53 MM1.S and MOLP-8 cells exposed to the IC_{50} of MI-63 for 48 hours. **B.** Transcript levels of ATG3 and ATG5 were studied in mutant and wild-type p53 myeloma cells exposed to MI-63 (*$p<0.005$). **C.** The impact of the autophagy inhibitors chloroquine (100 nM) and 3-methyladenine (1 μM) on the activity of MI-63 against mutant and wild-type p53 cell lines was studied using viability assays (*$p<0.005$). **D.** ATG5 expression was suppressed with a Lentiviral shRNA in RPMI 8226 cells, and the effect of MI-63 was then studied in comparison to control shRNA cells. **E.** Beclin-1 was depleted with an shRNA, and the median inhibitory concentration of MI-63 was determined in comparison with a control shRNA. **F.** Activation of autophagy and apoptosis in mutant p53 myeloma cells treated with MI-63 and/or autophagy inhibitors.

additive activity with other drugs. In MM1.S and MOLP-8 wt p53 cells, bortezomib alone and MI-63 alone showed single-agent activity, but the combinations showed additive to greater than additive effects in reducing myeloma cell viability (Figure S8A). Also, we tested the activity of a combination of MI-63 with the immunomodulatory agent lenalidomide, which does have direct anti-myeloma activity as a single agent *in vitro* [40]. As was the case for the combination with bortezomib, MI-63 with lenalidomide enhanced the reduction in viability induced by either agent alone (Figure S8B). Moreover, when MM1.S cells that had become resistant to lenalidomide [40,41] were exposed to MI-63, this agent was able to overcome this resistance (Figure S8C).

We also examined a combination of MI-63 with ABT-737, a BH3 mimetic inhibitor of B-cell lymphoma 2 (Bcl-2), Bcl-xL, and Bcl-w [48]. In wt p53 MM1.S and MOLP-8 cells, while both MI-63 and ABT-737 were able to reduce viability, the combination showed a greater effect than either agent alone (Figure 5A, left panel). Interestingly, this was also true in mut p53 RPMI 8226 and U266 cells (Figure 5A, right panel). By flow cytometry, the combination showed a strong increase in Annexin V staining in both MOLP-8 (Figure 5B, left panel) and U266 cells (Figure 5B, right panel), indicating that this was likely due to enhanced type I cell death, or apoptosis. Consistent with this possibility, Western blotting revealed increased activation of caspase-3 and cleavage of PARP in both MOLP-8 (Figure 5C, left panel) and U266 cells (Figure 5C, right panel).

Finally, we sought to examine the possibility that a combination of MI-63 and ABT-737 could show activity against primary patient samples, which were from bone marrow aspirates that were purified to obtain $CD138^+$ plasma cells. In all four tested samples (Figure 6, A–D), both MI-63 and ABT-737 showed an ability to reduce cellular viability as single agents. When combined, the two drugs both revealed synergistic activity as measured by an increased reduction in viability compared with either agent by itself (combination index 0.01, 0.46, 0.53 and 0.15, respectively). Notably, $CD138^-$ cells were also available from one patient (Figure 6A), and although some reduction in viability was seen with MI-63, ABT-737, and the combination, the magnitude was substantially less than that seen in $CD138^+$ plasma cells, suggesting that there may be some measure of a therapeutic index. These data support possible translation to the clinic of the regimen of an MDM2 inhibitor and a BH3 mimetic.

Discussion

Despite therapeutic advances that have improved the overall survival of myeloma patients, this plasma cell dyscrasia remains incurable, and is characterized clinically by multiple relapses, reduced benefit from subsequent treatments, and the development of refractory disease [4,5,6,7,8,9]. These facts support the need for continued research to identify novel targets and treatment approaches that can be used alone, or in combination with current standards of care, first in the relapsed and/or refractory setting, and eventually perhaps as part of initial therapy. The current data provide further support for the possibility that agents targeting the MDM2 E3 ubiquitin ligase, such as MI-63, could form part of our armamentarium against myeloma. This agent was shown to be active against *in vitro* and *in vivo* wt p53 myeloma models through a p53-dependent program (Figure 1) including PUMA, Bax, p21, and Noxa, leading to cell cycle arrest and apoptosis (Figure 2). While MI-63 and the Nutlins have a similar mechanism of action, they differ in that Nutlins bind MDM2 residues Phe-19, Trp-23, and Leu-26 in the p53 interacting domain, while MI-63 binds these and also Leu-22 [34,49,50]. This suggests the possibility that MI-63 could prove to be more potent than is the case for the Nutlins. Interestingly, recent studies from our group showed that resistance mechanisms were similar for both agents in models of myeloma and mantle cell lymphoma, including formation of point mutations in the p53 DNA binding and dimerization domains [51].

While the potency of MI-63 was reduced against mut p53 models, cell death could still be induced using ten-fold higher drug concentrations, which was associated with cell cycle arrest and type I programmed cell death (Figure 3). Under these conditions, MDM2 inhibition in a mut p53 background seemed to be accompanied by activation of autophagy (Figure 4). Since inhibition of autophagy protected myeloma cells from MI-63, this at first appeared to suggest that autophagy could be contributing to cell death [52,53]. However, additional studies revealed that the pharmacologic approaches which were used to inhibit autophagy also resulted in a reduction in type I cell death. These findings therefore argue in favor of cross-talk between these pathways [52,53], such as perhaps at the level of Beclin-1 and Bcl-2. Interestingly, wt p53 itself can in some models induce autophagy, in part through damage-regulated autophagy modulator [54,55], while in other models degradation of p53 through a pathway relying on MDM2 [56] induces autophagy. Additional studies will therefore be needed to determine the mechanism by which MDM2 inhibition leads to autophagy in a mut p53 background.

Rationally designed combination regimens often show increased activity against multiple myeloma compared with single agent approaches, and we were able to show that MI-63 did show enhanced efficacy when it was added to bortezomib (Figure S8). In this property, MI-63 is similar to Nutlin-3a, which has previously been shown to induce synergistic activity with bortezomib [31,32] against *in vitro* myeloma models, largely in association with a p53-mediated cell death program. One difference is that Nutlin-3a was inhibited by adhesion-mediated drug resistance [31], whereas MI-63 showed similar activity in the absence or presence of human bone marrow-derived stromal cells (Figure 1), possibly suggesting it may be a superior clinical candidate. We were also able for the first time to show that MDM2 inhibition could act synergistically in combination with the immunomodulatory agent lenalidomide, and could also overcome lenalidomide resistance (Figure S8). The mechanisms of lenalidomide resistance are under active investigation, and while initial studies showed that mutations of Cereblon might be responsible [18], sequencing of primary samples has shown that this likely occurs only in a small minority [57]. Interestingly, while p21 abundance is enhanced by lenalidomide in drug-sensitive plasma cells, in drug-resistant cells that express low

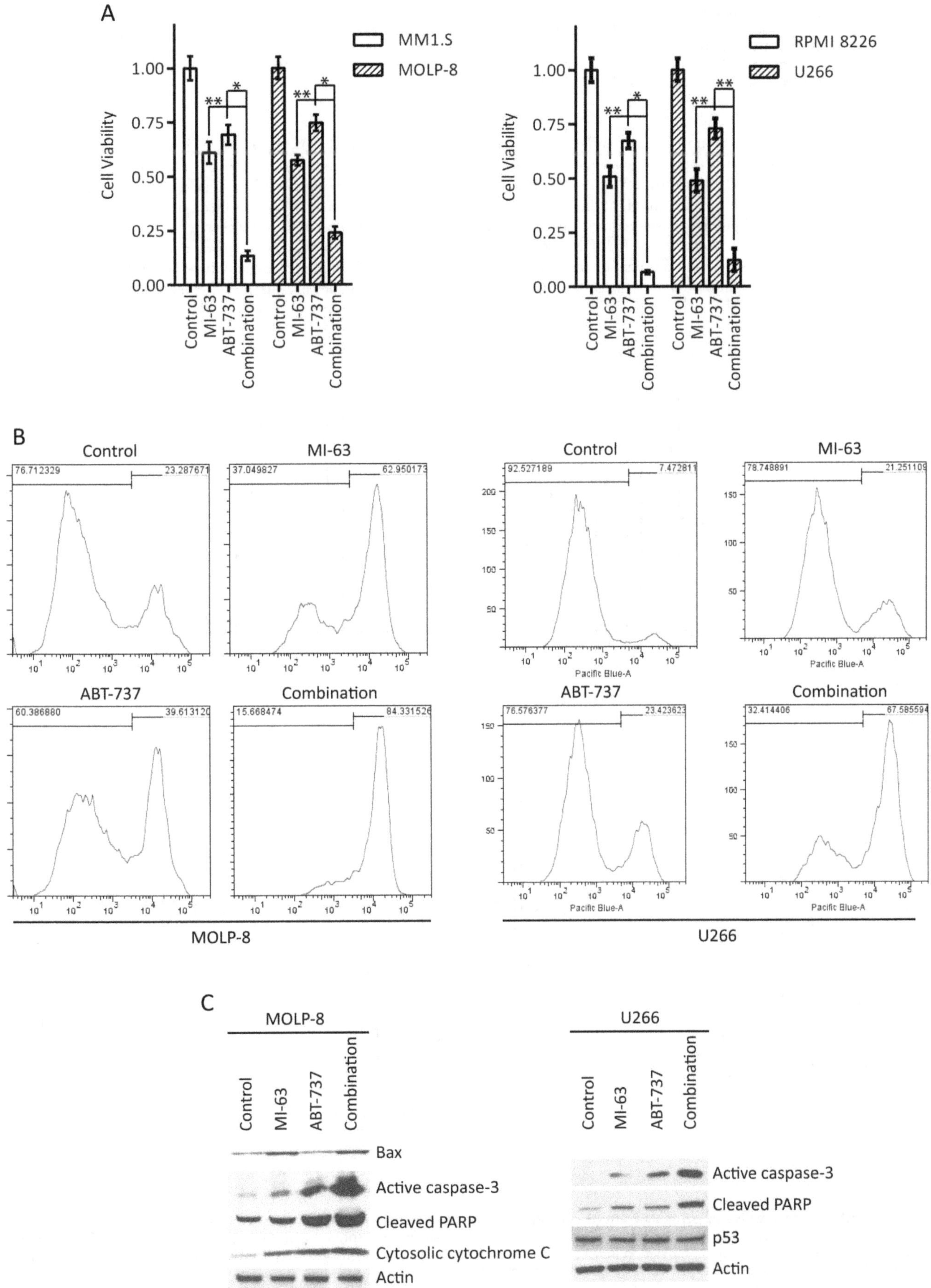
A
MM1.S
MOLP-8
RPMI 8226
U266
Cell Viability
1.00
0.75
0.50
0.25
0.00
Control
MI-63
ABT-737
Combination
B
Control
MI-63
ABT-737
Combination
76.712329
23.287671
37.049827
62.950173
60.386880
39.613120
15.668474
84.331526
92.527189
7.472811
78.748891
21.251109
76.576377
23.423623
32.414406
67.585594
Pacific Blue-A
MOLP-8
U266
C
MOLP-8
U266
Control
MI-63
ABT-737
Combination
Bax
Active caspase-3
Cleaved PARP
Cytosolic cytochrome C
Actin
p53

Figure 5. MI-63 acts synergistically with ABT-737. A. The combination of MI-63 and ABT-737 was studied in wild-type p53 MM1.S and MOLP-8 cells (left panel), and in mutant RPMI 8226 and U266 cells (right panel). Multiple doses of each drug were used for this experiment, with one representative condition shown. **p*<0.005, ** *p*<0.05. **B.** Apoptosis was studied by staining for Annexin V in both wild-type p53 (MOLP-8; left panel) and mutant p53 (U266; right panel) cells treated with vehicle, MI-63, ABT-737, or the combination. **C.** Abundance of important intermediates in type I programmed cell death was studied in MOLP8 and U266 cells by Western blotting.

levels of p21, neither lenalidomide nor pomalidomide substantially enhance p21 expression [19]. It is therefore tempting to speculate that it is this restoration of p21 levels by inhibition of MDM2, leading to transactivation of p21 by p53, that is at the center of the ability of an MDM2 inhibitor to overcome lenalidomide resistance, at least in a p53 wt background. If MDM2 inhibitors are translated to the clinic as part of combination regimens with proteasome inhibitors or immunomodulatory drugs, attention may need to be paid to the potential for additive myelosuppression. This conclusion is based on results from a proof of concept study in patients with liposarcomas of single-agent RG-7112, an inhibitor in the Nutlin family, which induced neutropenia and thrombocytopenia in 30% and 40%, respectively, of patients [58].

Finally, we sought to determine if the addition of a BH3 mimetic could enhance the activity of an MDM2 inhibitor, in part with the rationale that the p53-mediated activation of Bax could

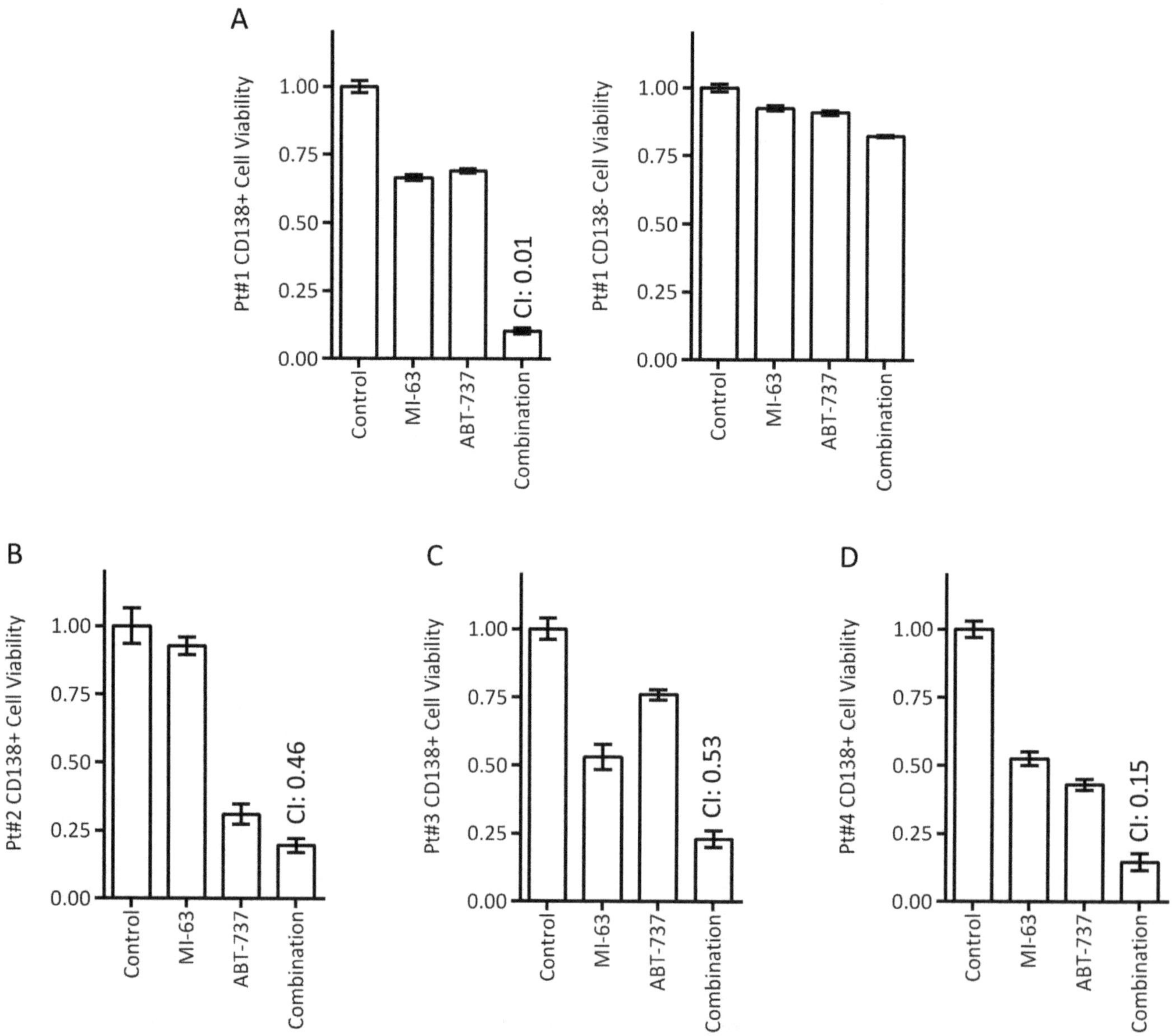

Figure 6. Combination studies in primary patient samples. A. The combination of MI-63 and ABT-737 was studied against CD138$^+$ primary plasma cells from a patient with multiple myeloma (left panel), and CD138$^-$ marrow cells (right panel). Note that multiple doses of each drug were used for this experiment to calculate combination indices, with one representative condition shown. **B–D.** Additional primary plasma cells isolated from unique patients were exposed to the combination of MI-63 and ABT-737.

be potentiated by blocking its interaction with Bcl-2. Consistent with this possibility, we did find that the combination of MI-63 and ABT-737 induced a greater reduction in cellular viability and induction of apoptosis than did either agent alone (Figure 5). This was accompanied by increased conversion of Bax and Bak to their active pro-apoptotic forms, as judged by conformation-specific antibodies (results not shown). Interestingly, the benefits of this combination may at least in part be due to possible off-target effects of MDM2 inhibitors. Indeed, the Nutlin class of drugs have been reported to also bind anti-apoptotic Bcl-2 family proteins, including Bcl-xL and Bcl-2 itself [59,60], though whether this is also the case for MI-63 is not known. Notably, enhanced activity was seen even in the mut p53 models, which again seemed to occur through type I programmed cell death (Figure 5). Thus, while some combinations based on an MDM2 inhibitor may be expected to benefit only those patients with wt p53, such as with a death receptor 5 agonist [61], a regimen of a BH3 mimetic and an MDM2 inhibitor could benefit patients with either wt or mut p53. This would be especially important since recent studies with p53-specific probes and sequencing have suggested that higher rates of p53 deletion may be present than previously thought [62,63,64], particularly at the time of relapse [64]. Moreover, p53 deletion and mutation are universally recognized as poor prognostic features in myeloma, and approaches that could help such patients would be very welcome. We are therefore working at this time to translate such a regimen to the clinic in the relapsed and/or refractory setting.

Supporting Information

Figure S1 Impact of MI-63 on the interactions between MDM2 and other proteins. MM1.S cells were treated with various doses of MI-63 for the indicated times, and cell extracts were subjected to immunoprecipitation with MDM2 antibodies, followed by Western blotting with antibodies specific to either p53 or MDM4.

Figure S2 p53 knock down in MM1.S cells. A. Impact of a Lentiviral-delivered shRNA targeting p53 compared to a control, non-targeting shRNA on p53 mRNA levels in MM1.S cells (*$p <$ 0.005). **B.** Western blotting shows the impact of these shRNAs on p53 protein expression.

Figure S3 Impact of stromal cells on the efficacy of MI-63 in MOLP-8 cells. The viability of MOLP-8 cells exposed to MI-63 either alone, or when propagated in co-culture with human-derived HS-5 stromal cells.

Figure S4 Proteomic studies of wild-type p53 myeloma cells exposed to MI-63. MM1.S and MOLP-8 cells were treated with MI-63 at its IC_{50} for 48 hours, and cell extracts were subjected to reverse phase protein array analysis. Changes are shown in selected proteins of interest. Error bars represent standard deviations of duplicate samples.

Figure S5 Suppression of MDM2 in U266 myeloma cells. U266 cell clones infected with one of two different shRNA constructs targeting MDM2 were isolated, and the reduction in MDM2 mRNA was evaluated by qPCR.

Figure S6 Proteomic studies of RPMI 8226 cells exposed to MI-63. RPMI 8226 cells were treated with MI-63 at its IC_{50} for 48 hours, and cell extracts were subjected to reverse phase protein array analysis. Changes are shown in selected proteins of interest. Error bars represent standard deviations of duplicate samples.

Figure S7 Knockdown of ATG5 and Beclin-1. A. Suppression of ATG5 in RPMI 8226 cells using a Lentiviral shRNA compared with a non-targeting control documented by Western blotting. **B.** Suppression of Beclin-1 in U266 cells using a Lentiviral shRNA compared with a non-targeting control documented by Western blotting.

Figure S8 MI-63 augments the activity of other approved anti-myeloma agents. A. MI-63 was combined with bortezomib in wild-type p53 MM1.S (left panel) and MOLP-8 (right panel) cells. Multiple doses of each drug were used with one representative condition shown (*$p<0.005$). **B.** MI-63 was combined with lenalidomide in wild-type p53 MM1.S (left panel) and MOLP-8 (right panel) cells. Multiple doses of each drug were used with one representative condition shown (*$p<0.005$). **C.** Cell viability was evaluated in lenalidomide-resistant MM1.S cells exposed to MI-63 for 48 hours, and compared to the efficacy of lenalidomide itself.

Acknowledgments

The authors would like to thank the MD Anderson Flow Cytometry and Cellular Imaging Core Facility, the RPPA Core Facility, and the Characterized Cell Line Core Facility.

Author Contributions

Conceived and designed the experiments: DG RZO. Performed the experiments: DG SW IK JH. Analyzed the data: DG RZO. Contributed reagents/materials/analysis tools: HW YD RJJ CCB JY SG. Wrote the paper: DG RZO.

References

1. Mahindra A, Hideshima T, Anderson KC (2010) Multiple myeloma: biology of the disease. Blood Rev 24 Suppl 1: S5–11.
2. Rajkumar SV (2011) Treatment of multiple myeloma. Nat Rev Clin Oncol 8: 479–491.
3. Siegel R, Naishadham D, Jemal A (2013) Cancer statistics, 2013. CA Cancer J Clin 63: 11–30.
4. Kumar SK, Rajkumar SV, Dispenzieri A, Lacy MQ, Hayman SR, et al. (2008) Improved survival in multiple myeloma and the impact of novel therapies. Blood 111: 2516–2520.
5. Brenner H, Gondos A, Pulte D (2009) Expected long-term survival of patients diagnosed with multiple myeloma in 2006–2010. Haematologica 94: 270–275.
6. Barlogie B, Attal M, Crowley J, van Rhee F, Szymonifka J, et al. (2010) Long-term follow-up of autotransplantation trials for multiple myeloma: update of protocols conducted by the intergroupe francophone du myelome, southwest oncology group, and university of arkansas for medical sciences. J Clin Oncol 28: 1209–1214.
7. Usmani SZ, Crowley J, Hoering A, Mitchell A, Waheed S, et al. (2013) Improvement in long-term outcomes with successive Total Therapy trials for multiple myeloma: are patients now being cured? Leukemia 27: 226–232.
8. Anderson KC (2012) The 39th David A. Karnofsky Lecture: bench-to-bedside translation of targeted therapies in multiple myeloma. J Clin Oncol 30: 445–452.
9. Kumar SK, Dispenzieri A, Lacy MQ, Gertz MA, Buadi FK, et al. (2013) Continued improvement in survival in multiple myeloma: changes in early mortality and outcomes in older patients. Leukemia.
10. Moreau P, Richardson PG, Cavo M, Orlowski RZ, San Miguel JF, et al. (2012) Proteasome inhibitors in multiple myeloma: 10 years later. Blood 120: 947–959.

11. Shah JJ, Orlowski RZ (2009) Proteasome inhibitors in the treatment of multiple myeloma. Leukemia 23: 1964–1979.
12. Orlowski RZ, Kuhn DJ (2008) Proteasome inhibitors in cancer therapy: lessons from the first decade. Clin Cancer Res 14: 1649–1657.
13. Hideshima T, Mitsiades C, Akiyama M, Hayashi T, Chauhan D, et al. (2003) Molecular mechanisms mediating antimyeloma activity of proteasome inhibitor PS-341. Blood 101: 1530–1534.
14. Hideshima T, Richardson P, Chauhan D, Palombella VJ, Elliott PJ, et al. (2001) The proteasome inhibitor PS-341 inhibits growth, induces apoptosis, and overcomes drug resistance in human multiple myeloma cells. Cancer Res 61: 3071–3076.
15. Pei XY, Dai Y, Grant S (2003) The proteasome inhibitor bortezomib promotes mitochondrial injury and apoptosis induced by the small molecule Bcl-2 inhibitor HA14-1 in multiple myeloma cells. Leukemia 17: 2036–2045.
16. Perez-Galan P, Roue G, Villamor N, Montserrat E, Campo E, et al. (2006) The proteasome inhibitor bortezomib induces apoptosis in mantle-cell lymphoma through generation of ROS and Noxa activation independent of p53 status. Blood 107: 257–264.
17. Ding WX, Ni HM, Chen X, Yu J, Zhang L, et al. (2007) A coordinated action of Bax, PUMA, and p53 promotes MG132-induced mitochondria activation and apoptosis in colon cancer cells. Mol Cancer Ther 6: 1062–1069.
18. Zhu YX, Braggio E, Shi CX, Bruins LA, Schmidt JE, et al. (2012) Cereblon expression is required for the antimyeloma activity of lenalidomide and pomalidomide. Blood 118: 4771–4779.
19. Lopez-Girona A, Mendy D, Ito T, Miller K, Gandhi AK, et al. (2012) Cereblon is a direct protein target for immunomodulatory and antiproliferative activities of lenalidomide and pomalidomide. Leukemia 26: 2326–2335.
20. Lu G, Middleton RE, Sun H, Naniong M, Ott CJ, et al. (2013) The Myeloma Drug Lenalidomide Promotes the Cereblon-Dependent Destruction of Ikaros Proteins. Science.
21. Gandhi AK, Kang J, Havens CG, Conklin T, Ning Y, et al. (2013) Immunomodulatory agents lenalidomide and pomalidomide co-stimulate T cells by inducing degradation of T cell repressors Ikaros and Aiolos via modulation of the E3 ubiquitin ligase complex CRL4. Br J Haematol.
22. Fahraeus R, Olivares-Illana V (2013) MDM2's social network. Oncogene.
23. Quesnel B, Preudhomme C, Oscier D, Lepelley P, Collyn-d'Hooghe M, et al. (1994) Over-expression of the MDM2 gene is found in some cases of haematological malignancies. Br J Haematol 88: 415–418.
24. Elnenaei MO, Gruszka-Westwood AM, A'Hernt R, Matutes E, Sirohi B, et al. (2003) Gene abnormalities in multiple myeloma; the relevance of TP53, MDM2, and CDKN2A. Haematologica 88: 529–537.
25. Pichiorri F, Suh SS, Rocci A, De Luca L, Taccioli C, et al. (2010) Downregulation of p53-inducible microRNAs 192, 194, and 215 impairs the p53/MDM2 autoregulatory loop in multiple myeloma development. Cancer Cell 18: 367–381.
26. Teoh G, Urashima M, Ogata A, Chauhan D, DeCaprio JA, et al. (1997) MDM2 protein overexpression promotes proliferation and survival of multiple myeloma cells. Blood 90: 1982–1992.
27. Escoubet-Lozach L, Lin IL, Jensen-Pergakes K, Brady HA, Gandhi AK, et al. (2009) Pomalidomide and lenalidomide induce p21 WAF-1 expression in both lymphoma and multiple myeloma through a LSD1-mediated epigenetic mechanism. Cancer Res 69: 7347–7356.
28. Vassilev LT, Vu BT, Graves B, Carvajal D, Podlaski F, et al. (2004) In vivo activation of the p53 pathway by small-molecule antagonists of MDM2. Science 303: 844–848.
29. Coutts AS, Boulahbel H, Graham A, La Thangue NB (2007) Mdm2 targets the p53 transcription cofactor JMY for degradation. EMBO Rep 8: 84–90.
30. Stuhmer T, Chatterjee M, Hildebrandt M, Herrmann P, Gollasch H, et al. (2005) Nongenotoxic activation of the p53 pathway as a therapeutic strategy for multiple myeloma. Blood 106: 3609–3617.
31. Ooi MG, Hayden PJ, Kotoula V, McMillin DW, Charalambous E, et al. (2009) Interactions of the Hdm2/p53 and proteasome pathways may enhance the antitumor activity of bortezomib. Clin Cancer Res 15: 7153–7160.
32. Saha MN, Jiang H, Jayakar J, Reece D, Branch DR, et al. (2010) MDM2 antagonist nutlin plus proteasome inhibitor velcade combination displays a synergistic anti-myeloma activity. Cancer Biol Ther 9: 936–944.
33. Zak K, Pecak A, Rys B, Wladyka B, Domling A, et al. (2013) Mdm2 and MdmX inhibitors for the treatment of cancer: a patent review (2011-present). Expert Opin Ther Pat 23: 425–448.
34. Ding K, Lu Y, Nikolovska-Coleska Z, Wang G, Qiu S, et al. (2006) Structure-based design of spiro-oxindoles as potent, specific small-molecule inhibitors of the MDM2-p53 interaction. J Med Chem 49: 3432–3435.
35. Shangary S, Qin D, McEachern D, Liu M, Miller RS, et al. (2008) Temporal activation of p53 by a specific MDM2 inhibitor is selectively toxic to tumors and leads to complete tumor growth inhibition. Proc Natl Acad Sci U S A 105: 3933–3938.
36. Jones RJ, Baladandayuthapani V, Neelapu S, Fayad LE, Romaguera JE, et al. (2011) HDM-2 inhibition suppresses expression of ribonucleotide reductase subunit M2, and synergistically enhances gemcitabine-induced cytotoxicity in mantle cell lymphoma. Blood 118: 4140–4149.
37. Kuhn DJ, Berkova Z, Jones RJ, Woessner R, Bjorklund CC, et al. (2012) Targeting the insulin-like growth factor-1 receptor to overcome bortezomib resistance in preclinical models of multiple myeloma. Blood 120: 3260–3270.
38. Yang L, Wang H, Kornblau SM, Graber DA, Zhang N, et al. (2011) Evidence of a role for the novel zinc-finger transcription factor ZKSCAN3 in modulating Cyclin D2 expression in multiple myeloma. Oncogene 30: 1329–1340.
39. Jones RJ, Gu D, Bjorklund CC, Kuiatse I, Remaley AT, et al. (2013) The novel anticancer agent JNJ-26854165 induces cell death through inhibition of cholesterol transport and degradation of ABCA1. J Pharmacol Exp Ther 346: 381–392.
40. Bjorklund CC, Ma W, Wang ZQ, Davis RE, Kuhn DJ, et al. (2011) Evidence of a role for activation of Wnt/beta-catenin signaling in the resistance of plasma cells to lenalidomide. J Biol Chem 286: 11009–11020.
41. Bjorklund CC, Baladandayuthapani V, Lin HY, Jones RJ, Kuiatse I, et al. (2013) Evidence of a role for CD44 and cell adhesion in mediating resistance to lenalidomide in multiple myeloma: therapeutic implications. Leukemia.
42. Tanimura S, Ohtsuka S, Mitsui K, Shirouzu K, Yoshimura A, et al. (1999) MDM2 interacts with MDMX through their RING finger domains. FEBS Lett 447: 5–9.
43. Hodge DR, Peng B, Cherry JC, Hurt EM, Fox SD, et al. (2005) Interleukin 6 supports the maintenance of p53 tumor suppressor gene promoter methylation. Cancer Res 65: 4673–4682.
44. Walker BA, Leone PE, Chiecchio L, Dickens NJ, Jenner MW, et al. (2010) A compendium of myeloma-associated chromosomal copy number abnormalities and their prognostic value. Blood 116: e56–65.
45. Avet-Loiseau H, Attal M, Moreau P, Charbonnel C, Garban F, et al. (2007) Genetic abnormalities and survival in multiple myeloma: the experience of the Intergroupe Francophone du Myelome. Blood 109: 3489–3495.
46. Chang H, Trieu Y, Qi X, Jiang NN, Xu W, et al. (2011) Impact of cytogenetics in patients with relapsed or refractory multiple myeloma treated with bortezomib: Adverse effect of 1q21 gains. Leuk Res 35: 95–98.
47. Wu YT, Tan HL, Shui G, Bauvy C, Huang Q, et al. (2010) Dual role of 3-methyladenine in modulation of autophagy via different temporal patterns of inhibition on class I and III phosphoinositide 3-kinase. J Biol Chem 285: 10850–10861.
48. Davids MS, Letai A (2012) Targeting the B-cell lymphoma/leukemia 2 family in cancer. J Clin Oncol 30: 3127–3135.
49. Lin J, Chen J, Elenbaas B, Levine AJ (1994) Several hydrophobic amino acids in the p53 amino-terminal domain are required for transcriptional activation, binding to mdm-2 and the adenovirus 5 E1B 55-kD protein. Genes Dev 8: 1235–1246.
50. Picksley SM, Vojtesek B, Sparks A, Lane DP (1994) Immunochemical analysis of the interaction of p53 with MDM2;–fine mapping of the MDM2 binding site on p53 using synthetic peptides. Oncogene 9: 2523–2529.
51. Jones RJ, Bjorklund CC, Baladandayuthapani V, Kuhn DJ, Orlowski RZ (2012) Drug resistance to inhibitors of the human double minute-2 E3 ligase is mediated by point mutations of p53, but can be overcome with the p53 targeting agent RITA. Mol Cancer Ther 11: 2243–2253.
52. White E (2012) Deconvoluting the context-dependent role for autophagy in cancer. Nat Rev Cancer 12: 401–410.
53. Choi AM, Ryter SW, Levine B (2013) Autophagy in human health and disease. N Engl J Med 368: 651–662.
54. Crighton D, Wilkinson S, O'Prey J, Syed N, Smith P, et al. (2006) DRAM, a p53-induced modulator of autophagy, is critical for apoptosis. Cell 126: 121–134.
55. Crighton D, Wilkinson S, Ryan KM (2007) DRAM links autophagy to p53 and programmed cell death. Autophagy 3: 72–74.
56. Tasdemir E, Maiuri MC, Galluzzi L, Vitale I, Djavaheri-Mergny M, et al. (2008) Regulation of autophagy by cytoplasmic p53. Nat Cell Biol 10: 676–687.
57. Thakurta A, Gandhi AK, Waldman MF, Bjorklund C, Ning Y, et al. (2013) Absence of mutations in cereblon (CRBN) and DNA damage-binding protein 1 (DDB1) genes and significance for IMiD therapy. Leukemia.
58. Ray-Coquard I, Blay JY, Italiano A, Le Cesne A, Penel N, et al. (2012) Effect of the MDM2 antagonist RG7112 on the P53 pathway in patients with MDM2-amplified, well-differentiated or dedifferentiated liposarcoma: an exploratory proof-of-mechanism study. Lancet Oncol 13: 1133–1140.
59. Ha JH, Won EY, Shin JS, Jang M, Ryu KS, et al. (2011) Molecular mimicry-based repositioning of nutlin-3 to anti-apoptotic Bcl-2 family proteins. J Am Chem Soc 133: 1244–1247.
60. Shin JS, Ha JH, He F, Muto Y, Ryu KS, et al. (2012) Structural insights into the dual-targeting mechanism of Nutlin-3. Biochem Biophys Res Commun 420: 48–53.
61. Surget S, Chiron D, Gomez-Bougie P, Descamps G, Menoret E, et al. (2012) Cell death via DR5, but not DR4, is regulated by p53 in myeloma cells. Cancer Res 72: 4562–4573.
62. Ortega MM, Melo MB, De Souza CA, Lorand-Metze I, Costa FF, et al. (2003) A possible role of the P53 gene deletion as a prognostic factor in multiple myeloma. Ann Hematol 82: 405–409.
63. Xiong W, Wu X, Starnes S, Johnson SK, Haessler J, et al. (2008) An analysis of the clinical and biologic significance of TP53 loss and the identification of potential novel transcriptional targets of TP53 in multiple myeloma. Blood 112: 4235–4246.
64. Drach J, Ackermann J, Fritz E, Kromer E, Schuster R, et al. (1998) Presence of a p53 gene deletion in patients with multiple myeloma predicts for short survival after conventional-dose chemotherapy. Blood 92: 802–809.

6

Risk of Multiple Myeloma in Rheumatoid Arthritis

Kaini Shen[1]ⓢ, Gufeng Xu[2]ⓢ, Qing Wu[3], Daobin Zhou[1], Jian Li[1]*

1 Department of Hematology, Peking Union Medical College Hospital, Chinese Academy of Medical Sciences and Peking Union Medical College, Beijing, People's Republic of China, **2** Zhejiang University, School of Medicine, Hangzhou, Zhejiang, People's Republic of China, **3** Division of Health Sciences Research, Mayo Clinic, Scottsdale, Arizona, United States of America

Abstract

Objectives: multiple myeloma is a malignant neoplasm of plasma cells mainly affecting elderly patients. Despite the wealth of information available on therapeutic strategies, the etiology and pathogenesis of myeloma remain unclear. In the current study, a meta-analysis was conducted to assess the possible association between rheumatoid arthritis and myeloma.

Methods: a literature search was conducted with PubMed, EMBASE and Web of Science for relevant studies. Additionally, we searched annual meeting abstracts of the American Society of Hematology from 2004 to 2013. Only original studies that investigated the association between rheumatoid arthritis and myeloma were included. In total, 8 case-control and 10 cohort studies were identified for analysis.

Results: the meta-estimate of the association between rheumatoid arthritis and myeloma was 1.14 (95% CI, 0.97–1.33) overall, with significant heterogeneity among studies. The relationship between myeloma and other autoimmune diseases was additionally examined from available data. Our results showed that myeloma risk is increased 1.31 to 1.65-fold in pernicious anemia and 1.36 to 2.30-fold in ankylosing spondylitis patients.

Conclusion: Rheumatoid arthritis does not appear to alter the risk of myeloma, while between-study heterogeneity analyses suggest caution in the interpretation of results. Pernicious anemia and ankylosing spondylitis may be potential risk factors for myeloma development. Future large-scale epidemiological studies with reliable exposure biomarkers are necessary to establish the possible contribution of autoimmune disorders to multiple myeloma.

Editor: Riccardo Dolcetti, IRCCS National Cancer Institute, Italy

Funding: This work was supported by National Public Health Grand Research Foundation (No. 201202017). The funders had no role in study design, data collection and analysis, decision to publish, or preparation of the manuscript.

Competing Interests: The authors have declared that no competing interests exist.

* E-mail: lijian@pumch.cn

ⓢ These authors contributed equally to this work.

Introduction

Multiple myeloma (MM) is one of the most common hematologic malignancies with poor prognosis, characterized by neoplastic proliferation of monoclonal plasma cells. The incidence of MM in developed countries is about 5–7 cases per 100 000 individuals [1]. Despite extensive research efforts over the last two decades, the risk factors of MM remain to be established. Numerous case-control and cohort studies to date have suggested that several environmental factors may be associated with the risk of MM, such as ionizing radiation [2], benzene [3] and agricultural occupation [4]. The relationship between autoimmune disease and hematopoietic malignancies was initially postulated in 1964 [5]. However, the issue of whether autoimmune diseases increase the incidence of MM remains controversial.

On the basis of animal models of MM, it is suggested that repeated antigenic stimulation of the immune system plays an important role in MM development [6,7]. A number of studies have confirmed an association of lymphoma with autoimmune conditions [8–12], including rheumatoid arthritis (RA), systemic lupus erythematosus (SLE), and autoimmune hemolytic anemia, although the underlying pathogenesis is unclear. Similarly, the relationship between MM and autoimmune disease has been a long-term subject of investigation, but inconsistent results have been obtained to date.

The main aim of this meta-analysis was to estimate the comparative risk of developing MM in RA patients versus the general population. Two additional goals were (1) to explore the variation in the association of RA and MM among subgroups of interest and (2) to investigate if there is an association between MM and other autoimmune diseases.

Methods

Search Strategy

A literature search was conducted with PubMed (from January 1, 1951), EMBASE (from January 1, 1955) and Web of Science (from January 1, 1970) using the following search terms: rheumatoid arthritis, autoimmune disease, etiology, epidemiology,

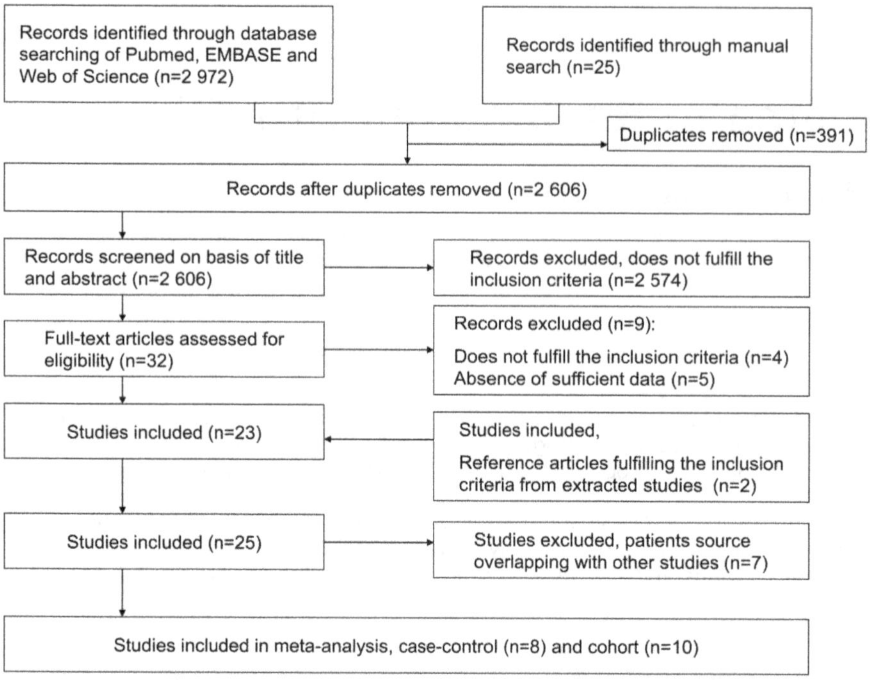

Figure 1. Flow diagram depicting the identification and selection of eligible case-control and cohort studies.

risk factors, multiple myeloma, cancer, malignancy. The final search strategy in PubMed was attached as appendix. The last literature search was performed on December 25, 2013. We also searched annual meeting abstracts of the American Society of Hematology from 2004 to 2013 to identify eligible unpublished data. All references cited in the retrieved articles were additionally reviewed to indentify additional eligible studies. Inclusion criteria were as follows: human participants without limitation of sex or geographic location, case-control or cohort studies, prior medical history of RA as exposure, MM as outcome, studies that reported relative risk (RR), standardized incidence ratio (SIR) or odds ratio (OR) of MM patients with prior history of RA, publication in English. In addition, the selection of cohort studies for inclusion was made regardless of specific RA management strategies. When duplicate reports for the same population and data source were eligible, we chose the original reports with the largest sample size. Case series, case reports, in vitro and animal studies were excluded. Eligibility assessment was performed independently by two reviewers, and disagreements resolved by consensus.

Data Extraction

Two authors performed data extraction independently, and any discrepancies were addressed by discussion and re-evaluation. We obtained information on the author, year of publication, country of origin, source of case, control and cohort, controlled factors, diagnosis criteria and treatment regimen for RA. Cohort size, number of cases, cohort duration, SIR and 95% confidence intervals (CIs) or sufficient data to allow calculation of these numbers were additionally necessary for cohort studies. For case-control studies, the exact numbers of cases and controls by RA, OR and 95% CIs were required. For the purpose of ascertaining the relationship between MM and other autoimmune diseases, related data were recorded, where available, according to the above extraction principles.

The Newcastle-Ottawa Scale (NOS), developed for evaluating the quality of nonrandomized studies [13], was used by two independent reviewers to assess the methodological quality of each study, and the scores subsequently used in subgroup analysis. A score of ≤5 was considered as relative low quality [14].

Statistical Analyses

In case-control studies, OR and 95% CIs for MM risk factors were directly extracted from original research papers or calculated when not provided. The primary outcome for cohort studies was SIR and corresponding 95% CI. In cases where SIRs were not specifically reported, calculations were made from the number of observed MM divided by the number of expected cases in the general population provided by authors, and 95% CI determined using the standard error of the natural logarithm of SIR, estimated from the inverse of the square root of the observed number of cases. The measure of interest was RR, estimated from ORs in case-control studies and SIRs in cohort studies. Since the incidence of MM is low, SIR and OR produce similar estimate of RR, thus we present all results as RR for simplicity [15–17]. Between-study heterogeneity was examined using a chi-square test of heterogeneity and I^2 measure of inconsistency. P-values less than 0.1 or the I^2 statistic greater than 50% were considered statistically significant [18]. Under these conditions, data were pooled based on the method of Dersimonian and Laird under a random effects model otherwise under fixed effects model. Two-tailed $p \leq 0.05$ was considered statistically significant for all analyses.

To evaluate publication bias, we constructed a funnel plot and applied Begg's test. Trim and Fill analysis was used to estimate the number of missing studies and their potential effects on outcomes. Sensitivity analyses were additionally conducted to ascertain the robustness of our findings. The influence of RA was examined by excluding studies restricted to elderly patients (≥65 years) or

Table 1. Characteristics of case-control studies enrolled in the meta-analysis.

Author	Year	Country	Sex	Controls	Cases		Controls		OR (95% CI)	Controlled Factors
					RA	Non-RA	RA	Non-RA		
Pearce NE	1986	New Zealand	M	Population	4	72	7	308	2.30 (0.60–8.00)	Age, registration year
Cohen HJ	1987	USA	M+F	Hospital	62	91	203	210	0.70 (0.48–1.03)	Age, gender, race, disease status
Boffetta P	1989	USA	M+F	Population	39	89	164	348	0.90 (0.60–1.50)	Age, gender, race, residence
Lewis DR	1994	USA	M+F	Population	64	509	241	1 890	0.80 (0.60–1.10)	Age, gender, race
Vlajinac HD	2003	Yugoslavia	M+F	Hospital	12	85	5	95	2.60 (0.90–7.60)	Age, gender, residence
Landgren O	2006	USA	F	Population	7	172	9	682	2.30 (0.80–6.50)	none
Anderson LA	2009	USA	M+F	Population	263	9 211	3 289	119 242	1.00 (0.90–1.10)	Gender, year of diagnosis, age at diagnosis
Lindqvist EK	2011	Sweden	M+F	Population	111	19 001	567	74 841	0.80 (0.60–0.90)	Age, gender, residence

Abbreviations: RA, rheumatoid arthritis; OR, odds ratio; CI, confidence intervals; M, male; F, female.

Table 2. Characteristics of cohort studies enrolled in the meta-analysis.

Author	Year	Country	Sex	Cohort Size	Number of MM	SIR (95% CI)	Follow-up Duration (PY)
Isomaki HA	1982	Finland	M+F	46 101	28	2.20 (1.52–3.19)	213 911
Mellemkjaer L	1996	Denmark	M+F	20 699	21	1.10 (0.70–1.70)	144 421
Kauppi M	1997	Finland	M+F	9 469	8	1.20 (0.50–2.30)	65 391
Thomas E	2000	England	M+F	26 623	38	1.66 (1.21–2.28)	151 987
Setoguchi S	2006	USA	M+F	7 830	19	2.00 (1.26–3.12)	33 410
Herrinton LJ	2008	USA	M+F	2 982	2	2.36 (0.28–8.50)	7 791
Brown LM	2008	USA	M	–	94	1.17 (0.94–1.45)	27 years
Parikh-Patel A	2009	USA	M+F	84 475	64	0.90 (0.70–1.15)	405 540
Hemminki K	2012	Sweden	M+F	72 309	81	0.88 (0.70–1.09)	731 954
Dreyer L	2013	Denmark	M+F	7 159	4	1.76 (0.66–4.69)	24 811

Abbreviations: M, male; F, female; MM, multiple myeloma; SIR, standardized incidence ratio; CI, confidence intervals; PY, person years.
–: Not mentioned.

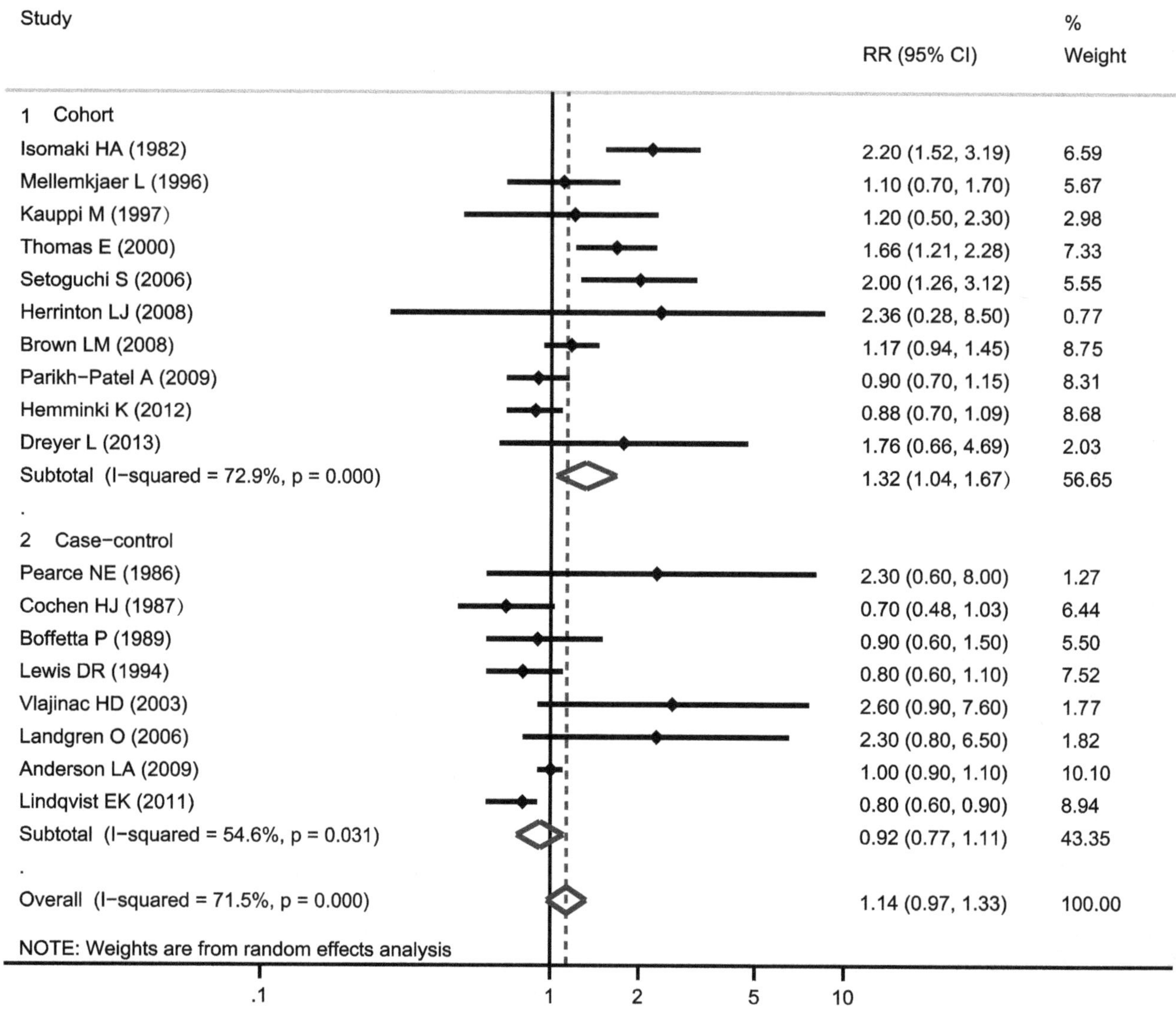

Figure 2. Forest plot of studies on multiple myeloma development risk in rheumatoid arthritis.

single-sex participants and those that failed to control important confounders. All meta-analyses were conducted with Stata 12.0.

Results

Abstract evaluation yielded thirty-two potential studies for analysis (Figure 1), of which five [19–23] were excluded, since they

Table 3. Sensitivity analysis of the association between multiple myeloma and rheumatoid arthritis according to different exclusion criteria.

Studies included	Studies (N)	RR (95% CI)	p value	I^2 (%)
All studies	18	1.14 (0.97–1.33)	<0.001	71.5
Studies without age restriction of participants[a]	17	1.09 (0.94–1.27)	<0.001	68.7
Studies with both male and female participants[b]	15	1.11 (0.94–1.32)	<0.001	74.1
Studies that controlled for important confounding factors[c]	16	1.11 (0.95–1.30)	<0.001	73.1

[a]Excludes the study by the group of Setoguchi [41].
[b]Excludes studies by the groups of Pearce [25], Landgren [36] and Brown [45].
[c]Excludes studies by the groups of Pearce [25] and Landgren [36].
Abbreviations: N, number; RR, relative risk; NS, not significant; CI, confidence interval.

Table 4. Meta-analysis of multiple myeloma incidence by subgroup.

	Subgroup	Analyses (N)	RR (95% CI)	p-value	I^2 (%)
Overall	Study design	Cohort (10)	1.32 (1.04–1.67)	<0.001	72.9
		Case-control (8)	0.92 (0.77–1.11)	0.031	54.6
	Publication year	Before 2000 (7)	1.10 (0.77–1.59)	<0.001	75.7
		After 2000 (11)	1.15 (0.96–1.37)	<0.001	71.3
	Study quality	NOS≤5 (13)	1.29 (1.02–1.64)	<0.001	72.7
		NOS>5 (5)	0.95 (0.79–1.14)	0.024	64.3
	Region[a]	USA (9)	1.02 (0.86–1.22)	0.008	61.4
		Europe (8)	1.30 (0.93–1.79)	<0.001	80.9
Cohort	Publication year	Before 2000 (3)	1.48 (0.90–2.45)	0.047	67.3
		After 2000 (7)	1.25 (0.96–1.61)	0.002	72.0
	Study quality	NOS≤5 (9)	1.36 (1.02–1.81)	<0.001	75.9
		NOS>5 (1)	1.17 (0.94–1.45)	–	–
	Region	USA (4)	1.25 (0.89–1.77)	0.017	70.4
		Europe (6)	1.37 (0.95–1.97)	<0.001	77.7
	Mean follow-up[b]	<5 years (5)	1.63 (0.97–2.74)	<0.001	80.4
		≥5 years (4)	1.17 (0.82–1.66)	0.015	71.2
Case-control	Publication year	Before 2000 (4)	0.81 (0.65–1.02)	0.352	8.1
		After 2000 (4)	1.02 (0.77–1.36)	0.021	69.1
	Study quality	NOS≤5 (4)	1.14 (0.71–1.83)	0.060	59.5
		NOS>5 (4)	0.88 (0.71–1.10)	0.046	62.5
	Region[a]	USA (5)	0.91 (0.74–1.11)	0.116	45.9
		Europe (2)	1.28 (0.41–3.96)	0.033	77.9
	Control type	Population (6)	0.92 (0.78–1.10)	0.088	47.8
		Hospital (2)	1.22 (0.34–4.36)	0.023	80.6

Abbreviations: N, number; M, male; F, female; RR, relative risk; NOS, Newcastle-Ottawa Scale.
[a]One case-control study conducted in New Zealand was excluded from analysis.
[b]One study with unknown mean follow-up duration was excluded from analysis.
–: Cannot be calculated.

failed to provide sufficient data for calculation. Twenty-three case-control and cohort studies were included after full text assessment. Another two publications [24,25] were incorporated after examining references from the extracted articles. Among the 25 studies, seven [12,26–31] were subsequently excluded for overlap in case or cohort resources. Consequently, our meta-analysis consisted of eight [24,25,32–37] case-control and ten [10,38–46] cohort studies.

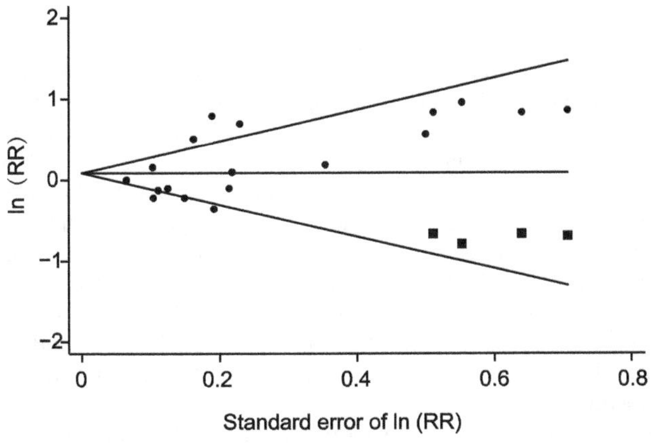

Figure 3. Funnel plot for case-control and cohort studies (dots: original data; squares: filled data).

All the studies published from 1982 to 2013 were performed in USA or Europe, except one case- control study from New Zealand [25]. There was slight overlap in the patient populations of two studies [38,40] from Finland. Landgren et al. [36] limited the study subjects to women, while the groups of Pearce [25] and Brown [45] mainly focused on the role of prior autoimmune disorders in male MM. The NOS scores varied from 5 to 7 in all case-control studies, with the exception of the reported score of 3 by Landgren and co-workers [36] as a result of unsatisfactory comparability. Since almost all the cohort studies used the expected cancer incidence calculated from national cancer rates as a comparison instead of the non-exposed cohort, NOS scores were relatively low, ranging from 4 to 5.

In the eight case-control studies, OR was all obtained from the published articles or calculated from the numbers of cases and controls by RA. In four cohort studies [10,38,43,44], the SIRs and 95% CIs were estimated from the number of observed MM and expected MM incidence provided by authors, while others were directly extracted from the original article. Only three studies [41,42,44] reported the type of treatment for RA before MM diagnosis. All important information is presented in Tables 1 and 2.

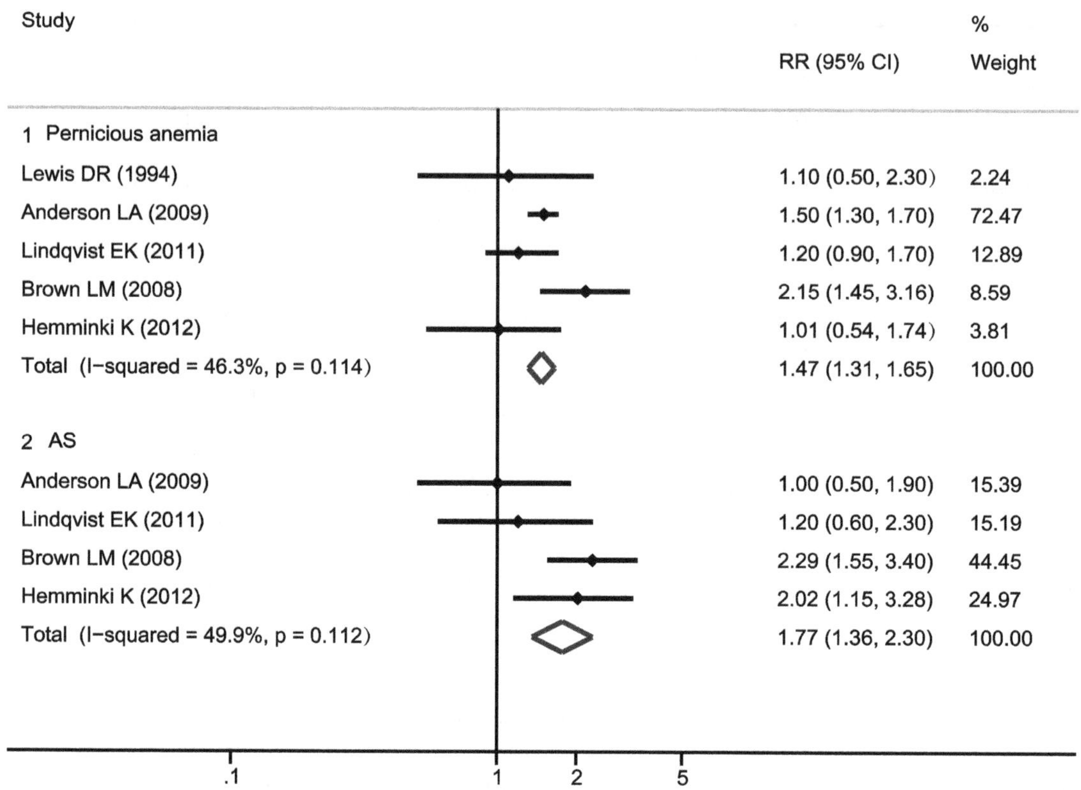

Figure 4. Forest plot of studies on multiple myeloma development risk in pernicious anemia and AS.

The RRs of MM for RA versus non-RA patients overall and by study design was presented (Figure 2). The random-effects pooled RRs for MM were 1.32 (95% CI, 1.04–1.67) for cohort studies and 0.92 (95% CI, 0.77–1.11) for case-control studies. Compared with non-RA patients, RA patients showed an RR of 1.14 (95% CI, 0.97–1.33) regardless of study type, possibly suggesting lack of association between RA and MM. However, overall analysis revealed significant between-study heterogeneity ($p<0.1$; $I^2=71.5\%$).

Sensitivity analysis was presented in Table 3. After excluding studies restricted to elderly patients (≥65 years) or single-sex participants and those that failed to adjust important factors, overall RR decreased slightly to 1.09, 1.11 and 1.11, respectively.

To investigate the source of heterogeneity, subset analysis by study design, publication year, study quality, geographic region, control type and average follow-up duration was conducted. Statistical association between RA and MM was only found to be significant in studies with relatively low quality (RR = 1.29, 95% CI, 1.02–1.64) and cohort studies with relatively low quality (RR = 1.36, 95% CI, 1.02–1.81). Overall, in studies with relatively higher quality according to NOS, as well as those published after 2000, RA was not associated with increase in MM risk (RR = 0.95, 95% CI, 0.79–1.14 and RR = 1.15, 95% CI 0.96–1.37, respectively). Notably, subgroup analyses failed to define the reason for heterogeneity (Table 4).

Publication bias in this meta-analysis was suspected as indicated from the funnel plot and Begg's test (p = 0.081). However, RR values remained similar after Trim and Fill correction for possible missing data (RR = 1.14, 95% CI 0.97–1.33 before Trim and Fill versus RR = 1.09, 95% CI 0.93–1.27 after Trim and Fill) (Figure 3).

The reported relevance of other autoimmune diseases, including pernicious anemia and ankylosing spondylitis (AS), in MM incidence is presented (Figure 4). Patients with pernicious anemia and AS displayed a 1.31- to 1.65-fold and 1.36- to 2.30-fold increase in MM risk, respectively. In contrast, MM development appeared to be unrelated to prior medical history of psoriasis (RR = 0.91, 95% CI, 0.78–1.05), SLE (RR = 1.18, 95% CI, 0.88–1.60), Sjögren syndrome (SS) (RR = 1.22, 95% CI 0.83–1.78) or polymyositis/dermatomyositis (RR = 1.37, 95% CI 0.86–2.17). The between-study heterogeneity analyses were all not statistically significant.

Discussion

Our meta-analysis results suggest that MM seems not more common in patients with a past history of RA, consistent with our sensitivity data. However, subgroup analysis revealed that RA patients are more likely to suffer from subsequent MM in cohort studies (RR = 1.32, 95% CI 1.04–1.67). Information on prior autoimmune diseases in case-control studies was mostly obtained from self-reports through interviews or questionnaires, while in cohort studies, investigators relied mainly on linkage records, which probably attributed to the differences between the two types of studies. Notably, subset analysis confirmed that statistical association between RA and MM was only significant in studies with NOS score≤5, further indicating that RA might not act as risk factor for MM.

A number of studies have explored whether repeated or chronic antigenic stimulation leads to hematopoietic malignancies. Some researchers [31] reported elevated risk for MM in patients with RA, while others [47,48] reached different conclusions. An antigenic stimulation hypothesis was proposed to explain the excessive risk of MM in patients with autoimmune diseases. Chronic immune stimulation resulting from autoimmune disorders, with its associated lymphocyte activation, tends to induce uncontrolled proliferation of malignant plasma cells, leading to MM [49]. Since no biologic marker has been developed that can effectively measure lifetime immune stimulation, this theory remains controversial. Meanwhile, evidence from previous studies indicates that increased risk could be a consequence of therapy, rather than the disease itself. For instance, higher risk of non-Hodgkin's lymphoma and MM has been reported following use of steroids [36,50], which are important for autoimmune disease treatment. Similarly, cytotoxic and immunosuppressive drugs may suppress immunodefense against malignant cells and lead to oncogenesis [51]. Moreover, there may be a common genetic or environmental susceptibility in autoimmune diseases and plasma cell tumors, or undiagnosed MM may manifest with clinical features that mimic connective tissue diseases. Taking our current results and the above studies into account, the credibility of the antigenic stimulation hypothesis is called into question.

Only one cohort study [39] investigated the effect of the duration of follow-up on the risk of MM and determined that the borderline excess of MM was confined to the early 4-year follow-up. Thomas [10] proposed that although increased risk of MM persisted for hematopoietic cancers throughout the follow-up period, the greatest excess was within the first 3 months after hospitalization. These findings could possibly indicate a common etiologic factor for RA and MM, or further prove the association confirmed in above two studies might be resulted from detection bias. With the current common application of anti-TNF drugs, concern has been raised about the risk of developing malignancy related with their use [52]. However, as implied from two studies mentioned earlier [41,44], there was no significant increase in the risk of MM among anti-TNF users. Considering the small number of reports available, further studies are warranted to account for this potential confounder when examining the relationship of autoimmune diseases and MM.

Meta-analysis results revealed that pernicious anemia is another risk factor for MM, consistent with several prior epidemiologic studies [53,54]. The related pathogenesis may involve immune alterations or chromosome abnormalities in the bone marrow of patients with pernicious anemia [54]. On the other hand, vitamin B12 deficiency caused by pernicious anemia may promote MM development by disrupting normal homeostasis for one-carbon metabolism [55]. The lack of association of MM with psoriasis, SLE, SS, and polymyositis/dermatomyositis raises the question of whether oncogenesis is dependent on the type of autoimmune disease. A number of studies evaluating the risk of MM in AS [45] and polymyalgia rheumatic [37] patients have reported positive associations, similar to our assessment of AS and MM. Assumptions such as whether an autoimmune disease resulting in MM is associated with disease activity, amount of autoantibody, and the extent of organ involvement should be examined. Although the current meta-analysis presents a more precise estimate of MM risk in RA patients than individual studies, significant heterogeneity remains a primary limitation of our study. Subgroup analyses failed to determine the source of heterogeneity. The diversity of subject sources and study methodologies may have led to inconsistencies. One such example is the study by Boffetta [33] including 282 patients that died from MM, meaning that they were likely to suffer from more severe diseases and past medical history obtained from their family members was possibly incomplete. Similarly, another study [41] was restricted to subjects older than 65 years whose disease spectrum may be distinct from that of the general population. The variable proportions of races in different studies may additionally contribute to significant heterogeneity. Moreover, misclassification of patients may have occurred in case-control studies, since no consistent diagnosis criteria were applied by investigators and most enrollments were dependent on reports and certificates, rather than specific laboratory data, similar to enrollment in cohort studies. As indicated in cohort studies, RA patients may develop MM after more than 20 years, in which case recall bias may exist in case-control studies.

Another limitation of this study is that certain articles had to be excluded, since no data on MM and RA were available, although their relationship was evaluated. Exclusion of such studies may have led to results bias. In spite of this, the possible bias might not be so evident, since why these data were not reported mostly lied in that authors found no specific association between RA and MM. Although publication bias was borderline significant as indicated by Begg's test, adjustment for possibly missing manuscripts yielded similar results, strongly supporting the robustness of our analyses.

Conclusion

Despite its limitations, our meta-analysis provides novel evidence for increased MM development risk in AS and pernicious anemia, although the underlying pathogenesis remains controversial. Notably, RA does not appear to alter the risk of MM, while between-study heterogeneity suggested caution in the interpretation of results. Further large-scale longitudinal studies containing details of risk factors and treatment information are necessary to determine the pathophysiological mechanism linking autoimmune diseases and MM. Moreover, identification of reliable exposure biomarkers of immune stimulation would be significantly beneficial.

Author Contributions

Conceived and designed the experiments: KNS GFX QW DBZ JL. Performed the experiments: KNS GFX QW JL. Analyzed the data: KNS GFX QW JL. Contributed reagents/materials/analysis tools: JL. Wrote the paper: KNS GFX QW.

References

1. Kyle RA, Therneau TM, Rajkumar SV, Larson DR, Plevak MF, et al. (2004) Incidence of multiple myeloma in Olmsted County, Minnesota - Trend over 6 decades. Cancer 101: 2667–2674.
2. Cuzick J (1981) Radiation-Induced Myelomatosis. New England Journal of Medicine 304: 204–210.
3. Infante PF (2006) Benzene exposure and multiple myeloma - A detailed meta-analysis of benzene cohort studies. Living In a Chemical World: Framing the Future In Light Of the Past 1076: 90–109.
4. Blair A, Zahm SH, Pearce NE, Heineman EF, Fraumeni JF (1992) Clues to Cancer Etiology from Studies of Farmers. Scandinavian Journal of Work Environment & Health 18: 209–215.

5. Lea AJ (1964) An association between the rheumatic diseases and the reticuloses. Ann Rheum Dis: 480–484.
6. Potter M (1986) Plasmacytomas in Mice. Seminars in Oncology 13: 275–281.
7. Radl J, Croese JW, Zurcher C, Van den Enden-Vieveen MH, de Leeuw AM (1988) Animal model of human disease. Multiple myeloma. Am J Pathol 132: 593–597.
8. Smedby KE, Vajdic CM, Falster M, Engels EA, Martinez-Maza O, et al. (2008) Autoimmune disorders and risk of non-Hodgkin lymphoma subtypes: a pooled analysis within the InterLymph consortium. Blood 111: 4029–4038.
9. Mellemkjaer L, Pfeiffer RM, Engels EA, Gridley G, Wheeler W, et al. (2008) Autoimmune disease in individuals and close family members and susceptibility to non-Hodgkin's lymphoma. Arthritis and Rheumatism 58: 657–666.
10. Thomas E, Brewster DH, Black RJ, Macfarlane GJ (2000) Risk of malignancy among patients with rheumatic conditions. International Journal of Cancer 88: 497–502.
11. Landgren O, Engels EA, Pfeiffer RM, Gridley G, Mellemkjaer L, et al. (2006) Autoimmunity and susceptibility to Hodgkin lymphoma: A population-based case-control study in Scandinavia. Journal of the National Cancer Institute 98: 1321–1330.
12. Gridley G, McLaughlin JK, Ekbom A, Klareskog L, Adami HO, et al. (1993) Incidence of Cancer among Patients with Rheumatoid-Arthritis. Journal of the National Cancer Institute 85: 307–311.
13. Wells G, Shea B, O'Connell D, Peterson J, Welch V, et al. (2011) The Newcastle-Ottawa Scale (NOS) for assessing the quality of nonrandomized studies in meta analyses. Ottawa, ON, Canada: Ottawa Hospital Research Institute. Available: http://www.ohri.ca/programs/clinical_epidemiology/oxford.asp. Accessed 28 December 2013.
14. Beranger R, Le Cornet C, Schuz J, Fervers B (2013) Occupational and Environmental Exposures Associated with Testicular Germ Cell Tumours: Systematic Review of Prenatal and Life-Long Exposures. Plos One 8.
15. Greenland S (1987) Quantitative Methods In the Review Of Epidemiologic Literature. Epidemiologic Reviews 9: 1–30.
16. Siristatidis C, Sergentanis TN, Kanavidis P, Trivella M, Sotiraki M, et al. (2013) Controlled ovarian hyperstimulation for IVF: impact on ovarian, endometrial and cervical cancer-a systematic review and meta-analysis. Human Reproduction Update 19: 105–123.
17. Larsson SC, Mantzoros CS, Wolk A (2007) Diabetes mellitus and risk of breast cancer: A meta-analysis. International Journal Of Cancer 121: 856–862.
18. Higgins JPT, Thompson SG, Deeks JJ, Altman DG (2003) Measuring inconsistency in meta-analyses. British Medical Journal 327: 557–560.
19. Doody MM, Linet MS, Glass AG, Friedman GD, Pottern LM, et al. (1992) Leukemia, lymphoma, and multiple myeloma following selected medical conditions. Cancer Causes Control 3: 449–456.
20. Bourguet CC, Logue EE (1993) Antigenic stimulation and multiple myeloma. A prospective study. Cancer 72: 2148–2154.
21. Prior P, Symmons DPM, Hawkins CF, Scott DL, Brown R (1984) Cancer Morbidity in Rheumatoid-Arthritis. Annals of the Rheumatic Diseases 43: 128–131.
22. Buchbinder R, Barber M, Heuzenroeder L, Wluka AE, Giles G, et al. (2008) Incidence of melanoma and other malignancies among rheumatoid arthritis patients treated with methotrexate. Arthritis & Rheumatism-Arthritis Care & Research 59: 794–799.
23. Chen YJ, Chang YT, Wang CB, Wu CY (2011) The Risk of Cancer in Patients With Rheumatoid Arthritis A Nationwide Cohort Study in Taiwan. Arthritis and Rheumatism 63: 352–358.
24. Anderson LA, Gadalla S, Morton LM, Landgren O, Pfeiffer R, et al. (2009) Population-based study of autoimmune conditions and the risk of specific lymphoid malignancies. International Journal of Cancer 125: 398–405.
25. Pearce NE, Smith AH, Howard JK, Sheppard RA, Giles HJ, et al. (1986) Case-Control Study of Multiple-Myeloma and Farming. British Journal of Cancer 54: 493–500.
26. Eriksson M (1993) Rheumatoid arthritis as a risk factor for multiple myeloma: a case-control study. Eur J Cancer 29A: 259–263.
27. Landgren O, Linet MS, McMaster ML, Gridley G, Hemminki K, et al. (2006) Familial characteristics of autoimmune and hematologic disorders in 8,406 multiple myeloma patients: A population-based case-control study. International Journal of Cancer 118: 3095–3098.
28. Askling J, Fored CM, Baecklund E, Brandt L, Backlin C, et al. (2005) Haematopoietic malignancies in rheumatoid arthritis: lymphoma risk and characteristics after exposure to tumour necrosis factor antagonists. Annals of the Rheumatic Diseases 64: 1414–1420.
29. Hemminki K, Li X, Sundquist K, Sundquist J (2008) Cancer risk in hospitalized rheumatoid arthritis patients. Rheumatology 47: 698–701.
30. Isomaki HA, Hakulinen T, Joutsenlahti U (1978) Excess risk of lymphomas, leukemia and myeloma in patients with rheumatoid arthritis. J Chronic Dis 31: 691–696.
31. Hakulinen T, Isomaki H, Knekt P (1985) Rheumatoid-Arthritis and Cancer Studies Based on Linking Nationwide Registries in Finland. American Journal of Medicine 78: 29–32.
32. Cohen HJ, Bernstein RJ, Grufferman S (1987) Role of Immune Stimulation in the Etiology of Multiple-Myeloma - a Case Control Study. American Journal of Hematology 24: 119–126.
33. Boffetta P, Stellman SD, Garfinkel L (1989) A Case-Control Study of Multiple-Myeloma Nested in the American-Cancer-Society Prospective-Study. International Journal of Cancer 43: 554–559.
34. Lewis DR, Pottern LM, Brown LM, Silverman DT, Hayes RB, et al. (1994) Multiple-Myeloma among Blacks and Whites in the United-States - the Role of Chronic Antigenic-Stimulation. Cancer Causes & Control 5: 529–539.
35. Vlajinac HD, Pekmezovic TD, Adanja BJ, Marinkovic JM, Kanazir MS, et al. (2003) Case-control study of multiple myeloma with special reference to diet as risk factor. Neoplasma 50: 79–83.
36. Landgren O, Zhang YW, Zahm SH, Inskip P, Zheng TZ, et al. (2006) Risk of multiple myeloma following medication use and medical conditions: A case-control study in Connecticut women. Cancer Epidemiology Biomarkers & Prevention 15: 2342–2347.
37. Lindqvist EK, Goldin LR, Landgren O, Blimark C, Mellqvist UH, et al. (2011) Personal and family history of immune-related conditions increase the risk of plasma cell disorders: a population-based study. Blood 118: 6284–6291.
38. Isomaki HA, Hakulinen T, Joutsenlahti U (1982) Excess risk of lymphomas, leukemia and myeloma in patients with rheumatoid arthritis. Annals of the Rheumatic Diseases 41: 34–36.
39. Mellemkjaer L, Linet MS, Gridley G, Frisch M, Moller H, et al. (1996) Rheumatoid arthritis and cancer risk. Eur J Cancer 32A: 1753–1757.
40. Kauppi M, Pukkala E, Isomaki H (1997) Elevated incidence of hematologic malignancies in patients with Sjogren's syndrome compared with patients with rheumatoid arthritis (Finland). Cancer Causes Control 8: 201–204.
41. Setoguchi S, Solomon DH, Weinblatt ME, Katz JN, Avorn J, et al. (2006) Tumor necrosis factor alpha antagonist use and cancer in patients with rheumatoid arthritis. Arthritis Rheum 54: 2757–2764.
42. Herrinton LJ, Liu L, Shoor S, Mines D (2008) Risk of lymphoproliferative cancer among patients with severe rheumatoid arthritis, 1996–2002. Ann Rheum Dis 67: 574–575.
43. Parikh-Patel A, White RH, Allen M, Cress R (2009) Risk of cancer among rheumatoid arthritis patients in California. Cancer Causes Control 20: 1001–1010.
44. Dreyer L, Mellemkjaer L, Andersen AR, Bennett P, Poulsen UE, et al. (2013) Incidences of overall and site specific cancers in TNF alpha inhibitor treated patients with rheumatoid arthritis and other arthritides - a follow-up study from the DANBIO Registry. Annals of the Rheumatic Diseases 72: 79–82.
45. Brown LM, Gridley G, Check D, Landgren O (2008) Risk of multiple myeloma and monoclonal gammopathy of undetermined significance among white and black male United States veterans with prior autoimmune, infectious, inflammatory, and allergic disorders. Blood 111: 3388–3394.
46. Hemminki K, Liu XD, Forsti A, Ji JG, Sundquist J, et al. (2012) Effect of autoimmune diseases on incidence and survival in subsequent multiple myeloma. Journal of Hematology & Oncology 5.
47. Gramenzi A, Buttino I, Davanzo B, Negri E, Franceschi S, et al. (1991) Medical History and the Risk of Multiple-Myeloma. British Journal of Cancer 63: 769–772.
48. Cuzick J, Destavola BL (1989) Autoimmune Disorders and Multiple-Myeloma. International Journal of Epidemiology 18: 283–283.
49. Symmons DPM (1988) Neoplasia in Rheumatoid-Arthritis. Journal of Rheumatology 15: 1319–1322.
50. Holly EA, Bracci PM (2003) Population-based study of non-Hodgkin lymphoma, histology, and medical history among human immunodeficiency virus-negative participants in San Francisco. American Journal of Epidemiology 158: 316–327.
51. Bachman TR, Sawitzke AD, Perkins SL, Ward JH, Cannon GW (1996) Methotrexate-associated lymphoma in patients with rheumatoid arthritis - Report of two cases. Arthritis and Rheumatism 39: 325–329.
52. Bongartz T, Sutton AJ, Sweeting MJ, Buchan I, Matteson EL, et al. (2006) Anti-TNF antibody therapy in rheumatoid arthritis and the risk of serious infections and malignancies: Systematic review and meta-analysis of rare harmful effects in randomized controlled trials (vol 295, pg 2275, 2006). Jama-Journal Of the American Medical Association 295: 2482–2482.
53. Hsing AW, Hansson LE, Mclaughlin JK, Nyren O, Blot WJ, et al. (1993) Pernicious-Anemia and Subsequent Cancer - a Population-Based Cohort Study. Cancer 71: 745–750.
54. Brinton LA, Gridley G, Hrubec Z, Hoover R, Fraumeni JF (1989) Cancer Risk Following Pernicious-Anemia. British Journal of Cancer 59: 810–813.
55. Friso S, Choi SW (2005) The potential cocarcinogenic effect of vitamin B12 deficiency. Clin Chem Lab Med 43: 1158–1163.

7

MYC Expression in Concert with BCL2 and BCL6 Expression Predicts Outcome in Chinese Patients with Diffuse Large B-Cell Lymphoma, not Otherwise Specified

Li-Xu Yan, Yan-Hui Liu*, Dong-Lan Luo, Fen Zhang, Yu Cheng, Xin-Lan Luo, Jie Xu, Jie Cheng, Heng-Guo Zhuang

Department of Pathology, Guangdong General Hospital, Guangdong Academy of Medical Science, Guangzhou, China

Abstract

Recent studies provide convincing evidence that a combined immunohistochemical or fluorescence *in situ* hybridization (FISH) score of MYC, BCL2, BCL6 proteins and *MYC* translocations predicted outcome in diffuse large B-cell lymphoma (DLBCL) patients treated with rituximab, cyclophosphamide, doxorubicin, vincristine, and prednisone (R-CHOP). However, by far, all these researches are based on Western populations. Therefore, we investigate the prognostic relevance of MYC-, BCL2- and BCL6-rearrangements and protein expression by immunohistochemistry and FISH from 336 *de novo* DLBCL, NOS treated with CHOP or R-CHOP. Breaks in *MYC* and *BCL6*, and fusion in *IGH/BCL2* were detected in 9.7%, 20.0%, and 11.1% of the cases, respectively, and were not significantly associated with clinical outcomes. Protein overexpression of MYC (≥40%), BCL2 (≥70%) and BCL6 (≥50%) was encountered in 51%, 51% and 36% of the tumors, respectively. On the basis of MYC, BCL2 and BCL6 expression, double-hit scores (DHSs) and triple-hit score (THS) were assigned to all patients with DLBCL. Patients with high MYC/BCL2 DHS, high MYC/BCL6 DHS and high THS had multiple adverse prognostic factors including high LDH level, poor performance status, advanced clinical stage, high International Prognostic Index (IPI) score, and non-germinal center B-cell. In univariate analysis, high MYC/BCL2 DHS, high MYC/BCL6 DHS and high THS were associated with inferior OS and PFS in both CHOP and R-CHOP cohorts ($P<0.05$). The highly significant correlations with OS and PFS were maintained in multivariate models that controlled for IPI ($P<0.05$). DLBCLs with high DHSs and high THS share the clinical features and poor prognosis of double-hit lymphoma ($P>0.05$). These data together suggest that the immunohistochemical DHSs and THS defined a large subset of DLBCLs with double-hit biology and was strongly associated with poor outcome in patients treated with R-CHOP or CHOP.

Editor: Luwen Zhang, University of Nebraska - Lincoln, United States of America

Funding: This work was supported by a National Natural Science Foundation of China (NSFC, http://www.nsfc.gov.cn/) (Grant No. 81172244). YL, FZ, JX, and HZ received the funding. The funders had no role in study design, data collection and analysis, decision to publish, or preparation of the manuscript.

Competing Interests: The authors have declared that no competing interests exist.

* Email: yanh_liu@163.com

Introduction

Diffuse large B-cell lymphoma (DLBCL) exhibits various morphologies, immunophenotypes, genetic aberrations, and clinical courses. These features vary across geographic regions, suggesting geographic heterogeneity as a characteristic of this type of lymphoma. DLBCL constitutes 31–34% of all non-Hodgkin lymphomas in Western countries, more than 40% in Asian countries and 45.8% in china [1,2].

The International Prognostic Index (IPI) has been confirmed to be a valid prognosticator for patients receiving standard chemotherapy [3]. However, there are considerable differences in outcome within each of risk groups, suggesting underlying biologic differences that are not encompassed by the IPI factor [4]. In addition, gene expression profiling has stratified DLBCL into prognostically different molecular subtypes based on cell of origin, including germinal center B-cell (GCB)-like, activated B-cell-like subtypes, and unclassified DLBCL [5,6]. However, these subtypes do not reliably predict the prognosis of individual patients [7]. Furthermore, gene expression profiling is not available in most clinical laboratories. An immunophenotypical subdivision of DLBCL, not otherwise specified (NOS) into GCB and non-germinal center B-cell (non-GCB) subgroups has been proposed as prognosis predictor by different groups [8]. However, in some studies this immunophenotypic subdivision do not correlate with prognosis [9,10], and does not currently determine therapy [11].

Recent studies provide convincing evidence that a DLBCL population characterized by the coexpression of MYC and BCL2 proteins by IHC has a poor prognosis with standard rituximab, cyclophosphamide, doxorubicin, vincristine, and prednisone (R-CHOP) immunochemotherapy [12–14]. More recently, Heike et al. [15] have reported that a combined immunohistochemical or fluorescence *in situ* hybridization (FISH)/immunohistochemical score, including MYC, BCL2, BCL6 protein expressions and *MYC* translocations, predicts outcome in DLBCL patients independent of the IPI following treatment with R-CHOP.

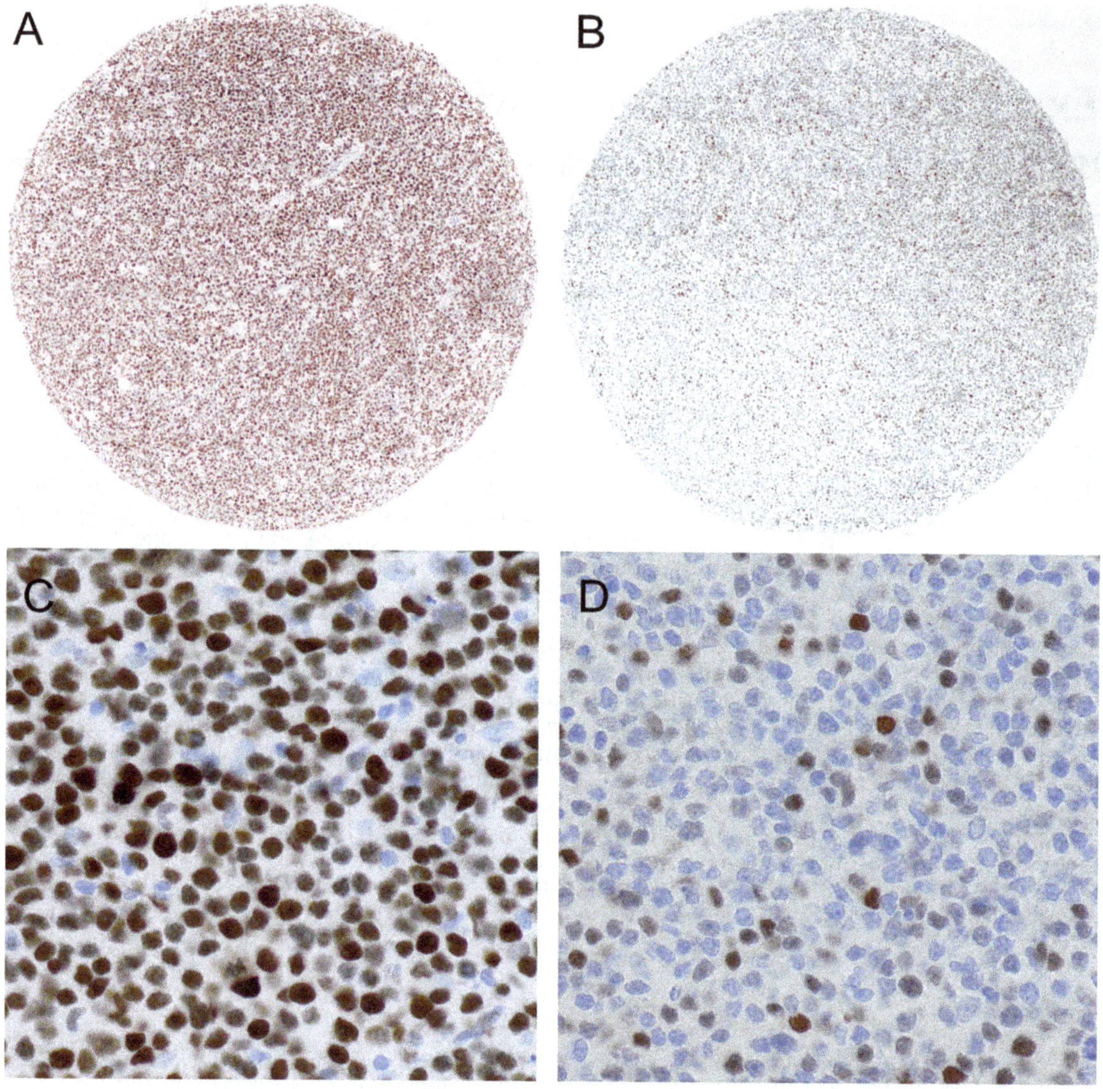

Figure 1. Tissue microarray based representative immunohistochemical analysis of MYC protein expression in DLBCL. The MYC staining pattern is distinctly nuclear. (A, C) DLBCL scored as having ≥40% MYC-positive lymphoma cells. (B, D) DLBCL scored as having <40% MYC-positive lymphoma cells. A and B original magnification, ×40. C and D original magnification, ×400.

DLBCL in China appears to have many characteristics different from those in Western countries; however, by far, all these researches are based on Western populations. In this study, therefore, we aimed to comprehensively assess the prognostic impact of protein expression patterns of MYC, BCL2, and BCL6 in concert with the chromosomal translocations targeting *MYC*, *BCL2*, and *BCL6* in a Chinese cohort of 336 *de novo* DLBCL, NOS patients treated with CHOP or R-CHOP.

Materials and Methods

Patient Selection

We studied 336 cases of *de novo* DLBCL, NOS from patients who were treated with 6 or 8 cycles of CHOP treatment with or without 8 applications of rituximab. Patients were selected based on the availability of baseline clinical and outcome data, and sufficient formalin-fixed paraffin-embedded (FFPE) tissue from the pre-treatment biopsy sample for representation in tissue microarrays (TMAs). The archived FFPE tissues were obtained from the Department of Pathology, Guangdong General Hospital between January 2000 and October 2012. A consensus diagnosis of DLBCL was confirmed by two expert pathologists according to 2008 World Health Organization (WHO) classification criteria [11]. Median follow-up time was 37 months (range, 1 to 145 months). The Research Ethics Committee of Guangdong General Hospital & Guangdong Academy of Medical Science reviewed and approved the study (No. GDREC2013122H) according to the principles expressed in the Declaration of Helsinki. The Research Ethics Committee specifically waived the need for informed consent for this project.

TMA Construction and Immunohistochemistry (IHC)

TMAs that contained three representative 2.0-mm cores from each tumor of the cases were prepared with a tissue microarrayer (Beecher Instruments, Silver Spring, MD). Immunohistochemical stainings were performed using Real Envision Kit (K5007, DAKO, Carpinteria, CA, USA) on two automated immunostaining instruments (Discovery XT, Ventana Medical Systems,

Table 1. Clinical and immunophenotypical characteristics of DLBCL, NOS patients.

	All patients (N = 336)		Patients with FISH data (n = 150)		
Characteristic	**No.**	**%**	**No.**	**%**	***P***
Male	195/336	58	86/150	57	0.885
Age, years median (range)	57 (7,87)		58 (7,86)		
LDH>upper limit of normal	129/336	38	59/150	39	0.844
ECOG PS ≥2[#]	51/336	15	29/150	19	0.254
Ann Arbor stage III/IV	156/336	46	68/150	45	0.823
Extranodal sites ≥2	57/336	17	22/150	15	0.526
IPI score[$]					
0 or 1	170/336	51	75/150	50	0.904
2	83/336	25	42/150	28	0.442
3	59/336	18	21/150	14	0.328
4 or 5	24/336	7	12/150	8	0.739
Extranodal involvement	235/336	70	100/150	67	0.471
Bone marrow involvement	36/336	11	12/150	8	0.354
Immunohistochemical subgroups					
CD5-positive DLBCL	15/336	4	11/150	7	0.194
GCB	90/336	27	47/150	31	0.303
non-GCB	231/336	69	92/150	61	0.110
High MYC expression	170/336	51	88/150	59	0.100
High BCL2 expression	171/336	51	84/150	56	0.298
High BCL6 expression	121/336	36	65/150	43	0.125
High Ki67 expression	176/336	52	92/150	61	0.067
R-CHOP	125/336	37	64/150	43	0.254
CHOP	211/336	63	86/150	57	0.254
Median follow-up time, months	37			27	
5-year OS	66			70	
5-year PFS	47			40	

P values were derived from Pearson's Chi-Square test. ECOG PS, Eastern Cooperative Oncology Group performance status.
[#]ECOG PS ranges from 0 to 4, where higher score indicates greater degree of impairment.
[$]IPI score ranges from 0 to 5, with 0 indicating absence of prognostic factors and 5 indicating presence of all prognostic factors.

Tucson, AZ, USA; Leica Bond-Max, Leica Biosystems, Germany) according to the manufacturer's instructions. Internal control cores were present in each TMA. Sections were subjected to staining protocols with the following antibodies: MYC (clone Y69; Epitomics, Burlingame, CA, USA), BCL2 (clone 124; DAKO, Glostrup, Denmark), BCL6 (clone PG-B6p; DAKO), and Ki67 (clone MIB1; DAKO; **Table S1**). All cases were scored semiquantitatively in 10% increments as previously reported [16] by two observers without knowledge of patient outcome or FISH results. Discrepant scoring of >10% was resolved using a multiheaded microscope to reach a consensus score.

Data were analyzed using MedCalc statistical software to determine the optimal survival cut-off points for dichotomizing expression of MYC protein (≥40%), BCL2 protein (≥70%), BCL6 protein (≥50%) and Ki67 index (≥90%). These cut points correspond to the maximum Chi-Square value of the Kaplan-Meier test for overall survival (OS) between groups above and below the cut-point threshold.

FISH

Interphase FISH was performed on TMAs of 150 cases from the same cohort as previously described [17]. The Vysis LSI *MYC* dual color, break apart rearrangement probe, the Vysis LSI *BCL6* dual color, break apart rearrangement probe and the Vysis LSI *IGH/BCL2* dual fusion translocation probe (Abbott Molecular, Abbott Park, IL) were used. FISH signals were analyzed using a fluorescence microscope (Olympus BX51, Tokyo, Japan) equipped with a DP72 camera and DP2-BSW software (Olympus, Tokyo, Japan). Patient cases with break-apart signals in >10% of nuclei were considered positive for the presence of a translocation. The signal distribution was evaluated by two independent observers (Dong-Lan Luo and Jie Cheng). In case of discordant results between the two observers, a third investigator (Jie Xu) was involved.

Statistical Analysis

Statistical analysis was prepared using the Statistical Package of MedCalc statistical software (version 12.7.4; MedCalc, Mariakerke, Belgium) and Social Sciences (SPSS, version 20.0; SPSS, Chicago, IL, USA). A receiver operating characteristic curves were constructed to estimate the optimal cut-off points for of MYC, BCL2 and BCL6 proteins as the predictors for OS. Pearson's Chi-Square test, Fisher's exact test, Correction for continuity and Spearman rank correlation analysis were used to determine

Table 2. Patient clinical and immunophenotypical characteristics of patients with DLBCL, NOS in relation to protein expressions.

Characteristic	All patients (n = 336)	MYC Low (n = 166)	MYC High (n = 170)	MYC *P*	BCL2 Low (n = 165)	BCL2 High (n = 171)	BCL2 *P*	BCL6 Low (n = 215)	BCL6 High (n = 121)	BCL6 *P*
	N (%)	N (%)	N (%)		N (%)	N (%)		N (%)	N (%)	
LDH>ULN	129 (38)	50 (30)	79 (46)	**0.002**	58 (35)	71 (42)	0.230	84 (39)	45 (37)	0.734
ECOG PS ≥2	51 (15)	19 (11)	32 (19)	0.060	17 (10)	34 (20)	**0.014**	34 (16)	17 (14)	0.665
Stage III/IV	156 (46)	70 (42)	86 (51)	0.122	75 (45)	81 (47)	0.725	108 (50)	48 (40)	0.062
Extranodal sites ≥2	57 (17)	29 (17)	28 (16)	0.807	27 (16)	30 (18)	0.773	39 (18)	18 (15)	0.444
IPI score of 3–5	83 (25)	33 (20)	50 (29)	**0.043**	36 (20)	51 (29)	0.056	59 (27)	24 (20)	0.121
Immunohistochemical subgroups										
CD5-positive	15 (4)	6 (4)	9(6)	0.658*	5 (2)	10 (7)	**0.001***	12 (6)	3 (3)	**0.004***
GCB	90 (27)	47 (28)	43 (25)	0.595#	59 (36)	31 (18)	**<0.001#**	45(21)	45 (37)	**0.002#**
non-GCB	231 (69)	113 (68)	118 (69)		101 (62)	130 (75)		158 (73)	73 (60)	

P values were derived from Pearson's Chi-Square test. Bold font indicates significance. ULN, upper limit of normal.
*P value CD5+ *vs.* GCB *vs.* non-GCB.
#P value GCB *vs.* non-GCB.

association and correlation between variables. Survival analyses were plotted using Kaplan-Meier curves and compared using the log-rank test. Univariate and Multivariate survival analyses were analyzed by Cox proportional hazards regression models. The results were considered statistically significant when two-sided $P<0.05$.

Results

Clinical and Immunophenotypical Characteristics

We studied the series of 336 DLBCL, NOS tumor samples by IHC on the TMAs using antibodies for MYC, BCL2, BCL6 and Ki67 (**Figure 1**). In addition, ten patient cases which could not be scored for technical reasons were also studied on the corresponding whole tissue sections from the original FFPE tumor blocks. Stainings of the four markers were reliably interpretable in all the 336 samples. The clinical and immunophenotypical characteristics of the DLBCL, NOS are provided in **Table 1**. DLBCL, NOS was immunophenotypically subdivided into CD5-positive, GCB and non-GCB subgroups according to the Hans classifier [8] and the 2008 WHO classification [11]. Fifteen DLBCL, NOS (4%) were of CD5-positive-subgroup, 90 (27%) of GCB-subgroup, and 231 (69%) of non-GCB-subgroup.

High Double-Hit Scores (DHSs) and Triple-Hit Score (THS) are Associated With High-Risk Clinicopathologic Parameters

One hundred and seventy tumors (51%) showed high MYC expression, 171 (51%) showed high BCL2 expression and 121 (36%) showed high BCL6 expression (**Table 1**). MYC overexpression was associated with high lactate dehydrogenase (LDH) level ($P=0.002$) and high IPI score ($P=0.043$; **Table 2**). BCL2 overexpression was associated with poor performance status ($P=0.014$; **Table 2**). However, no significant differences were observed with regard to clinical characteristics among low and high BCL6 groups.

Using the optimal survival cut-off points as described in Methods section, we assigned each patient a THS that ranged from 0 to 2. Each patient was given one point for each of the two markers (MYC and BCL2) expressed at or above the cut-off points, and one point for BCL6 expressed below the cut-off point. The DHSs of MYC/BCL2, MYC/BCL6 and BCL2/BCL6 were calculated as described previously [16]. Patients with high MYC/BCL2 DHS had multiple adverse clinical factors including high LDH level ($P=0.007$), poor performance status ($P=0.010$), and high IPI score ($P=0.038$; **Table 3**). Similarly, patients with high MYC/BCL2 DHS was associated with high LDH level, high clinical stage, and high IPI score ($P>0.05$). However, no significant differences were observed with regard to clinical factors included in **Table 3** among BCL2/BCL6 DHS 0, 1 and 2. Notably, patients with high THS had multiple adverse prognostic factors including high LDH level ($P=0.024$), poor performance status ($P=0.025$), high clinical stage ($P=0.008$), and high IPI score ($P=0.009$; **Table 3**).

One hundred and seventy-five tumors (52.1%) showed high Ki67 expression. No significant differences were observed with regard to LDH level, performance status, clinical stage, extranodal sites, IPI score, or immunohistochemical subgroups (GCB *vs.* non-GCB) among high Ki67 proliferation index and low Ki67 proliferation index groups.

High DHS and THS Show Non-GCB Predominance

The immunophenotypical characteristics of patients with DLBCL, NOS in relation to protein expressions are shown in

Table 3. Patient clinical and immunophenotypical characteristics of patients with DLBCL, NOS in relation to DHS and THS.

		MYC/BCL2				MYC/BCL6				BCL2/BCL6				MYC/BCL2/BCL6				
Characteristic	**All patients (n=336)**	**DHS 0 (n=90)**	**DHS 1 (n=151)**	**DHS 2 (n=95)**	*P*	**DHS 0 (n=57)**	**DHS 1 (n=173)**	**DHS 2 (n=106)**	*P*	**DHS 0 (n=65)**	**DHS 1 (n=156)**	**DHS 2 (n=115)**	*P*	**THS 0 (n=27)**	**THS 1 (n=131)**	**THS 2 (n=109)**	**THS 3 (n=69)**	*P*
	N (%)	**N (%)**	**N (%)**	**N (%)**		**N (%)**	**N (%)**	**N (%)**		**N (%)**	**N (%)**	**N (%)**		**N (%)**	**N (%)**	**N (%)**	**N (%)**	
LDH>ULN	129 (38)	28 (31)	52 (34)	49 (52)	**0.007**	17 (30)	61 (35)	51 (48)	**0.035**	23 (35)	57 (37)	49 (43)	0.512	7 (26)	47 (36)	38 (35)	37 (54)	**0.024**
ECOG PS ≥2	51 (15)	8 (9)	20 (13)	23 (24)	**0.010**	6 (11)	24 (14)	21 (20)	0.228	4 (6)	26 (17)	21 (18)	0.073	2 (7)	12 (9)	23 (21)	14 (20)	**0.025**
Stage III/IV	156 (46)	36 (40)	73 (48)	47 (49)	0.355	19 (33)	80 (46)	57 (54)	**0.044**	28 (43)	67 (43)	61 (53)	0.215	12 (44)	47 (36)	63 (58)	34 (49)	**0.008**
Extranodal sites ≥2	57(17)	13 (14)	30 (20)	14 (15)	0.440	8 (14)	31 (18)	18 (17)	0.795	11 (17)	23 (15)	23 (20)	0.522	4 (15)	20 (15)	22 (20)	11 (16)	0.751
IPI score of 3–5	83 (25)	14 (16)	39 (26)	30 (32)	**0.038**	7 (12)	43 (25)	33 (31)	**0.029**	11 (17)	36 (23)	36 (31)	0.081	3 (11)	23 (18)	36 (33)	21 (30)	**0.009**
Immunohistochemical subgroups																		
CD5-positive	15 (4)	2 (2)	7 (5)	6 (6)	NS*	3 (5)	3 (2)	9 (8)	NS*	0 (0)	8 (5)	7 (6)	NS*	0 (0)	5 (4)	4 (4)	6 (9)	NS*
GCB	90 (27)	29 (32)	48 (32)	13 (14)	**0.004**#	21 (37)	50 (29)	19 (18)	**0.034**#	33 (51)	38 (24)	19 (17)	**<0.001**#	12 (44)	47 (36)	21 (19)	10 (14)	**0.001**#
non-GCB	231 (69)	59 (66)	96 (63)	76 (80)		33 (58)	120 (69)	78 (74)		32 (49)	110 (71)	89 (77)		15 (56)	79 (60)	84 (77)	53 (77)	

P values were derived using Pearson's Chi-Square test. Bold font indicates significance.
*NS, not suitable for chi-square test among CD5+ *vs.* GCB *vs.* non-GCB, because more than 1/5 of the expected values were less than five.
#*P* value GCB *vs.* non-GCB.

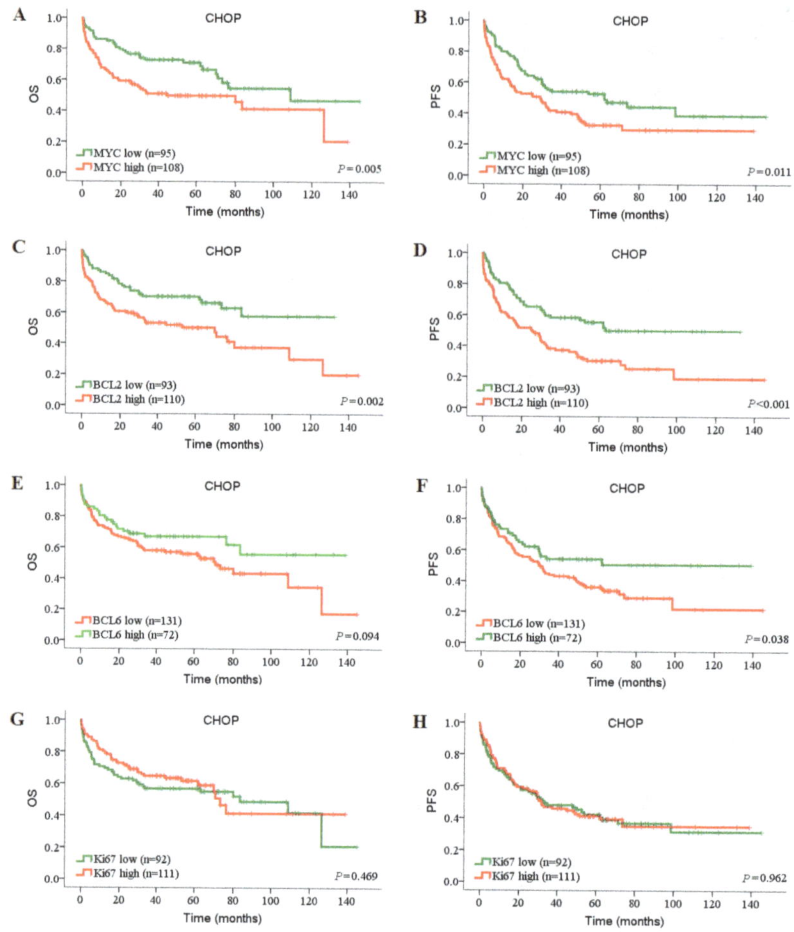

Figure 2. Prognostic impact of MYC, BCL2, BCL6 and Ki67 expression in DLBCL patients treated with CHOP. Patients' tumors were stained for (A, B) MYC, (C, D) BCL2, (E, F) BCL6, and (G, H) Ki67. The numbers of patients showing negative or positive stainings (MYC≥40%, BCL2≥70%, BCL6≥50%, Ki67≥90%), cut-off values, and *P* values are indicated.

Table 2. MYC expression demonstrated no correlation with immunohistochemical subgroups of DLBCL. Considering BCL2 and BCL6 expression individually, the high BCL2 expression group had a significantly higher frequency of non-GCB than the low BCL2 group (75% *vs.* 62%, $P<0.001$). However, low BCL6 expression group had a higher frequency of non-GCB than the high BCL6 group (73% *vs.* 60%, $P=0.002$).

MYC/BCL2 coexpression (DHS 2) correlated significantly with the non-GCB immunohistochemical subgroup ($P=0.004$; **Table 3**). Of total 336 cases of DLBCL, NOS, with MYC/BCL2 DHS 2, 76 (80%) were of the non-GCB-DLBCL. By contrast, only 96 (63%) of DLBCL with MYC/BCL2 DHS 1 were of the non-GCB-DLBCL, and 59 (66%) of DLBCL with MYC/BCL2 DHS 0 were of the non-GCB-DLBCL (**Table 3**). Similar results were found for MYC/BCL6, BCL2/BCL6 and MYC/BCL2/BCL6 coexpression.

FISH Studies and Double-Hit Lymphoma (DHL)

Initially, we created a pilot series of 336 DLBCL, NOS tumor samples spotted on TMAs. After IHC analysis, sufficient materials of 150 cases on the TMAs were available for complete FISH analysis. The clinical and immunophenotypical characteristics of the 150 patients are shown in **Table 1**. Of 150 DLBCL specimens hybridized, 144 (96%), 140 (93%) and 135 (90%) samples were successfully interpretable for the *MYC* and *BCL6* break-apart probes and the *IGH/BCL2* fusion probe used, respectively. *MYC*, *BCL6*, and *BCL2* gene translocations were observed in 9.7%, 20.0%, and 11.1% of the cases, respectively (**Figure S1**).

No significant corrections were observed between *MYC* and *BCL6* gene breaks and clinical characteristics, including LDH level, performance status, clinical stage, extranodal sites and IPI. Patients with high IPI score had higher *IGH/BCL2* fusion rate than those with low IPI score (28.6% *vs.* 7.4%; χ^2 test, correction for continuity, $P=0.006$). No correlations between gene translocations and immunohistochemical subgroups were seen (**Table S2**). The lack of significant differences in gene translocations between the GCB and the non-GCB DLBCL subgroups indicates that abnormalities of *MYC, BCL6 and BCL2* may be a more global phenomenon in Chinese DLBCL and not restricted to particular immunohistochemical subgroups. Breaks in *MYC* and *BCL6*, as well as fusion in *IGH/BCL2* did not predict OS and progression-free survival (PFS) in univariate and multivariate analyses in rituximab treated patients. We observed similar results for patients treated without rituximab.

We further investigated the double-hit lymphoma (DHL) in our series. One of 134 DLBCL (0.7%) had concurrent translocation of *MYC* and *BCL2*, 1/140 (0.7%) of *MYC* and *BCL6*, and 4/131 (3.1%) of *BCL2* and *BCL6*. Thus those were determined to have

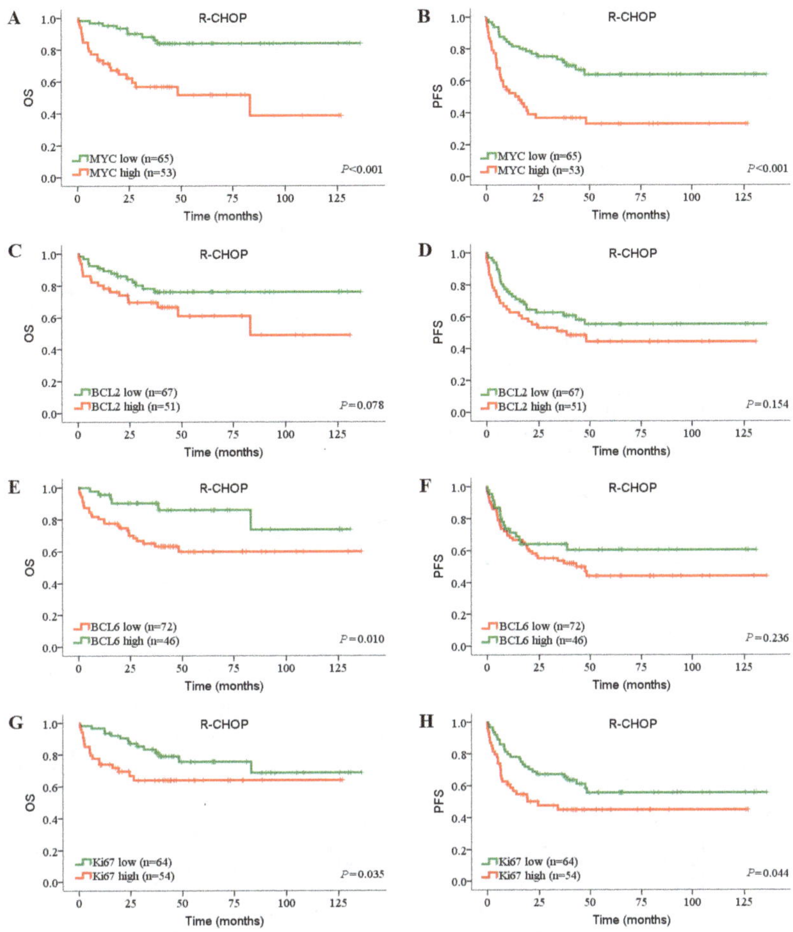

Figure 3. Prognostic impact of MYC, BCL2, BCL6 and Ki67 expression in DLBCL patients treated with R-CHOP. Patients' tumors were stained for (A, B) MYC, (C, D) BCL2, (E, F) BCL6, and (G, H) Ki67. The numbers of patients showing negative or positive stainings (MYC≥40%, BCL2≥ 70%, BCL6≥50%, Ki67≥90%), cut-off values, and *P* values are indicated.

DHL. No triple-hit lymphoma was detected. Given those low incidences, DHL data sets were pooled for subsequent analyses. These patients with DHL (by FISH) appeared to have more adverse clinical risk factors, including higher levels of LDH, worse performance status, and higher IPI scores than the patients without DHL (non-DHL) ($P>0.05$; **Table S3**). The lack of significance is probably due to low statistical power from small group sizes. However, BCL2 protein was expressed in a higher proportion of the DHL patients than the non-DHL patients with THS 0/1 ($P = 0.005$, **Table S3**). Three of 6 DHL patients were treated with R-CHOP. The 5-year OS rate of patients with DHL treated with R-CHOP or CHOP in this study (50%) was lower than that of the non-DHL patients (70%), although $P>0.05$ (**Figure S2**). Six but too few patient cases with DHL could not preclude any meaningful conclusions. However, the 5-year OS of the DHL patients was poor compared with outcome among non-DHL patients with THS 0/1 (50% *vs.* 83%; $P = 0.048$; **Figure S2**). When comparing the patients with DHL with non-DHL patients in the THS-2/3 group, no significant differences were found between clinical characteristics or survival, implying that patients with DHL and those non-DHL patients in the THS-2/3 group are clinically similar and indicating that they share the same unfavorable double-hit tumor biology (**Table S3; Figure S2**).

Protein Expressions Predict Corresponding Gene Translocations

To analyze the diagnostic performance of MYC, BCL2 and BCL6 protein expressions for corresponding gene translocations with the highest specificity and sensitivity, we used ROC curve analysis to determine the optimal cut-off values of the percentages of protein positive cells. The optimal cut-off values for MYC, BCL2 and BCL6 were ≥90%, ≥70% (equal to predetermined threshold) and ≥20%. The results signify that immunostaining for MYC, BCL2 and BCL6 appears to be an excellent test with high specificity for the presence of *MYC* breaks, *IGH/BCL2* fusion and *BCL6* breaks as detected by FISH (**Table S4**). High MYC expression showed correlation with *MYC* breaks in DLBCL, NOS (Spearman rank correlation analysis, Spearman's rho = 0.481, $P<0.001$), the GCB subgroup (Spearman's rho = 0.623, $P<0.001$) and the non-GCB subgroup (Spearman's rho = 0.556, $P<0.001$). High BCL6 expression showed correlation with *BCL6* breaks in DLBCL, NOS (Spearman's rho = 0.223, $P = 0.008$) and the non-GCB subgroup (Spearman's rho = 0.277, $P = 0.011$) but showed no significant correlation in the GCB subgroup. Inversely, high BCL2 expression showed correlation with *IGH/BCL2* fusion in and the GCB subgroup (Spearman's rho = 0.369, $P = 0.015$) but

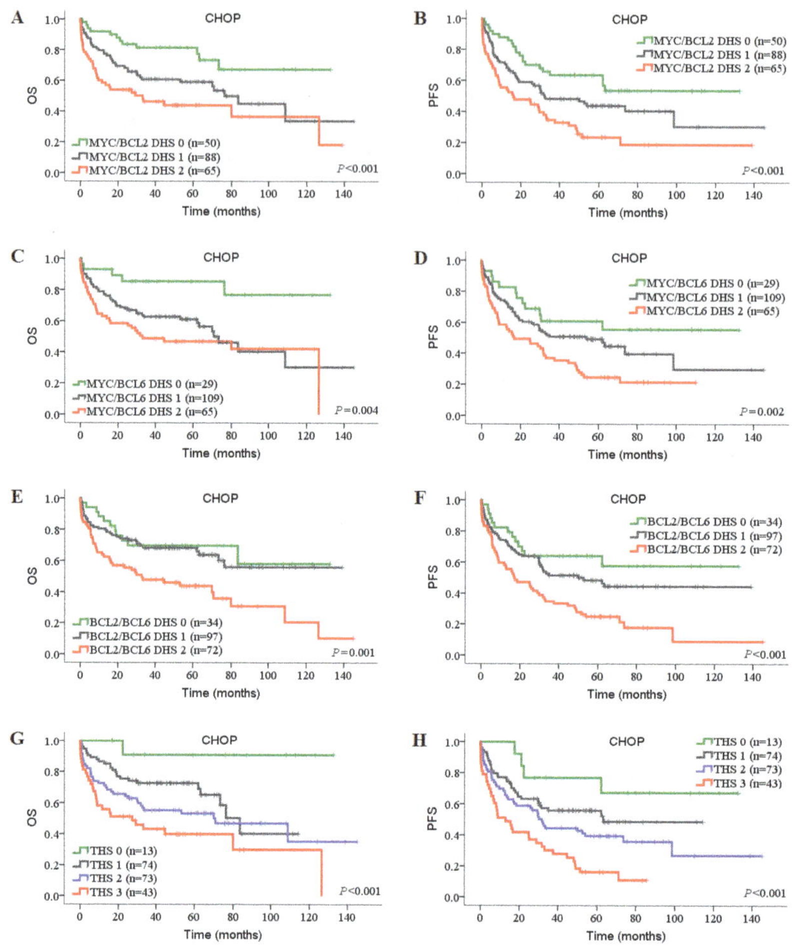

Figure 4. Prognostic impact of DHSs and THS in DLBCL patients treated with CHOP. (A, B) OS (A) and PFS (B) of patients with MYC/BCL2 DHS. (C, D) OS (C) and PFS (D) of patients with MYC/BCL6 DHS. (E, F) OS (E) and PFS (F) of patients with BCL2/BCL6 DHS. (G, H) OS (G) and PFS (H) of patients with MYC/BCL2/BCL6 THS. OS, overall survival; PFS, progression-free survival; DHS, double-hit score; THS, triple-hit score.

showed no significant correlation in DLBCL, NOS or the non-GCB subgroup. Chi-Square test for gene translocation and protein expression in are shown in **Table S5–S7**.

High DHSs and THS Predict Poor Prognosis in DLBCL, NOS

Because several recent studies have shown that prognostic value of biomarkers have changed significantly in rituximab era [18–20], we evaluated the candidate prognostic factors separately in the CHOP and R-CHOP cohorts. The survival curves showed that high MYC expression was significantly associated with inferior OS and PFS in both CHOP and R-CHOP cohorts ($P<0.05$, log-rank tests; **Figure 2A–B, Figure 3A–B**). High BCL2 expression, alone, was significantly associated with inferior OS and PFS in CHOP cohort (OS: $P=0.002$; PFS, $P<0.001$) but not in R-CHOP cohort (**Figure 2C–D, Figure 3C–D**). However, low BCL6 expression showed limited prognostic impact on inferior outcome in both CHOP and R-CHOP cohorts (PFS of CHOP cohort: $P=0.038$; OS of R-CHOP cohort: $P=0.010$; **Figure 2E–F, Figure 3E–F**). Interestingly, in contrast with BCL2, Ki67 was significantly associated with inferior OS and PFS in R-CHOP cohort (OS: $P=0.035$; PFS, $P=0.044$) but not in CHOP cohort (**Figure 2G–H, Figure 3G–H**).

Next, we investigated the prognostic impact of DHSs and THS on DLBCL patients in both CHOP and R-CHOP cohorts. In univariate analysis, high MYC/BCL2 DHS, high MYC/BCL6 DHS and high THS were associated with inferior OS and PFS in both CHOP and R-CHOP cohorts (**Table 4**; **Table 5**). In the CHOP cohort, compared with individual BCL2 and BCL6 protein, the negative prognostic impact of high BCL2 protein and low BCL6 protein was amplified when BCL2/BCL6 DHS was high (**Table 4; Figure 4E–F**). In the R-CHOP cohort, high BCL2 protein expression was only associated with inferior OS and PFS when MYC protein was coexpressed ($P<0.001$; **Table 5, Figure 5A–B**). BCL2/BCL6 DHS showed limited prognostic impact in R-CHOP cohort (univariate model: OS, $P=0.005$, PFS, $P=0.089$; multivariate model: OS, $P=0.006$, PFS, $P=0.132$).

In the CHOP cohort, multivariate Cox regression model that incorporated IPI, immunohistochemical subgroups (GCB *vs.* non-GCB), MYC, BCL2, and BCL6 proteins showed that IPI, MYC protein, and BCL2 protein maintained independent prognostic values for OS and PFS ($P<0.05$; **Table 6**). Also high MYC/BCL2 DHS, high MYC/BCL6 DHS, high BCL2/BCL6 DHS and high THS maintained independent prognostic values for OS and PFS (all $P<0.05$; **Table 6**).

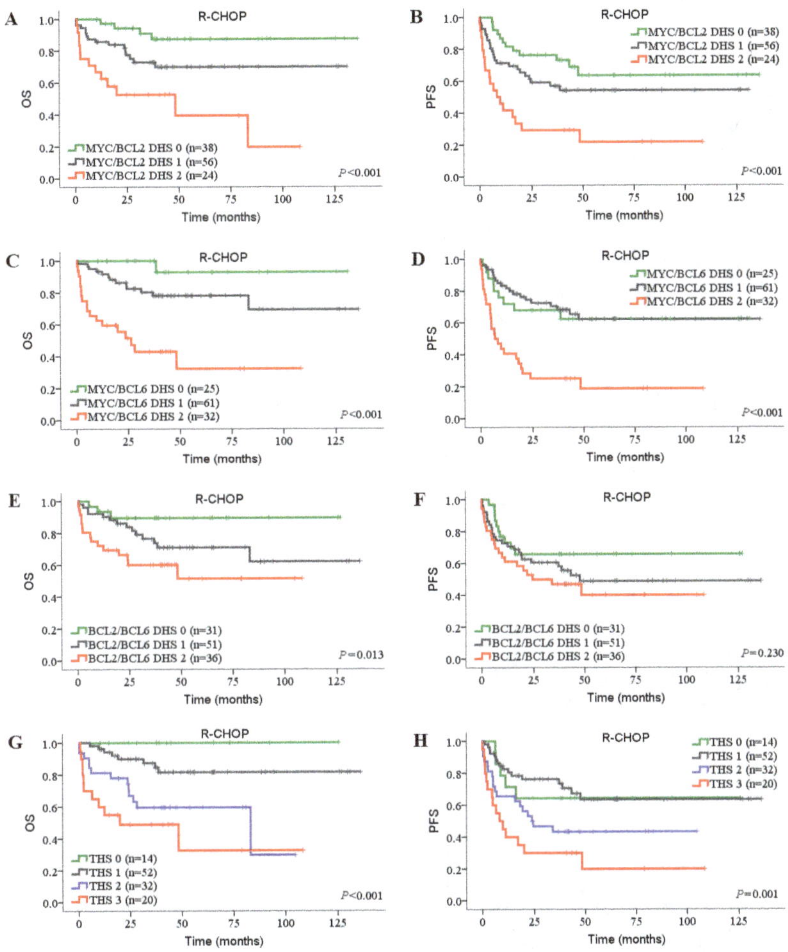

Figure 5. Prognostic impact of DHSs and THS in DLBCL patients treated with R-CHOP. (A, B) OS (A) and PFS (B) of patients with MYC/BCL2 DHS. (C, D) OS (C) and PFS (D) of patients with MYC/BCL6 DHS. (E, F) OS (E) and PFS (F) of patients with BCL2/BCL6 DHS. (G, H) OS (G) and PFS (H) of patients with MYC/BCL2/BCL6 THS. OS, overall survival; PFS, progression-free survival; DHS, double-hit score; THS, triple-hit score.

In the R-CHOP cohort, multivariate Cox regression model that incorporated IPI, MYC, BCL2, and BCL6 proteins showed that only high MYC protein maintained independent prognostic value for both inferior OS ($P<0.001$) and PFS ($P=0.001$), and low BCL6 protein for inferior OS ($P=0.019$; **Table 7**). Also high MYC/BCL2 DHS, high MYC/BCL6 DHS, and high THS maintained independent prognostic values for OS and PFS (all $P<0.05$). High BCL2/BCL6 DHS was independent prognostic value or OS ($P=0.006$; **Table 7**).

Immunohistochemical Subtyping and IPI Predict Survival in DLBCL Patients Treated With CHOP but Not With R-CHOP

For all DLBCL, NOS patients, rituximab significantly improved OS (72.9% *vs.* 56.2%, $P=0.011$; **Figure 6A**) but not PFS, although a trend was seen (54.2% *vs.* 40.9%, $P=0.135$; **Figure 6B**). In the GCB subgroup, the OS and PFS showed an increase in the R-CHOP group from survival curves (**Figure 6C–D**), but this was not significant. In the non-GCB subgroup, the patients receiving R-CHOP treatment showed a significantly improved OS than those who received CHOP (70.1% *vs.* 52.1%, $P=0.020$; **Figure 6E**). These findings were consistent with the results of previous studies in Chinese patients [20,21]. Importantly, these results indicated that the use of rituximab conferred a clinical benefit to non-GCB-DLBCL patients, frequently associated with poorer prognosis.

We further investigated the prognostic value of immunohistochemical subtyping in our series undergoing CHOP or R-CHOP treatment. For all patients, the GCB subgroup had superior OS and PFS than the non-GCB subgroup (OS: 71.1% *vs.* 58.9%, $P=0.047$; PFS: 62.2% *vs.* 39.4%, $P=0.002$; **Figure 7A–B**). In the CHOP cohort, the GCB subgroup had superior PFS than the non-GCB subgroup (57.6% *vs.* 34.0%, $P=0.012$; **Figure 7D**). However, the GCB lost its predictive value in patients treated with rituximab (**Figure 7E–F; Table 4**). These findings were consistent with the results of previous studies in both Chinese cohorts [19] and Western cohorts [22]. The IPI proved to be highly valuable for both all patients and CHOP-treated patients (**Figure 8A–D**). However, the IPI lost its predictive value in patients who were treated with rituximab which has improved prognosis significantly (**Figure 8E–F**). This result is consistent with previous studies [11,19] but inconsistent with some other studies [3,23].

Discussions

DLBCL, NOS constitutes 25–30% of adult non-Hodgkin lymphomas in Western countries [11] and a higher percentage

Table 4. Univariate Cox models for DLBCL, NOS patients treated with CHOP.

		OS			PFS		
Characteristic	**n#**	**HR**	**95% CI**	***P***	**HR**	**95% CI**	***P***
MYC protein low *vs.* High	203	1.83	1.19–2.82	**0.006**	1.60	1.11–2.31	**0.012**
BCL2 protein low *vs.* High	203	1.95	1.26–3.01	**0.003**	1.94	1.34–2.82	**0.001**
BCL6 protein low *vs.* High	203	0.68	0.43–1.07	0.096	0.66	0.44–0.98	**0.040**
High Ki67 protein low *vs.* High	203	0.86	0.56–1.30	0.470	0.99	0.69–1.42	0.962
MYC/BCL2 DHS 0 *vs.* 1 *vs.* 2	203	1.79	1.33–2.40	**<0.001**	1.67	1.30–2.14	**<0.001**
MYC/BCL6 DHS 0 *vs.* 1 *vs.* 2	203	1.71	1.24–2.37	**0.001**	1.63	1.23–2.16	**0.001**
BCL2/BCL6 DHS 0 *vs.* 1 *vs.* 2	203	1.70	1.24–2.34	**0.001**	1.73	1.32–2.28	**<0.001**
THS 0 *vs.* 1 *vs.* 2 *vs.* 3	203	1.70	1.33–2.18	**<0.001**	1.65	1.33–2.04	**<0.001**
GCB *vs.* Non-GCB	203	1.56	0.95–2.56	0.082	1.75	1.12–2.72	0.013
IPI score of 0–2 *vs.* 3–5	203	2.87	1.89–4.36	**<0.001**	2.21	1.52–3.19	**<0.001**
MYC break negative *vs.* positive	76	1.22	0.37–4.04	0.745	1.28	0.50–3.25	0.604
IGH/BCL2 fusion negative *vs.* positive	69	0.87	0.20–3.67	0.844	0.70	0.22–2.28	0.556
BCL6 break negative *vs.* positive	72	1.50	0.60–3.73	0.387	1.30	0.60–2.82	0.504

Bold font indicates significance. HR, hazard ratio; CI, confidence interval.
#Sample sizes differ due to complete data set per cox model.

Table 5. Univariate Cox models for DLBCL, NOS patients treated with R-CHOP.

		OS			PFS		
Characteristic	**n#**	**HR**	**95% CI**	***P***	**HR**	**95% CI**	***P***
MYC protein low *vs.* High	118	4.39	2.02–9.54	**<0.001**	2.87	1.66–4.99	**<0.001**
BCL2 protein low *vs.* High	118	1.86	0.92–3.73	0.083	1.47	0.86–2.51	0.157
BCL6 protein low *vs.* High	118	0.33	0.14–0.80	**0.014**	0.71	0.40–1.26	0.238
High Ki67 protein low *vs.* High	118	2.09	1.04–4.23	**0.040**	1.72	1.01–2.95	**0.047**
MYC/BCL2 DHS 0 *vs.* 1 *vs.* 2	118	2.76	1.66–4.60	**<0.001**	2.03	1.39–2.96	**<0.001**
MYC/BCL6 DHS 0 *vs.* 1 *vs.* 2	118	4.23	2.29–7.79	**<0.001**	2.25	1.47–3.45	**<0.001**
BCL2/BCL6 DHS 0 *vs.* 1 *vs.* 2	118	2.11	1.26–3.52	**0.005**	1.37	0.95–1.97	0.089
THS 0 *vs.* 1 *vs.* 2 *vs.* 3	118	2.54	1.70–3.81	**<0.001**	1.72	1.28–2.31	**<0.001**
GCB *vs.* non-GCB	118	1.67	0.69–4.06	0.259	1.97	0.96–4.03	0.064
IPI score of 0–2 *vs.* 3–5	118	1.76	0.79–3.92	0.167	1.74	0.91–3.30	0.093
MYC break negative *vs.* positive	57	0.52	0.07–3.98	0.529	1.19	0.42–3.41	0.740
IGH/BCL2 fusion negative *vs.* positive	55	1.74	0.48–6.36	0.402	0.90	0.32–2.59	0.851
BCL6 break negative *vs.* positive	57	1.04	0.29–3.81	0.948	1.27	0.59–2.73	0.550

Bold font indicates significance.
#Sample sizes differ due to complete data set per cox model.

Table 6. Multivariate Cox models for DBCL, NOS patients treated with CHOP (n = 203).

Characteristic	OS			PFS		
	HR	95% CI	*P**	HR	95% CI	*P**
IPI score of 0–2 *vs.* 3–5	2.78	1.83–4.23	**<0.001**	2.20	1.52–3.18	**<0.001**
GCB *vs.* non-GCB	1.26	0.74–2.13	0.397	1.49	0.94–2.37	0.092
MYC protein low *vs.* High	1.77	1.14–2.73	**0.010**	1.67	1.15–2.42	**0.007**
BCL2 protein low *vs.* High	1.66	1.05–2.63	**0.032**	1.63	1.10–2.41	**0.015**
BCL6 protein low *vs.* High	0.67	0.42–1.08	0.098	0.66	0.44–0.99	**0.042**
IPI score of 0–2 *vs.* 3–5	2.77	1.82–4.20	**<0.001**	2.20	1.52–3.18	**<0.001**
MYC/BCL2 DHS 0 *vs.* 1 *vs.* 2	1.76	1.30–2.38	**<0.001**	1.68	1.30–2.16	**<0.001**
IPI score of 0–2 *vs.* 3–5	2.86	1.88–4.34	**<0.001**	2.22	1.53–3.21	**<0.001**
MYC/BCL6 DHS 0 *vs.* 1 *vs.* 2	1.73	1.24–2.41	**0.001**	1.66	1.24–2.21	**0.001**
IPI score of 0–2 *vs.* 3–5	2.81	1.84–4.27	**<0.001**	2.14	1.48–3.11	**<0.001**
BCL2/BCL6 DHS 0 *vs.* 1 *vs.* 2	1.63	1.20–2.22	**0.002**	1.68	1.28–2.20	**<0.001**
IPI score of 0–2 *vs.* 3–5	2.79	1.84–4.25	**<0.001**	2.20	1.52–3.18	**<0.001**
THS 0 *vs.* 1 *vs.* 2 *vs.* 3	1.68	1.31–2.16	**<0.001**	1.67	1.34–2.06	**<0.001**

Bold font indicates significance.
*Cox regression enter method.

(37.9%) in Chinese [2]. The poor prognosis of DLBCL patients whose tumors overexpress either MYC or BCL2, or low express BCL6 is well established [24–27]. Recently, the negative prognostic impact of coexpression of MYC and BCL2 has been confirmed in DLBCL patients from Western populations treated with R-CHOP [16,23,28,29]. We have confirmed these data in larger series comprising DLBCL, NOS samples from 336 Chinese patients treated with either R-CHOP (n = 125) or CHOP (n = 211). Moreover, we have shown that combined immunohistochemical scores of MYC, BCL2 and BCL6 predict 5-year OS and 5-year PFS in DLBCL patients independent of the IPI following treatment with R-CHOP. Of note, we observed similar results for patients treated with CHOP (data not shown). In contrast, Johnson et al. reported that MYC overexpression predicted poor 3-year OS and event-free survival in R-CHOP-treated patients but not in CHOP-treated patients with unknown mechanism [15]. The contradictory findings may be due to population heterogeneity, different time-to-event end points and different second and/or third line treatments. Different populations treated uniformly within a prospective multicenter trial are needed to further consolidate the prognostic value of MYC combined with BCL2 and BCL6 protein. Importantly, our results

Table 7. Multivariate Cox models for DBCL, NOS patients treated with R-CHOP (n = 118).

Characteristic	OS			PFS		
	HR	95% CI	*P**	HR	95% CI	*P**
IPI score of 0–2 *vs.* 3–5	1.24	0.55–2.80	0.605	1.51	0.78–2.90	0.221
MYC protein low *vs.* High	4.12	1.86–9.10	**<0.001**	2.71	1.55–4.76	**0.001**
BCL2 protein low *vs.* High	1.48	0.71–3.07	0.293	1.35	0.77–2.36	0.303
BCL6 protein low *vs.* High	0.33	0.13–0.83	**0.019**	0.74	0.40–1.37	0.336
Ki67 protein low vs. High	1.71	0.83–3.51	0.144	1.49	0.86–2.57	0.151
IPI score of 0–2 *vs.* 3–5	1.34	0.59–3.03	0.483	1.56	0.81–2.97	0.181
MYC/BCL2 DHS 0 *vs.* 1 *vs.* 2	2.67	1.60–4.48	**<0.001**	1.97	1.35–2.88	**<0.001**
IPI score of 0–2 *vs.* 3–5	1.22	0.54–2.75	0.628	1.44	0.75–2.76	0.270
MYC/BCL6 DHS 0 *vs.* 1 *vs.* 2	4.14	2.23–7.68	**<0.001**	2.19	1.42–3.37	**<0.001**
IPI score of 0–2 *vs.* 3–5	1.50	0.67–3.34	0.326	1.61	0.84–3.07	0.151
BCL2/BCL6 DHS 0 *vs.* 1 *vs.* 2	2.07	1.23–3.50	**0.006**	1.33	0.92–1.94	0.132
IPI score of 0–2 *vs.* 3–5	1.30	0.58–2.91	0.522	1.49	0.78–2.85	0.223
THS 0 *vs.* 1 *vs.* 2 *vs.* 3	2.51	1.67–3.77	**<0.001**	1.69	1.25–2.29	**0.001**

Bold font indicates significance.
*Cox regression enter method.

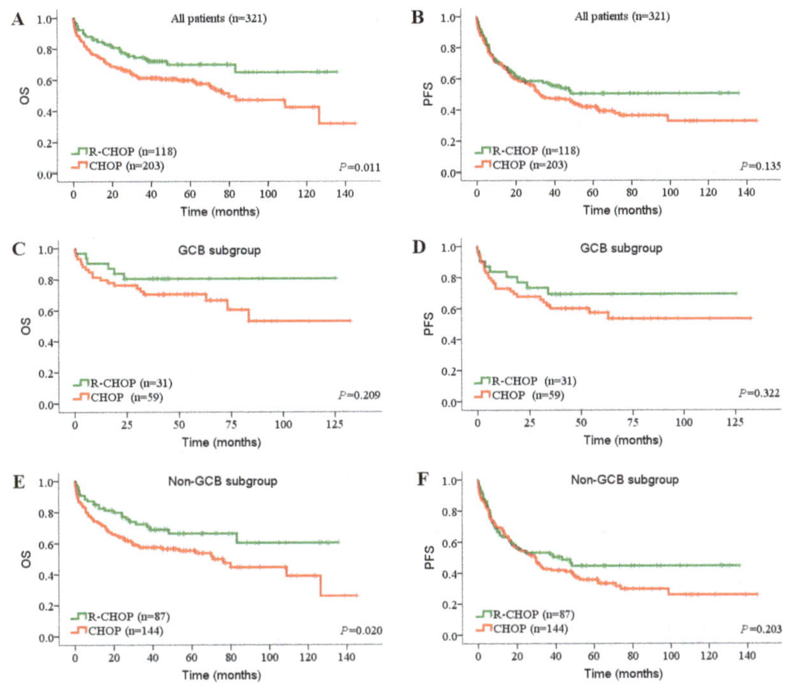

Figure 6. Prognostic impact of treatments in DLBCL risk-stratified according to immunohistochemical subgroups. (A, B) OS (A) and PFS (B) of all patients treated with CHOP or R-CHOP. (C, D) OS (C) and PFS (D) of patients treated with CHOP or R-CHOP in GCB subgroup. (E, F) OS (E) and PFS (F) of patients treated with CHOP or R-CHOP in non-GCB subgroup. OS, overall survival; PFS, progression-free survival; GCB, germinal center B-cell.

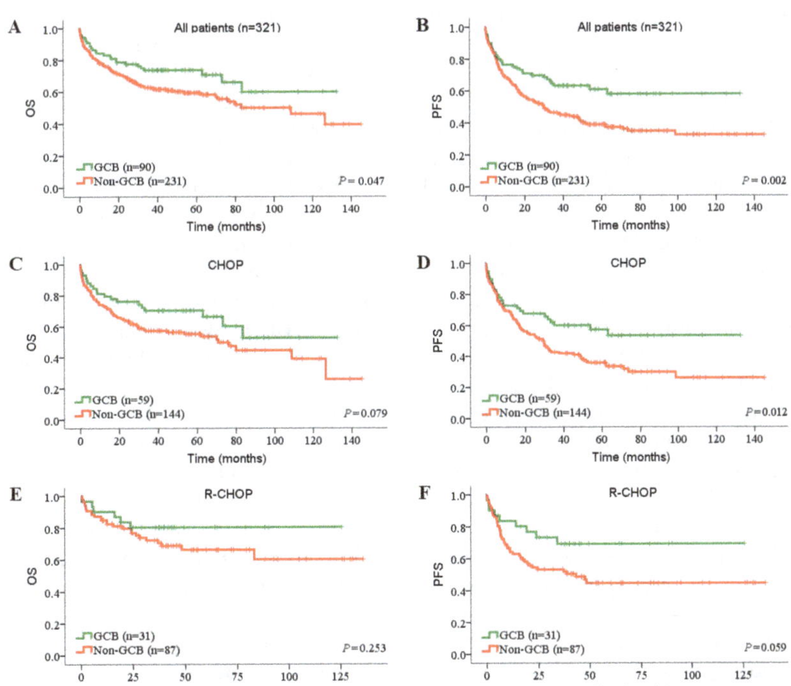

Figure 7. Prognostic impact of immunohistochemical subtypes in DLBCL risk-stratified according to treatments. (A, B) OS (A) and PFS (B) of all patients with GCB subtype or non-GCB subtype. (C, D) OS (C) and PFS (D) of CHOP-treated patients with GCB subtype or non-GCB subtype. (E, F) OS (E) and PFS (F) of R-CHOP-treated patients with GCB subtype or non-GCB subtype. OS, overall survival; PFS, progression-free survival; GCB, germinal center B-cell.

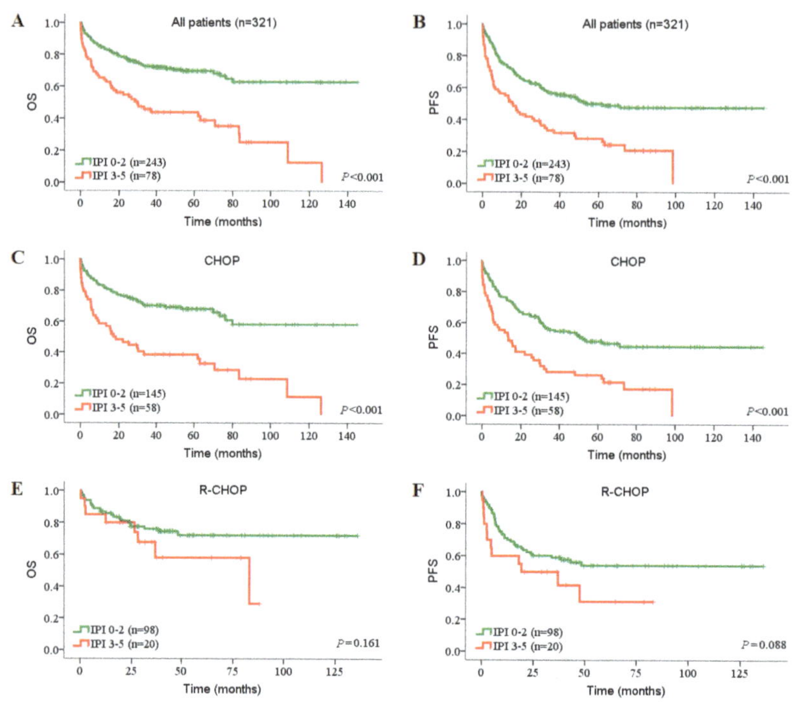

Figure 8. Prognostic impact of IPI in DLBCL risk-stratified according to treatments. (A, B) OS (A) and PFS (B) of all patients with IPI 0–2 or IPI 3–5. (C, D) OS (C) and PFS (D) of CHOP-treated patients with IPI 0–2 or IPI 3–5. (E, F) OS (E) and PFS (F) of R-CHOP-treated patients with IPI 0–2 or IPI 3–5. OS, overall survival; PFS, progression-free survival; IPI, International Prognostic Index.

indicated that addition of rituximab to standard chemotherapy eliminates the prognostic value of immunohistochemical subgroups (GCB and non-GCB), IPI, BCL2 protein, and BCL2/BCL6 DHS, but enhances the prognostic value of Ki67 in DLBCL.

We here have demonstrated that the analysis of MYC, BCL2 and BCL6 protein expression by IHC is feasible on TMAs in a highly reliable and reproducible manner. High DHSs and THS were associated with many high-risk clinicopathologic features, including high LDH level, poor performance status, advanced stage of disease, multiple extranodal sites of involvement, and high IPI score. Approximately one-third of DLBCL demonstrate MYC/BCL2 DHS 2, in keeping with the 29% and 28% frequency reported by Green et al [16] and Hu et al [29], respectively. By contrast, DHL characterized chromosomal translocations involving *MYC*, *BCL6* and *BCL2* is a rare disease, representing approximately 5% of all DLBCL cases in our study, indicating that, in addition to translocations, protein expression could be regulated by other mechanisms including other types of rearrangements, amplifications, mutation, or by miRNA-dependant mechanisms [30–32]. Thus, the findings in this study expand the spectrum of DLBCL, defined at the genetic level, by using IHC.

A number of investigators have attempted to use the immunohistochemical expression patterns as prognostic indicators in DLBCL [33,34]. Hans et al. reported that a combination of CD10, BCL6 and MUM1 expression could subdivide DLBCL patients into long- and short-term survivors [8]. However, contradictory results have been reported on the prognostic role of the Hans classifier [9,10,35]. Although non-GCB subgroup was correlated with inferior 5-year OS and PFS in BLBCL, when stratified by treatment non-GCB was only correlated inferior 5-year PFS in the CHOP cohort. Furthermore, non-GCB was not an independent survival predictor for DLBCL patients treated with CHOP, indicating that such algorithm was not a stable survival predictor for DLBCL especially for R-CHOP-treated patients. Consistent with previous reports [10,12,36,37], Chinese patients with DLBCL in our series had a much lower incidence of GCB subtype compared with those reported on Western populations [23,37,38]. These data support the notion that immunophenotypic subgroups in DLBCL vary according to the geographic factor.

Translocations of *MYC*, *BCL2* and *BCL6* in DLBCL have been consistently reported. Although the prognostic impact of *BCL2* and *BCL6* translocations has been disputed [13,15,22,39], there is consensus that *MYC* translocation is a worse prognostic marker in patients with DLBCL treated CHOP, both in combination with and without rituximab [4,17,40]. In our study, univariate and multivariate analyses disclosed that breaks in *MYC* and *BCL6*, as well as fusion in *BCL2* had no impact on survival in CHOP or R-CHOP cohorts.

In our study, *BCL6* breaks and *IGH/BCL2* fusion were observed in 20.0% and 11.1% of Chinese DLBCL cohort, respectively. While in Western cohorts, t(3;14)(q27;q32) involving *BCL6* and t(14;18)(q32;q21) involving IGH and *BCL2* have been found in 20–40% and 20–30%, respectively [15,41]. Consistent with previous studies [14,36,42], the incidence of *BCL-6* break and *IGH/BCL2* fusion were lower in DLBCL in Chinese population compared with Western populations. Similar to what has been previously described [43], we have found a higher frequency of *BCL6* translocations in non-GCB subgroup (25%) than in GCB subgroup (13%). In non-GCB subgroup, BCL6 translocations correlated significantly with high BCL6 expression level. However high BCL6 expression is more common in GCB subgroup, indicating that there may be other molecular mechanisms causing BCL6 over-expression in GCB subgroup. Relocation of an IGH transcriptional enhancer next to the BCL2 gene as a result of the t(14;18) translocation is thought to cause constitutive over-expression of BCL2 protein. In this study, high BCL2 expression showed correlation with *IGH/BCL2* fusion in GCB subgroup but not no correlation with *IGH/BCL2* fusion in GCB subgroup, indicating that BCL2 overexpression in GCB may be due to t(14;18) and in non-GCB is due to other molecular mechanisms. These findings suggest that GCB and non-GCB DLBCL subgroups are two different disease in molecular mechanisms causing the abnormal protein expression. Besides, the low incidence of *IGH/BCL2* fusion in Chinese cohort compared to the Western cohorts may be the possible reason for the lower incidence of GCB-DLBCL in China.

Moreover, our study demonstrate that immunostaining for MYC, BCL2 and BCL6, with the optimal cut off of 90%, 70% and 20%, predict the presence of *MYC* breaks, *IGH/BCL2* fusion and *BCL6* breaks as detected by FISH in DLBCL with high specificity (>90%). Therefore, all patients with protein aberrant expression should be tested for corresponding gene translocation by FISH. Our findings that high MYC and BCL2 protein expression predict gene translocations are consistent with previous studies [31,36]. However, Akyurek et al. reported that the level of BCL6 protein expression is not correlated with the presence or absence of *BCL6* rearrangement [22]. Different staining and scoring methodologies, cut-off values, and populations may cause this discrepancy. Although *MYC*, *BCL2* and *BCL6* translocations can be detected by FISH, FISH fails to detect gene deregulation caused by mechanisms other than translocation [4]. The availability of monoclonal antibodies that target the MYC, BCL2 and BCL6 protein, respectively, has been shown to predict the corresponding gene rearrangements by our and other independent groups and has been validated for use FFPE tissues [44], allowing for the study of large series of archived DLBCL samples for the protein expressions by IHC.

In conclusion, we show DHL in our series is a rare event and dose not predict survival in Chinese DLBCL, NOS. We confirm that DLBCL with high DHSs or THS characterize a subset of DLBCL patients with high-risk clinicopathologic features and inferior survival. Importantly, we report for the first time that high DHSs and THS are poor prognostic predictors independent of the IPI factor in the Chinese cohort that consisted of R-CHOP-treated patients and CHOP-treated patients. We further show that the incidence of non-GCB subtype in our series is higher than that in the Western populations reported by previous studies, and non-GCB subgroup is not a stable survival predictor for DLBCL, especially for R-CHOP-treated patients. Immunostaining for MYC, BCL2 and BCL6 proved to be an excellent test with high specificity (>90%) for the presence of *MYC* breaks, *IGH/BCL2* fusion and *BCL6* breaks as detected by FISH. Our data together suggest that the combinations of MYC, BCL2 and BCL6 protein expression assessed by IHC are reliable prognostic predictors and could be used in the future as prognostic markers for stratification of patients with DLBCL for novel therapies.

Supporting Information

Figure S1 Representative FISH analysis of *MYC*, *BCL2* and *BCL6* rearrangements in diffuse large B-cell lymphoma (DLBCL). (A) Split signals (orange and green) demonstrating presence of *MYC* break, and (C) *BCL6* break. Fusion signals (orange/green fusion) demonstrating presence of *IGH/BCL2* fusion. (A-C original magnification, ×1000). FISH, fluorescence *in situ* hybridization.

Figure S2 Prognostic impact of DHL in DLBCL. (A) OS and (B) PFS of patients with DHL, other patients without DHL (non-DHL), non-DHL with THS 0/1, and non-DHL with THS 2/3. OS, overall survival; PFS, progression-free survival; DHL, double-hit lymphoma; THS, triple-hit score.

Table S1 Immunohistochemical assays and methods.

Table S2 Gene translocation versus immunohistochemical subgroup comparison.

Table S3 Patient clinical and immunophenotypical characteristics of patients with DLBCL, NOS based on DHL status or THS.

Table S4 Diagnostic performance of protein candidates for gene translocations in DLBCL, NOS based on ROC curves analysis.

Table S5 Correlation between MYC protein expression and *MYC* break in DLBCL, NOS patients.

Table S6 Correlation between BCL6 protein expression and *BCL6* break in DLBCL, NOS patients.

Table S7 Correlation between BCL2 protein expression and *BCL2* break in DLBCL, NOS patients.

Author Contributions

Conceived and designed the experiments: YL LY. Performed the experiments: LY DL XL JC JX FZ YC. Analyzed the data: LY YL HZ DL. Contributed reagents/materials/analysis tools: FZ YC. Contributed to the writing of the manuscript: LY YL.

References

1. Krol AD, le Cessie S, Snijder S, Kluin-Nelemans JC, Kluin PM, et al. (2003) Primary extranodal non-Hodgkin's lymphoma (NHL): the impact of alternative definitions tested in the Comprehensive Cancer Centre West population-based NHL registry. Ann Oncol 14: 131–139.
2. Li XQ, Li GD, Gao ZF, Zhou XG, Zhu XZ (2011) The relative frequencies of lymphoma subtypes in China:a nationwide study of 10002 cases by the Chinese Lymphoma Study Group. Ann Oncol 22: iv141.
3. Ziepert M, Hasenclever D, Kuhnt E, Glass B, Schmitz N, et al. (2010) Standard International prognostic index remains a valid predictor of outcome for patients with aggressive CD20+ B-cell lymphoma in the rituximab era. J Clin Oncol 28: 2373–2380.
4. Pfreundschuh M (2012) Growing importance of MYC/BCL2 immunohistochemistry in diffuse large B-cell lymphomas. J Clin Oncol 30: 3433–3435.
5. Alizadeh AA, Eisen MB, Davis RE, Ma C, Lossos IS, et al. (2000) Distinct types of diffuse large B-cell lymphoma identified by gene expression profiling. Nature 403: 503–511.
6. Rosenwald A, Wright G, Chan WC, Connors JM, Campo E, et al. (2002) The use of molecular profiling to predict survival after chemotherapy for diffuse large-B-cell lymphoma. N Engl J Med 346: 1937–1947.
7. Hussain AR, Uddin S, Ahmed M, Al-Dayel F, Bavi PP, et al. (2013) Phosphorylated IkappaBalpha predicts poor prognosis in activated B-cell lymphoma and its inhibition with thymoquinone induces apoptosis via ROS release. PLoS One 8: e60540.
8. Hans CP, Weisenburger DD, Greiner TC, Gascoyne RD, Delabie J, et al. (2004) Confirmation of the molecular classification of diffuse large B-cell lymphoma by immunohistochemistry using a tissue microarray. Blood 103: 275–282.

9. Gutierrez-Garcia G, Cardesa-Salzmann T, Climent F, Gonzalez-Barca E, Mercadal S, et al. (2011) Gene-expression profiling and not immunophenotypic algorithms predicts prognosis in patients with diffuse large B-cell lymphoma treated with immunochemotherapy. Blood 117: 4836–4843.
10. Toda H, Sato Y, Takata K, Orita Y, Asano N, et al. (2013) Clinicopathologic analysis of localized nasal/paranasal diffuse large B-cell lymphoma. PLoS One 8: e57677.
11. Swerdlow SH, Campo E, Harris NL, Jaffe ES, Pileri SA, et al. (2008) WHO Classification of Tumours of Haematopoietic and Lymphoid Tissues: Lyon, France, IARC Press.
12. Shiozawa E, Yamochi-Onizuka T, Takimoto M, Ota H (2007) The GCB subtype of diffuse large B-cell lymphoma is less frequent in Asian countries. Leuk Res 31: 1579–1583.
13. Klapper W, Stoecklein H, Zeynalova S, Ott G, Kosari F, et al. (2008) Structural aberrations affecting the MYC locus indicate a poor prognosis independent of clinical risk factors in diffuse large B-cell lymphomas treated within randomized trials of the German High-Grade Non-Hodgkin's Lymphoma Study Group (DSHNHL). Leukemia 22: 2226–2229.
14. Chen PM, Yang MH, Yu IT, Lin JT, Lin YC, et al. (2002) Low incidence of BCL-6 gene alterations for diffuse large B-cell lymphomas in Taiwan Chinese. Cancer 94: 2635–2644.
15. Horn H, Ziepert M, Becher C, Barth TF, Bernd HW, et al. (2013) MYC status in concert with BCL2 and BCL6 expression predicts outcome in diffuse large B-cell lymphoma. Blood 121: 2253–2263.
16. Green TM, Young KH, Visco C, Xu-Monette ZY, Orazi A, et al. (2012) Immunohistochemical double-hit score is a strong predictor of outcome in patients with diffuse large B-cell lymphoma treated with rituximab plus cyclophosphamide, doxorubicin, vincristine, and prednisone. J Clin Oncol 30: 3460–3467.
17. Savage KJ, Johnson NA, Ben-Neriah S, Connors JM, Sehn LH, et al. (2009) MYC gene rearrangements are associated with a poor prognosis in diffuse large B-cell lymphoma patients treated with R-CHOP chemotherapy. Blood 114: 3533–3537.
18. Feugier P, Van Hoof A, Sebban C, Solal-Celigny P, Bouabdallah R, et al. (2005) Long-term results of the R-CHOP study in the treatment of elderly patients with diffuse large B-cell lymphoma: a study by the Groupe d'Etude des Lymphomes de l'Adulte. J Clin Oncol 23: 4117–4126.
19. Lu HY, Song LX (2012) [Impact of immunochemotherapy on prognostic factors in diffuse large B-cell lymphoma patients]. Zhongguo Shi Yan Xue Ye Xue Za Zhi 20: 315–319.
20. Huang Y, Ye S, Cao Y, Li Z, Huang J, et al. (2012) Outcome of R-CHOP or CHOP regimen for germinal center and nongerminal center subtypes of diffuse large B-cell lymphoma of Chinese patients. ScientificWorldJournal 2012: 897178.
21. Xia ZG, Xu ZZ, Zhao WL, Zhao SQ, Ding F, et al. (2010) The prognostic value of immunohistochemical subtyping in Chinese patients with de novo diffuse large B-cell lymphoma undergoing CHOP or R-CHOP treatment. Ann Hematol 89: 171–177.
22. Akyurek N, Uner A, Benekli M, Barista I (2012) Prognostic significance of MYC, BCL2, and BCL6 rearrangements in patients with diffuse large B-cell lymphoma treated with cyclophosphamide, doxorubicin, vincristine, and prednisone plus rituximab. Cancer 118: 4173–4183.
23. Perry AM, Alvarado-Bernal Y, Laurini JA, Smith LM, Slack GW, et al. (2014) MYC and BCL2 protein expression predicts survival in patients with diffuse large B-cell lymphoma treated with rituximab. Br J Haematol.
24. Iqbal J, Greiner TC, Patel K, Dave BJ, Smith L, et al. (2007) Distinctive patterns of BCL6 molecular alterations and their functional consequences in different subgroups of diffuse large B-cell lymphoma. Leukemia 21: 2332–2343.
25. Kluk MJ, Chapuy B, Sinha P, Roy A, Dal Cin P, et al. (2012) Immunohistochemical detection of MYC-driven diffuse large B-cell lymphomas. PLoS One 7: e33813.
26. Visco C, Tzankov A, Xu-Monette ZY, Miranda RN, Tai YC, et al. (2013) Patients with diffuse large B-cell lymphoma of germinal center origin with BCL2 translocations have poor outcome, irrespective of MYC status: a report from an International DLBCL rituximab-CHOP Consortium Program Study. Haematologica 98: 255–263.
27. Thompson RC, Vardinogiannis I, Gilmore TD (2013) The sensitivity of diffuse large B-Cell lymphoma cell lines to histone deacetylase inhibitor-induced apoptosis is modulated by BCL-2 family protein activity. PLoS One 8: e62822.
28. Johnson NA, Slack GW, Savage KJ, Connors JM, Ben-Neriah S, et al. (2012) Concurrent expression of MYC and BCL2 in diffuse large B-cell lymphoma treated with rituximab plus cyclophosphamide, doxorubicin, vincristine, and prednisone. J Clin Oncol 30: 3452–3459.
29. Hu S, Xu-Monette ZY, Tzankov A, Green T, Wu L, et al. (2013) MYC/BCL2 protein coexpression contributes to the inferior survival of activated B-cell subtype of diffuse large B-cell lymphoma and demonstrates high-risk gene expression signatures: a report from The International DLBCL Rituximab-CHOP Consortium Program. Blood 121: 4021–4031; quiz 4250.
30. Valentino C, Kendrick S, Johnson N, Gascoyne R, Chan WC, et al. (2013) Colorimetric in situ hybridization identifies MYC gene signal clusters correlating with increased copy number, mRNA, and protein in diffuse large B-cell lymphoma. Am J Clin Pathol 139: 242–254.
31. Green TM, Nielsen O, de Stricker K, Xu-Monette ZY, Young KH, et al. (2012) High levels of nuclear MYC protein predict the presence of MYC rearrangement in diffuse large B-cell lymphoma. Am J Surg Pathol 36: 612–619.
32. Leucci E, Cocco M, Onnis A, De Falco G, van Cleef P, et al. (2008) MYC translocation-negative classical Burkitt lymphoma cases: an alternative pathogenetic mechanism involving miRNA deregulation. J Pathol 216: 440–450.
33. de Jong D, Rosenwald A, Chhanabhai M, Gaulard P, Klapper W, et al. (2007) Immunohistochemical prognostic markers in diffuse large B-cell lymphoma: validation of tissue microarray as a prerequisite for broad clinical applications–a study from the Lunenburg Lymphoma Biomarker Consortium. J Clin Oncol 25: 805–812.
34. Veelken H, Vik Dannheim S, Schulte Moenting J, Martens UM, Finke J, et al. (2007) Immunophenotype as prognostic factor for diffuse large B-cell lymphoma in patients undergoing clinical risk-adapted therapy. Ann Oncol 18: 931–939.
35. Mitchell KA, Finn WG, Owens SR (2008) Differences in germinal centre and non-germinal center phenotype in gastric and intestinal diffuse large B-cell lymphomas. Leuk Lymphoma 49: 1717–1723.
36. Chen Y, Han T, Iqbal J, Irons R, Chan WC, et al. (2010) Diffuse large B-cell lymphoma in Chinese patients: immunophenotypic and cytogenetic analyses of 124 cases. Am J Clin Pathol 133: 305–313.
37. Chen Z, Du Z, Chen J, Chen Z, Bao Y, et al. (2011) Prognostic evaluation of immunohistochemical profiles in diffuse large B-cell lymphoma: a Chinese study. Med Oncol 28: 241–248.
38. Gupta M, Maurer MJ, Wellik LE, Law ME, Han JJ, et al. (2012) Expression of Myc, but not pSTAT3, is an adverse prognostic factor for diffuse large B-cell lymphoma treated with epratuzumab/R-CHOP. Blood 120: 4400–4406.
39. van Imhoff GW, Boerma EJ, van der Holt B, Schuuring E, Verdonck LF, et al. (2006) Prognostic impact of germinal center-associated proteins and chromosomal breakpoints in poor-risk diffuse large B-cell lymphoma. J Clin Oncol 24: 4135–4142.
40. Barrans S, Crouch S, Smith A, Turner K, Owen R, et al. (2010) Rearrangement of MYC is associated with poor prognosis in patients with diffuse large B-cell lymphoma treated in the era of rituximab. J Clin Oncol 28: 3360–3365.
41. Hummel M, Bentink S, Berger H, Klapper W, Wessendorf S, et al. (2006) A biologic definition of Burkitt's lymphoma from transcriptional and genomic profiling. N Engl J Med 354: 2419–2430.
42. Biagi JJ, Seymour JF (2002) Insights into the molecular pathogenesis of follicular lymphoma arising from analysis of geographic variation. Blood 99: 4265–4275.
43. Chen YW, Hu XT, Liang AC, Au WY, So CC, et al. (2006) High BCL6 expression predicts better prognosis, independent of BCL6 translocation status, translocation partner, or BCL6-deregulating mutations, in gastric lymphoma. Blood 108: 2373–2383.
44. Gurel B, Iwata T, Koh CM, Jenkins RB, Lan F, et al. (2008) Nuclear MYC protein overexpression is an early alteration in human prostate carcinogenesis. Mod Pathol 21: 1156–1167.

8

The Deficiency of Tumor Suppressor *Prep1* Accelerates the Onset of *Meis1- Hoxa9* Leukemogenesis

Leila Dardaei, Livia Modica, Giorgio Iotti, Francesco Blasi*

Fondazione Istituto FIRC di Oncologia Molecolare (IFOM), Milan, Italy

Abstract

Prep1 and Meis1 ortholog TALE transcription factors have opposing roles in tumorigenesis: *Meis1* serves as an oncogene, Prep1 as a tumor suppressor. We now report that, *Meis1* overexpression in primary *Prep1*-deficient (*Prep1*$^{i/i}$) embryonic hematopoietic cells increases self-renewal potential of cells *in vitro* but not *in vivo*, whereas leukemia is instead obtained when *Meis1* is combined with another oncogene, *HoxA9*. *Prep1*$^{i/i}$ *Meis1-HoxA9*-generated leukemic cells are less differentiated and grow more aggressively after the second passage in the mouse. These data indicate that *Prep1* represents a barrier to the transforming activity of *Meis1 in vitro*, but its absence is not sufficient to induce early leukemogenesis. On the other hand, the *Prep1*$^{i/i}$ background appears to favor the insurgence of mutations that cause a more aggressive *Meis1-HoxA9*-generated leukemia. Indeed, the *Prep1*$^{i/i}$ leukemic cells upregulate the Polycomb protein Bmi-1 and expectedly down-regulate the *Ink4a/Arf* locus products. Finally, an important feature contributed by the *Prep1*$^{i/i}$ background is the post-transcriptional increase in Meis1 protein level.

Editor: Antimo Migliaccio, II Università di Napoli, Italy

Funding: Leila Dardaei was supported by FUV (Fondazione Umberto Veronesi) fellowship. This work was supported by grants from AIRC (Italian Association for Cancer Research), Cariplo, and the Italian Ministry of Health to FB. The funders had no role in study design, data collection and analysis, decision to publish or preparation of the manuscript.

Competing Interests: The authors have declared that no competing interests exist.

* E-mail: francesco.blasi@ifom.eu

Introduction

Prep1 (Pbx-regulating protein 1) and Meis1 (Myeloid ecotropic insertion site 1) are ortholog TALE (three amino acids loop extension) homeodomain transcription factors that competitively interact with the Hox co-factor Pbx (pre-B-cell leukemia homeobox) and with Hox proteins [1,2], but play opposite roles in tumorigenesis. In primary hematopoietic progenitors, *Meis1* overexpression is unable on its own to transform, but cooperates in the oncogenic activity by accelerating *HoxA9*-induced leukemia [3,4]. On the other hand, in immortalized mouse embryo fibroblasts, *Meis1* alone is able to transform but only in the absence of *Prep1* [5].

Prep1 exerts a tumor suppressive function in mice and man [6]. In fact, 40% of the few hypomorphic *Prep1*$^{i/i}$ mutant mice (expressing 3–10% of the protein) that survive embryonic lethality [7], develop tumors or pretumoral lesions at late stages in life [6]. In addition, *Prep1* haploinsufficiency (*Prep1*$^{+/-}$) sharply accelerates the death rate of *EμMyc* transgenic mice [8]. Finally, a large percent of human tumors expresses no or reduced Prep1 [6].

Hox homeodomain-containing transcription factors are involved in normal hematopoiesis and leukemogenesis [9,10,11,12]. Their DNA-binding selectivity and specificity is very limited, but is increased by the interaction with Pbx, Meis and Prep cofactors [1,13,14]. *Hox* genes promote leukemogenesis by either overexpression or forming chimeric proteins by fusing with other genes [15,16,17,18]. In particular, *HoxA9* is a key regulator of hematopoiesis that has oncogenic functions in leukemogenesis [12]. Its overexpression directly induces leukemia after a long latency [19]. However, *HoxA9* selective collaboration with *Meis1*, but not with *Prep1*, drastically lowers the latency of acute myeloid leukemia (AML) onset in mice [19]. *HOXA9* and *MEIS1* are also expressed in more than 80% of human AML and their expression level is correlated with poor prognosis [20,21].

Here, we have studied the impact of *Prep1* genotype on *Meis1-HoxA9* induced transformation of hematopoietic cells and subsequent AML induction in mice. We show that, *Meis1* on its own is unable to induce leukemia in primary fetal liver (FL) cells hypomorphic for *Prep1 expression* (*Prep1*$^{i/i}$). However, the absence of *Prep1* favors the *in vitro* immortalization and self-renewal of FL cells induced by *Meis1* or *HoxA9*, whereas *in vivo* it accelerates the rate of appearance of *Meis1-HoxA9*-induced AML but only after two passages in the mouse. As also shown in transformed *Prep1*$^{i/i}$ MEFs [5], the *Prep1*$^{i/i}$ phenotype leads to increased Meis1 protein level in leukemic cells through a post-transcriptional mechanism. Moreover, *Prep1*$^{i/i}$ leukemic cells upregulate Polycomb protein Bmi-1, which results in a decreased expression of Ink4a/Arf cell cycle regulators, p16^{Ink4a} and p19^{Arf}, which are known to regulate stem cell potential and proliferation [22]. Overall, the absence of *Prep1* induces a more aggressive leukemia, which may depend on its tumor suppressive function that is based on preventing DNA damage accumulation [23]. Moreover, the less differentiated and highly proliferative phenotypes of *Prep1*$^{i/i}$ leukemias may result from the upregulation of Meis1.

Results

Meis1 Overexpression in the Absence of Prep1 Induces Serial Transplantation Activity of Mouse Fetal Liver Cells

To determine whether *Prep1* can exert a tumor suppressive role in leukemia induction, we first compared the transformation rate of *Prep1*$^{i/i}$ and WT fetal liver (FL) cells overexpressing the oncogenic *Meis1* **(Figure 1A)**. E14.5 *Prep1*$^{i/i}$ and WT FL cells were retrovirally transduced with *Meis1*-GFP and sorted by FACS (fluorescence-activated cell sorting) for GFP expression. The GFP positive cells were then plated in methylcellulose **(Figure 1A)**. The ability of FL cells to successfully proliferate and form colonies in methylcellulose upon serial transplantations is normally used to define neoplastic transformation in hematopoietic cells [24]. Serial plating in methylcellulose showed that *Meis1*-overexpression induced self-renewal capacity *in vitro* in *Prep1*$^{i/i}$, but not in WT FL cells **(Figure 1B)**, an indication of immortalization and neoplastic transformation [24].

When FL cells were transduced with the *HoxA9* oncogene and selected with puromycin, both *Prep1*$^{i/i}$ and WT cells were capable of inducing sustained replating, although the efficiency was higher with *Prep1*$^{i/i}$ cells **(Figure 1C)**. When both *Meis1* and *HoxA9* oncogenes were used, both *Prep1*$^{i/i}$ and WT cell were capable of inducing sustained replating **(Figure 1D)** and again the efficiency was higher with *Prep1*$^{i/i}$ cells. Thus the absence of *Prep1* is sufficient to induce self-renewal capacity in primary hematopoietic cells. In addition, the absence of *Prep1* appeared to increase the efficacy of both *HoxA9* and of the *Meis1* and *HoxA9* combination.

The Prep1$^{i/i}$ Mutation Provides a Genetic Background that Causes a More Aggressive Leukemic Phenotype Upon Transformation with Meis1 and HoxA9

Since *Prep1* exerts a tumor suppressive function [6], we tested whether the absence of *Prep1* would allow *Meis1* to induce AML *in vivo* without *HoxA9* overexpression. As shown in **Figure 1E** *Meis1* overexpression in either *Prep1*$^{i/i}$ or WT cells was unable to

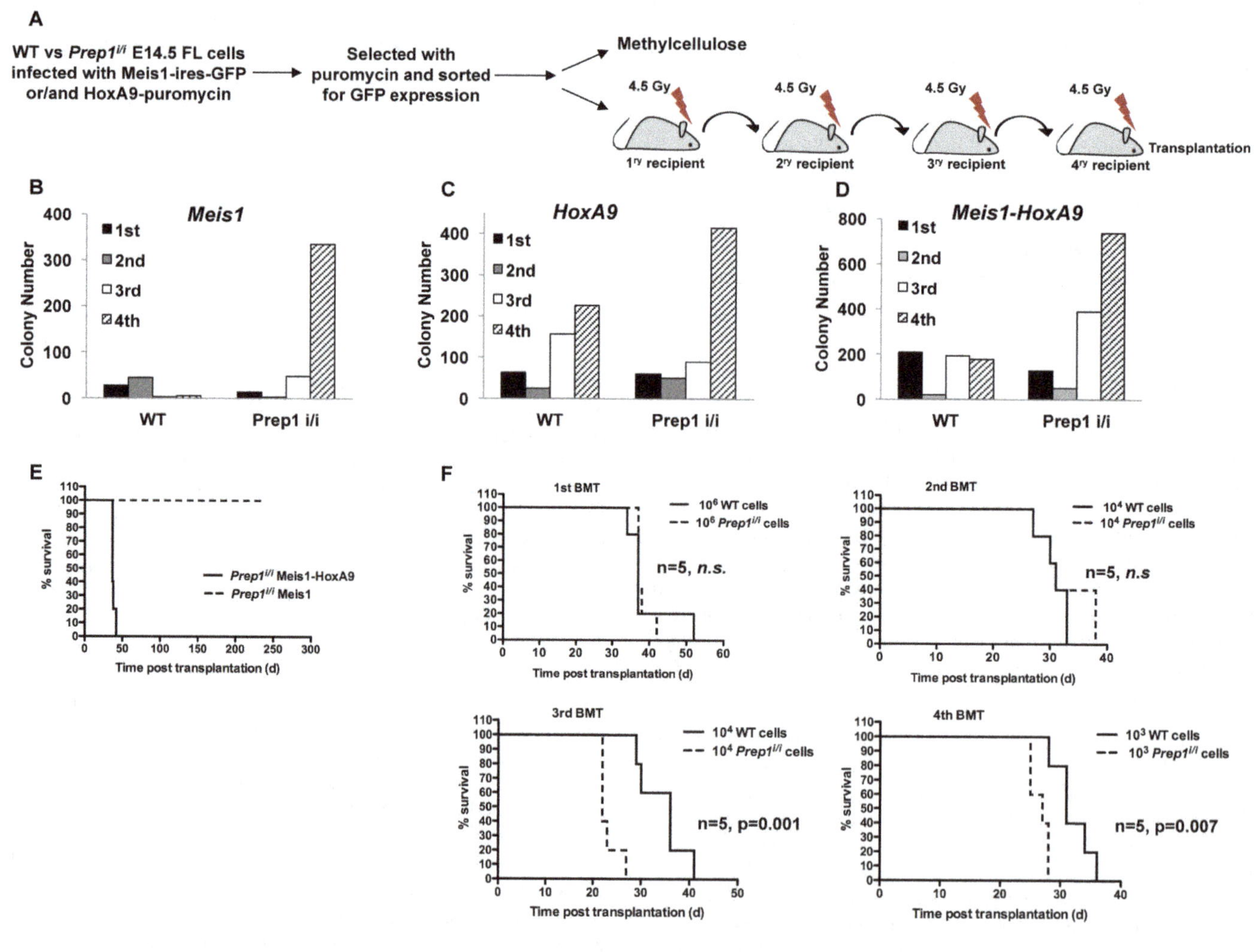

Figure 1. *Prep1* absence accelerates *Meis1-HoxA9* induced myeloid transformation and leukemogenesis. (**A**) Overview of the experimental strategy. FL cells taken from 14.5 WT or *Prep1*$^{i/i}$ embryos were transduced with *Meis1* (**B**) or *HoxA9* (**C**) or co-transduced with both oncogenes (**D**) and serially plated in methylcellulose cultures every 7day. Results are shown as colony numbers per 5×10^4 plated cells for each round of culture. (**E**) Survival curves are shown for cohorts of mice transplanted with 1×10^6 of *Prep1*$^{i/i}$ FL cells transduced with either *Meis1* or *Meis1-HoxA9*. Five mice for each group were used. (**F**) Survival curves are shown for cohorts of mice serially transplanted with the indicated numbers of WT or *Prep1*$^{i/i}$ FL cells co-transduced with *Meis1* and *HoxA9*. Five mice per group were used. In the 1st and 2nd Bone marrow transplantation (BMT), the difference between the survival of the mice transplanted with either WT or *Prep1*$^{i/i}$ transduced cells was not significant (n.s.). However, in the 3rd and 4th BMTs the p-values of mice survival transplanted with either WT or *Prep1*$^{i/i}$ transduced cells were significant ($p = 0.001$ and $p = 0.007$, respectively).

induce AML in mice. Thus the absence of *Prep1* is sufficient to induce *Meis1*-dependent self-renewal *in vitro*, but not AML *in vivo*.

We then tested the role of the *Prep1* genotype on the leukemogenic potential of *Meis1-HoxA9* combination. Regardless of the *Prep1*$^{i/i}$ or WT genotype, *Meis1-HoxA9*-transduced FL cells induced AML with a similar latency in the primary recipients (**Figure 1F**). We then serially transferred the leukemia by transplanting bone marrow (BM) cells. Upon the third bone marrow transplantation (BMT), *Prep1*$^{i/i}$ cells promoted AML in recipient mice about 30% earlier than WT cells (**Figure 1F**) and this property was maintained in subsequent transplantations.

The fact that *Prep1*$^{i/i}$ cells induced AML acceleration only after the second transplantation indicates that *Prep1*-deficient cells acquire an aggressive phenotype with the time, probably because of the accumulation of further genetic or epigenetic events. This is in agreement with a primary defect of *Prep1*$^{i/i}$ cells to maintain genomic stability [23].

The Level of Meis1 Protein in Meis1-HoxA9-transduced Cells is Higher in Prep1-deficent than in WT Cells

Prep1 overexpression decreases Meis1 half-life in mouse embryonic fibroblasts, and hence reduces its protein level by competing for Pbx1 [5]. To test whether an opposite effect takes place in leukemic cells lacking Prep1, we measured the percent and the signal intensity of GFP-positive cells in *Prep1*$^{i/i}$ and WT leukemic BM cells of serially transplanted mice. Since *Meis1* is GFP-tagged the percent of GFP-positive cells and the intensity of the signal represent the frequency and the level of Meis1 in these cells, respectively. The percent of Meis1-GFP positive cells was identical in the two genotypes, indicating equal transduction efficiency in the *Prep1*$^{i/i}$ and WT cells (**Figure 2A**). However, a clear difference between the two genotypes was observed in terms of *Meis1*-GFP signal intensity (**Figure 2C**). Meis1-GFP mean fluorescence intensity, and hence Meis1 protein level, was significantly higher in *Prep1*$^{i/i}$ cells compared to WT (**Figure 2D**). Moreover, we also checked the FLAG-Meis1 protein level by immuno-blotting, and found it to be higher in the *Prep1*$^{i/i}$ leukemic than in WT cells (**Figure 2E**). However, the *Meis1* mRNA expression level measured by qRT-PCR did not show any significant difference between *Prep1*$^{i/i}$ and WT leukemic cells (**Figure 2F**). Overall these results suggest that, like in MEFs, the absence of *Prep1* in hematopoietic cells leads to stabilization of Meis1 with subsequent increase of its protein level.

The Prep1$^{i/i}$ Mutation causes a Less Differentiated and Highly Proliferative Meis1-HoxA9-dependent Leukemias

Flow cytometric immunophenotyping of the leukemias arisen in two sets of mice transplanted with WT or *Prep1*$^{i/i}$ *Meis1-HoxA9*-transduced cells, demonstrated that they all were donor-derived as about 90% of the cells expressed GFP (**Figure 2A**) and displayed Mac-1 and Gr-1 myeloid cell surface antigens (**Figure 2B**). However, *Prep1*$^{i/i}$ leukemias were less differentiated than WT, exhibiting a higher percent of c-Kit-positive cells (**Figure 3A**) and a higher frequency of c-Kit and Gr-1 co-expressing cells (**Figure 3B**). The less differentiated phenotype of *Prep1*$^{i/i}$ leukemic bone marrow cells was not limited to the primary recipient but was constantly observed in secondary and tertiary recipients (**Figure 3A and 3B**).

The difference between differentiation states of *Prep1*$^{i/i}$ and WT leukemic cells might be both a direct and indirect effect of the absence of Prep1. Indeed, the increased c-Kit expression might be consequent to the higher Meis1 expression induced by the absence of *Prep1*, since *Meis1* has been shown to quantitatively regulate the differentiation arrest of *MLL*-leukemic cells [22].

A direct comparison of the cell cycle profiles of *Prep1*$^{i/i}$ and WT leukemic BM cells induced by *Meis1-HoxA9* showed that more *Prep1*$^{i/i}$ leukemic cells accumulated in S/G2/M than WT, whereas their number was reduced in G0–G1 (**Figure 4A**). These differences became more evident in the second and third transplantation (**Figure 4A**). We have therefore measured the level of various cell cycle regulators in leukemic cells coming from the two genetic backgrounds. Indeed, the higher cycling rate of *Prep1*-deficient leukemic BM cells correlated with a higher expression of the Polycomb group gene *Bmi-1* (both at the mRNA and protein level) (**Figure 4B and 4C**), which plays a profound role in cell cycle regulation and maintenance of hematopoietic and leukemic stem cells self-renewal, through transcriptional repression of the *Ink4a/Arf* locus [25]. Indeed, the high level of Bmi-1 in *Prep1*$^{i/i}$ leukemic cells correlates with a significant reduction of the p16^{Ink4a} and p19^{Arf} tumor suppressors (**Figure 4B**). The impairment of the Bmi-1/Ink4a/Arf axis may explain the less differentiated and highly cycling state of *Prep1*$^{i/i}$ leukemic cells. A direct connection between leukemic cells proliferation, *Meis1-HoxA9* and *Bmi-1* has already been established [26].

Discussion

The *Hox* genes specify cell identity in embryonic development and are involved in several adult processes including hematopoiesis. Likewise, three amino acid loop extension (TALE) proteins, the most important Hox cofactors, are essential in embryonic and adult development including hematopoiesis [12]. For instance, *Pbx1*$^{-/-}$ embryos die because of severe hematopoietic defects [27]. *Meis1*$^{-/-}$ embryos exhibit profound hemorrhage and lack megakaryocytes [28]. Both *Pbx1* and *Meis1* are required for the maintenance of long-term hematopoietic stem cells [29,30]. *Prep1* is also implicated in the maintenance of embryonic long-term repopulating hematopoietic stem cells [7] and in adult T cell lymphopoiesis [31].

Consistently, the deregulation of *Hox* and *Meis1* is associated with a number of malignancies including leukemogenesis [12]. However, the *Prep1* function in leukemogenesis is still unexplored. Here we show that in the absence of Prep1 (*Prep1*$^{i/i}$), FL cells are immortalized and transformed by *Meis1* as shown by serial replating assays *in vitro*. Why these cells do not progress to AML in mice remains to be established. In the presence of the *Prep1*$^{i/i}$ phenotype, replating efficiency of *Meis1*-transduced cells was as high as with *HoxA9* (**Figure 1B and C**), and the co-overexpression of the two oncogenes had an additive effect (**Figure 1D**).

We have previously shown in MEFs that *Prep1* inhibits *Meis1* oncogenicity by destabilizing and hence reducing its protein level [5]. Indeed, the absence of *Prep1* leads to increased *Meis1* protein also in hematopoietic cells, and this level increases in the subsequent transplantations of the leukemic cells (**Figure 2**). Increased Meis1 is bound to affect the self-renewal of transduced cells, since *Meis1* quantitatively regulates the leukemic stem cell frequency [32], and the aggressiveness of the leukemias, as Meis1 regulates the latency of *MLL* leukemias [22]. Thus it is likely that the progressively higher level of Meis1 in the serial transplantations explains the increased serial replating efficiency, and the increased oncogenic potency.

The absence of *Prep1* has a clear effect on the progression of the *Meis1-HoxA9* dependent AML. *Prep1*$^{i/i}$ AML displays a more aggressive phenotype than WT AML only after two passages in the mouse. Also this phenotype therefore can be put in connection with the increased Meis1 level. However, it may also depend on

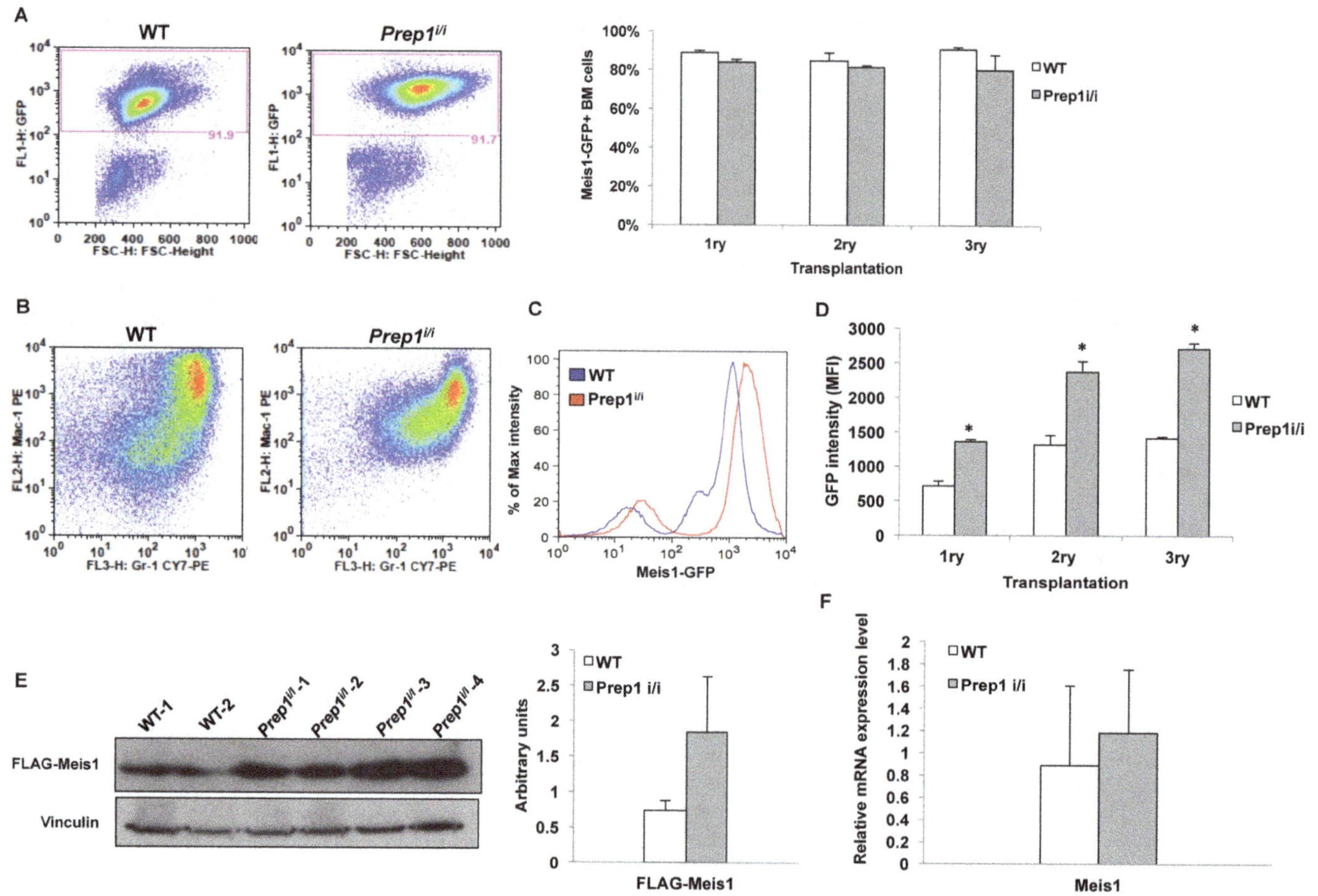

Figure 2. ***Meis1*** **expression is higher in** ***Prep1$^{i/i}$*** **leukemic cells compared to WT.** (**A**) FACS plot represent the Meis1-GFP-positive cells percent in WT and *Prep1$^{i/i}$* leukemic BM cells (left side). Bar graph shows the summary of Meis1-GFP-positive *Prep1$^{i/i}$* and WT BM cells taken from serially transplanted leukemic mice (right side). Error bars indicate SEM. (**B**) FACS plots represent the Mac-1 and Gr-1 positive cells on GFP-positive cell populations from WT and *Prep1$^{i/i}$* leukemic BM. (**C**) Representative FACS plots of Meis1-GFP expression in *Prep1$^{i/i}$* and WT leukemic BM cells co-transduced with *Meis1*-GFP and *HoxA9*. (**D**) *Meis1*-GFP mean fluorescence intensity of *Prep1$^{i/i}$* and WT BM cells taken from serially transplanted leukemic mice is shown as a graph. *p-value <0.05. Error bars indicate SEM. (**E**) 30 µg of total lysates of leukemic *Prep1$^{i/i}$* and WT BM cells was analyzed by immunoblotting using anti-FLAG antibody. Vinculin was used as loading control. Densitometric analysis was performed using ImageJ64. (**F**) Bar graph shows *Meis1* transcript level measured by real-time PCR in *Prep1$^{i/i}$* and WT leukemic bone marrow cells from serially transplanted mice. Error bars show SD.

the occurrence of novel mutations. This possibility is in line with *Prep1* being required to maintain genomic stability [23]. Novel mutations would accelerate the onset of the AML after the second bone marrow transplantation (BMT). Regardless of the number of BMTs, the leukemic cells arisen from *Prep1$^{i/i}$* *Meis1-HoxA9*-transduced cells are less differentiated and have a higher percent of cycling cells. These phenotypes become more evident with increasing serial transplantations. The absence of *Prep1* might act indirectly to affect the differentiation and proliferation of leukemic cells through the increase of Meis1 (**Figure 2**). *Meis1* positively regulates the differentiation arrest and the proliferation potential of leukemic cells [22,33]. For instance in *MLL*, *Meis1* induces cell proliferation by regulating the expression of *Bmi-1* [22] which encodes a Polycomb group epigenetic repressor protein that regulates the proliferation of normal and leukemic hematopoietic stem cells by silencing cell cycle regulators p16^{Ink4a} and p19^{Arf} [25]. We also find that the highly proliferative state of *Prep1$^{i/i}$* leukemic cells is associated with the increased expression of *Bmi-1* and the subsequent repression p16^{Ink4a} and p19^{Arf} tumor suppressors (**Figure 4B and 4C**).

The Bmi-1 repression of *INK4a/Arf* locus may explain the highly cycling status of *Prep1$^{i/i}$* leukemic cells. It remains to be established why the *Prep1$^{i/i}$*-dependent aggressiveness of *Meis1-HoxA9* leukemia appears only at a later stage.

Materials and Methods

Mice

Prep1$^{i/i}$ mice and embryos have been described [7]. Recipient mice (C57Bl6J background, which were CD45.2^{+}) were purchased from Charles River and maintained in a specific pathogen free animal facility and housed according to institutional guidelines for a maximum of 1 week before experiments were performed. All animal experiments were performed in accordance with Institutional Animal Care and Use Committee of IFOM and approved by the Italian Ministry of Health (project #110/11). All animal handlings (transplantation, sacrifice etc.,) were in accordance with the guidelines established by EU (directive 2010/63/EU).

Topical anesthesia (ELMA cream) applied to the site 30 minutes prior to intravenous injection of cells. Mice were monitored 3 times per week for three weeks. Starting from 4th week, they were

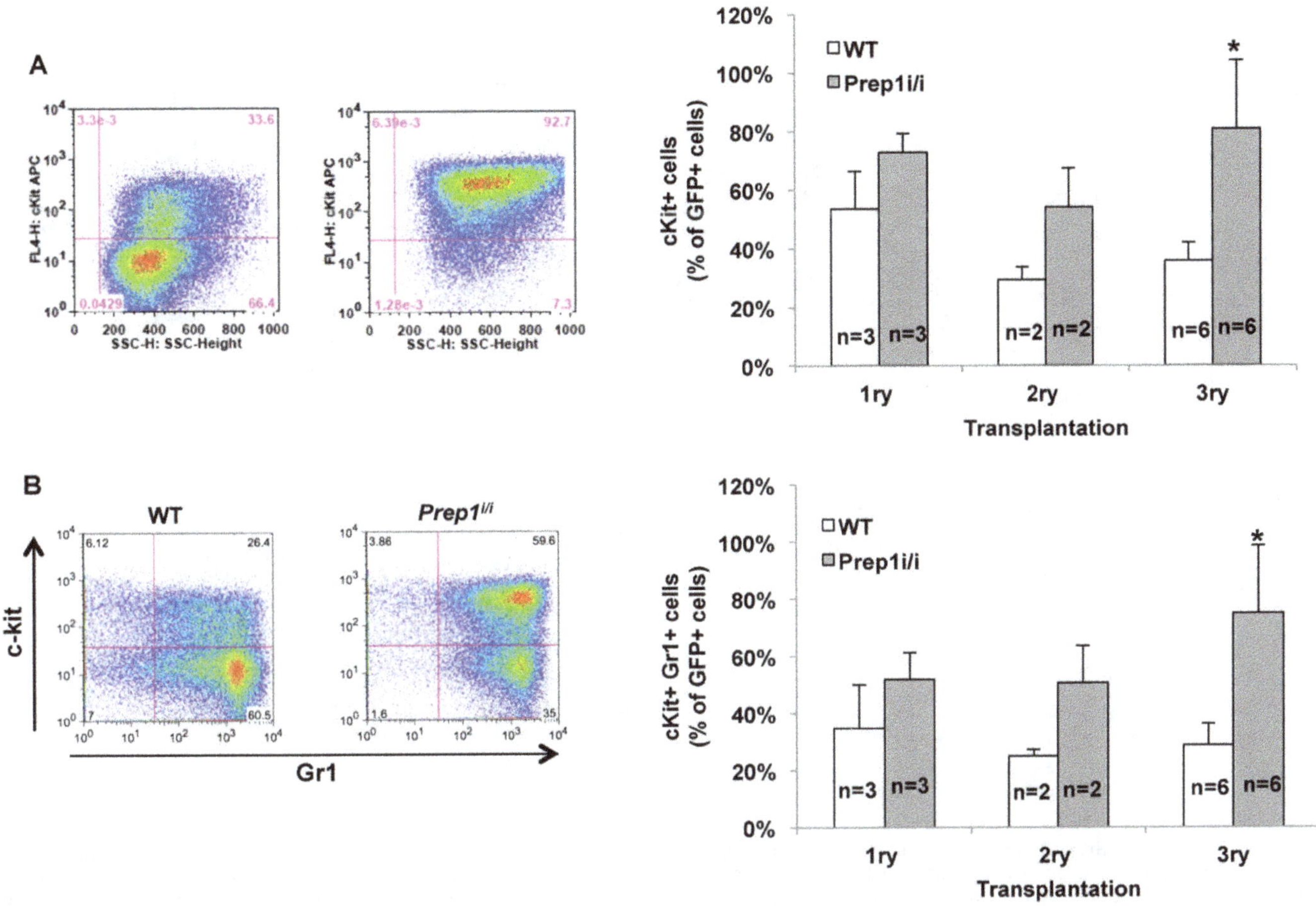

Figure 3. In vitro characterization of *Prep1^{i/i}* and WT leukemic cells. (**A**) FACS plots show c-Kit expression on GFP-positive cells in leukemic WT or *Prep1^{i/i}* BM cells (right side). Bar graph represents the percent of c-Kit positive cells on GFP-positive population on BM cells from different BMTs (left side). Error bars indicate SD. *p-value <0.001. (**B**) FACS profiles show c-Kit and Gr-1 expressions on BM from mice with AML induced by transplantation of *Prep1^{i/i}* or WT cells overexpressing *Meis1-HoxA9* (left side). Bar graph shows the percent of cells co-expressing c-Kit and GR-1 on BM from serially transplanted mice. Error bars represent SD. *p-value <0.001. The number of the mice analyzed for each group is shown on the graph.

monitored daily. Monitoring for disease was carried out by palpation and observation. Humane endpoints were used to minimize animal suffering when the following distressing signs were observed: 20% weight loss compared to pre-transplantation weight, difficulty to eat, drink, move and enlarged spleen. Mice were euthanized by inhalation of high concentration of CO_2.

Plasmids and Retroviral Infection

pMSCVpuro-HA-*HoxA9* was obtained by cloning HA-tagged *HoxA9* cDNA into XhoI/EcoRI restriction sites of pMSCV-puro retroviral vector. MSCV-IRES-GFP carrying FLAG-tagged-*Meis1* was obtained by cloning FLAG-tagged-*Meis1* cDNA into EcoRI restriction site of the vector. Phoenix-Eco (ATCC CRL-3214) cell line was used to produce FLAG-*Meis1-GFP* and HA-*HoxA9* expressing retroviruses. The preparation of single cell suspensions from E14.5 FLs has been described [34]. FL cells were pre-stimulated in 4-cytokine transduction medium (IMDM medium supplemented with 20% heat inactivated fetal bovine serum (FBS), 50 ng/mL SCF, 20 ng/mL IL-6, 10 ng/mL IL-3, and 10 ng/mL FLT3l) overnight to induce cell proliferation in order to improve the efficiency of infection. Pre-stimulated FLs were infected with FLAG-*Meis1-GFP*, HA-*HoxA9* or both in retronectin (Takara, 33.3 μg/mL) coated non-tissue culture treated plate (Falcon; 6-well plate polystyrene) in the presence of 4 μg/mL polybrene overnight. 48 h after infection FLAG-*Meis1-GFP* expressing cells were sorted for GFP-positive cells using FACS, and selected with 1 μg/mL puromycin for 3days (for HA-*HoxA9* expression). All cytokines used in this study were purchased from R & D systems (Minneapolis, USA).

In vivo Transplantation and Leukemogenic Assay

8 to 12 weeks old syngeneic recipient mice were sub-lethally irradiated (4.5 Gy), and indicated numbers of retrovirally transduced FL cells were injected into the tail vein of recipient mice. Indicated numbers of unfractionated bone marrow (BM) cells from primary leukemic mice were serially transplanted into secondary, tertiary, and quaternary recipients. Mice regularly were monitored for signs of leukemia.

Flow Cytometry Analysis

Leukemic BM cells harvested by flushing femurs and tibias were stained with the following conjugated monoclonal antibodies: c-Kit (2B8 clone), Gr-1 (RB6-8C5 clone), and Mac-1 (M1/70 clone). FLAG-*Meis1-GFP* expression was analyzed by FACS and expression of aforementioned antibodies were assessed on the GFP-positive cell population. Cells co-stained with anti-Mac–1 and anti-Gr-1 were considered as a myeloid lineage. Data were collected using a FACSCalibur cytometer (BD Biosciences, San

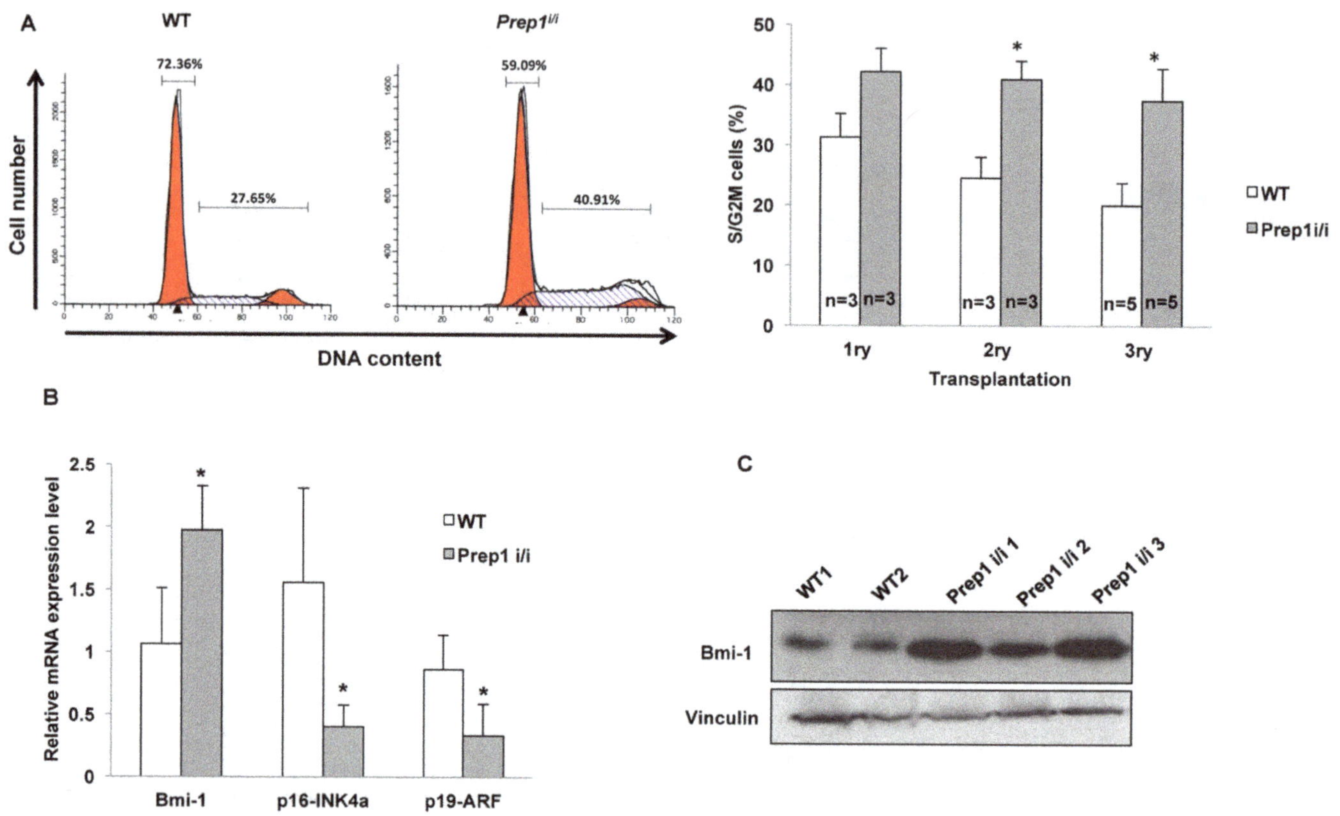

Figure 4. *Prep1*-deficient cells show altered cell cycle activity in *Meis1-HoxA9* leukemia. (**A**) Cell cycle profile of WT or *Prep1*$^{i/i}$ leukemic BM cells (right side) performed by flow cytometry. Bar graph summarizes data from cell cycle analysis of leukemic BM cells coming from primary, secondary and tertiary transplanted mice. Error bars indicate the SD. *p-value <0.01. The number of the mice analyzed for each group is shown on the graph. (**B**) mRNA expression level of the indicated transcripts in leukemic BM cells coming from seven mice transplanted with either WT or *Prep1*$^{i/i}$ *Meis1-HoxA9*-transduced cells. Levels were normalized to the GAPDH expression. Error bars indicate SD. *p-value <0.001 (**C**) Immunoblot represents the Bmi-1 protein level in the total lysate of *Meis1-HoxA9*-transduced leukemic WT or *Prep1*$^{i/i}$ BM cells. Vinculin was used as loading control.

Jose, CA) and analyzed using FlowJo (Tree Star) software. Antibodies were purchased from eBioscience (San Diego, CA) or BD (BD Pharmingen).

In vitro Colony Formation Assay

Indicated numbers of *Meis1*, *HoxA9* or *Meis1-HoxA9* transduced FL cells were seeded into 35 mm plates in cytokine-supplemented methylcellulose medium (MethoCult, M3434; STEMCELL Technologies) and incubated at 37°C in 5% CO_2. Colonies were scored on day 7 of culturing. All colonies were collected from the plate and cells were resuspended, counted and replated (50000 cells/replicate) for a total of 4 platings.

Cell Cycle Analysis

DNA content analysis was performed by propidium iodide (PI) staining and analyzed by FACS. 1×10^6 BM cells from leukemic mice were fixed in 75% cold ethanol for 1 h. Cells were then washed twice with PBS plus 1% BSA, and stained in 1 ml PI (50 μg/mL) supplemented with RNase (250 μg/mL) solution for 3 h at room temperature. Data were collected using a FACSCalibur cytometer (BD Biosciences, San Jose, CA) and analyzed using ModFit LT 3.2 software.

Western Blot Analysis

Western blot analysis was performed following standard procedures. Bone marrow cells were directly lysed in 2X sample buffer and equal amount of the cell lysates were separated in a 10% SDS-PAGE using electrophoresis. The following antibodies were used to detect the proteins of interest: anti-FLAG (clone-M2, Sigma-Aldrich, St-Louis, USA), anti-Bmi-1 (clone-F6, Millipore Massachusetts, USA) and anti-Vinculin (Sigma-Aldrich, St-Louis, USA) antibodies. The ImageJ64 software was used to normalize the results.

Real-time Quantitative PCR

Total RNA was isolated from *Prep1*$^{i/i}$ and WT leukemic BM cells using RNeasy mini kit (QIAGEN, Netherlands) according to the manufacture's instructions. 500 ng of total RNA was retro-transcribed in buffer containing dN_6-hexamer random primers, dNTPs, RNase OUT, and SuperScript III reverse transcriptase (Invitrogen, Carlsbad, USA). Primers (Table 1) were ordered from Sigma-Aldrich (St-Louis, USA) and Real-time PCR was performed with SYBR Green I master (Roche, Germany) on a LightCycler 480 system (Roche, Germany). GAPDH was used as control to normalize results. For all experiments, reverse-transcriptase minus controls were performed.

Statistical Analyses

The serial transplantation data were analyzed by *GraphPad Prism* software (Version 5.04) to identify significant differences between groups. All other statistical analyses were done by two-tailed

Table1. List of primers used for Real-time PCR.

Gene	Forward primer	Reverse primer
GAPDH	CTCTTCCACCTTCGA	GTCCACCACCCTGTTGCTGTA
Meis1	GTTGTCCAAGCCATCACCTT	ATCCACTCGTTCAGGAGGAA
Bmi-1	CAACCAGAATCAAGATCACTG	CCATTGGCAGCATCAGCTGAC
$P16^{Ink4a}$	GAACTCTTTCGGTCGTACC	CCAGCGTGTCCAGGAAG
$P19^{Arf}$	GCTCTGGCTTTCGTGAACATG	TCGAATCTGCACGTAGTTGAG

Student's *t* test, and values are expressed as means ± SEM or ± SD. Differences were regarded as significant at p-value <0.05.

Acknowledgments

The authors are grateful to all members of the IFOM mouse and flow cytometry facilities.

Author Contributions

Conceived and designed the experiments: LD FB. Performed the experiments: LD LM GI. Analyzed the data: LD LM FB. Wrote the paper: LD FB.

References

1. Moens CB, Selleri L (2006) Hox cofactors in vertebrate development. Dev Biol 291: 193–206.
2. Longobardi E, Penkov D, Mateos D, De Florian G, Torres M, et al. (2013) Biochemistry of the tale transcription factors PREP, MEIS, and PBX in vertebrates. Developmental dynamics: an official publication of the American Association of Anatomists.
3. Moskow JJ, Bullrich F, Huebner K, Daar IO, Buchberg AM (1995) Meis1, a PBX1-related homeobox gene involved in myeloid leukemia in BXH-2 mice. Mol Cell Biol 15: 5434–5443.
4. Nakamura T, Largaespada DA, Shaughnessy JD Jr, Jenkins NA, Copeland NG (1996) Cooperative activation of Hoxa and Pbx1-related genes in murine myeloid leukaemias. Nat Genet 12: 149–153.
5. Dardaei L, Longobardi E, Blasi F (2014) Prep1 and Meis1 competition for Pbx1 binding regulates protein stability and tumorigenesis. Proceedings of the National Academy of Sciences of the United States of America 111: E896–905.
6. Longobardi E, Iotti G, Di Rosa P, Mejetta S, Bianchi F, et al. (2010) Prep1 (pKnox1)-deficiency leads to spontaneous tumor development in mice and accelerates EmuMyc lymphomagenesis: a tumor suppressor role for Prep1. Mol Oncol 4: 126–134.
7. Ferretti E, Villaescusa JC, Di Rosa P, Fernandez-Diaz LC, Longobardi E, et al. (2006) Hypomorphic mutation of the TALE gene Prep1 (pKnox1) causes a major reduction of Pbx and Meis proteins and a pleiotropic embryonic phenotype. Mol Cell Biol 26: 5650–5662.
8. Iotti G, Mejetta S, Modica L, Penkov D, Ponzoni M, et al. (2012) Reduction of Prep1 levels affects differentiation of normal and malignant B cells and accelerates Myc driven lymphomagenesis. PloS one 7: e48353.
9. Keung YK, Cobos E, Morgan D, Whitehead RP, Tonk V (1997) Double minute chromosomes and myelodysplastic syndrome: a case report and literature review. Cancer Genet Cytogenet 97: 94–96.
10. Pineault N, Helgason CD, Lawrence HJ, Humphries RK (2002) Differential expression of Hox, Meis1, and Pbx1 genes in primitive cells throughout murine hematopoietic ontogeny. Experimental hematology 30: 49–57.
11. Grier DG, Thompson A, Kwasniewska A, McGonigle GJ, Halliday HL, et al. (2005) The pathophysiology of HOX genes and their role in cancer. J Pathol 205: 154–171.
12. Alharbi RA, Pettengell R, Pandha HS, Morgan R (2013) The role of HOX genes in normal hematopoiesis and acute leukemia. Leukemia 27: 1000–1008.
13. Berthelsen J, Zappavigna V, Ferretti E, Mavilio F, Blasi F (1998) The novel homeoprotein Prep1 modulates Pbx-Hox protein cooperativity. EMBO J 17: 1434–1445.
14. Jacobs Y, Schnabel CA, Cleary ML (1999) Trimeric association of Hox and TALE homeodomain proteins mediates Hoxb2 hindbrain enhancer activity. Mol Cell Biol 19: 5134–5142.
15. Abate-Shen C (2002) Deregulated homeobox gene expression in cancer: cause or consequence? Nat Rev Cancer 2: 777–785.
16. Calvo KR, Sykes DB, Pasillas MP, Kamps MP (2002) Nup98-HoxA9 immortalizes myeloid progenitors, enforces expression of Hoxa9, Hoxa7 and Meis1, and alters cytokine-specific responses in a manner similar to that induced by retroviral co-expression of Hoxa9 and Meis1. Oncogene 21: 4247–4256.
17. Borrow J, Shearman AM, Stanton VP Jr, Becher R, Collins T, et al. (1996) The t(7;11)(p15;p15) translocation in acute myeloid leukaemia fuses the genes for nucleoporin NUP98 and class I homeoprotein HOXA9. Nature genetics 12: 159–167.
18. Rawat VP, Thoene S, Naidu VM, Arseni N, Heilmeier B, et al. (2008) Overexpression of CDX2 perturbs HOX gene expression in murine progenitors depending on its N-terminal domain and is closely correlated with deregulated HOX gene expression in human acute myeloid leukemia. Blood 111: 309–319.
19. Thorsteinsdottir U, Kroon E, Jerome L, Blasi F, Sauvageau G (2001) Defining roles for HOX and MEIS1 genes in induction of acute myeloid leukemia. Mol Cell Biol 21: 224–234.
20. Kawagoe H, Humphries RK, Blair A, Sutherland HJ, Hogge DE (1999) Expression of HOX genes, HOX cofactors, and MLL in phenotypically and functionally defined subpopulations of leukemic and normal human hematopoietic cells. Leukemia 13: 687–698.
21. Serrano E, Lasa A, Perea G, Carnicer MJ, Brunet S, et al. (2006) Acute myeloid leukemia subgroups identified by pathway-restricted gene expression signatures. Acta Haematol 116: 77–89.
22. Wong P, Iwasaki M, Somervaille TC, So CW, Cleary ML (2007) Meis1 is an essential and rate-limiting regulator of MLL leukemia stem cell potential. Genes Dev 21: 2762–2774.
23. Iotti G, Longobardi E, Masella S, Dardaei L, De Santis F, et al. (2011) Homeodomain transcription factor and tumor suppressor Prep1 is required to maintain genomic stability. Proc Natl Acad Sci U S A 108: E314–322.
24. Zeisig BB, Milne T, Garcia-Cuellar MP, Schreiner S, Martin ME, et al. (2004) Hoxa9 and Meis1 are key targets for MLL-ENL-mediated cellular immortalization. Mol Cell Biol 24: 617–628.
25. Lessard J, Sauvageau G (2003) Bmi-1 determines the proliferative capacity of normal and leukaemic stem cells. Nature 423: 255–260.
26. van Gosliga D, Schepers H, Rizo A, van der Kolk D, Vellenga E, et al. (2007) Establishing long-term cultures with self-renewing acute myeloid leukemia stem/progenitor cells. Experimental hematology 35: 1538–1549.
27. DiMartino JF, Selleri L, Traver D, Firpo MT, Rhee J, et al. (2001) The Hox cofactor and proto-oncogene Pbx1 is required for maintenance of definitive hematopoiesis in the fetal liver. Blood 98: 618–626.
28. Hisa T, Spence SE, Rachel RA, Fujita M, Nakamura T, et al. (2004) Hematopoietic, angiogenic and eye defects in Meis1 mutant animals. EMBO J 23: 450–459.
29. Ficara F, Murphy MJ, Lin M, Cleary ML (2008) Pbx1 regulates self-renewal of long-term hematopoietic stem cells by maintaining their quiescence. Cell stem cell 2: 484–496.
30. Azcoitia V, Aracil M, Martinez AC, Torres M (2005) The homeodomain protein Meis1 is essential for definitive hematopoiesis and vascular patterning in the mouse embryo. Dev Biol 280: 307–320.
31. Penkov D, Di Rosa P, Fernandez Diaz L, Basso V, Ferretti E, et al. (2005) Involvement of Prep1 in the alphabeta T-cell receptor T-lymphocytic potential of hematopoietic precursors. Mol Cell Biol 25: 10768–10781.
32. Kahlina K, Goren I, Pfeilschifter J, Frank S (2004) p68 DEAD box RNA helicase expression in keratinocytes. Regulation, nucleolar localization, and functional connection to proliferation and vascular endothelial growth factor gene expression. J Biol Chem 279: 44872–44882.
33. Argiropoulos B, Yung E, Xiang P, Lo CY, Kuchenbauer F, et al. (2010) Linkage of the potent leukemogenic activity of Meis1 to cell-cycle entry and transcriptional regulation of cyclin D3. Blood 115: 4071–4082.
34. Morrison SJ, Hemmati HD, Wandycz AM, Weissman IL (1995) The purification and characterization of fetal liver hematopoietic stem cells. Proceedings of the National Academy of Sciences of the United States of America 92: 10302–10306.

9

A Gene Panel, Including *LRP12*, is Frequently Hypermethylated in Major Types of B-Cell Lymphoma

Nicole Bethge[1,2], Hilde Honne[2,3], Kim Andresen[2,3], Vera Hilden[1,2], Gunhild Trøen[4], Knut Liestøl[2,5], Harald Holte[2,6], Jan Delabie[4], Guro E. Lind[2,3], Erlend B. Smeland[1,2]*

1 Department of Immunology, Institute for Cancer Research, Oslo University Hospital, Oslo, Norway, **2** Centre for Cancer Biomedicine, University of Oslo, Oslo, Norway, **3** Department of Cancer Prevention, Institute for Cancer Research, Oslo University Hospital, Oslo, Norway, **4** Department of Pathology, Oslo University Hospital, Oslo, Norway, **5** Department of Informatics, University of Oslo, Oslo, Norway, **6** Department of Oncology, The Norwegian Radium Hospital, Oslo University Hospital, Oslo, Norway

Abstract

Epigenetic modifications and DNA methylation in particular, have been recognized as important mechanisms to alter gene expression in malignant cells. Here, we identified candidate genes which were upregulated after an epigenetic treatment of B-cell lymphoma cell lines (Burkitt's lymphoma, BL; Follicular lymphoma, FL; Diffuse large B-cell lymphoma, DLBCL activated B-cell like, ABC; and germinal center like, GCB) and simultaneously expressed at low levels in samples from lymphoma patients. Qualitative methylation analysis of 24 candidate genes in cell lines revealed five methylated genes (*BMP7, BMPER, CDH1, DUSP4* and *LRP12*), which were further subjected to quantitative methylation analysis in clinical samples from 59 lymphoma patients (BL, FL, DLBCL ABC and GCB; and primary mediastinal B-cell lymphoma, PMBL). The genes *LRP12* and *CDH1* showed the highest methylation frequencies (94% and 92%, respectively). *BMPER* (58%), *DUSP4* (32%) and *BMP7* (22%), were also frequently methylated in patient samples. Importantly, all gene promoters were unmethylated in various control samples (CD19+ peripheral blood B cells, peripheral blood mononuclear cells and tonsils) as well as in follicular hyperplasia samples, underscoring a high specificity. The combination of *LRP12* and *CDH1* methylation could successfully discriminate between the vast majority of the lymphoma and control samples, emphasized by receiver operating characteristic analysis with a c-statistic of 0.999. These two genes represent promising epigenetic markers which may be suitable for monitoring of B-cell lymphoma.

Editor: Joseph S. Pagano, The University of North Carolina at Chapel Hill, United States of America

Funding: This work was supported by grants from the South-Eastern Norway Regional Health Authority (ES: no. 39232, funding NB as PhD and GEL: no. 39535), and The Norwegian Cancer Society (ES: no. 33260 and GEL: PR-2008-0163). In addition, this work was partly supported by the Research Council of Norway through its Centres of Excellence funding scheme, project number 179571. The funders had no role in study design, data collection and analysis, decision to publish, or preparation of the manuscript.

Competing Interests: A US provisional patent application entitled "Methods and biomarkers for detection of hematological cancers" (61824278/INVEN-33229/US-1/PRO) has been filed covering the investigated genes as biomarkers for detection and monitoring of hematological cancer. GEL and EBS are listed as two of the inventors.

* Email: ebs@rr-research.no

Introduction

B-cell lymphoma comprises diverse neoplasms that are typed according to different B-cell developmental stages [1]. Chromosomal translocations involving the immunoglobulin (Ig) gene loci and oncogenes, such as *MYC*, *BCL1* and *BCL2*, are typical for B-cell lymphoma. In addition, a broad pattern of other acquired genetic changes have been described, although considerable heterogeneity exists even within each lymphoma type [2]. During the past decades it has become evident that alterations in the methylome can be found in nearly all cancer types [3,4] and this is now considered to be important in the pathogenesis of most cancer types [5]. DNA promoter hypermethylation has been described in a variety of genes and represents one important mechanism for the loss of tumor suppressor gene activity [6,7]. Inactivation of tumor suppressor genes by methylation has also been shown in lymphoma, e.g. the cyclin-dependent kinase inhibitors *CDKN2A* and *CDKN2B* [8], the TP53 homologue *TP73* and the death-associated protein kinase *DAPK1* [9]. Recently, several large-scale studies have been used to discover additional aberrantly methylated genes in lymphoma, although at various frequencies [10,11]. Interestingly, some of the these hypermethylated genes have been shown to predict the outcome of therapy [12], and it was recently shown that DLBCL with hypermethylation of the *MGMT* promoter had a favorable outcome [13].

The aim of this study was to identify novel methylated genes and to analyze their promoter methylation status in major types of B-cell lymphomas (diffuse large B cell-, follicular- and Burkitt's lymphoma).

Methods

Primary samples

DNA from 59 patients diagnosed with B-cell lymphoma (germinal center B cell–like (GCB) (n = 16) and activated B cell–like (ABC)

Table 1. Methylation status of candidate genes in 12 B-cell lymphoma cell lines.

cell line/gene	BL (n = 3; %)	DLBCL ABC (n = 3; %)	DLBCL GCB (n = 3; %)	FL (n = 3; %)	all types combined
BMPER	100%	100%	100%	100%	100%
CDH1	100%	100%	100%	100%	100%
LRP12	100%	100%	100%	100%	100%
DUSP4	100%	100%	100%	66%	92%
CCL22	100%	66%	66%	100%	83%
CLU	100%	66%	66%	100%	83%
NPY1R	100%	100%	66%	66%	83%
BCL2L10	100%	66%	66%	66%	75%
PTPRG	100%	33%	66%	100%	75%
UCHL1	66%	100%	66%	66%	75%
SGPP2	66%	33%	66%	100%	67%
BMP7	0%	100%	0%	66%	42%
HBEGF	66%	33%	33%	0%	33%
BCL2	33%	0%	0%	0%	8%
PRKAR2B	0%	0%	33%	0%	8%
CALR	0%	0%	0%	0%	0%
GPSM2	0%	0%	0%	0%	0%
ICOSLG	0%	0%	0%	0%	0%
KLF13	0%	0%	0%	0%	0%
MAP3K3	0%	0%	0%	0%	0%
MAPK81P3	0%	0%	0%	0%	0%
MYBL1	0%	0%	0%	0%	0%
SNX22	0%	0%	0%	0%	0%
XRCC4	0%	0%	0%	0%	0%

Only candidate genes which have a CpG island in their promoter region have been analyzed by MSP. Candidate genes for each lymphoma type have been analyzed in 12 B-cell lymphoma cell lines (three cell lines per type). Genes have been sorted by the combined methylation frequency (brackets) across all lymphoma cell lines. A cell line has been considered as methylated when it was partially or fully methylated. Abbreviations: BL, Burkitt's lymphoma; DLBCL ABC, activated B-cell like diffuse large B-cell lymphoma; DLBCL GCB, germinal centre B-cell like diffuse large B-cell lymphoma; and FL, follicular lymphoma.

(n = 18) subtypes of diffuse large B cell lymphoma (DLBCL), primary mediastinal B-cell lymphoma (PMBL) (n = 6), follicular lymphoma (FL) (n = 12) and Burkitt's lymphoma (BL) (n = 7)) were included in the study. In addition, DNA from several non-malignant sources, which are referred to as control samples (n = 49) were included as well; i.e. normal B cells isolated from buffy coat with CD19$^+$ Dynabeads (Invitrogen), $n = 20$; peripheral blood mononuclear cells, $n = 10$; and tonsils, $n = 10$; in addition to follicular hyperplasia samples; $n = 9$. The 59 patients included in this study were observed for on average 36 months (median value) after diagnosis. During this time, eight out of the 59 patients (14%) died.

Ethical statement

The study was approved by the Regional Committees for Medical and Health Research Ethics, Region Eastern Norway (S-05145) and was performed in accordance with the Declaration of Helsinki. Informed consent was signed by all patients included in this study.

Epigenetic treatment of lymphoma cell lines

Twelve B-cell lymphoma cell lines (BL: BL41, Raji and Ramos (Deutsche Sammlung von Microorganismen und Zellkulturen Gmbh; DSMZ); DLBCL ABC: HLY-1 (T.Saati), OciLy3, and OciLy10 (L. Staudt); DLBCL GCB: OciLy7 and SUDHL4 (L. Staudt), SUDHL6 (DSMZ); and FL: K422, SC-1 and ROS50 (DSMZ) were cultured with and without a combination of epigenetic drugs; the demethylating reagent 5-aza-2′deoxycytidine (aza; 1 µM for 72 h) and the histone deacetylase inhibitor trichostatin A (TSA; 0.5 µM added the last 12 h). Culturing conditions are described in File S1.

Gene expression profiling

A stepwise approach was applied to identify potentially methylated target genes. Epigenetic drug treated cell lines and their untreated counterparts were analyzed with the Applied Biosystems Human Genome Survey Microarray following manufacturer's protocol. Post-processing and normalization was performed with the R-script "ABarray" and Bioconductor (GSE46064). Furthermore, gene expression data from 480 B-cell lymphomas were available from the Leukemia Lymphoma Molecular Profiling Project (LLMPP) (BL $n = 24$, GSE 4732 [14]; DLBCL ABC $n = 168$, GSE10846 [15]; DLBCL GC $n = 97$, GSE10846 [15]; FL $n = 191$, unpublished). The gene expression profile of each lymphoma type was compared to the average expression of the remaining B-cell lymphoma types. We selected candidate genes by the following criteria; gene expression of B-cell lymphoma patients had to be at least 2-fold downregulated in one B-cell lymphoma type compared to the other types. At the same

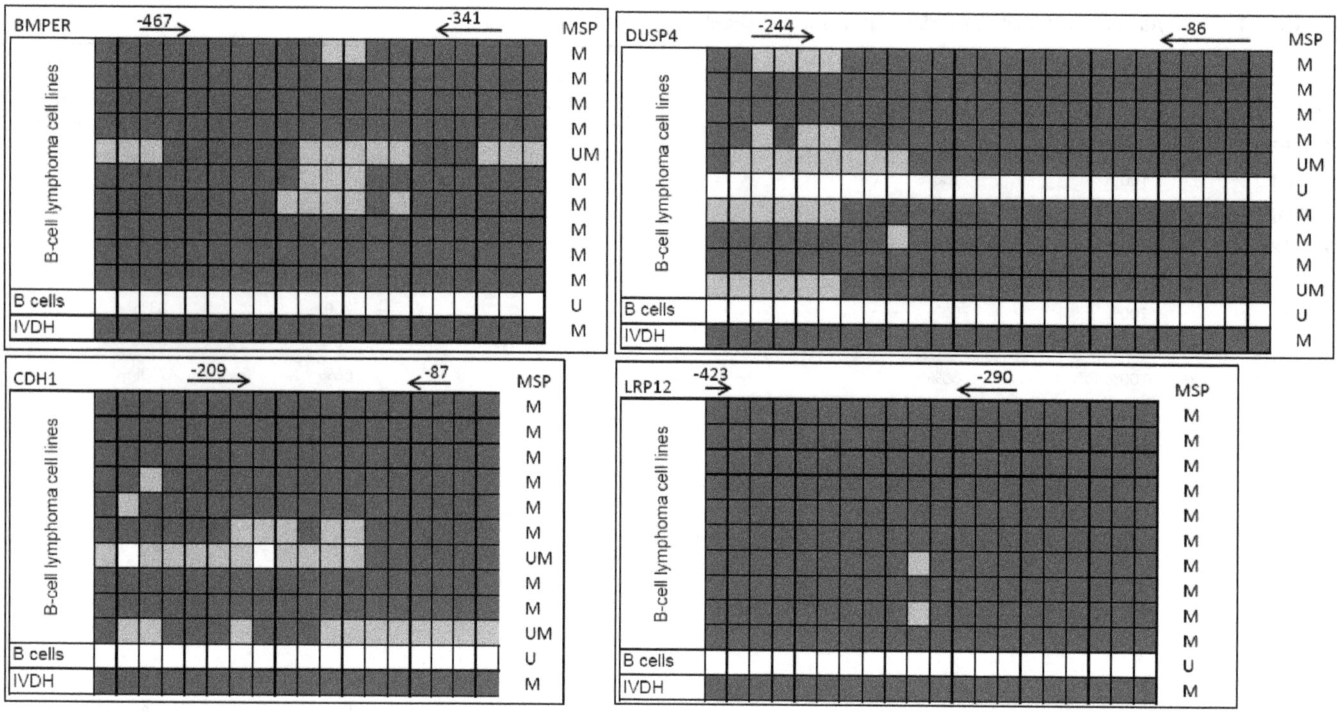

Figure 1. Bisulfite sequencing of individual CpG sites in the promoter regions of *BMPER, CDH1, DUSP4* and *LRP12.* CpG sites are represented by a box, a methylated site is symbolized by a dark grey box, a partially methylated CpG site is colored in gray and a white box represents an unmethylated CpG site. MSP-primer binding sites are indicated with an arrow above the CpG site. The distance from transcription start to the first base of the primer is indicated by the number above the arrow.

time, the genes had to be at least 0.5-fold upregulated after epigenetic drug treatment of cell lines representing the same type of lymphoma. Furthermore, the average response of epigenetic drug treatment of cell lines of the given lymphoma type should be 0.5-fold higher compared to the average response of the remaining cell lines.

Analysis of promoter methylation status in cell lines

Genes harboring a CpG-Island in their promoter region (CpG-Island Searcher Software, [16]), were analyzed by methylation specific PCR (MSP) in B-cell lymphoma cell lines and CD19$^+$ B-cells. MSP was performed as previously described [17] and each reaction was run twice for an independent validation. All primers amplifying methylated or unmethylated loci were designed using the Methyl Primer Express 1.0 (Applied Biosystems; sequences listed in Table S1 in File S1). DNA from B-cell lymphoma cell lines and CD19$^+$ B-cells was isolated with the AllPrep DNA/RNA/protein Kit from Qiagen. For each sample, 1.3 µg DNA was bisulfite treated with the EpiTect bisulfite kit (Qiagen).

Direct bisulfite sequencing

Primers for bisulfite sequencing were designed using Methyl Primer Express 1.0 (Applied Biosystems) to amplify the respective MSP primer binding sites for each gene of interest (Primer sequences are provided in Table S1 in File S1). Bisulfite sequencing was performed as previously described [17]. By comparing the peak height of the cytosine signal with the sum of the cytosine and thymine peak height signals, the approximate amount of methyl cytosine of each CpG site was calculated. CpG sites with ratio between: 0 and 0.20 were scored as unmethylated, 0.21 to 0.80 were scored as partially methylated, whereas 0.81 to 1.0 was considered to be fully methylated.

Quantitative methylation-specific polymerase chain reaction (qMSP)

Primers and probes for qMSP, which bind bisulfite treated and methylated DNA, were designed with the Primer Express 3.0 Software (Applied Biosystems; assays listed in Table S1 in File S1). All qMSP reactions were performed in triplicates using a 7900HT Fast Real-Time PCR System (Applied Biosystems) and analyzed with the sequence detector system 2.3 (Applied Biosystems), as previously described [17]. Briefly, normalization for DNA input was performed using the ALU-C4 as a reference gene [18], and the quantity of methylated DNA in each sample was determined using a standard curve of bisulfite treated universal methylated DNA (Chemicon, Millipore).

Statistics

Statistical analyses were carried out using GraphPad Prism 6 (GraphPad Software, Inc, San Diego, CA, USA). A Mann-Whitney test was used to compare the PMR values of the candidate genes between the various sample groups testes. A Fisher's exact test was used for analyzing potential differences in the number of methylated samples between the test and validation series. All P-values were derived from two-sided tests, and $P \leq 0.05$ was considered to be statistically significant. Finally, Receiver operating characteristics (ROC) curve analyses were used to evaluate the performance of the methylation biomarkers.

Table 2. Methylation frequency of the analyzed lymphoma samples.

Patients/genes		BL	DLBCL ABC	DLBCL GCB	FL	PMBL	All types combined
Test series	BMP7	0/7 (0%)	3/10 (30%)	3/10 (30%)	2/10 (20%)	n.a.	8/37 (22%)
	BMPER	n.a.	6/10 (60%)	7/10 (70%)	5/10 (50%)	n.a.	18/30 (60%)
	CDH1	n.a.	9/10 (90%)	9/10 (90%)	10/10 (100%)	n.a.	28/30 (93%)
	DUSP4	n.a.	n.a.	n.a.	n.a.	n.a.	n.a.
	LRP12	n.a.	10/10 (100%)	7/10 (70%)	10/10 (100%)	n.a.	27/30 (90%)
Validation series	BMP7	n.a.	n.a.	n.a.	n.a.	n.a.	n.a.
	BMPER	n.a.	5/8 (63%)	4/6 (67%)	0/2 (0%)	3/6 (50%)	12/22 (55%)
	CDH1	n.a.	7/8 (88%)	6/6 (100%)	2/2 (100%)	5/6 (84%)	20/22 (91%)
	DUSP4	n.a.	4/8 (50%)	0/6 (0%)	2/2 (100%)	1/6 (17%)	7/22 (32%)
	LRP12	n.a.	8/8 (100%)	6/6 (100%)	2/2 (100%)	6/6 (100%)	22/22 (100%)

Gene promoters have been analyzed by qMSP in five different lymphoma types. The methylation frequency is given in brackets for each lymphoma type and as a combination of all lymphoma types (last column). Abbreviations: BL, Burkitt's lymphoma; DLBCL ABC, activated B-cell like diffuse large B-cell lymphoma; DLBCL GCB, germinal centre B-cell like diffuse large B-cell lymphoma; FL, follicular lymphoma; n.a., not analyzed; and PMBL, primary mediastinal B-cell lymphoma.

Results

Identification of genes upregulated after epigenetic treatment of B-cell lymphoma cell lines and expressed at a low level in lymphoma patients

We analyzed the top 24 candidate genes, which were upregulated after epigenetic treatment of cell lines and simultaneously expressed at low levels in lymphoma samples of the corresponding type. These candidates were analyzed by MSP in 12 B-cell lymphoma cell lines and CD19+ peripheral blood B cells from healthy donors. The gene promoters of *BMPER, CDH1* and *LRP12* were methylated in all analyzed B-cell lymphoma cell lines across all subtypes (Table 1). In addition, the following genes had a high promoter methylation frequency *DUSP4* (92%); *CCL22, CLU and NPY1R* (83%); *BCL2L10, PTPRG* and *UCHL1* (75%). Of note, *BMP7* was methylated in all three DLBCL ABC cell lines and in two of three FL cell lines, but not in cell lines derived from BL or DLBCL GCB (Table 1). It was the only gene showing a subtype-specific methylation pattern in DLBCL cell lines.

Bisulfite sequencing of the *BMP7-, BMPER-, CDH1-, DUSP4-* and *LRP12*-promoter

Before designing qMSP primers and probes, we used direct bisulfite sequencing to analyze the methylation status of individual CpG sites in the promoter regions of the five most promising candidates (*BMP7, BMPER, CDH1, DUSP4* and *LRP12*). In general, the bisulfite sequencing confirmed complete bisulfite conversion since all non-methylated cytosines were converted to thymine. All cell lines, which showed partial or complete methylation as assessed by MSP, revealed partially or fully methylated CpG-sites in the region for MSP-primer binding. Furthermore, B cells from healthy donors were confirmed to be negative for promoter CpG-island methylation by bisulfite sequencing (Figure 1, *BMP7* can be found in Figure S1 in File S1).

DNA methylation analysis of lymphoma and healthy donor samples

We next analyzed *BMPER, CDH1, DUSP4* and *LRP12* promoter methylation in clinical samples by qMSP in a test and validation series. The lymphoma patients included in the test series showed methylation frequencies of 93%, 90% and 60% for *CDH1, LRP12* and *BMPER*, respectively. Due to a limited access to patient material, *DUSP4* was only analyzed in the validation series. The analyzed control samples showed low PMR values, ranging from 0–3.7%. We used the highest PMR value obtained from the analyzed control samples to set a threshold (4%) for scoring methylation positive samples. For the test and validation series, no statistically significant differences were seen for neither the number of methylated tumors nor for the level of PMR values (Table S2 in file S1). The promoter methylation of *LRP12, CDH1, BMPER* and *DUSP4* was 100%, 91%, 55%, and 32% across all analyzed lymphoma types included in the validation series, respectively (Table 2 and Figure 2). For *BMPER, CDH1* and *LRP12* statistically significant differences in the PMR values were seen between several of the lymphoma groups analyzed, as well as in comparison with the control samples (Table S2 in file S1).

The *BMP7*-promoter methylation status was analyzed by qMSP in 37 lymphoma samples and $CD19^+$ B-cells from 10 healthy donors. The promoter methylation of *BMP7* was 0%, 20%, 30% and 30% in BL, FL, DLBCL ABC and DLBCL GCB, respectively. Thus, the subtype specific methylation pattern seen in DLBCL cell lines could not be confirmed in patient samples. The promoter of *BMP7* showed no methylation in control samples

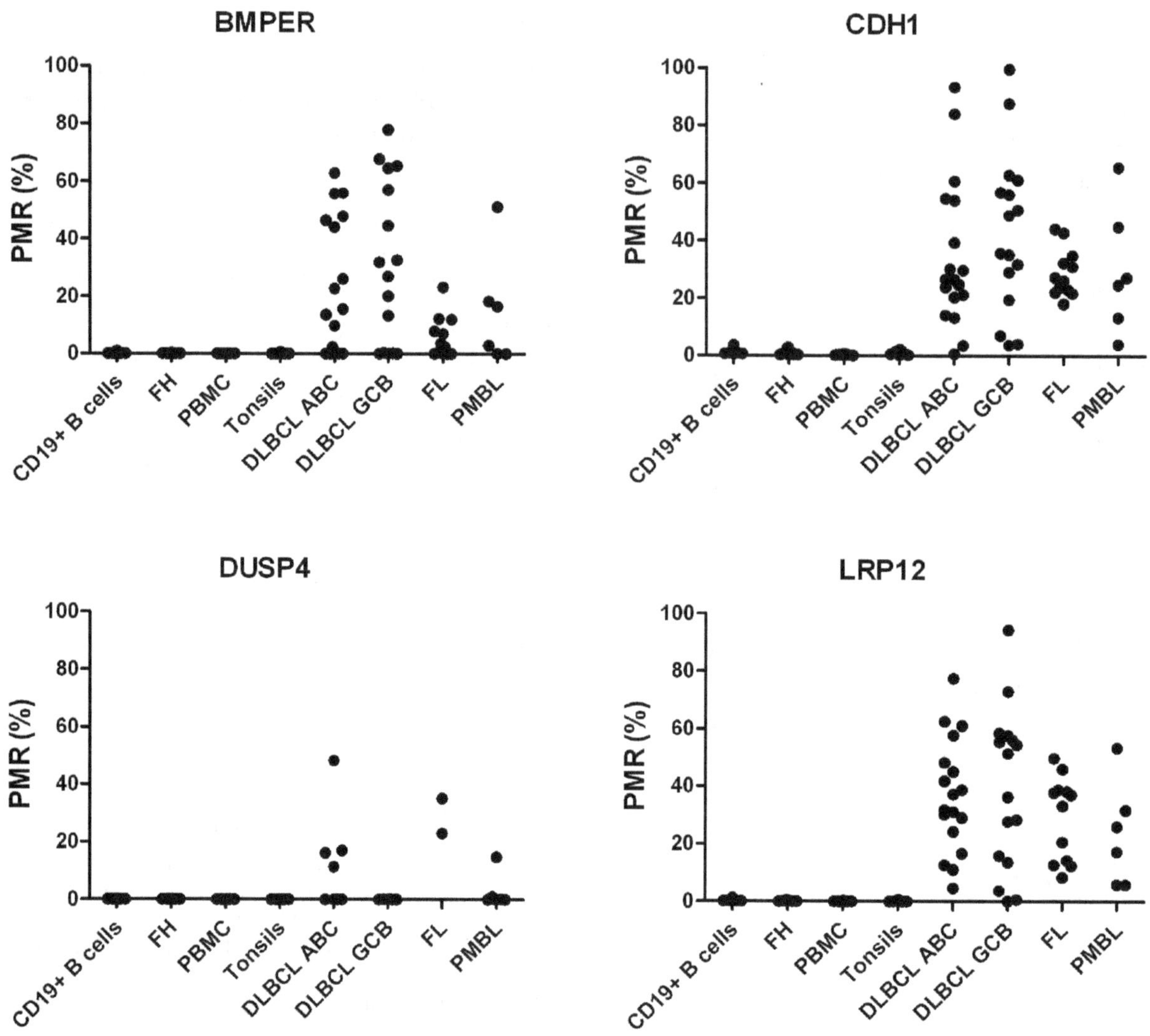

Figure 2. Methylation status of *BMPER, CDH1, DUSP4* and *LRP12* assessed by qMSP. Percent promoter methylation in control samples (CD19+ B cells, PMBC, tonsils); follicular hyperplasia samples (FH) and lymphoma patient samples. Each dot represents one sample. Abbreviations: BL, Burkitt's lymphoma; DLBCL ABC, activated B-cell like diffuse large B-cell lymphoma; DLBCL GCB, germinal centre B-cell like diffuse large B-cell lymphoma; FL, follicular lymphoma; and PMBL, primary mediastinal B-cell lymphoma; PMR, percent methylated reference.

(Figure S2 in file S1). Interestingly, *DUSP4* was methylated in 50% of DLBCL ABC and showed no methylation in DLBCL GCB.

Receiver Operating Characteristics (ROC) curves

We used the PMR values obtained for lymphomas and healthy controls from the qMSP analysis as input in the receiver operating characteristics (ROC) curves. *BMP7, BMPER, CDH1, DUSP4* and *LRP12* showed an individual area under the curve (AUC) of 0.70, 0.83, 0.99, 0.74 and 0.99 (Figure 3a). By combining the panel (by summarizing the PMR values) we could discriminate all lymphoma samples (BL, DLBCL ABC, DLBCL GCB, FL and PMBL), except one, from the various control samples (B cells, PBMC and tonsils) and follicular hyperplasia as shown by an AUC of 0.999 (Figure 3b).

Discussion

In the present study we identified genes frequently methylated in B-cell lymphoma by a stepwise approach. Genes, which were upregulated after epigenetic drug treatment of a panel of B-cell lymphoma cell lines and expressed at a low level in lymphoma patient samples, were subjected to promoter methylation analyses in cell lines. Frequently methylated genes were further analyzed in clinical samples. We focused on major types of B-cell lymphoma (BL, DLBCL ABC, DLBCL GCB, FL and PMBL) and demonstrated that the gene promoters of *LRP12 (94%), CDH1 (92%)*, and *BMPER* (58%) were methylated at a high frequency, whereas *DUSP4* and *BMP7* showed lower methylation frequencies (32% and 22%, respectively). Combined, these genes could successfully discriminate the vast majority (98%) of lymphoma samples from controls and follicular hyperplasia samples, as shown by receiver operating characteristics with an AUC of 0.999.

We found *LPR12* and *CDH1* to be the most frequently methylated genes in our study. Of note, *CDH1* has previously been shown to be frequently methylated in various cancer types [19,20], including lymphoma [21,22] and leukemia [23,24] and functions as a tumor suppressor by inhibiting proliferation and invasion [25]. However, to the best of our knowledge, this is the

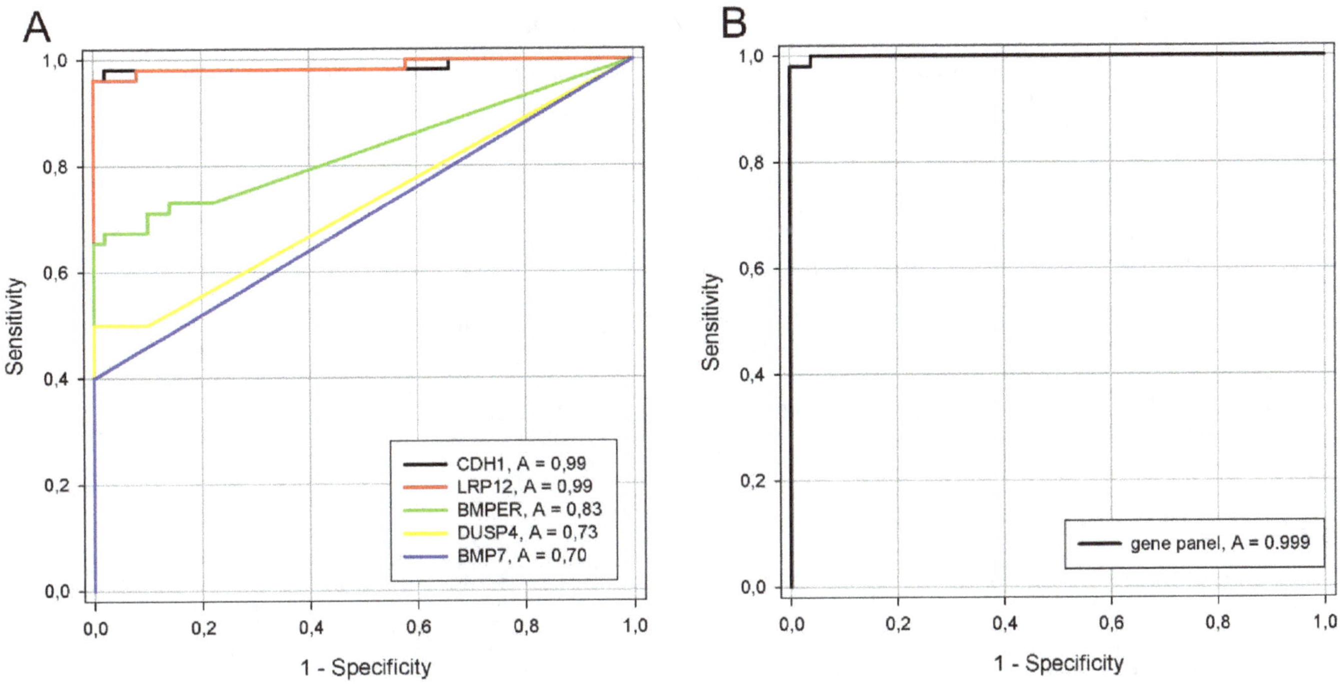

Figure 3. Receiver Operating Characteristics (ROC) curves for individual and combined markers in lymphoma patients versus healthy donors. The area under the ROC curve (AUC) represents how accurate the individual and combined biomarkers can discriminate between lymphoma and control samples. A) Lymphoma patients versus controls for individual genes. B) Lymphoma patients versus controls for the combined gene panel.

first time *BMPER*, *BMP7*, *DUSP4* and *LRP12* are reported to be methylated in lymphoma. From previous studies, *DUSP4* and *BMP7* are known to be methylated in gliomas [26] and gastric- and prostate cancer [27,28], respectively. Even though large scale methylation studies have been performed on different lymphoma types increasing the knowledge about methylated genes, we were able to discover novel methylated genes using a cell line based approach and studying FL, DLBCL and BL at the same time. This is in contrast to other studies focusing mainly on one lymphoma type [10,11].

Alterations of the TGF-β/BMP signaling pathways are frequently found in human cancer [29]. In addition, TGF-β often acts as a tumor suppressor during early stages of carcinogenesis; however, at later stages it may act as a tumor promoter [30]. Interestingly, three of the methylated genes identified in the present study are related to these signaling pathways. The *LRP12 gene*, that had the highest methylation frequency, encodes a low density lipoprotein receptor-related protein. A role in signal transduction is proposed, since the cytoplasmic c-terminus of this protein can interact among others with SARA (Smad anchor receptor activation), which is reported to interact with the TGF-β and BMP pathways [31]. Moreover, the gene *BMPER*, which encodes for BMP endothelial cell precursor-derived regulator, was frequently methylated in our lymphoma samples. BMPER is a secreted factor, which modulates BMP activity, showing both pro- and anti-BMP effects [32,33]. In addition, *BMP7*, which is methylated in 23% of the analyzed patients, as well as *BMP6*, which previously has been reported to be frequently methylated in lymphoma [12], are members of the TGF-β superfamily of cytokines. In concordance with other cancer types the TGF-β-receptor II has also been reported to be methylated in B-cell lymphoma cell lines [34–36]. Taken together, the data presented here indicates that alterations within the TGF-β and/or BMP signaling in lymphoma could be due to promoter hypermethylation-induced downregulation of essential TGF-β/BMP signaling pathway components.

The usage of a DNA methylation based biomarker in either primary biopsies or various body fluids has already been shown for several cancer types [37]. Of note, detection of *DLC1* methylation in primary lymphoma biopsies and plasma samples from the same patients, showed a concordance of 80% [38], indicating a possible use of plasma analyses as well. These data are encouraging, but further studies are needed to establish the degree of methylation in cell free circulating DNA of lymphoma patients. The *LRP12* and *CDH1* genes have a great potential as DNA methylation biomarkers for lymphoma, since these were able to discriminate with a high sensitivity and specificity lymphoma patients from the various control samples and follicular hyperplasia. In addition, DNA methylation is an early event in tumor development; a DNA methylation based biomarker could be used to monitor lymphoma patients for relapse. Furthermore, biomarkers, which can predict the response to therapy are of great value and has been shown for various methylated genes [39–42]. Of note, epigenetic modifications are reversible, and the therapeutic effects of demethylating agents in hematological malignancies have been shown *in vitro* experiments and clinical trials [21]. Markers for monitoring the dose-response of such agents to minimize side-effects would be appreciated. The methylation status of the genes we present here could be used for these purposes and should be validated in larger studies.

In this study, we did not identify genes that were methylated in a lymphoma type or subtype specific pattern in patient samples, although the *BMP7* gene promoter was methylated in DLDCL ABC and not DLBCL GCB cell lines. This shows that the methylation pattern in cell lines not always reflects the methylation status in patient samples and underscores the need for validation.

Interestingly, when we examined the methylation status of *DUSP4*, which was highly methylated across the various cell lines, we discovered that it was methylated in 50% of DLBCL ABC but was unmethylated in all DLBCL GCB. The possibility of *DUSP4* methylation as an additional biomarker for differentiating between the two DLBCL subtypes should be further investigated. Of interest, the *DUSP4* gene product dephosphorylates and thereby inactivates MAPKs, which are involved in regulation of growth and proliferation. Further, by blocking the MAPK cascade, *DUSP4* could act as a candidate tumor suppressor gene [26].

Taken together, we identified several genes (*BMPER, BMP7, CDH1, DUSP4* and *LRP12*) which were frequently methylated in major lymphoma types. In a future perspective, the hypermethylated *CDH1* and *LRP12* gene promoters could be used in a blood-based test to differentiate lymphoma patients from healthy donors and follicular hyperplasia.

Acknowledgments

The gene expression data from lymphoma samples were obtained from published data from the Lymphoma/Leukemia Molecular Profiling Project, headed by L.M. Staudt, National Cancer Institute, USA. The Bioinformatics Core Facility, Oslo University Hospital assisted with the analysis of the gene expression data.

Author Contributions

Conceived and designed the experiments: ES GL. Performed the experiments: NB H. Honne VH. Analyzed the data: NB H. Holte H. Honne JD KA KL GL. Contributed reagents/materials/analysis tools: GT H. Holte JD. Contributed to the writing of the manuscript: NB ES GL.

References

1. Shaffer AL, Rosenwald A, Staudt LM (2002) Lymphoid Malignancies: the dark side of B-cell differentiation. Nat Rev Immunol 2: 920–933. 10.1038/nri953.
2. De S, Shaknovich R, Riester M, Elemento O, Geng H, et al. (2013) Aberration in DNA Methylation in B-Cell Lymphomas Has a Complex Origin and Increases with Disease Severity. PLoS Genet 9: e1003137. doi:10.1371/journal.pgen.1003137.
3. Esteller M (2007) Cancer epigenomics: DNA methylomes and histone-modification maps. Nat Rev Genet 8: 286–298. 10.1038/nrg2005.
4. Ting AH, McGarvey KM, Baylin SB (2006) The cancer epigenome: components and functional correlates. Genes & Development 20: 3215–3231.
5. Jones PA, Baylin SB (2007) The Epigenomics of Cancer. Cell 128: 683–692. doi: DOI: 10.1016/j.cell.2007.01.029.
6. Herman JG, Baylin SB (2003) Gene Silencing in Cancer in Association with Promoter Hypermethylation. N Engl J Med 349: 2042–2054.
7. Jones PA, Baylin SB (2002) The fundamental role of epigenetic events in cancer. Nat Rev Genet 3: 415–428. 10.1038/nrg816.
8. Herman JG, Civin CI, Issa JP, Collector MI, Sharkis SJ, et al. (1997) Distinct Patterns of Inactivation of p15INK4B and p16INK4A Characterize the Major Types of Hematological Malignancies. Cancer Res 57: 837–841.
9. Mulero-Navarro S, Esteller M (2008) Epigenetic biomarkers for human cancer: The time is now. Critical Reviews in Oncology/Hematology 68: 1–11. doi: DOI: 10.1016/j.critrevonc.2008.03.001.
10. O'Riain C, O'Shea DM, Yang Y, Le Dieu R, Gribben JG, et al. (2009) Array-based DNA methylation profiling in follicular lymphoma. Leukemia 3(10):1858–66.doi:10.1038/leu.
11. Shaknovich R, Geng H, Johnson NA, Tsikitas L, Cerchietti L, et al. (2010) DNA methylation signatures define molecular subtypes of diffuse large B cell lymphoma. Blood 116.20: e81.
12. Daibata M, Nemoto Y, Bandobashi K, Kotani N, Kuroda M, et al. (2007) Promoter Hypermethylation of the Bone Morphogenetic Protein-6 Gene in Malignant Lymphoma. Clin Cancer Res 13: 3528–3535.
13. Uccella S, Cerutti R, Placidi C, Marchet S, Carnevali I, et al. (2009) MGMT methylation in diffuse large B-cell lymphoma: validation of quantitative methylation-specific PCR and comparison with MGMT protein expression. Journal of Clinical Pathology 62: 715–723.
14. Dave SS, Fu K, Wright GW, Lam LT, Kluin P, et al, the Lymphoma/Leukemia Molecular Profiling Project (2006) Molecular Diagnosis of Burkitt's Lymphoma. N Engl J Med 354: 2431–2442.
15. Alizadeh AA, Eisen MB, Davis RE, Ma C, Lossos IS, et al. (2000) Distinct types of diffuse large B-cell lymphoma identified by gene expression profiling. Nature 403: 503–511. 10.1038/35000501.
16. Takai D, Jones PA (2002) Comprehensive analysis of CpG islands in human chromosomes 21 and 22. Proceedings of the National Academy of Sciences of the United States of America 99: 3740–3745.
17. Andresen K, Boberg KM, Vedeld HM, Honne H, Hektoen M, et al. (2012) Novel target genes and a valid biomarker panel identified for cholangiocarcinoma. Epigenetics 7: 1249–1257.
18. Weisenberger DJ, Campan M, Long TI, Kim M, Woods C, et al. (2005) Analysis of repetitive element DNA methylation by MethyLight. Nucl Acids Res 33: 6823–6836.
19. Sudo M, Chong JM, Sakuma K, Ushiku T, Uozaki H, et al. (2004) Promoter hypermethylation of E-cadherin and its abnormal expression in Epstein-Barr virus-associated gastric carcinoma. Int J Cancer 109: 194–199.
20. Sebova K, Zmetakova I, Bella V, Kajo K, Stankovicova I, et al. (2011) RASSF1A and CDH1 hypermethylation as potential epimarkers in breast cancer. Cancer Biomarkers 10: 13–26.
21. Amara K, Trimeche M, Ziadi S, Laatiri A, Hachana M, et al. (2008) Prognostic significance of aberrant promoter hypermethylation of CpG islands in patients with diffuse large B-cell lymphomas. Ann Oncol 19: 1774–1786.
22. Huang Q, Su X, Ai L, Li M, Fan CY, et al. (2007) Promoter hypermethylation of multiple genes in primary gastric lymphoma. Leukemia and Lymphoma 48: 1988–1996.
23. Corn PG, Smith BD, Ruckdeschel ES, Douglas D, Baylin SB, et al. (2000) E-cadherin expression is silenced by 5' CpG island methylation in acute leukemia. Clin Cancer Res 6: 4243–4248.
24. Melki JR, Vincent PC, Brown RD, Clark SJ (2000) Hypermethylation of E-cadherin in leukemia. Blood 95: 3208–3213.
25. Berx G, van Roy F (2009) Involvement of Members of the Cadherin Superfamily in Cancer. Cold Spring Harbor Perspectives in Biology; 10.1101/cshperspect.a0031291.
26. Waha A, Felsberg J, Hartmann W, Von dem Knesebeck A, Mikeska T, et al. (2010) Epigenetic Downregulation of Mitogen-Activated Protein Kinase Phosphatase MKP-2 Relieves Its Growth Suppressive Activity in Glioma Cells. Cancer Res 70: 1689–1699.
27. Yamashita S, Tsujino Y, Moriguchi K, Tatematsu M, Ushijima T (2006) Chemical genomic screening for methylation-silenced genes in gastric cancer cell lines using 5-aza-2-deoxycytidine treatment and oligonucleotide microarray. Cancer Science 97: 64–71. 10.1111/j.1349-7006.2006.00136.x.
28. Kron K, Pethe V, Briollais L, Sadikovic B, Ozcelik H, et al. (2009) Discovery of Novel Hypermethylated Genes in Prostate Cancer Using Genomic CpG Island Microarrays. PLoS ONE 4: e4830. doi:10.1371/journal.pone.0004830.
29. Levy L, Hill CS (2006) Alterations in components of the TGF-β superfamily signaling pathways in human cancer. Cytokine & Growth Factor Reviews 17: 41–58.
30. Inman GJ (2011) Switching TGFβ from a tumor suppressor to a tumor promoter. Current Opinion in Genetics & Development 21: 93–99.
31. Garnis C, Coe BP, Zhang L, Rosin MP, Lam WL (2004) Overexpression of LRP12, a gene contained within an 8q22 amplicon identified by high-resolution array CGH analysis of oral squamous cell carcinomas. Oncogene 23: 2582–2586.
32. Helbing T, Volkmar F, Goebel U, Heinke J, Diehl P, et al. (2010) Krüppel-like factor 15 regulates BMPER in endothelial cells. Cardiovascular Research 85: 551–559.
33. Kelley R, Ren R, Pi X, Wu Y, Moreno I, et al. (2009) A concentration-dependent endocytic trap and sink mechanism converts Bmper from an activator to an inhibitor of Bmp signaling. The Journal of Cell Biology 184: 597–609.
34. Pinto M, Oliveira C, Cirnes L, Carlos Machado J, Ramires M, et al. (2003) Promoter methylation of TGFα receptor I and mutation of TGFα receptor II are frequent events in MSI sporadic gastric carcinomas. J Pathol 200: 32–38.
35. Chen G, Ghosh P, Osawa H, Sasaki CY, Rezanka L, et al. (2007) Resistance to TGF-α correlates with aberrant expression of TGF-α receptor II in human B-cell lymphoma cell lines. Blood 109: 5301–5307.
36. de Carvalho Fc, Colleoni GWB, Sampaio Almeida MS, Carvalho AL, Vettore AL (2009) TGFα R aberrant methylation is a potential prognostic marker and therapeutic target in multiple myeloma. Int J Cancer 125: 1985–1991.
37. Shivapurkar N, Gazdar AF (2010) DNA Methylation Based Biomarkers in Non-Invasive Cancer Screening. Current Molecular Medicine 10: 123–132.
38. Shi H, Guo J, Duff DJ, Rahmatpanah F, Chitima-Matsiga R, et al. (2007) Discovery of novel epigenetic markers in non-Hodgkin's lymphoma. Carcinogenesis 28: 60–70.
39. Esteller M, Gaidano G, Goodman SN, Zagonel V, Capello D, et al. (2002) Hypermethylation of the DNA Repair Gene O6-Methylguanine DNA Methyltransferase and Survival of Patients With Diffuse Large B-Cell Lymphoma. J Natl Cancer Inst 94: 26–32.

40. Syed N, Coley HM, Sehouli J, Koensgen D, Mustea A, et al. (2011) Polo-like Kinase Plk2 Is an Epigenetic Determinant of Chemosensitivity and Clinical Outcomes in Ovarian Cancer. Cancer Res 71: 3317–3327.
41. Iorns E, Turner NC, Elliott R, Syed N, Garrone O, et al. (2008) Identification of CDK10 as an Important Determinant of Resistance to Endocrine Therapy for Breast Cancer. Cancer Cell 13: 91–104.
42. Ibanez de Caceres I, Cortes-Sempere M, Moratilla C, hado-Pinilla R, Rodriguez-Fanjul V, et al. (2010) IGFBP-3 hypermethylation-derived deficiency mediates cisplatin resistance in non-small-cell lung cancer. Oncogene 29: 1681–1690.

10

Serum Levels of Interleukin-9 Correlate with Negative Prognostic Factors in Extranodal NK/T-Cell Lymphoma

Jing Zhang[1,2,3]ⓢ, Wei-da Wang[1,2]ⓢ, Qi-rong Geng[1,2], Liang Wang[1,2], Xiao-qin Chen[1,2], Cheng-cheng Liu[1,2], Yue Lv[1,2]*

1 Department of Hematologic Oncology, Sun Yat-Sen University Cancer Center, Guangzhou, Guangdong, P. R. China, **2** State Key Laboratory of Oncology in South China, Guangzhou, Guangdong, P. R. China, **3** Department of Medical Oncology, Hubei Cancer Hospital, Wuhan, Hubei, P. R. China

Abstract

Interleukin-9 (IL-9) is more functionally diverse than previously expected, especially with regards to lymphomagenesis. However, the relationship between IL-9 and the clinicopathological features of extranodal NK/T-cell lymphoma is less well established. Patients with this lymphoma in Sun Yat-Sen University Cancer Center between January 2003 and March 2013 were systematically reviewed in an intention-to-treat analysis. Baseline serum IL-9 levels were determined using sandwich enzyme-linked immunosorbent assays. A total of seventy-four patients were enrolled in this study. The mean concentration of serum IL-9 for all patients was 6.48 pg/mL (range: 1.38–51.87 pg/mL). Age, B symptoms and local lymph node involvement were found to be related to high serum IL-9 levels. Patients with low IL-9 levels tended to have higher rates of complete remission. Notably, the median progression-free survival (PFS) and overall survival (OS) were longer in the low IL-9 level group than in the high IL-9 level group (PFS: 68.7 months vs. 28.3 months, $P<0.001$; OS: 86 months vs. 42.8 months, $P=0.001$). Multivariate analysis revealed independent prognostic factors for PFS. Similarly, high IL-9 levels ($P=0.003$) and old age ($P=0.007$) were independently predictive of shorter OS. Serum IL-9 is closely related to several clinical features, such as age, B symptoms and local lymph node involvement. It can also be a significant independent prognostic factor for extranodal NK/T-cell lymphoma, which suggests a role for IL-9 in the pathogenesis of this disease and offers new insight into potential therapeutic strategies.

Editor: Masaru Katoh, National Cancer Center, Japan

Funding: This work was supported by the following funds: National Natural Science Foundation of China (contract/grant numbers 30471976 and 81272620) and Science and Technology projects of Guangdong Province (contract/grant numbers 2010B031600233 and 2010A090200019). The funders had no role in study design, data collection and analysis, decision to publish, or preparation of the manuscript.

Competing Interests: The authors have declared that no competing interests exist.

* E-mail: lvyue@sysucc.org.cn

ⓢ These authors contributed equally to this work.

Introduction

Extranodal NK/T-cell lymphoma (ENKTL) is more prevalent in Asia than in Western countries [1,2]. According to a recent large survey [3], it is the second most common lymphoma subtype in China and is only inferior to diffuse large B-cell lymphoma. It is characterized by vascular damage, zonal tumor cell death and prominent tissue necrosis. Many studies have suggested the involvement of cytokines in these pathological changes, such as CXCL9, CXCL10 [4,5], and interleukin-9 (IL-9) [6].

IL-9 has attracted renewed interest since its expression was identified in multiple T helper (Th) cell subsets (including Th2, Th9, Th17), regulatory T cells (Treg) and natural killer (NK)/T cells [7]. Several studies have indicated that IL-9 may promote oncogenesis during Hodgkin's Lymphoma (HL) and large cell anaplastic lymphoma [8–10] in addition to its significant regulatory role in allergy and autoimmunity [11–13]. Dysregulation of the Janus kinase (JAK)/signal transducer and activator of transcription (STAT) pathway may be responsible for the oncogenesis of IL-9 *in vitro* and *in vivo* [14–16].

Correlations have been found between IL-9 levels and negative prognostic factors, including advanced stage, B-symptoms (including weight loss >10%, fever, drenching night sweats), low blood hemoglobin and elevated erythrocyte sedimentation rates in HL [8]. Nagato T *et al.* also reported that IL-9 was present in biopsy samples and serum from patients with ENKTL and played an important role in the disease, possibly via an autocrine mechanism [6]. These results suggest that IL-9 may be associated with the clinicopathological features of ENKTL, although little is known about the relationship between them. To clarify this problem, we measured IL-9 levels in the serum of patients with ENKTL and explored the clinical significance of serum IL-9 during ENKTL.

Methods

Ethics statement

This study was approved by the Institutional Review Board of Sun Yat-Sen University Cancer Center, and written informed consent was obtained from all healthy volunteers and patients prior to treatment. Additionally, this study was conducted in accordance with the Helsinki Declaration.

Eligibility criteria

This study used a retrospective cohort study design. Patients with nasal ENKTL who received chemotherapy, radiotherapy or both in Sun Yat-Sen University Cancer Center between January 2003 and March 2013 were systematically reviewed in an intention-to-treat analysis. All eligible cases were selected consecutively. Eligibility criteria for inclusion in this study were as follows: (1) pathologically confirmed diagnosis of ENKTL according to the World Health Organization classification; (2) positive for CD3, CD56, cytotoxic molecules, and Epstein-Barr virus by in situ hybridization and negative for CD20; (3) primary symptoms and the bulk of the tumor localized to the nasal cavity; (4) no previous anti-tumor treatments; (5) available serum samples obtained before the primary treatment and stored at −80°C; (6) complete follow-up results. The exclusion criteria were: (1) prior or concomitant malignant tumors; (2) any co-existing medical problems of sufficient severity to prevent full compliance with standard antitumor therapy protocols; (3) other subtypes of non-Hodgkin lymphoma (NHL), including myeloid/NK cell precursor acute leukemia, blastic NK cell lymphoma/precursor NK cell lymphoblastic leukemia, aggressive NK cell leukemia, and peripheral T cell lymphoma.

All enrolled patients underwent standard Ann Arbor staging with history, physical examination, nasopharyngeal endoscopy, whole body positron emission tomography/computed tomography (PET/CT) scans, CT scans or magnetic resonance imaging of the involved organs of the head and neck and CT scans of the chest, abdomen and pelvis. Complete blood counts and serum biochemistry were routinely examined.

Treatment

Patients received one of the following initial treatment modalities: (1) chemotherapy followed by involved-field radiotherapy; (2) chemotherapy alone; (3) radiotherapy alone. The following chemotherapy regimens were included: (1) CHOP (cyclophosphamide, doxorubicin, vincristine, prednisone); (2) EPOCH (etoposide, doxorubicin, vincristine, cyclophosphamide, prednisone); (3) alternating triple therapy (ATT): CHOP-B (CHOP plus bleomycin), IMVP-16 (ifosfamide, methotrexate, etoposide), DHAP (dexamethasone, cisplatin, cytarabine); (4) GELOX (gemcitabine, oxaliplatin, L-asparaginase) or modified GELOX [17]; (5) others: CHOP-L (CHOP plus L-asparaginase), DeVIC (dexamethasone, etoposide, ifosfamide, carboplatin). Patients received at least one cycle and a maximum of eight cycles of initial chemotherapy. Involved-field radiotherapy of 50–60 Gy was delivered in daily fractions of 1.8–2.0 Gy with five fractions each week. The treatment response was assessed according to the standardized response criteria for non-Hodgkin lymphomas [18]. After the completion of treatment, patients were followed by their ambulatory oncologists. The follow-up interval was based on the regular standard. Overall survival (OS) was measured from the time of diagnosis until death from any cause. Progression-free survival (PFS) was measured from the time of diagnosis until disease progression, relapse, or death from any cause or until the last follow-up.

ELISA

Serum IL-9 levels were determined using sandwich enzyme-linked immunosorbent assay (ELISA) kits (Human IL-9 Platinum ELISA; Bender MedSystems, Vienna, Austria). All venous blood samples were drawn from ten healthy volunteers and from patients at diagnosis. The samples were centrifuged at 4°C, and serum was collected and quickly frozen at −80°C until further assay. A routine ELISA method was performed according to the manufacturer's protocol. The limit of detection of human IL-9 was 0.5 pg/mL. All samples were analyzed in duplicate, experiments were repeated three times, and the results are presented as the means ± standard deviations.

Statistical analysis

Differences in the mean values were tested using the non-parametric Mann-Whitney U-test. The cut off concentration of serum IL-9 for survival analysis was determined using the receiver operating characteristics (ROC) curve analysis. The correlation between serum IL-9 levels and complete remission (CR) rates was performed using the Chi-square test. Univariate analyses of the effects of several pretreatment characteristics upon survival, including IL-9, were performed using the Kaplan-Meier method and log-rank test. Multivariate analysis was performed using the Cox proportional-hazards regression technique to define the prognostic significance of selected variables, including IL-9. A two-sided *P* value <0.05 was considered statistically significant. All statistical analyses were performed using PASW Statistics 18.0 software (Apache Software Foundation, Forest Hill, MD).

Results

Patient characteristics and serum IL-9 content at baseline

A total of seventy-four patients were enrolled in this study. The clinical characteristics are listed in Table 1. The ratio of males to females was 3.11:1, with a median age of 42.5 years. Seventy-one patients (95.9%) had a good performance status (Eastern Cooperative Oncology Group 0–1), and B symptoms occurred in more than half of the patients. Sixty-two patients (83.7%) had stage I-II disease, and the remaining patients had stage III-IV disease. Most patients were assigned to the low-risk group with an International Prognostic Index (IPI) score of 0-1. However, nearly half the patients were grouped in the high-risk group according to the Korean Prognostic Index (KPI) score.

The mean concentration of serum IL-9 for all patients was 6.48 pg/mL (range: 1.38–51.87 pg/mL) with a median of 3.12 pg/mL. Serum IL-9 was detected in six of ten healthy volunteers, and the average concentration was 0.56 pg/mL (range: 0–1.23 pg/mL), which was significantly lower than that of ENKTL patients ($P<0.001$, Fig. 1A).

Correlation between serum IL-9 levels and clinical features

To explore the correlation between serum IL-9 levels and prognostic factors, the IL-9 content at baseline was compared according to the clinical features of all patients (Table 2). The IL-9 levels for patients >60 years, with B symptoms and with local lymph node involvement were significantly higher than for those ≤60 years ($P=0.042$), without B symptoms ($P=0.009$), or without local lymph node involvement ($P=0.011$, Fig. 1B–D). Other clinical factors, such as male ($P=0.316$), poor performance status ($P=0.125$), elevated LDH ($P=0.995$), advanced stages ($P=0.084$), high IPI ($P=0.125$) or KPI score ($P=0.284$), low lymphocyte counts ($P=0.250$) and high monocyte counts ($P=0.724$), were not significantly associated with high serum IL-9 concentrations.

Cut-off value for serum IL-9

To identify an optimal cut-off point for survival outcomes, the ROC curve analysis was selected. The most discriminative cut-off concentration of serum IL-9 was 3.49 pg/mL with an area under the curve (AUC) value of 0.799 [95% confidence interval (CI) 0.688–0.909, $P<0.001$] (Fig. 2). The sensitivity and specificity of

Table 1. Clinical characteristics at baseline.

Characteristics	No.	%
Gender, male	**56**	**75.7**
Age, y		
Median (range)	42.5 (13–76)	
≤60	63	85.1
ECOG performance status		
0	28	37.8
1–2	46	62.2
B symptoms	39	52.7
Serum LDH (Elevated)	23	31.1
LN involvement	39	52.7
Ann Arbor stage		
I	32	43.2
II	30	40.5
III–IV	12	16.3
IPI		
0–1	61	82.4
2–5	13	17.6
KPI		
0	15	20.3
1	27	36.5
2	16	21.6
3–4	16	21.6
Lymphocytes (<normal)	23	31.1
Monocytes (>normal)	41	55.4
Pretreatment serum IL-9		
Mean concentration, pg/mL (range)	6.48 (1.38–51.87)	

Abbreviations: ECOG, Eastern Cooperative Oncology Group; LDH, lactate dehydrogenase; LN, local lymph node; IPI, international prognostic index; KPI, Korean prognostic index.

the dichotomized IL-9 levels (≤3.49 pg/mL vs. >3.49 pg/mL) were 74.5% and 73.7%, respectively.

Treatment response and survival

The treatment response was evaluated in each patient: 55 of 74 (74.3%) achieved CR, 8 of 74 (10.8%) achieved partial response, 5 of 74 (6.8%) showed stable disease, and 6 patients (8.1%) showed progressive disease. The CR rates of patients with IL-9 levels ≤ 3.49 pg/mL and >3.49 pg/mL were 83.3% and 57.7%, respectively ($P=0.016$).

Within a median follow-up time of 17.7 months, the 3-year PFS and OS for all patients were 53.3% (95% CI 45.8%–60.8%) and 68.4% (95% CI 61.8%–75%), respectively (Fig. 3). Univariate analysis revealed that young age, (≤60 years), no local lymph node involvement, early stage, and low serum IL-9 levels (≤3.49 pg/mL) could significantly predict longer PFS (Table 3, Fig. 4). The 3-year PFS (68.7%) was much higher in patients with low IL-9 content (≤3.49 pg/mL) than in those with high IL-9 content (> 3.49 pg/mL) (28.3%, $P<0.001$). In the subgroup with stage I–II disease, low serum IL-9 concentrations were still predictive of better PFS (data not shown). In terms of OS, only age and serum IL-9 levels were predictive for 3-year survival rates. Ann Arbor stage and KPI scores lost their prognostic roles for OS. For patients of no more than 60 years, the 3-year OS was 78.9%, but it was fairly low in patients older than 60 years (21.8%, $P<0.001$, Fig. 5A). In addition, the 3-year OS was as high as 86% for patients with low IL-9 levels. However, the 3-year OS was only 42.8% in those with high IL-9 levels ($P=0.001$, Fig. 5B).

Multivariate analysis

The clinical factors that were statistically significant predictors of the PFS were included in the multivariate analysis. Multivariate analysis revealed that the independent prognostic factors for PFS were serum IL-9 concentration ($P=0.001$; relative risk, 3.541; 95% CI 1.626–7.714) and age ($P=0.025$; relative risk, 1.029; 95% CI 1.004–1.056). Similarly, high IL-9 levels ($P=0.003$; relative risk, 4.377; 95% CI 1.628–11.766) and old age ($P=0.007$; relative risk, 1.043; 95% CI 1.012–1.076) were independently predictive of shorter OS (Table 4).

Discussion

IL-9 was first described in the late 1980s as an emerging cytokine with pleiotropic functions in the immune system [19]. It

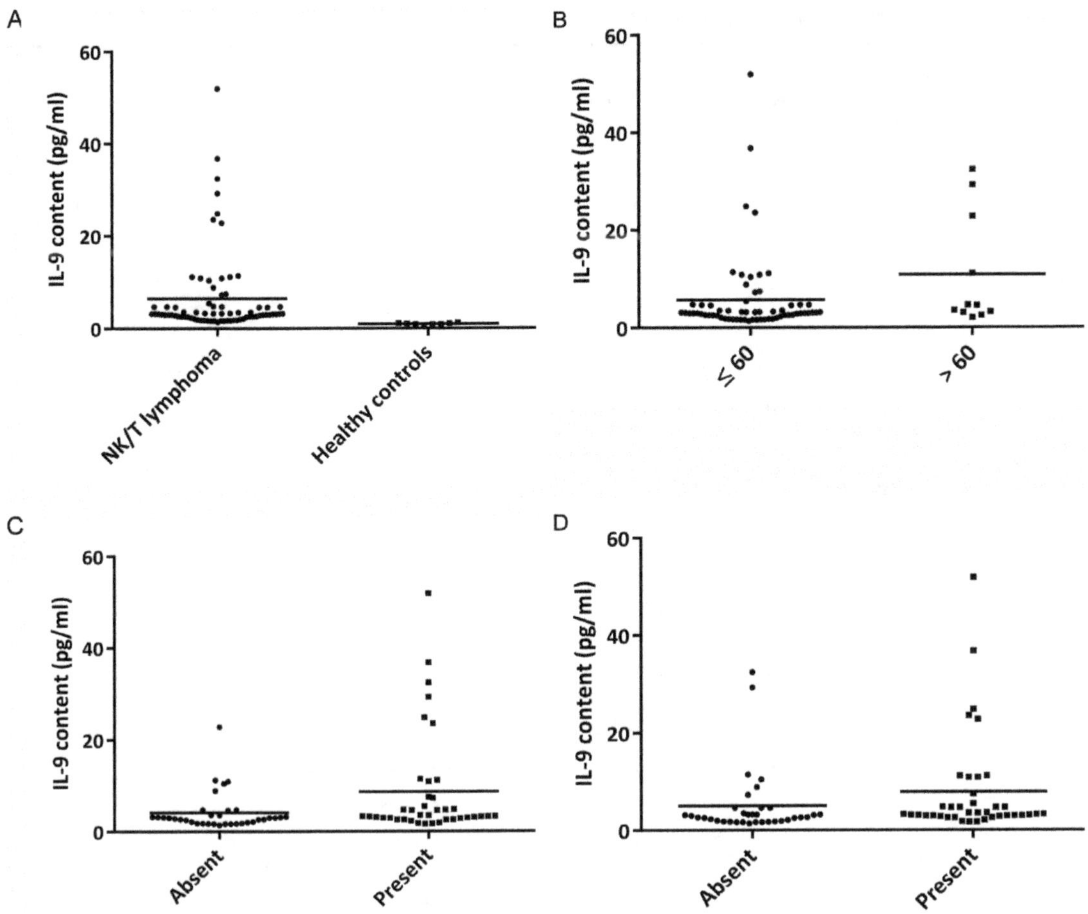

Figure 1. Correlation between serum IL-9 levels and clinical features. A: Serum IL-9 levels were significantly higher in patients with ENKTL than in healthy volunteers ($P<0.001$). B: Serum IL-9 levels in patients >60 years were significantly higher than in those ≤60 years ($P=0.042$). C: Serum IL-9 levels in patients with B symptoms were significantly higher than in those without B symptoms ($P=0.009$). D: Serum IL-9 levels in patients with local lymph node involvement were significantly higher than in those without local lymph node involvement ($P=0.011$).

demonstrated pro-inflammatory activity and played a key role in the pathogenesis of atopic diseases and asthma [20–22]. Its activities are mediated via a heterodimeric receptor complex formed by the IL-9Rα chain, which associates with JAK1 and the IL-2Rγ chain, also known as γc (common γ chain), which associates with JAK3 [23]. JAK3 mutations are involved in the pathogenesis of NK/T cell lymphoma [24,25]. With the detection of more immune targets and increased expression, IL-9 may be far more functionally diverse than previously expected, especially on lymphomagenesis. *In vitro*, IL-9 was able to stimulate JAK3-dependent survival of ALK+ anaplastic large-cell lymphoma cells [9] and protect thymic lymphoma cells from dexamethasone-induced apoptosis [26]. *In vivo*, nucleophosmin-ALK expression during transgenic IL-9 expression led to the development of murine plasmacytoma, plasmoblastic/anaplastic lymphoma and precursor T-lymphoblastic lymphoma [27]. IL-9R was markedly overexpressed in diffuse large B-cell lymphoma tissues compared to their counterparts, and it was associated with several adverse prognostic parameters [28]. IL-9 was also expressed in two of six cases of large cell anaplastic lymphoma and in 6 of 13 cases of Hodgkin's disease by northern blot analysis or in situ hybridization [10]. Fischer M *et al.* detected IL-9 in serum samples and found a novel correlation between increased serum IL-9 levels, HL and clinical features [8]. Additionally, Kelleher K *et al.* reported that IL-9 was constitutively expressed in human T-cell leukemia virus-I-transformed human T cells, implying a possible correlation between IL-9 expression and T cell lymphoma/leukemia [29].

ENKTL was previously known as lethal midline granuloma because, macroscopically, the tumor looked like a necrotic granuloma, and the disease showed an aggressive and lethal course [30,31]. Histologically, ENKTL is characterized by angiocentric and polymorphous lymphoreticular infiltrates, known as polymorphic reticulosis [31,32]. Previous studies indicated that many cytokines might be responsible for its pathological features. TNF-α induced by Epstein-Barr virus could lead to the observed necrosis [33]. The monokine induced by interferon-γ (IFN-γ), and the IFN-γ-inducible protein-10 play important roles in the pathogenesis of tissue necrosis and vascular damage associated with certain EBV-positive lymphoproliferative processes [4,5]. Furthermore, Yang *et al.* reported that IL-9 induced by EBV-encoded small RNA acted as an autocrine growth factor for EBV-infected T cells [34]. Furthermore, several studies have mentioned the role of IL-9 in ENKTL. For example, IL-9 was specifically expressed by nasal NK/T-cell lymphoma cell lines, where it acted as an autocrine growth factor, suggesting that the IL-9 signaling pathway may be a new therapeutic target for NK/T-cell lymphoma [6]. However, few studies have focused on the

Table 2. The differences of serum IL-9 levels in various clinical factors.

Factors	No.	Average	Range	*P* value
Gender				
Male	56	7.02	1.38–51.87	0.316
Female	18	4.78	1.62–23.52	
Age				
≤60	63	5.71	1.38–51.87	0.042
>60	11	10.85	2.08–32.4	
ECOG performance status				
0	28	4.61	1.38–22.8	0.125
1–2	46	7.61	1.62–51.87	
B symptoms				
Absent	35	4.1	1.38–22.8	0.009
Present	39	8.61	1.62–51.87	
Serum LDH				
Normal	51	5.61	1.62–32.4	0.995
>normal	23	8.39	1.38–51.87	
LN involvement				
Absent	35	4.98	1.38–32.4	0.011
Present	39	7.82	1.66–51.87	
Ann Arbor stage				
I	32	5.17	1.38–32.4	0.084
II	30	7.76	1.62–51.87	
III–IV	12	6.74	1.69–24.82	
IPI				
0–1	62	6.38	1.38–51.87	0.125
2–5	12	6.99	2.62–24.82	
KPI				
0	15	5.16	1.38–32.4	0.284
1	27	5.74	1.62–29.28	
2	16	4.59	1.66–11.12	
3–4	16	10.84	1.69–51.87	
Lymphocytes				
Normal	51	7.56	1.38–51.87	0.25
<normal	23	4.07	1.62–23.52	
Monocytes				
Normal	33	6.4	1.38–32.4	0.724
>normal	41	6.54	1.62–51.87	

Abbreviations: ECOG, Eastern Cooperative Oncology Group; LDH, lactate dehydrogenase; LN, local lymph node; IPI, international prognostic index; KPI, Korean prognostic index.

relationship between IL-9 levels and clinical manifestations of ENKTL.

In the present study, we measured serum IL-9 levels in healthy volunteers and patients with ENKTL. We found that IL-9 was fairly low in the healthy controls (average concentration: 0.56 pg/mL), but it showed a relative higher level in patients with ENKTL, with a mean value of 6.48 pg/mL. Age, B symptoms and local lymph node involvement were correlated with high serum IL-9 levels. Due to its role in recruiting non-malignant infiltrating cells, IL-9 makes a crucial contribution to tumor survival, migration and metastasis [35]. Thus, it is easy to explain the correlation between IL-9 and B symptoms and local lymph node involvement. However, it remains unclear why IL-9 levels were also associated with age. According to the ROC curve analyses, 3.49 pg/mL was an optimal cut-off value for distinguishing between poor outcomes. Patients with low IL-9 levels (≤3.49 pg/mL) tended to have higher CR rates (83.3%) than those with high IL-9 levels (> 3.49 pg/mL) (57.7%) ($P=0.016$). Specifically, the median PFS and OS in the low IL-9 level group were clearly longer than those in the high IL-9 level group (PFS: 68.7 months vs. 28.3 months, $P<0.001$; OS: 86 months vs. 42.8 months, $P=0.001$). Multivariate analysis also indicated that IL-9 was an independent prognostic

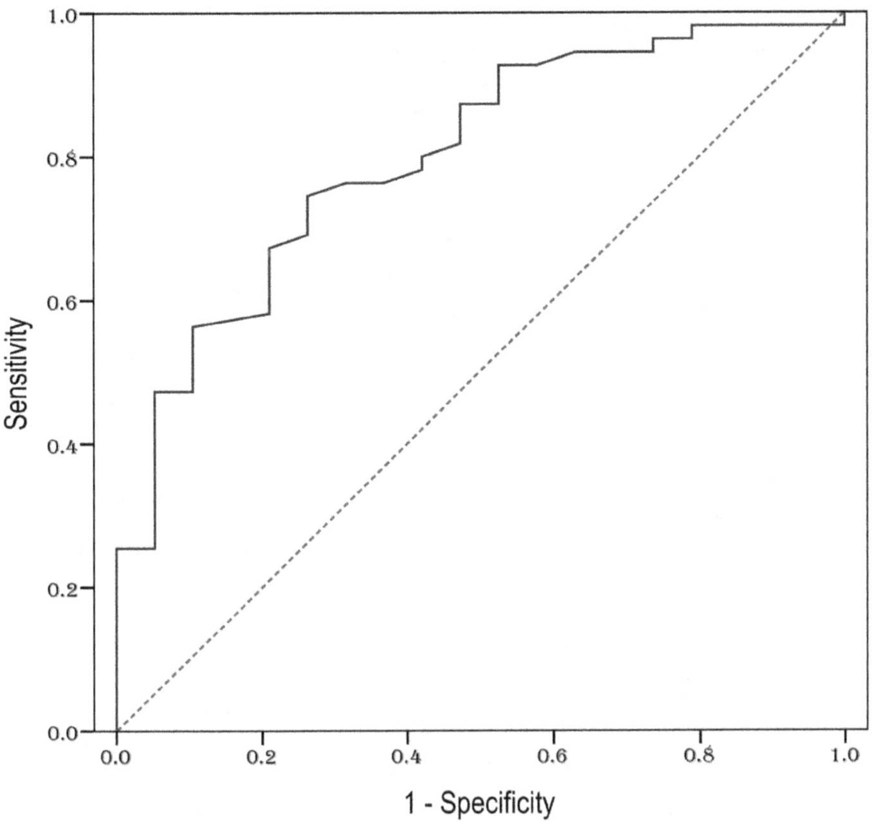

Figure 2. ROC curve analysis for the optimal cut-off point of serum IL-9. The most discriminative cut-off concentration of serum IL-9 was 3.49 pg/mL with an AUC value of 0.799. The sensitivity and specificity were 74.5% and 73.7%, respectively.

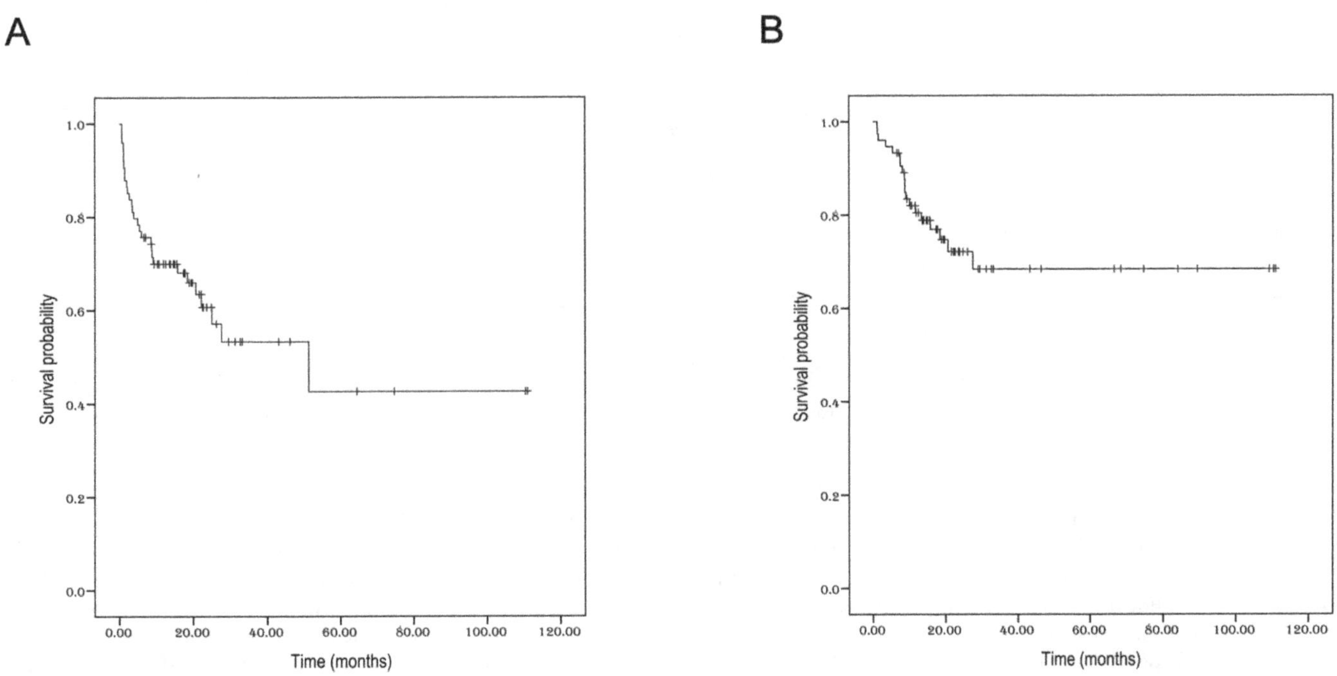

Figure 3. The survival for all patients. A: Progression-free survival. B: Overall survival.

Table 3. The 3-year survival rates according to various clinical factors.

Factors	3-y PFS (%)	95% CI	*P*	3-y OS (%)	95% CI	*P*
Gender			0.117			0.118
Male	45.3	36.4–54.2		61.9	53.7–70.1	
Female	77.8	68–87.6		88.1	80.2–96	
Age			0.011			<0.001
≤60	60	51.8–68.2		78.9	71.8–85.3	
>60	21.8	8.4–35.2		21.8	8.4–35.2	
ECOG performance status			0.109			0.152
0	60.4	48.5–72.3		76.7	66.8–86.6	
1–2	52	43.6–60.4		63.9	55.7–72.1	
B symptoms			0.122			0.285
Absent	66.8	57.5–76.1		77.9	70.4–85.4	
Present	43	32.8–53.2		61.2	51.5–70.9	
Serum LDH			0.455			0.202
Normal	57.3	48.8–65.8		70.5	62.7–78.3	
>normal	44.7	29.6–59.8		68	58–78	
LN involvement			0.005			0.071
Absent	70.8	61.7–79.9		78.3	70.2–86.4	
Present	35.2	23.7–46.7		58.7	48.3–69.1	
Ann Arbor stage			0.042			0.304
I	68.3	58.6–78		76.2	67.4–85	
II	41.3	27.9–54.7		61.7	50.4–73	
III–IV	41.7	27.5–55.9		66.7	53.1–80.3	
IPI			0.067			0.053
0–1	55.9	47.6–64.2		70.8	63.6–78	
2–5	41.7	27.5–55.9		58.3	44.1–72.5	
KPI			0.064			0.251
0	66	51.9–80.1		73.5	60–87	
1	67.9	58.2–77.6		75.3	66.3–84.3	
2	34.4	9.4–59.4		53.5	30.6–76.4	
3–4	20.1	4.5–35.7		59.1	46.1–72.1	
Lymphocytes			0.286			0.217
Normal	49.3	40.8–57.8		62.5	54.4–70.6	
<normal	62.6	47–78.2		86.7	47.3–93.8	
Monocytes			0.432			0.861
Normal	51.6	41.5–61.7		69	60.1–77.9	
>normal	53.5	42.4–64.6		67.3	57.4–77.2	
Serum IL-9			<0.001			0.001
≤3.49	68.7	59.4–78		86	80.6–91.4	
>3.49	28.3	18.4–38.2		42.8	31.9–53.7	

Abbreviations: PFS, progression-free survival; OS, overall survival; ECOG, Eastern Cooperative Oncology Group; LDH, lactate dehydrogenase; LN, local lymph node; IPI, international prognostic index; KPI, Korean prognostic index

factor for PFS and OS. All these data confirmed that serum IL-9 was closely correlated with certain clinical features, treatment response and prognosis in ENKTL, implying a significant role for IL-9 in the pathogenesis and development of this disease. Nevertheless, IL-9 can lead to either a favorable or unfavorable clinical prognosis depending on the tumor. Lu Y *et al.* elucidated the role of Th9 cells and the γ chain family member IL-9 in a B16 melanoma mouse model, and they found that Th9-derived IL-9 inhibited tumor progression [36]. This was also supported by Purwar R *et al.*, who indicated that the generation of IL-9-mediated immune responses may have an important role in the treatment of melanoma and other solid tumors [37]. The inconsistent roles of IL-9 in tumors may be partly attributed to different immune effects or single nucleotide polymorphisms

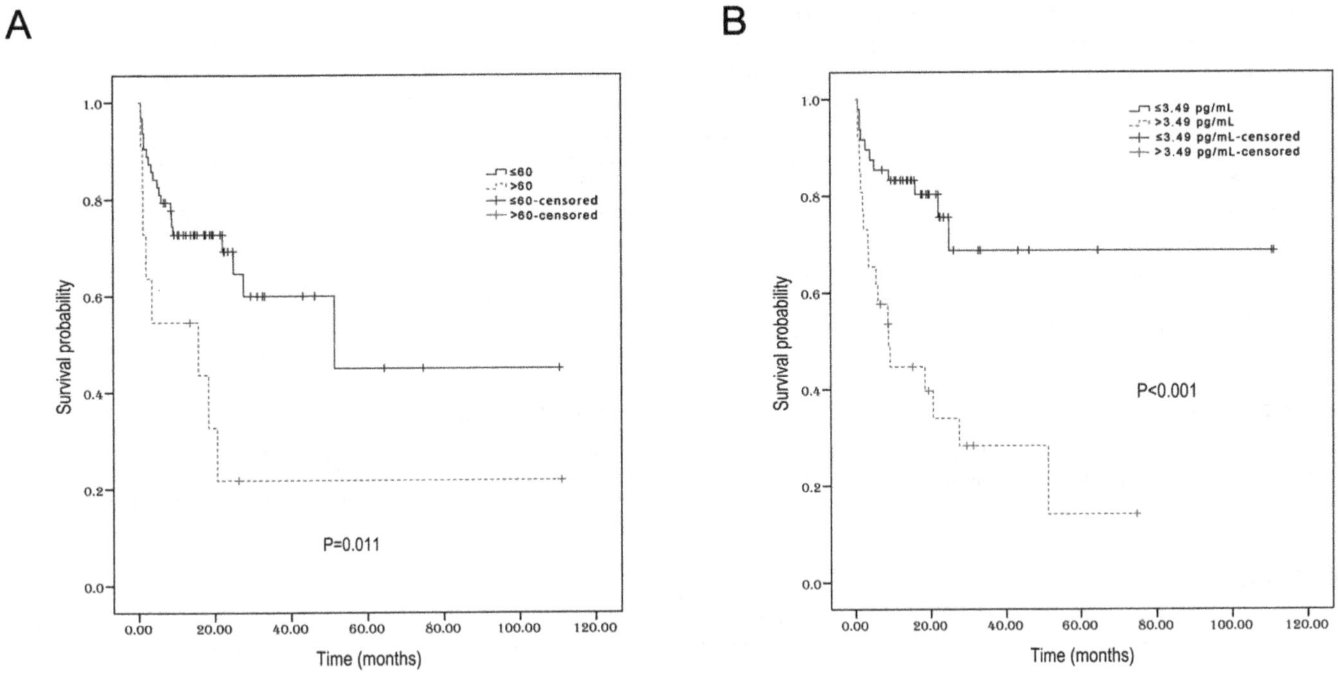

Figure 4. The progression-free survival according to age (A) and serum IL-9 levels (B).

[38,39]. Thus, the exact molecular mechanisms of IL-9 in the pathogenesis and development of ENKTL need to be further clarified.

In conclusion, this is the first study that confirms the close relationship of IL-9 with several clinical features of ENKTL, including age, B symptoms and local lymph node involvement. Serum IL-9, which can be easily measured in clinical practice, may be a significant independent prognostic factor for this disease. These results suggest a role for IL-9 in the pathogenesis of ENKTL and offer new insight into potential therapeutic strategies.

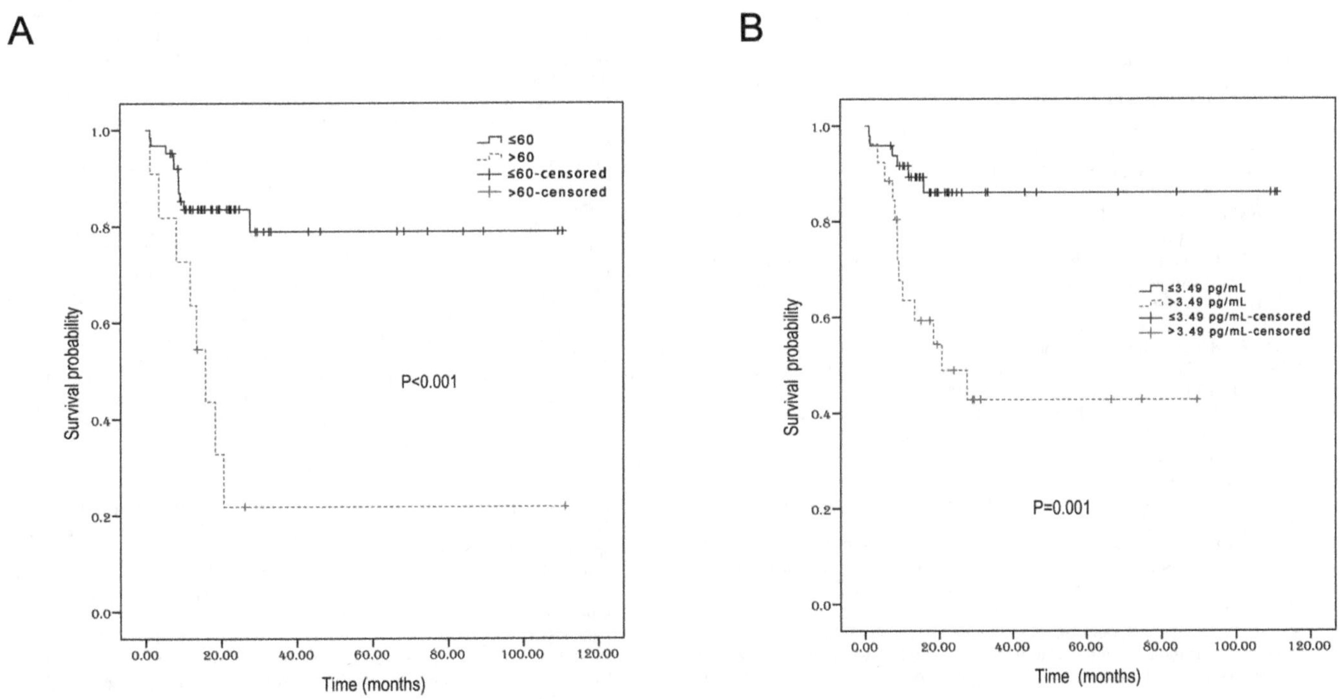

Figure 5. The overall survival according to age (A) and serum IL-9 levels (B).

Table 4. Multivariate analysis of prognostic factors for survival.

	PFS			OS		
Parameters	*P*	**RR**	**95% CI**	*P*	**RR**	**95% CI**
Age >60 years	0.025	1.029	1.004–1.056	0.007	1.043	1.012–1.076
LN involvement	0.107	2.650	0.810–8.668	0.386	1.867	0.456–7.654
Serum IL-9 (>3.49 pg/mL)	0.001	3.541	1.626–7.714	0.003	4.377	1.628–11.766
Ann Arbor stage (I vs. II vs. III–IV)	0.945	0.979	0.535–1.791	0.972	1.013	0.496–2.068

Abbreviations: PFS, progression-free survival; OS, overall survival; LN, local lymph node.

Acknowledgments

We thank all the investigators, including the physicians, nurses, pathologists, and laboratory technicians in this study.

Author Contributions

Conceived and designed the experiments: YL JZ. Performed the experiments: JZ QRG LW CCL. Analyzed the data: WDW CCL. Contributed reagents/materials/analysis tools: JZ XQC LW. Wrote the paper: JZ WDW.

References

1. Au WY, Weisenburger DD, Intragumtornchai T, Nakamura S, Kim WS, et al. (2009) Clinical differences between nasal and extranasal natural killer/T-cell lymphoma: a study of 136 cases from the International Peripheral T-Cell Lymphoma Project. Blood 113: 3931–3937.
2. Lee J, Suh C, Park YH, Ko YH, Bang SM, et al. (2006) Extranodal natural killer T-cell lymphoma, nasal-type: a prognostic model from a retrospective multicenter study. J Clin Oncol 24: 612–618.
3. Sun J, Yang Q, Lu Z, He M, Gao L, et al. (2012) Distribution of lymphoid neoplasms in China: analysis of 4,638 cases according to the World Health Organization classification. Am J Clin Pathol 138: 429–434.
4. Moriai S, Takahara M, Ogino T, Nagato T, Kishibe K, et al. (2009) Production of interferon-{gamma}-inducible protein-10 and its role as an autocrine invasion factor in nasal natural killer/T-cell lymphoma cells. Clin Cancer Res 15: 6771–6779.
5. Teruya-Feldstein J, Jaffe ES, Burd PR, Kanegane H, Kingma DW, et al. (1997) The role of Mig, the monokine induced by interferon-gamma, and IP-10, the interferon-gamma-inducible protein-10, in tissue necrosis and vascular damage associated with Epstein-Barr virus-positive lymphoproliferative disease. Blood 90: 4099–4105.
6. Nagato T, Kobayashi H, Kishibe K, Takahara M, Ogino T, et al. (2005) Expression of interleukin-9 in nasal natural killer/T-cell lymphoma cell lines and patients. Clin Cancer Res 11: 8250–8257.
7. Noelle RJ, Nowak EC (2010) Cellular sources and immune functions of interleukin-9. Nat Rev Immunol 10: 683–687.
8. Fischer M, Bijman M, Molin D, Cormont F, Uyttenhove C, et al. (2003) Increased serum levels of interleukin-9 correlate to negative prognostic factors in Hodgkin's lymphoma. Leukemia 17: 2513–2516.
9. Qiu L, Lai R, Lin Q, Lau E, Thomazy DM, et al. (2006) Autocrine release of interleukin-9 promotes Jak3-dependent survival of ALK+ anaplastic large-cell lymphoma cells. Blood 108: 2407–2415.
10. Merz H, Houssiau FA, Orscheschek K, Renauld JC, Fliedner A, et al. (1991) Interleukin-9 expression in human malignant lymphomas: unique association with Hodgkin's disease and large cell anaplastic lymphoma. Blood 78: 1311–1317.
11. Li H, Nourbakhsh B, Ciric B, Zhang GX, Rostami A (2010) Neutralization of IL-9 ameliorates experimental autoimmune encephalomyelitis by decreasing the effector T cell population. J Immunol 185: 4095–4100.
12. Cheng G, Arima M, Honda K, Hirata H, Eda F, et al. (2002) Anti-interleukin-9 antibody treatment inhibits airway inflammation and hyperreactivity in mouse asthma model. Am J Respir Crit Care Med 166: 409–416.
13. Steenwinckel V, Louahed J, Orabona C, Huaux F, Warnier G, et al. (2007) IL-13 mediates in vivo IL-9 activities on lung epithelial cells but not on hematopoietic cells. J Immunol 178: 3244–3251.
14. Demoulin JB, Van Snick J, Renauld JC (2001) Interleukin-9 (IL-9) induces cell growth arrest associated with sustained signal transducer and activator of transcription activation in lymphoma cells overexpressing the IL-9 receptor. Cell Growth Differ 12: 169–174.
15. Shang Y, Kakinuma S, Amasaki Y, Nishimura M, Kobayashi Y, et al. (2008) Aberrant activation of interleukin-9 receptor and downstream Stat3/5 in primary T-cell lymphomas in vivo in susceptible B6 and resistant C3H mice. In Vivo 22: 713–720.
16. Demoulin JB, Uyttenhove C, Lejeune D, Mui A, Groner B, et al. (2000) STAT5 activation is required for interleukin-9-dependent growth and transformation of lymphoid cells. Cancer Res 60: 3971–3977.
17. Wang L, Wang ZH, Chen XQ, Li YJ, Wang KF, et al. (2013) First-line combination of gemcitabine, oxaliplatin, and L-asparaginase (GELOX) followed by involved-field radiation therapy for patients with stage IE/IIE extranodal natural killer/T-cell lymphoma. Cancer 119: 348–355.
18. Cheson BD, Horning SJ, Coiffier B, Shipp MA, Fisher RI, et al. (1999) Report of an international workshop to standardize response criteria for non-Hodgkin's lymphomas. NCI Sponsored International Working Group. J Clin Oncol 17: 1244.
19. Hultner L, Druez C, Moeller J, Uyttenhove C, Schmitt E, et al. (1990) Mast cell growth-enhancing activity (MEA) is structurally related and functionally identical to the novel mouse T cell growth factor P40/TCGFIII (interleukin 9). Eur J Immunol 20: 1413–1416.
20. Nicolaides NC, Holroyd KJ, Ewart SL, Eleff SM, Kiser MB, et al. (1997) Interleukin 9: a candidate gene for asthma. Proc Natl Acad Sci U S A 94: 13175–13180.
21. Levitt RC, McLane MP, MacDonald D, Ferrante V, Weiss C, et al. (1999) IL-9 pathway in asthma: new therapeutic targets for allergic inflammatory disorders. J Allergy Clin Immunol 103: S485–491.
22. Shimbara A, Christodoulopoulos P, Soussi-Gounni A, Olivenstein R, Nakamura Y, et al. (2000) IL-9 and its receptor in allergic and nonallergic lung disease: increased expression in asthma. J Allergy Clin Immunol 105: 108–115.
23. Knoops L, Renauld JC (2004) IL-9 and its receptor: from signal transduction to tumorigenesis. Growth Factors 22: 207–215.
24. Koo GC, Tan SY, Tang T, Poon SL, Allen GE, et al. (2012) Janus kinase 3-activating mutations identified in natural killer/T-cell lymphoma. Cancer Discov 2: 591–597.
25. Bouchekioua A, Scourzic L, de Wever O, Zhang Y, Cervera P, et al. (2014) JAK3 deregulation by activating mutations confers invasive growth advantage in extranodal nasal-type natural killer cell lymphoma. Leukemia 28: 338–348.
26. Renauld JC, Vink A, Louahed J, Van Snick J (1995) Interleukin-9 is a major anti-apoptotic factor for thymic lymphomas. Blood 85: 1300–1305.
27. Lange K, Uckert W, Blankenstein T, Nadrowitz R, Bittner C, et al. (2003) Overexpression of NPM-ALK induces different types of malignant lymphomas in IL-9 transgenic mice. Oncogene 22: 517–527.
28. Lv X, Feng L, Fang X, Jiang Y, Wang X (2013) Overexpression of IL-9 receptor in diffuse large B-cell lymphoma. Int J Clin Exp Pathol 6: 911–916.
29. Kelleher K, Bean K, Clark SC, Leung WY, Yang-Feng TL, et al. (1991) Human interleukin-9: genomic sequence, chromosomal location, and sequences essential for its expression in human T-cell leukemia virus (HTLV)-I-transformed human T cells. Blood 77: 1436–1441.
30. Kassel SH, Echevarria RA, Guzzo FP (1969) Midline malignant reticulosis (so-called lethal midline granuloma). Cancer 23: 920–935.
31. Eichel BS, Harrison EG Jr, Devine KD, Scanlon PW, Brown HA (1966) Primary lymphoma of the nose including a relationship to lethal midline granuloma. Am J Surg 112: 597–605.
32. Harris NL, Jaffe ES, Stein H, Banks PM, Chan JK, et al. (1994) A revised European-American classification of lymphoid neoplasms: a proposal from the International Lymphoma Study Group. Blood 84: 1361–1392.
33. Jaffe ES, Chan JK, Su IJ, Frizzera G, Mori S, et al. (1996) Report of the Workshop on Nasal and Related Extranodal Angiocentric T/Natural Killer Cell Lymphomas. Definitions, differential diagnosis, and epidemiology. Am J Surg Pathol 20: 103–111.
34. Yang L, Aozasa K, Oshimi K, Takada K (2004) Epstein-Barr virus (EBV)-encoded RNA promotes growth of EBV-infected T cells through interleukin-9 induction. Cancer Res 64: 5332–5337.

35. Lv X, Wang X (2013) The role of interleukin-9 in lymphoma. Leuk Lymphoma 54: 1367–1372.
36. Lu Y, Hong S, Li H, Park J, Hong B, et al. (2012) Th9 cells promote antitumor immune responses in vivo. J Clin Invest 122: 4160–4171.
37. Purwar R, Schlapbach C, Xiao S, Kang HS, Elyaman W, et al. (2012) Robust tumor immunity to melanoma mediated by interleukin-9-producing T cells. Nat Med 18: 1248–1253.
38. Li H, Rostami A (2010) IL-9: basic biology, signaling pathways in CD4+ T cells and implications for autoimmunity. J Neuroimmune Pharmacol 5: 198–209.
39. Yang XR, Pfeiffer RM, Wheeler W, Yeager M, Chanock S, et al. (2009) Identification of modifier genes for cutaneous malignant melanoma in melanoma-prone families with and without CDKN2A mutations. Int J Cancer 125: 2912–2917.

11

The use of Novel Drugs can Effectively Improve Response, Delay Relapse and Enhance Overall Survival in Multiple Myeloma Patients with Renal Impairment

Katarina Uttervall[1,2]*, Adil D. Duru[1], Johan Lund[1,2], Johan Liwing[1], Gösta Gahrton[1], Erik Holmberg[3], Johan Aschan[4], Evren Alici[1,2], Hareth Nahi[1,2]

1 Department of Medicine, Karolinska Institutet Huddinge, Stockholm, Sweden, **2** Hematology Center, Karolinska University Hospital Huddinge, Stockholm, Sweden, **3** Department of Oncology, Institute of Clinical Sciences, Sahlgrenska Academy at University of Gothenburg, Sweden, **4** Janssen-Cilag AB, Sollentuna, Sweden

Abstract

Background: Renal impairment is a common feature in multiple myeloma and is considered a poor prognostic factor.

Aim: To determine the impact of novel drugs (i.e. bortezomib, lenalidomide and thalidomide) in the treatment of myeloma patients with renal impairment. The primary endpoint was overall survival and secondary endpoints were time to next treatment and response.

Methods: The study population included all patients diagnosed with treatment-demanding multiple myeloma January 2000 to June 2011 at 15 Swedish hospitals. Renal impairment was defined as an estimated glomerular filtration rate under 60 mL/min/1.73 m^2.

Result: The study population consisted of 1538 patients, of which 680 had renal impairment at diagnosis. The median overall survival in patients with renal impairment was 33 months, which was significantly shorter than 52 months in patients with normal renal function ($P<0.001$). Novel agents in first line improved overall survival (median 60 months) in non-high-dose treated patients with renal impairment (n = 143) as compared to those treated with conventional cytotoxic drugs (n = 411) (median 27 months) ($P<0.001$). In the multivariate analysis up front treatment with bortezomib was an independent factor for better overall survival in non-high-dose treated renally impaired patients. High-dose treated renally impaired patients had significantly better median overall survival than non-high-dose ones (74 versus 26 months) and novel drugs did not significantly improve survival further in these patients. Patients with renal impairment had both a shorter median time to next treatment and a lower response rate than those with normal renal function. However, novel drugs and high dose treatment lead to a significantly longer time to next treatment and the use of novel agents significantly improved the response rate of these patients.

Conclusion: High dose treatment and novel drugs, especially bortezomib, can effectively overcome the negative impact of renal impairment in patients with multiple myeloma.

Editor: Hiromu Suzuki, Sapporo Medical University, Japan

Funding: Swedish cancer society, Swedish Research Council, Cancer Foundation in Sweden, Janssen-Cilag AB, Celgene lifetime achievement award. The funder provided support in the form of salaries for authors Johan Liwing and Johan Aschan, but did not have any additional role in the study design, data collection and analysis, decision to publish, or preparation of the manuscript. The specific roles of these authors are articulated in the 'author contributions' section.

Competing Interests: Co-author Johan Liwing and Johan Aschan are employed by Janssen-Cilag AB. Gösta Gahrton has received Celgene lifetime achievement award last year.

* Email: katarina.uttervall@ki.se

Introduction

Although the five-year survival for multiple myeloma (MM) patients has gradually increased over the last decades, especially with the use of high-dose chemotherapy and novel agents such as protease inhibitors and immunomodulatory drugs (IMiDs), MM is still considered incurable by conventional means. For the majority of patients the goal of therapy i.e. prolonged survival and preventing progression is related to the quality of response to initial therapy and depth of remissions reached [1,2].

Renal impairment (RI) is a relatively common feature of MM both at diagnosis and in relapsed/refractory MM [3]. With the use of conventional chemotherapy, it has been shown in several studies that renal impairment at diagnosis correlates to inferior survival [4,5], significant morbidity and increased early death rate.

The current gold standard for the treatment of patients less than 65 years of age is high-dose chemotherapy (HDT) followed by autologous stem cell transplantation [6]. However, the use of alkylators during induction treatment is associated with low response rate in patients with MM and RI [7]. Dexamethasone alone or in combination with cyclophosphamide is superior to melphalan containing regimens, because the latter are more dependent on renal elimination [7]. The addition of novel agents such as bortezomib has resulted in a substantial increase in the number of patients responding to therapy when compared to conventional therapy. Bortezomib is a proteasome inhibitor that promotes apoptosis, prevents DNA repair and inhibits proliferation [8] and it is effective in both newly diagnosed MM and relapsed/refractory MM [9]. It can be administered at the full-approved dose and schedule in patients with impaired renal function, because neither the pharmacokinetics nor the primary metabolic pathway of bortezomib are affected by renal impairment [10,11]. Moreover, other novel agents such as the IMiDs lenalidomide and thalidomide increase the susceptibility of tumor cells to lymphocyte-mediated immunosurveillance, which leads to enhanced cytotoxicity towards previously tolerated tumor cells [12,13]. However, lenalidomide is mainly excreted by the kidney [14] while thalidomide pharmacokinetics is not affected by renal function [15]. Currently there are limited data for the efficacy of IMiDs in patients with MM and RI.

The objective of this study is to understand the impact of RI on response to treatment, time to next treatment (TTNT) and most importantly survival in the era of novel agents (i.e. bortezomib, lenalidomide and thalidomide). In this retrospective study, we demonstrate that the use of novel drugs, especially bortezomib can effectively improve response, increase TTNT and enhance overall survival (OS) in multiple myeloma patients with renal impairment.

Materials and Methods

Study population

Consecutive patients diagnosed with MM between January 2000 and June 2011 at 7 university clinics, 5 regional centers and 3 local hospitals in Sweden were included. All patients were identified from the Swedish Cancer Registry, which covers 96.3% of all individuals with malignant disease [16]. Patients were excluded if they had non-treatment demanding disease (watch and wait), plasma cell leukemia or solitary plasmacytoma. All data were collected from the hospitals' electronic medical records and, in the case of death, from the national death registry. The study has received ethical approval from the Regional Ethical Vetting Board in Stockholm, Sweden. No informed consent was obtained because this was not required by the ethical committee. The patient information was anonymized and de-identified prior to analysis.

For each patient data regarding age, sex, type of myeloma and extent of bone disease as well as laboratory measurements of calcium, hemoglobin, β2-microglobulin, albumin and creatinine were collected at the time of diagnosis. Serum M-protein and urine M-protein values were collected at baseline and every significant change in the M-protein level was noted. In general, these proteins were measured on a monthly basis or at the start of every treatment cycle. For each treatment line the types of drugs given for MM were noted, with specific start and stop dates for each drug or drug combination. In the case of allogeneic stem cell transplantation the date was recorded and the patient was censored in all analysis after this date.

The estimated glomerular filtration rate (eGFR) was calculated using the Modification of Diet in Renal Disease (MDRD) formula: eGFR in mL/min/1.73 $m^2 = 186.3\times(\text{S-creatinine}/88.4)^{-1.154}\times(\text{age})^{-0.203}$ (×0.742 if female) [17]. Renal function was classified according to National Kidney Foundation Kidney Disease Outcomes Quality Initiative (KDOQI) chronic kidney disease classification [18] (Table 1). In this study RI was defined as eGFR <60 mL/min/1.73 m^2.

The study population was divided according to Fig. 1.

To evaluate renal response, all MM patients from our hospital were selected. Patients with a GFR <50 ml/min were identified and for these patients all serum creatinine values were gathered from diagnosis until death or end of follow up. The patients were also followed regarding changes in body weight. This cohort was divided into those receiving bortezomib and those receiving other drug combinations (control group). The control group consisted of different treatment regimes: melphalan-based, cyclophosphamide-based, VAD-based (vincristine, adriamycin and prednisone), IMiDs-based and other single drugs or drug combinations.

Definition of endpoints

Near complete response was defined as an undetectable M-protein in the blood and urine by standard electrophoresis but was not always confirmed by immunofixation since it was not required in clinical practice. Very good partial response (VGPR) was defined as at least 90% reduction of M-protein or a decrease to <200 mg/24 h in the urine M-protein levels. Partial response (PR) was defined as a 50% reduction in M-protein. No response (NR) was defined as less than 50% reduction of M-protein. Progress was considered when M-protein increased by 25% in serum and/or urine, absolute increases of ≥5 g/L in serum, or ≥200 mg/24 hours in urine [19]. Time to next treatment was defined as the time between the start date of the current treatment line and the start date of the next treatment line, death or last follow-up. OS was calculated from the start of the treatment until death or last follow-up.

Renal response was assessed according to the criteria suggested by Ludwig et al and the International Myeloma Group as either a complete response (CRrenal) defined as an improvement of GFR from <50 mL/min at baseline to ≥60 mL/min; a partial response (PRrenal) defined as an improvement of GFR from <15 mL/min at baseline to 30–59 mL/min; a minimal response (MRrenal) defined as an improvement of GFR from <15 mL/min at baseline to 15–29 mL/min or from 15–29 mL/min to 30–59 mL/min; or other, when there was no renal response or the response did not reach a MR renal criteria [20,21].

Statistical methods

The Mann-Whitney test for uncorrelated means was performed to investigate possible differences between two independent

Table 1. Classification of renal function according to National Kidney Foundation Kidney Disease Outcomes Quality Initiative.

Stage	Estimated glomerular filtration rate (mL/min/1.73 m^2)
1	≥90
2	60–89
3	30–59
4	15–29
5	<15

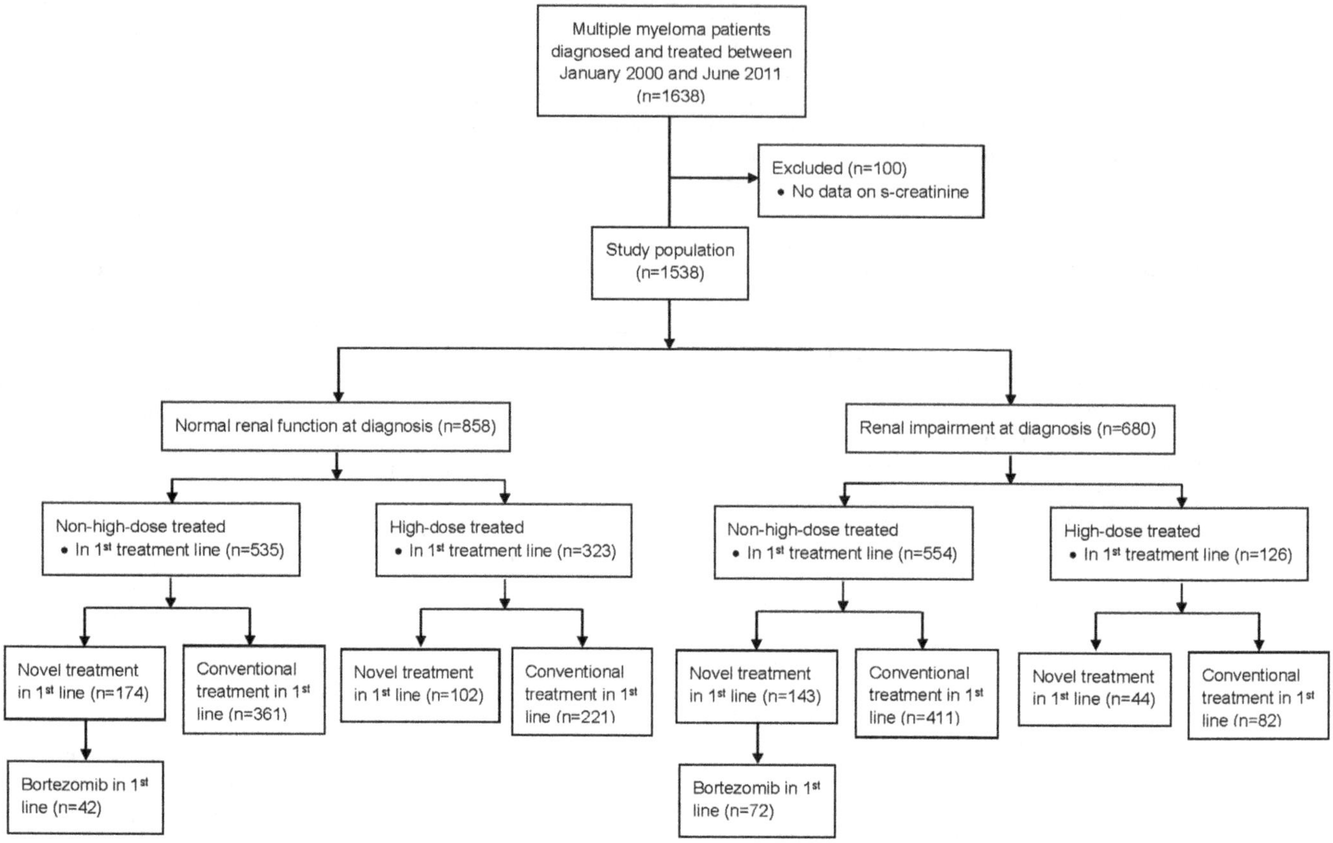

Figure 1. Patients enrolled in this study.

groups. In order to evaluate the variables in contingency tables, the Fisher's Exact Test was performed. Cox regression analyses were used to identify predictive factors and life table curves were calculated according to Kaplan-Meier and compared using log-rank tests. In addition, descriptive statistics were used to characterize the data. A probability value (P) of <0.05 was considered as significant.

Results

Patients enrolled in this study

The patients enrolled in this study were divided according to Fig. 1.

The median age at diagnosis was 73 years and 51% of the patients were male. The most common subtype was IgG (53%) followed by IgA (21%), Bence Jones (21%) and other (3%); 63% of the patients had RI stage 3, 21% stage 4 and 17% stage 5. Population characteristics are shown in (Tables 2–3).

Of the 1538 patients 556 came from our hospital. Of these 95 patients had a GFR <50 mL/min at diagnosis.

Overall survival in patients with or without renal impairment

Patients with RI at diagnosis had a significantly worse median OS than those without RI (Fig. 2A). Further, there was a clear correlation between the degree of RI and OS (Fig. 2B).

In the non-HDT group the existence of renal failure correlated with impaired OS (25 versus 37 months, $P<0.001$). Novel drugs in 1st line significantly improved the median OS in this group (Fig. 3A). The difference was still highly significant ($P<0.001$) after correction for age, calcium, hemoglobin and albumin in multivariate analysis. The same improvement was seen when analyzing only the bortezomib treated patients (Fig. 3B). Both the univariate and the multivariate analysis showed that bortezomib treatment was an independent factor affecting OS (Tables S1 and S2). On the other hand, no significant difference in median OS was observed among the patients treated with novel agents in 1st line when comparing the RI patients to those with normal renal function (Fig. 4A). When analyzing only the bortezomib treated patients, the same tendency was seen (Fig. 4B).

On the other hand, in the HDT eligible patients with RI, the median OS was 74 months compared to 91 months for HDT-patients without RI and there was no significant difference in OS between those treated with novel agents and those treated with conventional cytotoxic drugs ($P = 0.96$).

Novel agents improved response to treatment among the patients with renal impairment

Non-RI patients had a higher response rate than the RI patients: 74% reached at least PR after 1st line treatment compared to 65%. However, after using novel agent in the 1st treatment line 85% of the RI patients reached at least PR, which can be compared to 56% for the RI patients treated with conventional agents. Of the bortezomib treated patients 85% reached at least PR after the 1st treatment line (Fig. 5).

Renal response

Of the patients treated with bortezomib in 1st line 11 of 12 (92%) improved their GFR (≥MRrenal) compared to 57 of 83

Table 2. Population characteristics for all patients comparing those with and without renal impairment.

		HDT			Non-HDT		
		Renal impairment			Renal impairment		
		Yes	No	*P*	Yes	No	*P*
No. of patients		224	258		456	600	
Mean age		58	59	0.76	76	75	0.66
Type of MM, %							
	IgG	50.0	59.3		54.8	62.8	
	IgA	25.0	26.0		19.3	21.8	
	BJ	19.2	8.9		21.9	10.2	
	Others	4.9	5.0		2.4	4.7	
	Missing	0.9	0.8		1.5	0.5	
Laboratory values at diagnosis, mean							
	Albumin, g/L	32	34	0.006	33	34	0.005
	Hb, g/L	100	114.2	<0.001	102	114	<0.001
	Ca, mmol/L	2.6	2.4	<0.001	2.6	2.4	<0.001
	β2μ, mg/L	9.5	3.3	<0.001	8.1	3.3	<0.001
Stage of renal function, %							
	1	0	34.6		0	33.3	
	2	0	65.4		0	66.7	
	3	57.8	0		65.1	0	
	4	22.9	0		18.9	0	
	5	19.3	0		16.0	0	
Novel drugs, %							
	Yes	25.6	36.2		30.5	28.0	
	No	74.4	63.8		69.5	72.0	

The HDT patients are those that at some point have received high-dose treatment, irrespective of treatment line and the non-HDT those that have not. Patients classified has having received novel drugs implies that they have received this treatment in one or more treatment lines.

HDT, high-dose treated; non-HDT, non-high-dose treated; MM, multiple myeloma; novel drugs, bortezomib, lenalidomide or thalidomide; IgG, immunoglobulin G; IgA, immunoglobulin A; BJ, Bence Jones; Hb, hemoglobin; Ca, calcium; β2μ, beta-2-mikroglobulin.

Table 3. Population characteristics for patients with renal impairment treated with novel agents.

		HDT with renal impairment			Non-HDT with renal impairment		
		Novel treatment			Novel treatment		
		Yes	No	*P*	Yes	No	*P*
No. of patients		57	166		135	308	
Mean age		59	58	0.62	75	75	0.67
Type of MM, %							
	IgG	49.1	50		53.3	55.8	
	IgA	31.6	22.9		17.8	19.8	
	BJ	15.8	20.5		25.2	20.5	
	Other	3.5	5.4		2.2	2.3	
	Missing	0	1.2		1.5	1.6	
Laboratory values, mean							
	Albumin, g/L	30	33	0.03	33	32	0.76
	Hb, g/L	98	100	0.46	102	101	0.70
	Ca, mmol/L	2.5	2.6	0.34	2.6	2.6	0.24
	B2M, mg/L	10.2	9.2	0.72	8.3	8.0	0.78
	Creatinine	314	238	0.04	295	217	0.002
Stage of renal function, %							
	3	52.6	59.6		60	67.2	
	4	21.1	23.5		18.5	19.2	
	5	26.3	16.9		21.5	13.6	

The HDT patients are those that at some point have received high-dose treatment, irrespective of treatment line and the non-HDT those that have not. Patients classified has having received novel drugs implies that they have received this treatment in one or more treatment lines.

HDT, high-dose treated; non-HDT, non-high-dose treated; MM, multiple myeloma; IgG, immunoglobulin G; IgA, immunoglobulin A; BJ, Bence Jones; Hb, hemoglobin; Ca, calcium; β2μ, beta-2-mikroglobulin.

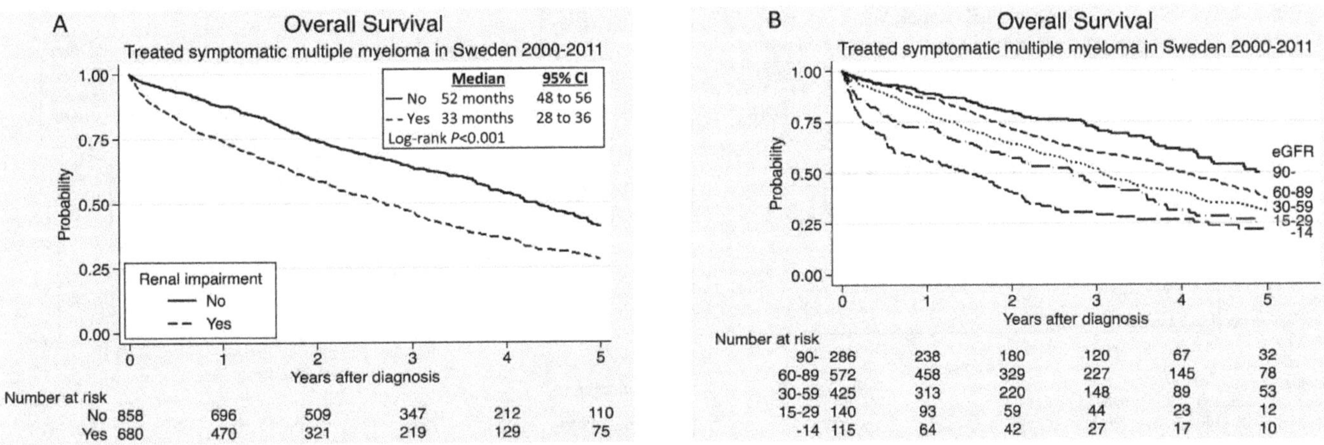

Figure 2. Overall survival in symptomatic multiple myeloma patients. (A) Patients presenting with renal impairment compared to those with normal renal function. (B) Patients divided into five groups according to the chronic kidney disease classification.

patients (69%) in the control group ($P=0.049$). Four of the 12 (33%) bortezomib treated patients and 38 of 83 patients (46%) in the control group reached CRrenal after 1st treatment line.

Novel agents and HDT prolonged time to next treatment

RI implied a shorter median TTNT after 1st line (13 versus 20 months, $P<0.001$). However, TTNT between 2nd and 3rd treatment lines was not affected by renal function at diagnosis, neither among the HDT-patients nor among the non-HDT-patients (Fig. 6A–B).

Additionally, the non-HDT patients with RI had a median TTNT after 1st line of 11 months, compared to 14.5 months for patients without RI ($P<0.001$). Novel drugs prolonged the TTNT after 1st line in these patients (Fig. 6C) and bortezomib treatment lead to a significant improvement of TTNT after adjusting for age, calcium, hemoglobin and albumin ($P=0.02$) (Fig. 6D).

On the contrary, the HDT population with RI had a median TTNT after 1st line of 30 months compared to patients without RI who had a median TTNT of 35 months ($P=0.159$) and novel agents in 1st line did not affect median TTNT in this population (Fig. 6E).

Discussion

Our main finding is that novel agents, especially bortezomib, are associated with survival benefits in MM patients with RI in a real life setting. By using novel agents the OS among RI patients not eligible for HDT was significantly improved from a median 21 to 60 months. Bortezomib-based regimens also improved the median OS to 60 months and was an independent factor to enhance OS in non-HDT patients with RI ($P=0.02$). Moreover, the difference in survival between those with and without RI vanished with the use of novel agents. The median TTNT between the 1st and 2nd treatment lines in non-HDT patients with RI was more than doubled by the use of novel agents. However, the same effect on TTNT was not seen in the HDT group.

Renal impairment is a frequent complication of MM and has been associated with poor outcome. The present study investigated the impact of RI on survival and myeloma response in a large cohort of MM patients treated in a real life setting; all consecutive cases were obtained from the Swedish Cancer Registry. The data in this study derive from several different hospitals, not only referral centers. Therefore, we believe that our population

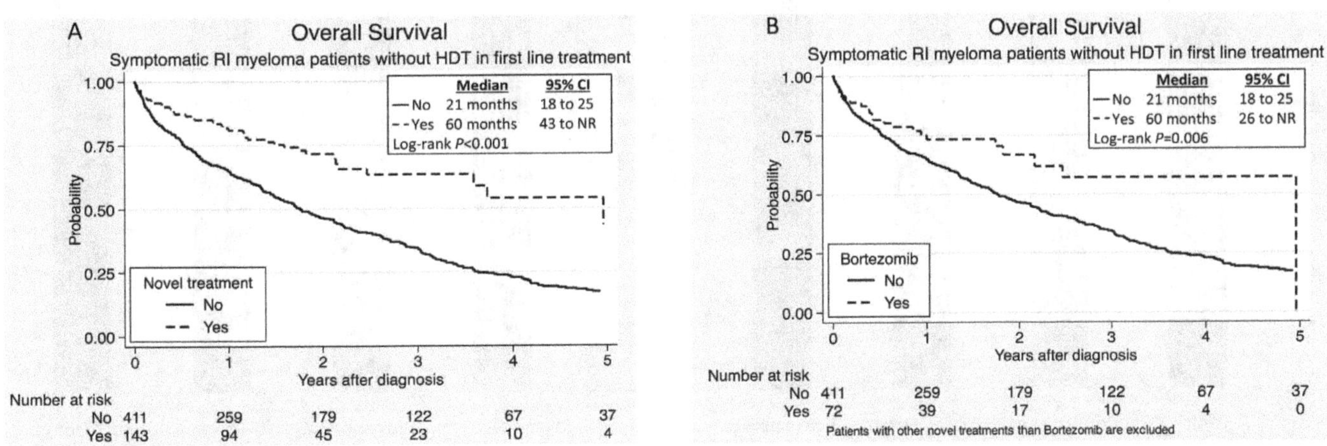

Figure 3. Overall survival for non-high-dose treated (non-HDT) patients with renal impairment. (A) Patients treated with novel agents (bortezomib, thalidomide or lenalidomide) compared to conventional agents in the 1st treatment line. (B) Patients treated with bortezomib compared to conventional agents in the 1st treatment line.

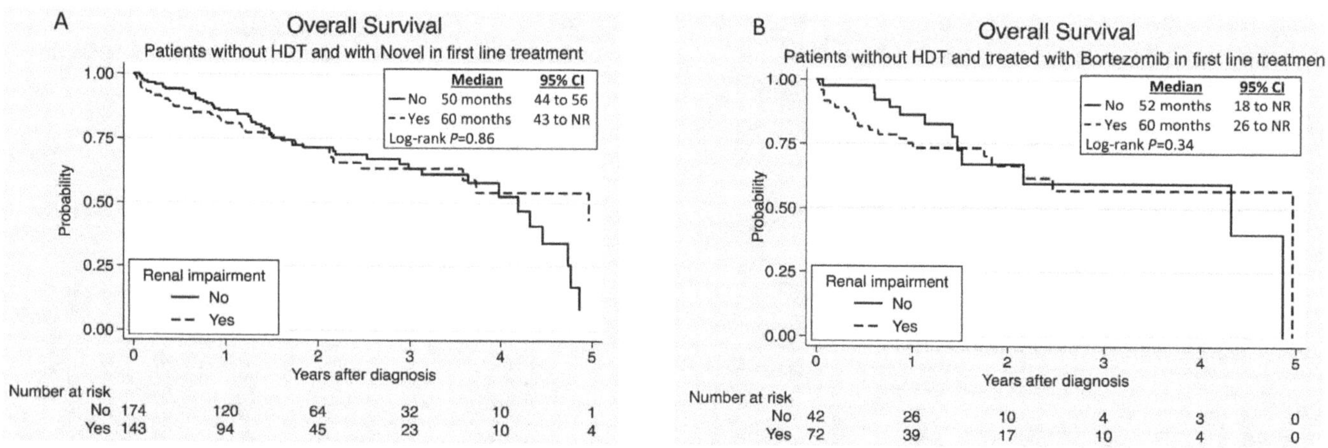

Figure 4. Overall survival in non-high-dose treated (non-HDT) patients with and without renal impairmet treated with novel agents. (A) Patients with renal impairment compared to those without renal impairment after the use of novel agents (bortezomib, lenalidomide or thalidomide) in the 1st treatment line. (B) Patients with renal impairment compared to those without renal impairment after the use of bortezomib in the 1st treatment line.

represents the full spectrum of different MM patients and we consider the study representative for the whole Swedish MM population.

One reason for the improved OS in RI patients with novel agents is a better disease control [22]. We found a clear improvement of responses when using novel agents compared to the use of conventional agents. In line with the study by Dimopoulos et al [23] we have observed that among RI patients treated with novel agents in the 1st treatment line 85% obtained more than PR. This was significantly better than for those treated with conventional drugs (66%). Interestingly, more than half of the patients with RI treated with bortezomib-based regimens reached at least VGPR (55%) even though the amount of patients reaching at least PR was the same (85%).

We found that renal response occurred more frequently in patients treated with bortezomib compared to conventional agents and this result corresponds with earlier studies [24,25]. Renal response is correlated to improved myeloma response [25] and improved OS [26]. When renal response coincides with myeloma response the outcome is improved compared to when renal

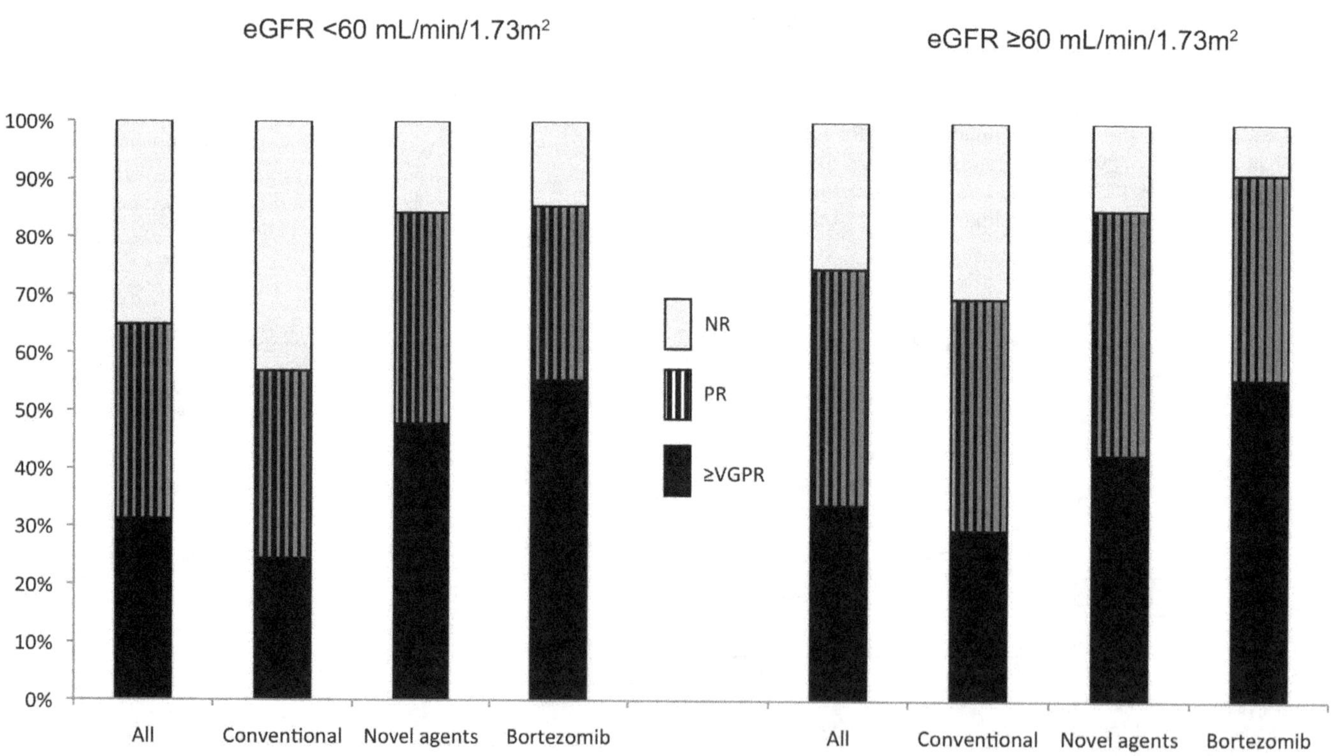

Figure 5. Response distribution after the 1st treatment line in patients with and without renal impairment. Comparing the population treated with novel agents (bortezomib, lenalidomide or thalidomide) to the population treated with conventional agents. (A) Patients with renal impairment. (B) Patients without renal impairment. NR, no response; PR, partial response; ≥VGPR, at least very good partial response.

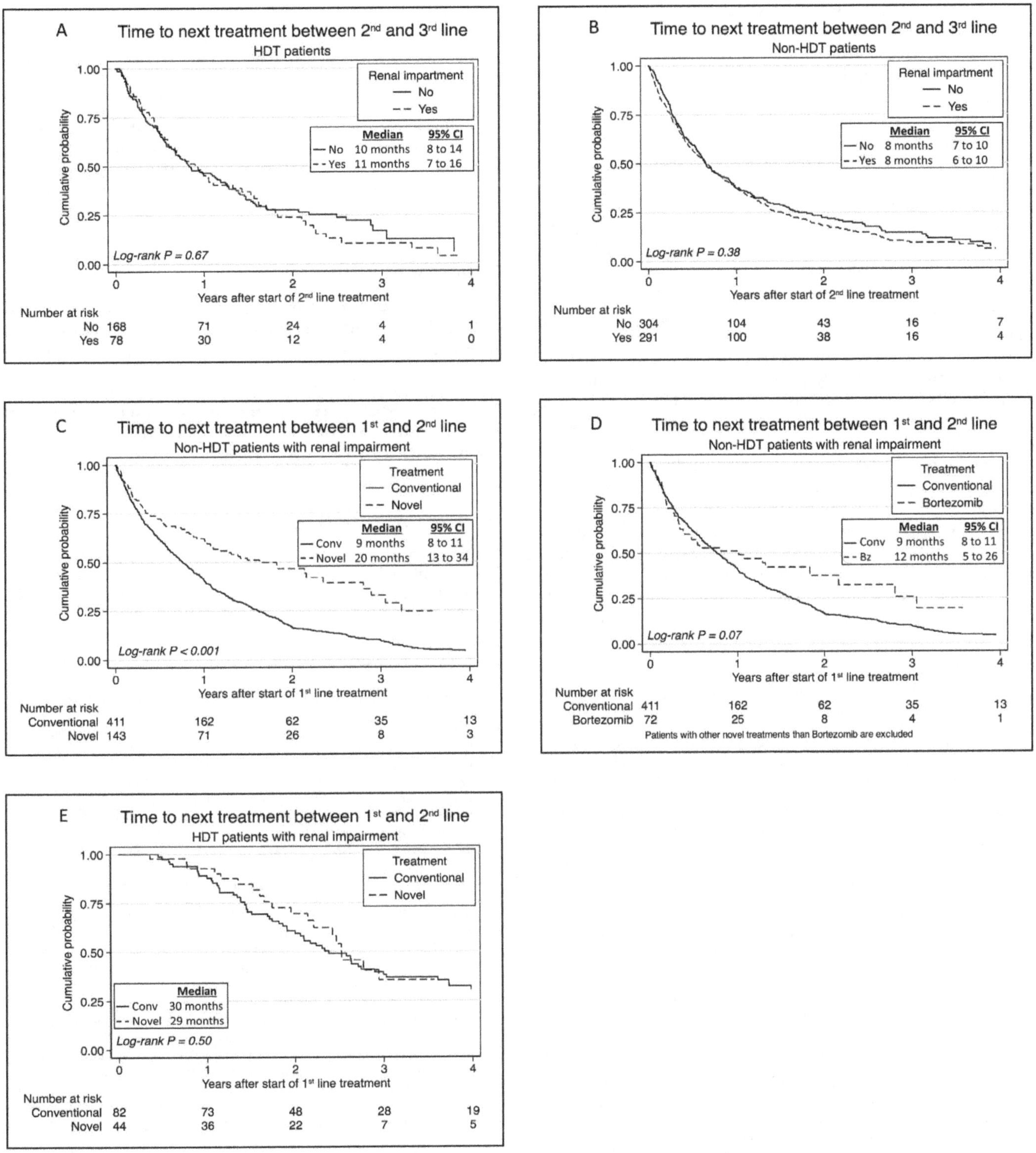

Figure 6. Time to next treatment in patients with and without renal impairment at diagnosis. (A) In high-dose treated (HDT) patients with and without renal impairment after 2nd line of therapy. (B) In non-HDT patients with and without renal impairment after 2nd line of therapy. (C) Non-HDT patients with renal impairment treated with novel agents (bortezomib, lenalidomide or thalidomide) in the 1st line compared to those treated with conventional agents (Conv.). (D) Non-HDT-patients with renal impairment treated with bortezomib (Bz) in the 1st line compared to those treated with conventional agents. (E) HDT-patients with renal impairment treated with novel agents (bortezomib, lenalidomide or thalidomide) in the 1st line compared to to those treated with conventional agents.

response and myeloma response occur separately [26]. However, renal response can also occur in patients not experiencing a myeloma response [24,25].

Since this is a retrospective study with data from 15 different hospitals it is influenced by center specific clinical routines. This includes measurement of response, which was mostly done monthly but sometimes every 6–8 weeks. These variations might affect time to progression and progression free survival. However, treatments were started when the physician considered the relapse to be treatment demanding and this is why we consider data on TTNT to be more reliable than time to progression and progression free survival. Since it is more likely that patients treated at university clinics could be included in clinical trials than those treated at local hospitals, it is also impossible to avoid some degree of selection bias in the choice of treatment. One weakness of this study is the lack of information about concomitant diseases, thus making it impossible to correct for comorbidity. However, the results were stratified according to age, sex, type of MM and important laboratory values at diagnosis in an attempt to cover the majority of possible differences between the groups.

Nevertheless, our results concur with earlier studies. A subgroup analysis of patients with RI enrolled in the VISTA study (bortezomib plus melphalan and prednisone versus melphalan and prednisone to previously untreated patients) reports a higher myeloma response rate as well as a longer time to progression and a better OS in the bortezomib plus melphalan and prednisone group [24]. A recent study reports that even though the incidence and severity of RI at diagnosis have been unchanged during the last 20 years the survival among these patients has improved significantly since the introduction of novel agents in 2000. The survival has improved even more after 2005 when the use of bortezomib increased. This indicates an advantage of bortezomib-based therapy, even though the correlation could not be verified [22]. A study analyzing the effect of novel agents on newly diagnosed MM patients with RI found that RI was not independently associated with inferior survival [27]. An earlier study of MM patients presenting with RI (the majority of which had received earlier MM treatment) observed an overall response rate of 80% in previously untreated patients and 58% in relapsed/refractory patients after bortezomib treatment [28].

In conclusion, the use of novel agents such as IMiDs and most importantly bortezomib, improves OS in MM patients with RI leading to the same median OS regardless the existence of RI. We therefore conclude that novel agents can overcome the negative impact of RI and improve the outcome of MM treatment.

Supporting Information

Table S1 Univariate analysis of factors affecting overall survival in multiple myeloma patients with renal impairment. Both HDT and non-HDT patients are included.

Table S2 Multivariate analysis of factors affecting overall survival in non-HDT patients treated with bortezomib in 1st treatment line.

Author Contributions

Conceived and designed the experiments: KU HN. Analyzed the data: EA HN. Contributed reagents/materials/analysis tools: KU J. Lund. Contributed to the writing of the manuscript: KU AD J. Lund J. Liwing GG EH JA EA HN.

References

1. Chanan-Khan AA, Giralt S (2010) Importance of achieving a complete response in multiple myeloma, and the impact of novel agents. J Clin Oncol 28: 2612–2624.
2. Dingli D, Pacheco JM, Nowakowski GS, Kumar SK, Dispenzieri A, et al. (2007) Relationship between depth of response and outcome in multiple myeloma. Journal of clinical oncology : official journal of the American Society of Clinical Oncology 25: 4933–4937.
3. Alexanian R, Barlogie B, Dixon D (1990) Renal failure in multiple myeloma. Pathogenesis and prognostic implications. Archives of internal medicine 150: 1693–1695.
4. Abbott KC, Agodoa LY (2001) Multiple myeloma and light chain-associated nephropathy at end-stage renal disease in the United States: patient characteristics and survival. Clinical nephrology 56: 207–210.
5. Rayner HC, Haynes AP, Thompson JR, Russell N, Fletcher J (1991) Perspectives in multiple myeloma: survival, prognostic factors and disease complications in a single centre between 1975 and 1988. The Quarterly journal of medicine 79: 517–525.
6. Harousseau JL, Shaughnessy J Jr, Richardson P (2004) Multiple myeloma. Hematology/the Education Program of the American Society of Hematology American Society of Hematology Education Program: 237–256.
7. Dimopoulos MA, Kastritis E, Rosinol L, Blade J, Ludwig H (2008) Pathogenesis and treatment of renal failure in multiple myeloma. Leukemia 22: 1485–1493.
8. Laubach J, Richardson P (2011) Hematology: Bortezomib and dexamethasone induction for multiple myeloma. Nature reviews Clinical oncology 8: 8–10.
9. Dimopoulos MA, Terpos E, Chanan-Khan A, Leung N, Ludwig H, et al. (2010) Renal impairment in patients with multiple myeloma: a consensus statement on behalf of the International Myeloma Working Group. Journal of clinical oncology : official journal of the American Society of Clinical Oncology 28: 4976–4984.
10. Pekol T, Daniels JS, Labutti J, Parsons I, Nix D, et al. (2005) Human metabolism of the proteasome inhibitor bortezomib: identification of circulating metabolites. Drug metabolism and disposition: the biological fate of chemicals 33: 771–777.
11. Uttamsingh V, Lu C, Miwa G, Gan LS (2005) Relative contributions of the five major human cytochromes P450, 1A2, 2C9, 2C19, 2D6, and 3A4, to the hepatic metabolism of the proteasome inhibitor bortezomib. Drug metabolism and disposition: the biological fate of chemicals 33: 1723–1728.
12. Chang DH, Liu N, Klimek V, Hassoun H, Mazumder A, et al. (2006) Enhancement of ligand-dependent activation of human natural killer T cells by lenalidomide: therapeutic implications. Blood 108: 618–621.
13. Wu L, Adams M, Carter T, Chen R, Muller G, et al. (2008) Lenalidomide enhances natural killer cell and monocyte-mediated antibody-dependent cellular cytotoxicity of rituximab-treated CD20+ tumor cells. Clin Cancer Res 14: 4650–4657.
14. Chen N, Lau H, Kong L, Kumar G, Zeldis JB, et al. (2007) Pharmacokinetics of lenalidomide in subjects with various degrees of renal impairment and in subjects on hemodialysis. J Clin Pharmacol 47: 1466–1475.
15. Eriksson T, Höglund P, Turesson I, Waage A, Don BR, et al. (2003) Pharmacokinetics of thalidomide in patients with impaired renal function and while on and off dialysis. J Pharm Pharmacol 55: 1701–1706.
16. Barlow L, Westergren K, Holmberg L, Talbäck M (2009) The completeness of the Swedish Cancer Register: a sample survey for year 1998. Acta Oncol 48: 27–33.
17. Levey AS, Bosch JP, Lewis JB, Greene T, Rogers N, et al. (1999) A more accurate method to estimate glomerular filtration rate from serum creatinine: a new prediction equation. Modification of Diet in Renal Disease Study Group. Annals of internal medicine 130: 461–470.
18. (2002) Part 4. Definition and classification of stages of chronic kidney disease. American journal of kidney diseases : the official journal of the National Kidney Foundation 39: S46–S75.
19. Blade J, Samson D, Reece D, Apperley J, Bjorkstrand B, et al. (1998) Criteria for evaluating disease response and progression in patients with multiple myeloma treated by high-dose therapy and haemopoietic stem cell transplantation. Myeloma Subcommittee of the EBMT. European Group for Blood and Marrow Transplant. British journal of haematology 102: 1115–1123.
20. Dimopoulos MA, Terpos E, Chanan-Khan A, Leung N, Ludwig H, et al. (2010) Renal impairment in patients with multiple myeloma: a consensus statement on behalf of the International Myeloma Working Group. J Clin Oncol 28: 4976–4984.
21. Ludwig H, Adam Z, Hajek R, Greil R, Tothova E, et al. (2010) Light chain-induced acute renal failure can be reversed by bortezomib-doxorubicin-dexamethasone in multiple myeloma: results of a phase II study. J Clin Oncol 28: 4635–4641.
22. Dimopoulos MA, Delimpasi S, Katodritou E, Vassou A, Kyrtsonis MC, et al. (2014) Significant improvement in the survival of patients with multiple myeloma presenting with severe renal impairment after the introduction of novel agents. Ann Oncol 25: 195–200.
23. Dimopoulos MA, Roussou M, Gkotzamanidou M, Nikitas N, Psimenou E, et al. (2013) The role of novel agents on the reversibility of renal impairment in newly diagnosed symptomatic patients with multiple myeloma. Leukemia 27: 423–429.
24. Dimopoulos MA, Richardson PG, Schlag R, Khuageva NK, Shpilberg O, et al. (2009) VMP (Bortezomib, Melphalan, and Prednisone) is active and well tolerated in newly diagnosed patients with multiple myeloma with moderately

impaired renal function, and results in reversal of renal impairment: cohort analysis of the phase III VISTA study. J Clin Oncol 27: 6086–6093.

25. Roussou M, Kastritis E, Christoulas D, Migkou M, Gavriatopoulou M, et al. (2010) Reversibility of renal failure in newly diagnosed patients with multiple myeloma and the role of novel agents. Leuk Res 34: 1395–1397.
26. Dimopoulos MA, Roussou M, Gavriatopoulou M, Zagouri F, Migkou M, et al. (2009) Reversibility of renal impairment in patients with multiple myeloma treated with bortezomib-based regimens: identification of predictive factors. Clin Lymphoma Myeloma 9: 302–306.
27. Eleftherakis-Papapiakovou E, Kastritis E, Roussou M, Gkotzamanidou M, Grapsa I, et al. (2011) Renal impairment is not an independent adverse prognostic factor in patients with multiple myeloma treated upfront with novel agent-based regimens. Leukemia & lymphoma 52: 2299–2303.
28. Dimopoulos MA, Roussou M, Gavriatopoulou M, Zagouri F, Migkou M, et al. (2009) Reversibility of renal impairment in patients with multiple myeloma treated with bortezomib-based regimens: identification of predictive factors. Clinical lymphoma & myeloma 9: 302–306.

12

Effects of ^{28}Si Ions, ^{56}Fe Ions, and Protons on the Induction of Murine Acute Myeloid Leukemia and Hepatocellular Carcinoma

Michael M. Weil[1]*, F. Andrew Ray[1], Paula C. Genik[1], Yongjia Yu[2], Maureen McCarthy[2], Christina M. Fallgren[1], Robert L. Ullrich[2]

1 Colorado State University, Fort Collins, Colorado, United States of America, **2** University of Texas Medical Branch, Galveston, Texas, United States of America

Abstract

Estimates of cancer risks posed to space-flight crews by exposure to high atomic number, high-energy (HZE) ions are subject to considerable uncertainty because epidemiological data do not exist for human populations exposed to similar radiation qualities. We assessed the carcinogenic effects of 300 MeV/n ^{28}Si or 600 MeV/n ^{56}Fe ions in a mouse model for radiation-induced acute myeloid leukemia and hepatocellular carcinoma. C3H/HeNCrl mice were irradiated with 0.1, 0.2, 0.4, or 1 Gy of 300 MeV/n ^{28}Si ions, 600 MeV/n ^{56}Fe ions or 1 or 2 Gy of protons simulating the 1972 solar particle event (1972SPE) at the NASA Space Radiation Laboratory. Additional mice were irradiated with ^{137}Cs gamma rays at doses of 1, 2, or 3 Gy. All groups were followed until they were moribund or reached 800 days of age. We found that ^{28}Si or ^{56}Fe ions do not appear to be substantially more effective than gamma rays for the induction of acute myeloid leukemia. However, ^{28}Si or ^{56}Fe ion irradiated mice had a much higher incidence of hepatocellular carcinoma than gamma ray irradiated or proton irradiated mice. These data demonstrate a clear difference in the effects of these HZE ions on the induction of leukemia compared to solid tumors, suggesting potentially different mechanisms of tumorigenesis. Also seen in this study was an increase in metastatic hepatocellular carcinoma in the ^{28}Si and ^{56}Fe ion irradiated mice compared with those exposed to gamma rays or 1972SPE protons, a finding with important implications for setting radiation exposure limits for space-flight crew members.

Editor: Eric Y. Chuang, National Taiwan University, Taiwan

Funding: This work was supported by grant NNX09AM08G from the National Aeronautics and Space Administration (www.nasa.gov/exploration/humanresearch/) to RLU. The funders had no role in study design, data collection and analysis, decision to publish, or preparation of the manuscript.

Competing Interests: The authors have declared that no competing interests exist.

* Email: michael.weil@colostate.edu

Introduction

The effects of HZE (high Z, high energy) ions found in the space environment on cancer risks to space-flight crews are not well understood because few people have been exposed to space radiation [1–6]. In the absence of human exposure data, results from animal studies utilizing simulated space radiation are a key component to risk modeling. The most complete data set is for Harderian gland tumors in the mouse. These data indicate a substantial increase in risks for tumor induction over gamma ray exposure for a number of HZE ions at low doses followed by a bend-over/plateau. To estimate the relative biological effectiveness (RBE) of these ions a linear dose response model over the 0 to 0.5 Gy dose range has been used. A more recent analysis has suggested that a continuously bending dose response provides a better fit to the data [7]. From this analysis it was argued that the continuously bending curve indicated a role for non-targeted effects involved in the pathogenesis of Harderian gland tumors following exposure to both HZE ions and fission spectrum neutrons. Because humans lack Harderian glands, the applicability of these results to human risks has been an important question. With a few exceptions, other investigators have also provided evidence for a substantial increase in risks for the induction of other epithelial tumors following exposure to HZE ions compared to gamma rays with RBE values ranging from approximately 10 to greater than 50 [8].

We have recently described results of a study examining the induction of acute myeloid leukemia (AML) and hepatocellular carcinoma (HCC) in male CBA mice following exposure to either ^{137}Cs gamma rays or 1 GeV/n ^{56}Fe ions [9]. The RBE for the induction of AML was very low (essentially 1), a result that contributed to the use of a smaller maximum quality factor function for leukemia in the NASA model for space cancer risk [10,11]. However, the study found a substantial RBE (about 50) for the induction of HCC. Furthermore, the dose response for HCC showed a large increase in the incidence of tumors over the dose range from 0 to 0.4 Gy followed by a bend-over between 0.4 and 1 Gy, similar to that previously described for Harderian gland tumors in mice [12–14] and mammary tumors in Sprague Dawley rats [15]. However, the dose response for AML was essentially linear and similar to that observed for gamma rays.

Additional studies have now been conducted in our laboratories extending these investigations to include an examination of the carcinogenic effects of ^{137}Cs gamma rays compared to 600 MeV/

Table 1. Incidences of AML and HCC as a function of dose and radiation quality.

Radiation Quality	Dose in cGy (Initial Animal Numbers)	Frequency of AML (incidence ± SE[a])	Frequency of HCC (Incidence ± SE)
None	0 (300)	1/280 (0.36 ± 0.36)	46/280 (16.5 ± 2.5)
300 MeV/n ^{28}Si	10 (300)	6/298 (2.0 ± 0.8)	124/298 (41.6 ± 4.7)
	20 (300)	10/290 (3.4 ± 1.1)	150/290 (51.7 ± 3.0)
	40 (200)	7/189 (3.7 ± 1.4)	82/189 (43.4 ± 3.6)
	100 (200)	8/185 (4.3 ± 2.1)	78/185 (42.2 ± 3.6)
600 MeV/n ^{56}Fe	10 (300)	5/288 (1.7 ± 0.8)	109/288 (37.8 ± 4.6)
	20 (300)	13/295 (4.4 ± 1.7)	143/295 (48.4 ± 2.9)
	40 (200)	1/189 (0.5 ± 0.5)	83/189 (43.9 ± 2.9)
	100 (200)	3/180 (1.6 ± 0.9)	74/180 (41.7 ± 3.7)
^{137}Cs Gamma Rays	100 (400)	10/386 (2.6 ± 0.8)	54/386 14.0 ± 1.8
	200 (300)	19/276 (6.9 ± 1.5)	47/276 (17.0 ± 2.3)
	300 (100)	15/98 (15.3 ± 3.9)	23/98 (23.0 ± 4.3)
1972SPE Protons	100 (400)	10/392 (2.6 ± 0.8)	51/392 (13.0 ± 1.7)
	200 (300)	17/287 (5.9 ± 1.4)	49/287 (17.1 ± 2.2)

[a]As calculated assuming binomial distribution.

n ^{56}Fe ions, 300MeV/n ^{28}Si ions, and protons with energies simulating the 1972 solar particle event (1972SPE). For these studies we used male C3H mice that, as in the case of CBA mice, have been shown to be susceptible to the induction of AML following radiation exposure and to spontaneous HCC. The results of the present study confirm our previous observations with 1 GeV/n ^{56}Fe ions of a low RBE for AML and a very high RBE for HCC. No significant differences were observed between the effects of ^{137}Cs gamma rays and 1972SPE protons with respect to the induction of either AML or HCC. In addition to the substantial quantitative differences in the effectiveness of HZE ions compared to either gamma rays or protons on the induction of HCC, we also observed qualitative differences as measured by an increase in the frequency of metastases from tumors arising in ^{28}Si and ^{56}Fe ion irradiated mice compared with those from gamma ray or proton irradiated mice.

Materials and Methods

Mice, Irradiations, and Morbidity Monitoring

Eight to ten-week-old male C3H/HeNCrl mice were purchased from Charles River Laboratories and shipped to the Brookhaven National Laboratory (BNL) for irradiation. Upon arrival they were acclimated for at least 2 days prior to being irradiated with 0.1, 0.2, 0.4, or 1 Gy of 300 MeV/n ^{28}Si ions (LET = 64 keV/μm), 600 MeV/n ^{56}Fe ions (LET = 181 keV/μm) or 1 or 2 Gy of 1972SPE protons (30 MeV to 80 MeV) at the NASA Space Radiation Laboratory at BNL. Additional mice were irradiated at BNL with ^{137}Cs gamma rays at doses of 1, 2, or 3 Gy. Numbers of animals used were based on our previous study described above. Male mice were selected because they have a higher incidence of radiation-induced AML than female mice. Control mice were sham-irradiated at BNL under the same conditions as the irradiated groups. Because of the large numbers of animals in each group, each dose group consisted of two cohorts irradiated approximately 12 months apart. Doses selected were based on previous studies [9]. The mice were not anesthetized during irradiation or any part of the study. Details of the irradiation conditions have been described previously [9]. Briefly, mice were loaded headfirst into 50 ml polypropylene centrifuge tubes with 8–10 predrilled 1/8 inch holes in the bottom. Ten tubes were then placed into a foam holder affixed perpendicular to the beam trajectory. The proton beam was delivered at 6 different energies, from 30 MeV to 80 MeV, in 10 MeV increments. The total dose was made up of partial doses for each energy, the dominant one being the 30 MeV dose, which makes up more than 90% of the total. The dose distribution was determined by scaling down the depth-dose spectrum from an SPE based on several recorded ones, from that expected in a 30 cm diameter water cylinder (man) to a 3 cm cylinder (mouse). The energy distribution which would yield that particular depth-dose spectrum was approximated with the 6 said energy bins, and the dose for each was fixed. Six separate setup and calibration files were created for each energy, so the beam could be delivered to the target stand sequentially without moving the targets in and out of the beam for each change. Before reaching the target, the beam transverses a large ion chamber previously calibrated with a NIST-traceable calibration chamber. The large chamber is used to automatically cut the beam when the desired dose is reached. The range for the majority of the SPE1972 proton beam is less than 9 mm and the width of a mouse is just under 3 cm.

The numbers of animals in each dose group are shown in Table 1. Mice were shipped to the Animal Resource Center at the University of Texas Medical Branch (UTMB) 3 to 5 days post-irradiation. At UTMB animals were housed 5 per cage in ventilated cage racks using Harlan Sani-chip bedding and maintained on an Harlan 7912 diet and autoclaved reverse osmosis purified water *ad libitum* throughout the study.

Animals were monitored daily and palpated weekly. They were euthanized when moribund and/or displaying signs and symptoms of AML, HCC or other neoplasms or when they reached 800 days of age. Dead, moribund, or symptomatic animals were necropsied and tissues (lung, liver, spleen, other tumors or pathologies) taken for histological evaluation. All necropsies and histological examinations were performed blinded. The large majority of animals were necropsied promptly enough to allow collection of tissues suitable for evaluation and diagnosis. AML were diagnosed using H&E stained tissue sections in addition to immunohistochemistry for myeloperoxidase using an anti-myeloperoxidase antibody at a concentration of 1:200 (Thermo Scientific catalogue number RB-373-A). Liver tumors were classified as adenomas or adenocarcinomas [16] other types of liver tumors were seen occasionally but at a low frequency, and there was no apparent relationship between these tumors and radiation dose.

Ethics Statement

All animal work was approved by the Institutional Animal Care and Use Committees at UTMB and BNL (OAW Animal Welfare Assurance Numbers A3314-01 and A3106-01) under protocols 0906043 and 393 respectively. Both facilities are AAALAC accredited. Euthanasia was by carbon dioxide inhalation.

Statistical Analyses

For evaluation of the proportion of animals contracting either AML or HCC as a function of dose and radiation type a multinomial logistic regression was used and odds ratios calculated to test for significant differences in risks among the radiation and control groups and between the various radiation types using the chi-square test. The relative biological effectiveness (RBE) was calculated using a weighted linear regression model to determine the linear slopes for the ^{28}Si ion, ^{56}Fe ion, 1972SPE proton, and gamma ray dose responses. Linear slopes (y) of the gamma ray and 1972SPE proton AML and HCC dose responses were determined over the dose range of 0 to 2 Gy compared with 0 to 1 Gy for the ^{28}Si ion and ^{56}Fe ion AML dose responses, and 0 to 0.2 Gy for the ^{28}Si ion and ^{56}Fe ion HCC dose responses. The ratios of these slopes were used to determine the RBE values ($Z = x/y$).

For determining significance of differences in the frequency of metastasis between controls and radiation groups and between radiation types a chi-square test was used.

Results

Although a variety of sporadic neoplasms were observed in irradiated and control animals, only AML and HCC were found to increase significantly as a function of radiation dose. The data with respect to dose response and RBE estimates for these two neoplasms are described below.

Acute myeloid leukemia

The incidences of AML as a function of dose and radiation type are shown in Table 1 and presented graphically in Figure 1. The time of appearance of these neoplasms ranged from 300 to 600 days with a median of 450–500 days of age. This range and median is similar to that previously reported previously for CBA mice [9,17]. The dose response for the incidence of AML following exposure to gamma rays is also quite similar to that observed for both CBA and RFM mice [9,18]. To determine whether there were significant differences between risks for induction of AML for the various radiation types, odds ratios were calculated and the significance of differences among groups was determined using the chi-square test. These analyses used the 0 to 2 Gy dose range for gamma rays and protons for comparison with the data over the 0 to 1 Gy dose range for the high LET radiations. Based on the results of these analyses over these dose ranges there were no significant differences between any of the radiation types.

The relative biological effectiveness (RBE) was calculated using a weighted linear regression model to determine the linear slopes for the ^{28}Si ion, ^{56}Fe ion, 1972SPE proton, and gamma ray dose responses. Linear slopes of the gamma ray and 1972SPE proton AML and HCC dose responses were determined over the dose range of 0 to 2 Gy compared with 0 to 1 Gy for the ^{28}Si ion and ^{56}Fe ion AML dose responses, and 0 to 0.2 Gy for the ^{28}Si ion and ^{56}Fe ion HCC dose responses. These data are shown in Tables 2 and 3. RBE values of approximately 1 or less were observed for 300 MeV/n ^{28}Si ions, 600 MeV/n ^{56}Fe, and 1972SPE protons when compared to ^{137}Cs gamma ray exposures. These data are consistent with our previous studies examining AML induction by 1GeV/n ^{56}Fe ions for which an RBE of essentially 1 was also obtained. It should be noted that there is an increase in the incidence of AML at the 0.2 Gy dose over that observed at other doses. This results in an apparent hump in the dose response. For ^{56}Fe ions there was also a substantial decrease at 0.4 Gy. However, it is not appropriate to over interpret such detailed results in an observational study. This is especially the case in situations when the numbers of tumors in each dose group are relatively small and an increase or decrease of one or two tumors in any dose group can have a large impact on tumor incidence for that group. In this regard, we considered the possibility that the 0.2 Gy and 0.4 ^{56}Fe ion results were outliers. However, for the sake of completeness multiple RBEs were determined for each HZE ion based on initial slope ratios calculated through 2 Gy for gamma rays and through 0.2, 0.4 or 1.0 Gy for the HZE ions (data not shown). The preponderance of the data supports an RBE of approximately 1,

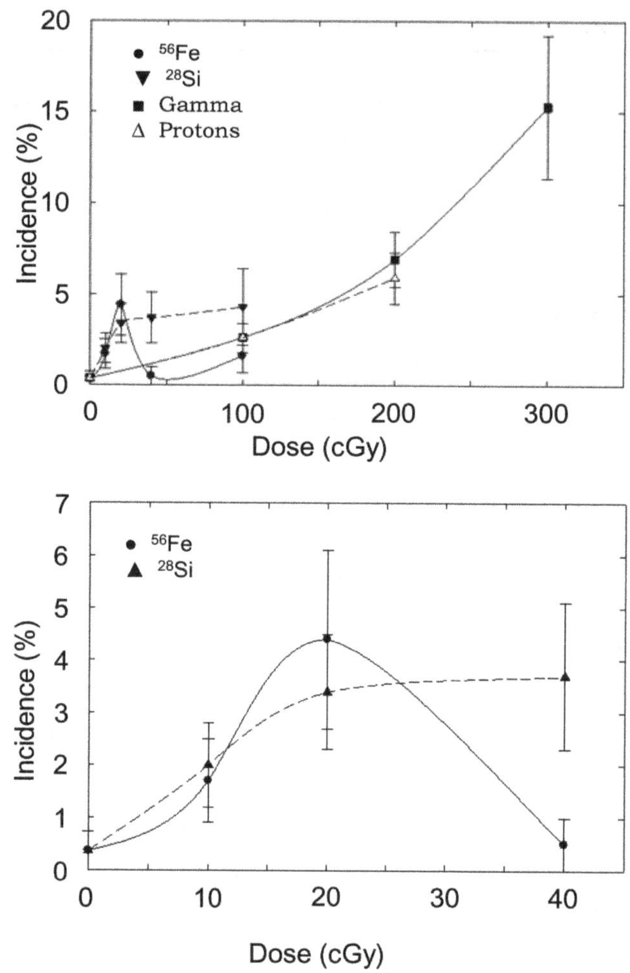

Figure 1. Incidence (%) of AML following exposure to 300 MeV/n ^{28}Si (▼); 600 MeV/n ^{56}Fe (•); ^{137}Cs gamma rays (o); or 1972SPE protons (♦). The dose response over the 0-3 Gy dose range (top). The dose response over the 0–0.4 Gy dose range (bottom).

Table 2. Slopes determined using weighted linear regression for the induction of AML or HCC as a function of radiation quality[a].

Cancer Type	Radiation	α	c	R^2
AML	600 MeV/n ^{56}Fe 0 to 1 Gy	0.008 ± 0.015	0.61 ± 0.71	0.083
	300 MeV/n ^{28}Si 0 to 1 Gy	0.047 ± 0.017	0.71 ± 0.47	0.712
	γ-rays 0 to 2 Gy	0.037 ± 0.008	0.22 ± 0.56	0.910
	1972SPE Protons 0 to 2 Gy	0.026 ± 0.003	0.34 ± 0.15	0.989
HCC	600 MeV/n ^{56}Fe 0 to 0.2 Gy	1.61 ± 0.31	18.2 ± 4.0	0.964
	300 MeV/n ^{28}Si 0 to 0.2 Gy	1.77 ± 0.44	18.9 ± 5.6	0.943
	γ-rays 0 to 2 Gy	0.024 ± 0.014	14.1 ± 2.6	0.596
	1972SPE Protons 0 to 0.2 Gy	0.004± 0.022	15.2 ± 2.8	0.025

[a]Fit as $I = \alpha D + c$.

although it could be as high as 5 if the analyses were limited to data over 0 to 0.2 Gy. However, such an approach is not warranted based on the present data. To use this approach the current results would need to be confirmed in follow-up studies.

Hepatocellular carcinoma

The time of appearance of HCC was later than that for AML with a range of 300 to 800 days of age and a median of approximately 650 days for control and irradiated groups. This median time of appearance was not substantially different as a function of dose or radiation type. The incidence of HCC by dose and radiation type is shown in Table 1 and presented graphically in Figure 2. There was only a very slight increase in the incidence of HCC with increasing dose of gamma rays with the dose response for proton irradiated mice being similar. Analysis of these data based on chi-square analysis from calculated odds ratios as described in the methods section found no statistically significant increase in risks for gamma rays or protons compared to controls. Because of the steep dose response for HZE ion-induced HCC the calculations were limited to the 0.2 Gy dose range. As shown previously for 1 GeV/n ^{56}Fe ions in CBA mice, there is a large, statistically significant increase in the risks of HCC over the 0 to 0.2 Gy dose range for both ^{28}Si and ^{56}Fe ions compared to gamma rays and protons over the 0 to 2 Gy dose range ($p < 0.008$ and 0.004 respectively) based on chi-square analysis from calculated odds ratios. RBE values derived from the slope ratios (Tables 2 and 3) in the range of 65 to 70 were obtained, with that for 300 MeV/n ^{28}Si ions being slightly but not significantly higher than that for 600 MeV/n ^{56}Fe ions. Importantly with respect to risk, while somewhat higher than the RBE reported for 1 GeV/n ^{56}Fe ions, the data are consistent with previous results indicating a more convex shaped dose response curve with the maximum incidence in the 0.2 to 0.4 Gy dose range and very high RBE values following irradiation with HZE ions in this energy range.

Metastatic HCC

During histological examination some of the HCC were found to have metastasized to the lung. Because of speculation about qualitative as well as quantitative differences between HZE ion and gamma ray induced tumors [19], we decided to determine whether there were differences in the frequency of metastases among the various radiation groups. Since the numbers of metastases were relatively low in any given dose group and the frequencies of these metastases were evenly distributed among dose groups with no apparent dose response relationship, we pooled the data and compared the overall frequencies of metastases as a function of radiation type. These data are shown in Figure 3. Based on chi-square analysis the frequency of lung metastases was significantly higher in both the ^{28}Si and ^{56}Fe ion groups when compared to gamma ray or proton irradiation ($p < 0.05$). No significant differences in metastasis frequencies were found between spontaneous tumors and those arising in gamma ray and proton irradiated mice. It should be noted that lungs were not systematically examined for metastases. However, all apparent tumors in the lungs were taken for diagnosis. In those instances when the lung appeared to be tumor free by gross examination, the right lobe of the lung was systematically taken for examination for occult tumors. Therefore, these results are likely to underestimate the actual metastatic frequencies. Since necropsy technicians and the histopathologist were blinded to the radiation histories of the individual mice, it is unlikely that the data are biased with respect to any particular radiation type. Further, the frequencies of metastases for each radiation type were consistent in both irradiation cohorts which means that the results for

Table 3. RBE values (± S.D) for 300 MeV/n ^{28}Si, 600 MeV/n ^{56}Fe, and 1972SPE protons.

Cancer Type	Radiation	RBE
AML 0–1 Gy dose range	600 MeV/n ^{56}Fe	0.2 ± 0.4
	300 MeV/n ^{28}Si	1.2 ± 0.5
	1972SPE Protons	0.7 ± 0.2
HCC 0–0.2 Gy dose range	600 MeV/n ^{56}Fe	67 ± 41
	300 MeV/n ^{28}Si	74 ± 47
	1972SPE Protons	1 ± 10

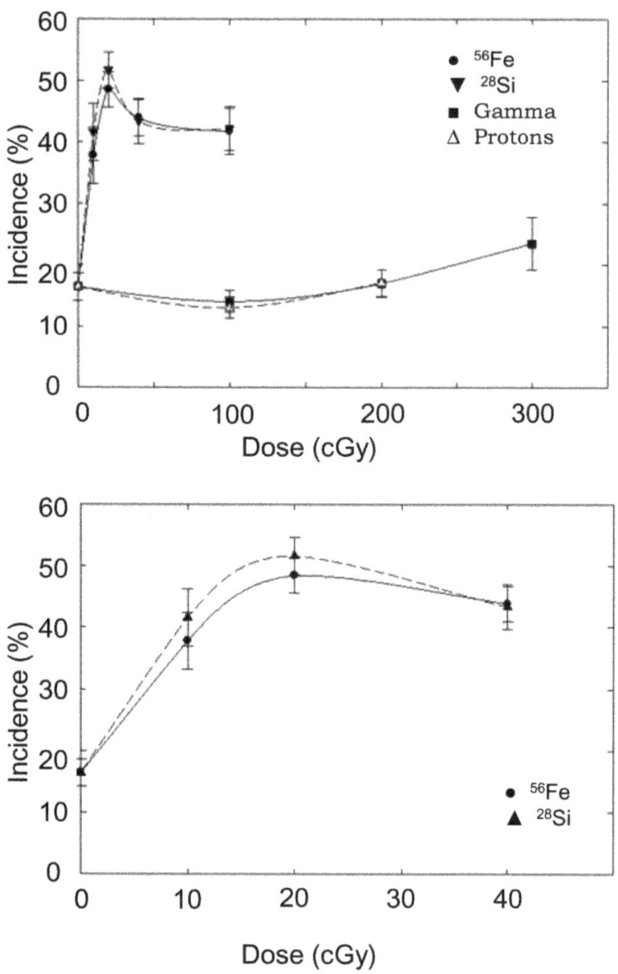

Figure 2. Incidence (%) of HCC following exposure to 300 MeV/n ^{28}Si (▼); 600 MeV/n ^{56}Fe (•); ^{137}Cs gamma rays (o); or 1972SPE protons (♦). The dose response over the 0–3 Gy dose range (top). The dose response over the 0–0.4 Gy dose range (bottom).

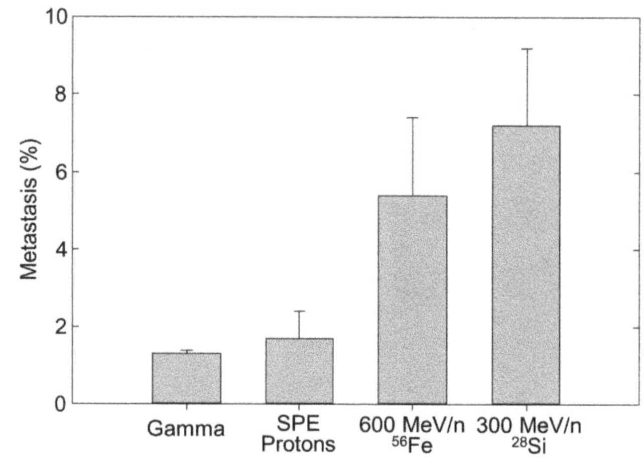

Figure 3. Incidence (%) of HCC with metastases to the lung as a function of radiation type.

metastatic frequencies were consistent in two groups of animals irradiated at different times. There was no apparent effect with respect to time of appearance of the primary liver tumor and the probability of metastasis. Therefore, we believe these data to be a true representation of increased metastatic frequency differences among groups.

Discussion

This study has extended previous data for the induction of AML and HCC as a function of dose to include the effects of 300 MeV/n ^{28}Si ions, 600 MeV/n ^{56}Fe ions, and 1972SPE protons. The similar leukemogenic effects of gamma rays and 1972SPE protons in the present study are consistent with the finding by Clapp et al [20] that 60 MeV/n protons were just slightly less effective than 250 kVp X-rays for AML induction in RF mice. An RBE of 1 in this study over the dose range of 0–1 Gy for 300 MeV/n ^{28}Si and 600 MeV/n ^{56}Fe ions as compared to gamma rays was also consistent with our previous finding of an RBE of approximately 1 for 1 GeV/n ^{56}Fe ions in CBA mice [9].

As with previous data for effects of 1 GeV/n ^{56}Fe ions, we observed a steep dose response for the induction of HCC at low doses (0–0.2 Gy) of 300 MeV/n ^{28}Si and 600 MeV/n ^{56}Fe ions followed by a bend-over/plateau, i.e., a convex shaped dose response. While irradiation with 300 MeV/n ^{28}Si ions or 600 MeV/n ^{56}Fe ions resulted in a sharp increase in the incidence of HCC, irradiation with ^{137}Cs gamma rays or 1972SPE protons had very little effect on incidence. Importantly, there was no significant difference between the effects of gamma rays and 1972SPE protons indicating an RBE of approximately 1 for 1972SPE protons. As a result of the substantial differences in the dose responses, calculated RBE values for 300 MeV/n ^{28}Si and 600 MeV/n ^{56}Fe ions were very high (in the range of 60–70). Such high values are consistent with our previous results for HCC following irradiation with 1 GeV/n ^{56}Fe ions. Similar dose responses have also been reported for Harderian gland tumors in mice, mammary tumors in both mice and rats, and lung tumors in mice following irradiation with fission spectrum neutrons [21,22]. The reason for this steep dose response with very high frequencies of HCC and other epithelial tumors at doses as low as 0.1 Gy (in some instance as low as 0.025 Gy) is a matter of speculation and is of considerable interest with respect to mechanisms and to evaluation of risks in humans. One factor which might play an important role in determining the form of the dose response after irradiation with HZE and which could be responsible for the apparent bend-over at doses in the range of 0.2 to 0.4 Gy is dose distribution alone. If a single hit were sufficient for cell transformation after irradiation with 300 MeV/n ^{28}Si and with 600 MeV/n or 1 GeV/n ^{56}Fe ions then a linear dose response followed by a plateau or bend-over for tumor induction would be predicted based on the probability of an hepatocyte being traversed as a function of dose. To examine this idea the relationship between the probability of an hepatocyte being traversed by either a ^{28}Si ion or a ^{56}Fe ion and the probability of HCC as a function of dose was examined and the data are shown in figures 4A and B. These data clearly demonstrate that at low doses the probability of a cell traversal is lower than the probability of the induction of HCC. Based on this it would appear that the dose response for the induction of HCC following exposure to HZE ions is more complex than simply a matter of dose distribution. This conclusion is supported by earlier microbeam studies on cellular effects following single cell irradiation *in vitro* [23,24].

A more attractive hypothesis, which is supported by several lines of evidence, is that irradiation with HZE ions and other high LET radiations such as fission neutrons results in non-targeted effects

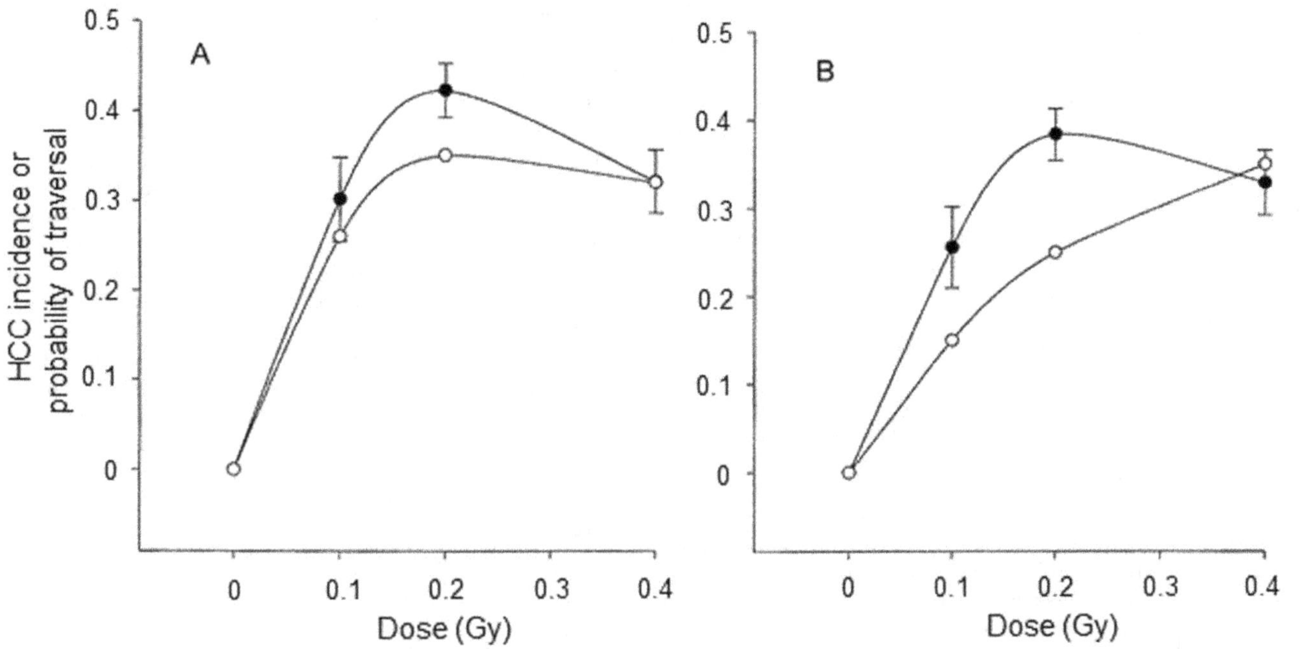

Figure 4. The probability for development of HCC corrected for background (solid line) with Abbott's correction [34] and the probability of a single traversal of a 50 μm² hepatocyte nucleus (dashed line) with a 300 MeV/n ^{28}Si ion (A) or 600 MeV/n ^{56}Fe ion (B).

(NTE) on neighboring non-irradiated cells involving changes in the microenvironment that serve to promote tumor development and progression.

With respect to tumor induction following high LET radiation exposure Cucinotta and Chappell [7] have modeled the dose response relationships for the induction of Harderian gland tumors following irradiations with a range of HZE ions over a broad spectrum of LETs comparing a linear model with a model factoring in NTE such as the release of clastogenic factors, the increased expression of cytokines and up-regulation of inflammatory pathways, and genomic instability. Their analysis demonstrated empirically that the NTE model provided a better fit to the dose response data, especially at low doses, than did a classical biophysical model for which an initial linear slope would be predicted. More direct support for such an NTE model and for effects on progression following high LET radiations come from animal studies of the carcinogenic processes involved in the development of mouse mammary cancer following exposure to fission spectrum neutrons [25]. In addition, Datta et al [19] have shown that heavy ion radiation exposure results in higher intestinal tumor frequency and greater β-catenin activation than gamma radiation in $Apc^{Min/+}$ mice. Further, Cheema et al [26] demonstrated that HZE ion exposure is more effective than an equitoxic dose of γ-ray radiation in increasing levels of metabolites indicative of persistent (2 month post-exposure) inflammation.

Beyond radiation-induced cancer the role of the microenvironment has been shown to be a major factor in carcinogenic processes in general [27]. Of particular importance is up-regulation of inflammatory pathways and increased expression of cytokines. Such effects have the potential to increase the probability of initiation, the probability of progression of these initiated cells to the neoplastic phenotype, and the probability of metastasis. Of particular importance in this regard is chronic inflammation. Importantly, subclinical inflammation may be as important as frank inflammation in increasing cancer risks.

The role of inflammation in the development of liver cancer is well documented. In humans, inflammation is a primary driver of liver cancer and a common feature of three major causes of hepatocellular carcinoma: infection with hepatitis B virus or hepatitis C virus; alcoholic cirrhosis; and obesity [28–30]. Animal models of liver cancer development including mechanistic studies on the induction and progression of preneoplastic foci have made a major impact on the current understanding of the neoplastic process. Results from these animal models also support an important role for inflammatory processes in the pathogenesis of liver cancer.

The increased frequency of lung metastases supports the hypothesis that qualitative as well as quantitative differences exist for radiation effects on neoplastic processes following irradiation with the HZE ions used in this study. Such qualitative differences are consistent with the NTE model and would, in fact, be predicted by a number of studies suggesting that changes in the tissue microenvironment associated with up-regulation of cytokines and inflammatory pathways increases the probability of tumor progression [27]. Importantly, this NTE model appears to apply to tumor induction for the HZE ions used in this study but not for gamma ray or proton irradiation for which a more biophysically based model appears to apply.

The finding of increased metastases from HZE ion-induced HCC is important because current NASA radiation exposure limits for space-flight crew members are based on not exceeding a 3% risk of fatal cancer at the upper 95% confidence interval [10]. If HZE ion-induced cancers are more metastatic, and consequently more lethal, the incidence to mortality ratio for spontaneous tumors used to predict cancer deaths in the current NASA risk model may be inappropriate and the radiation exposures now permitted may be excessive [31].

As described above, the data reported here confirm a low HZE ion RBE for the induction of AML over a dose range of 0 to 1 Gy with a potential RBE of 3 to 5 over the 0 to 0.2 Gy dose range.

The data also confirm a very high RBE for the induction of HCC over the 0 to 0.2 Gy dose range. The difference in RBE values for leukemogenesis compared with HCC is a matter of speculation. One possible explanation is related to apparent differences in the pathways involved and the degree to which target cell intrinsic effects as opposed to tissue microenvironment may contribute to the pathogenesis of AML versus solid tumors. It is thought that only a few steps are required for the development of murine AML and that it is principally driven by an initial deletion in chromosome 2 with the dose response for this alteration predominating with respect to the shape of the AML dose response. Because of this, the interplay between the induction of chromosome 2 deletions and killing of target cells is a major factor in determining dose response relationships and by definition RBE. It should be pointed out that this does not preclude an important role for the microenvironment in radiation leukemogenesis, particularly the hematopoietic niche. Evidence for the strong role played by chromosome 2 aberrations in murine AML comes from a study of Darakashan et al [32] who demonstrated that a primary factor in multiple strain differences (including C3H mice) in sensitivity to AML is sensitivity to chromosome 2 aberrations. How this may apply to risks in humans is not known, but what is known is that a large proportion of radiation-induced AML arising as second cancers in patients treated with radiotherapy involve chromosomal deletions in chromosomes 5 and/or 7 [33]. On the other hand, based on current data, the mechanistic pathways involved in the development of epithelial tumors appear to be much more complex with a larger role for the interplay of cellular alterations and changes in cell signaling, cell-cell interactions, and other effects on the microenvironment which are likely to act to promote the neoplastic process and the progression of altered cells toward the neoplastic phenotype. Several studies examining radiation-induced cancer provide strong direct evidence for such a model. The increase in numbers of metastases in the HZE ion-induced cancers in this study would also tend to support such an effect on tumor progression. Such effects may play a particularly important role at low doses at which only a small proportion of target cells are traversed.

Based on the above discussion, it might be predicted that a majority of epithelial cancers induced by high LET ions would have a similar NTE associated dose response and high RBE values. On the other hand tumors, both leukemias and epithelial cancers, for which early cellular events and cell killing play a predominant role in the neoplastic process would tend to have dose responses more compatible with biophysical models with lower RBE values when compared to gamma rays. Whether such predictions hold and what factors are involved in effects on progression in those tumors for which NTE play a major role will require additional systematic studies to test these hypotheses. Clearly these are important questions with respect to our ability to estimate human risks using model systems. Once such factors can be identified studies to determine if similar events take place in human tissues and organs would facilitate a more direct approach to risk assessment.

Acknowledgments

We wish to thank Dr. Adam Rusek for his help in describing the dosimetry of the 1972SPE proton simulations, the staff at the NASA Space Radiation Laboratory for dosimetry and irradiation services, and the staff of the Brookhaven Laboratory Animal Facility (Brookhaven National Laboratory) for excellent animal care. We also wish to thank Dr. Reid Landes for advice on statistical analysis.

Author Contributions

Conceived and designed the experiments: MMW FAR RLU. Performed the experiments: MMW FAR PCG YY MM CMF RLU. Analyzed the data: MMW RLU. Contributed to the writing of the manuscript: MMW FAR PCG YY MM CMF RLU. Designed the database: MMW FAR.

References

1. Cucinotta FA, Durante M (2006) Cancer risk from exposure to galactic cosmic rays: implications for space exploration by human beings. Lancet Oncol 7: 431–435.
2. Cucinotta FA, Durante M (2009) Risk of Radiation Carcinogenesis. In: McPhee JC, Charles JB, editors. Human health and performance risks of space exploration missions. NASA SP-2009-3405. Houston: National Aeronautics and Space Administration. pp.119–170.
3. Durante M, Cucinotta FA (2008) Heavy ion carcinogenesis and human space exploration. Nat Rev Cancer 8: 465–472.
4. ICRP (2013) Assessment of radiation exposure of astronauts in space. ICRP Publication 123. Oxford: Elsevier.
5. NCRP (2006) Information needed to make radiation protection recommendations for space missions beyond low-earth orbit. NCRP Report No. 153. Bethesda: National Council for Radiation Protection and Measurements.
6. THESEUS (2012) Cluster 3: Space Radiation Report. Available: http://www.theseus-eu.org/. Accessed 2014 Jun 1.
7. Cucinotta FA, Chappell LJ (2010) Non-targeted effects and the dose response for heavy ion tumor induction. Mutat Res 687: 49–53.
8. Bielefeldt-Ohmann H, Genik PC, Fallgren CM, Ullrich RL, Weil MM (2012) Animal studies of charged particle-induced carcinogenesis. Health Phys 103: 568–576.
9. Weil MM, Bedford JS, Bielefeldt-Ohmann H, Ray FA, Genik PC, et al. (2009) Incidence of acute myeloid leukemia and hepatocellular carcinoma in mice irradiated with 1 GeV/nucleon (56)Fe ions. Radiat Res 172: 213–219.
10. Cucinotta FA, Kim MY, Chappell LJ (2011) Space radiation cancer risk projections and uncertainties- 2010. NASA/TP-2011-216155. Washington, DC: National Aeronautics and Space Administration.
11. Cucinotta FA, Kim MY, Chappell LJ (2013) Space radiation cancer risk projections and uncertainties - 2012. NASA/TP-2013-217375. Washington, DC: National Aeronautics and Space Administration.
12. Alpen EL, Powers-Risius P, Curtis SB, DeGuzman R (1993) Tumorigenic potential of high-Z, high-LET charged-particle radiations. Radiat Res 136: 382-391.
13. Alpen EL, Powers-Risius P, Curtis SB, DeGuzman R, Fry RJ (1994) Fluence-based relative biological effectiveness for charged particle carcinogenesis in mouse Harderian gland. Adv Space Res 14: 573–581.
14. Fry RJ, Powers-Risius P, Alpen EL, Ainsworth EJ (1985) High-LET radiation carcinogenesis. Radiat Res Suppl 8: S188–S195.
15. Dicello JF, Christian A, Cucinotta FA, Gridley DS, Kathirithamby R, et al. (2004) In vivo mammary tumourigenesis in the Sprague-Dawley rat and microdosimetric correlates. Phys Med Biol 49: 3817–3830.
16. Turusov VS, Mohr U (1994) Pathology of tumours in laboratory animals. Lyon: International Agency for Research on Cancer.
17. Mole RH, Papworth DG, Corp MJ (1983) The dose-response for x-ray induction of myeloid-leukemia in male CBA/H mice. British Journal of Cancer 47: 285–291.
18. Ullrich RL, Preston RJ (1987) Myeloid leukemia in male RFM mice following irradiation with fission spectrum neutrons or gamma rays. Radiat Res 109: 165–170.
19. Datta K, Suman S, Kallakury BV, Fornace AJ Jr (2013) Heavy ion radiation exposure triggered higher intestinal tumor frequency and greater beta-catenin activation than gamma radiation in APC(Min/+) mice. PLoS One 8: e59295.
20. Clapp NK, Darden EB Jr, Jernigan MC (1974) Relative effects of whole-body sublethal doses of 60-MeV protons and 300-kVp X-rays on disease incidences in RF mice. Radiat Res 57: 158–186.
21. Ullrich RL, Jernigan MC, Storer JB (1977) Neutron carcinogenesis. Dose and dose-rate effects in BALB/c mice. Radiat Res 72: 487–498.
22. Ullrich RL (1983) Tumor induction in BALB/c female mice after fission neutron or gamma irradiation. Radiat Res 93: 506–515.
23. Fournier C, Zahnreich S, Kraft D, Friedrich T, Voss KO, et al. (2012) The fate of a normal human cell traversed by a single charged particle. Sci Rep 2: 643.
24. Miller RC, Randers-Pehrson G, Geard CR, Hall EJ, Brenner DJ (1999) The oncogenic transforming potential of the passage of single alpha particles through mammalian cell nuclei. Proc Natl Acad Sci U S A 96: 19–22.
25. Shuryak I, Brenner DJ, Ullrich RL (2011) Radiation-induced carcinogenesis: mechanistically based differences between gamma-rays and neutrons, and interactions with DMBA. PLoS One 6: e28559.

26. Cheema AK, Suman S, Kaur P, Singh R, Fornace AJ, et al. (2014) Long-term differential changes in mouse intestinal metabolomics after gamma and heavy ion radiation exposure. PLoS One 9: e87079.
27. Grivennikov SI, Greten FR, Karin M (2010) Immunity, inflammation, and cancer. Cell 140: 883–899.
28. Alzahrani B, Iseli TJ, Hebbard LW (2014) Non-viral causes of liver cancer: does obesity led inflammation play a role? Cancer Lett 345: 223–229.
29. Orman ES, Odena G, Bataller R (2013) Alcoholic liver disease: pathogenesis, management, and novel targets for therapy. J Gastroenterol Hepatol 28 Suppl 1: 77–84.
30. Shlomai A, de Jong YP, Rice CM (2014) Virus associated malignancies: The role of viral hepatitis in hepatocellular carcinoma. Semin Cancer Biol 26: 78–88.
31. Cucinotta FA (2014) Space radiation risks for astronauts on multiple International Space Station missions. PLoS One 9: e96099.
32. Darakhshan F, Badie C, Moody J, Coster M, Finnon R, et al. (2006) Evidence for complex multigenic inheritance of radiation AML susceptibility in mice revealed using a surrogate phenotypic assay. Carcinogenesis 27: 311–318.
33. Smith SM, Le Beau MM, Huo D, Karrison T, Sobecks RM, et al. (2003) Clinical-cytogenetic associations in 306 patients with therapy-related myelodysplasia and myeloid leukemia: the University of Chicago series. Blood 102: 43–52.
34. Finney D J (1947) Probit analysis: a statistical treatment of the sigmoid response curve. Cambridge: Cambridge University Press.

13

Loss of Function of TET2 Cooperates with Constitutively Active KIT in Murine and Human Models of Mastocytosis

Serena De Vita[1], Rebekka K. Schneider[2], Michael Garcia[1], Jenna Wood[1], Mathilde Gavillet[1], Benjamin L. Ebert[2], Alexander Gerbaulet[3], Axel Roers[3], Ross L. Levine[4], Ann Mullally[2], David A. Williams[1]*

1 Division of Hematology/Oncology, Boston Children's Hospital, Harvard Medical School, Boston, Massachusetts, United States of America, **2** Division of Hematology, Department of Medicine, Brigham and Women's Hospital, Harvard Medical School, Boston, Massachusetts, United States of America, **3** Institute for Immunology, Medical Faculty Carl Gustav Carus, Dresden University of Technology, Dresden, Germany, **4** Human Oncology and Pathogenesis Program, and Leukemia Service, Department of Medicine, Memorial Sloan-Kettering Cancer Center, New York, New York, United States of America

Abstract

Systemic Mastocytosis (SM) is a clonal disease characterized by abnormal accumulation of mast cells in multiple organs. Clinical presentations of the disease vary widely from indolent to aggressive forms, and to the exceedingly rare mast cell leukemia. Current treatment of aggressive SM and mast cell leukemia is unsatisfactory. An imatinib-resistant activating mutation of the receptor tyrosine kinase KIT (*KIT D816V*) is most frequently present in transformed mast cells and is associated with all clinical forms of the disease. Thus the etiology of the variable clinical aggressiveness of abnormal mast cells in SM is unclear. *TET2* appears to be mutated in primary human samples in aggressive types of SM, suggesting a possible role in disease modification. In this report, we demonstrate the cooperation between *KIT D816V* and loss of function of TET2 in mast cell transformation and demonstrate a more aggressive phenotype in a murine model of SM when both mutations are present in progenitor cells. We exploit these findings to validate a combination treatment strategy targeting the epigenetic deregulation caused by loss of TET2 and the constitutively active KIT receptor for the treatment of patients with aggressive SM.

Editor: Halvard Boenig, German Red Cross Blood Service Frankfurt, Germany

Funding: This work was supported by grant NIH 5R01DK062757-11 to D.A.W. and by an American Italian Cancer Foundation (AICF) postdoctoral fellowship to S.D.V. The funders had no role in study design, data collection and analysis, decision to publish, or preparation of the manuscript.

Competing Interests: The authors have declared that no competing interests exist.

* E-mail: DAWilliams@childrens.harvard.edu

Introduction

Systemic mastocytosis (SM) is a clonal disease of the mast cell lineage with clinical presentations ranging from mild forms to more aggressive disease [1]. The current classification of SM includes 5 subtypes: indolent SM (ISM), smoldering SM (SSM), SM with an associated hematologic non-mast cell-lineage disease (SM-AHNMD), aggressive SM (ASM), and mast cell leukemia (MCL) [2,3]. Most cases of SM are mild and respond to symptomatic therapy with antihistamines and inhibitors of mast cell degranulation. Management of aggressive types of disease, where mast cells infiltrate multiple organs (including skin, lymph nodes, spleen, liver, lungs, heart and bone marrow) is more challenging and is approached with chemotherapy or other targeted therapeutic interventions.

In adults, most cases of SM are associated with the presence of activating mutations in the receptor tyrosine kinase *c-KIT* (KIT), which binds to stem cell factor (SCF or KIT ligand), a known trophic factor for mast cells.

By far the most frequent *KIT* mutation in mastocytosis is a substitution of aspartic acid to valine at position 816 *(KIT D816V)* that leads to constitutive activation of the receptor [4,5]. The presence of the *KIT D816V* mutation does not appear to correlate with a specific subtype of the disease and does not contribute to the disease prognosis. Moreover, this mutation is imatinib-resistant [6,7] and targeted therapy with second-generation tyrosine kinase inhibitors (TKIs) has shown variable success [8,9], although promising preliminary data have been obtained with midostaurin (PKC412) [10].

Additional cooperating events may contribute to the pathogenesis and/or the phenotype of SM [11,12,13]. Mutations in *TET2* have been reported in as many as 40% of *KIT D816V*-positive SM cases [11,12]. TET2 is an enzyme that catalyzes the conversion of 5-methylcytosine (5-mC) to 5-hydroxymethylcytosine (5-hmC) and further modified cytosines, regulating gene expression at the cellular level [14,15]. Loss-of-function mutations in *TET2* have been reported in a variety of hematological malignancies including acute myeloid leukemias (AMLs), chronic myelomonocytic leukemia (CMML), myeloproliferative neoplasms (MPNs), myelodysplastic syndromes (MDS) and lymphoid malignancies [16,17,18]. In mouse models, loss of one or both copies of *Tet2* has been shown to contribute to the pathogenesis of hematological malignancies by increasing the self-renewal capacity of the hematopoietic stem cell compartment and expanding the immature pool of myeloid and lymphoid progenitors [19,20,21].

In SM, the coexistence of mutations in *TET2* and the *KIT D816V* lesion have recently been suggested to lead to a more aggressive type of disease and an overall worse prognosis, although the effect on mast cell biology was not properly analyzed [22]. In the current study, we investigate the biological relevance of loss of

TET2 in the context of *KIT D816V* associated mast-cell disease both *in vivo* in a mouse model and *in vitro* in human cells. We demonstrate that mutations in both loci cooperate in the mast cell lineage to cause an aggressive type of mastocytosis. Furthermore, we show that Tet2 loss-of-function makes *KIT D816V*-positive mastocytosis amenable to combination therapy with epigenetic modifiers and TKIs.

Methods

Ethics statement

This study was carried out in strict accordance with the recommendations in the Guide for the Care and Use of Laboratory Animals of the National Institutes of Health. The Institutional Animal Care and Use Commitee at Boston Children's Hospital approved all of the animal care procedures and experiments (authorization no. 11-03-1894R).

Mice

Kit D814V^{Fl} mice have been previously described [23]. The *Kit D814V* transgene is expressed upon Cre-mediated excision of the loxP-flanked transcriptional stop element in adult mice. Tet2$^{Fl/Fl}$ mice have been described elsewhere [19]. These mice were crossed to Kit D814^{Fl} mice to generate Tet2$^{Fl/WT}$;Kit D814V double transgenic animals, and to Mx1-Cre [24] or Mcpt5-Cre [25] mice to generate Tet2$^{Fl/WT}$;Mx1-Cre and Tet2$^{Fl/WT}$;Mcpt5-Cre double transgenic animals. Tet2$^{Fl/WT}$;Kit D814V were then crossed to Tet2$^{Fl/WT}$;Mx1-Cre or Tet2$^{Fl/WT}$;Mcpt5-Cre mice and their progeny were used for subsequent experiments. In mice carrying the Mx1-Cre allele, Cre expression was induced by 3 i.p. injections of 250 µg polyinosine-polycytidylic acid (pI:C) every second day to activate expression of the transgenic *Kit D814V* and deletion of one or both *Tet2* alleles. Mice were treated with pI:C at 4 weeks of age. All mice used in this study were backcrossed for at least 5 generation and maintained on a C57/BL6 background. All mice were housed in the experimental animal facility at Boston Children's Hospital and were provided free access to food and water.

Experimental procedures

For survival studies, starting one week after the last pI:C injection, mice were monitored every other day to detect early signs of leukemia. Whenever ruffled fur, reduced movements or hind limb paralysis were noticed, mice were bled by retro-orbital bleeding, and humanely euthanized using carbon dioxide, followed by cervical dislocation. Of the experimental cohorts reported in leukemia studies, all mice were humanely euthanized when they met any of the humane endpoints listed above. One mouse in the primary leukemic mice cohort was lost at follow-up and found dead before humane euthanasia could be performed. WBC counts couldn't be obtained for this animal.

For survival studies and for determination of peripheral blood chimerism, mice underwent retro-orbital bleeding after anesthesia with isofluorane. Following this procedure, animals were treated with eye lubricant to minimize their discomfort.

Cell lines

The human mast cell leukemia cell line HMC-1.2 (carrying the *KIT G560V* and the *KIT D816V* activating mutations) was a kind gift from Dr. JH Butterfield (Mayo Clinic, Rochester, MN) [26]. HMC-1.2 were grown in RPMI supplemented with 10% fetal bovine serum (FBS), 2 mM glutamine, 100 U/mL penicillin and 0.1 mg/mL streptomycin in a humidified incubator with 5% CO_2 at 37°C. Fresh HMC-1.2 cells were thawed from an original stock every 8 weeks, and cells were periodically checked for the presence of metachromatic granules and for expression of the KIT receptor [27].

Derivation of BMMCs

Bone marrow-derived mast cells (BMMCs) were generated from low density BM cells by four weeks of culture in RPMI supplemented with 10% fetal bovine serum (FBS), 2 mM glutaminè, 100 U/mL penicillin, 0.1 mg/mL streptomycin and 10 ng/mL of mouse recombinant IL-3 (PeproTech, Rocky Hill, NJ) in a humidified incubator with 5% CO_2 at 37°C.

Giemsa staining

Giemsa staining was performed on skin and stomach sections from diseased animals using standard protocols. Slides were evaluated by photomicroscopy using the Spot Advance software from Spot^{TM} Imaging Solutions, (Sterling Heights, MI) on an Eclipse E400 microscope from Nikon (Melville, NY). Images were taken using a 20× objective.

Cell proliferation and apoptosis

Apoptosis was evaluated using the Annexin V-APC flow kit from BD Biosciences (San Jose, CA). Cells were counterstained with 7-AAD (Invitrogen, Carlsbad, CA). For proliferation assays, cells were cultured in the presence of 5-bromo-2′-deoxy-uridine (BrdU) for 4 hours then fixed, permeabilized, and stained using the APC BrdU Flow Kit (BD Biosciences), following the manufacturer's instructions. Data were acquired on a LSR II flow cytometer (BD Biosciences). For cell growth, cells were plated in 96-well plates at 10,000 cells/well and lysed at the indicated time point with CellTiter-Glo Luminescent Cell Viability Assay reagent (Promega, Madison, WI). Luminescence was read using a DTX 880 plate reader from Beckman Coulter (Brea, CA). Cell growth was normalized to 5 days post-transduction.

Statistical analysis

Datasets were compared by two-tailed *t* tests and *P* values less than .05 were considered statistically significant.

Results

Knock down of TET2 increases proliferation of a *KIT D816V* positive human mast cell leukemia cell line

To model the cooperation between loss of function of TET2 and the *KIT D816V* mutation *in vitro*, we knocked down (KD) TET2 in a human mast cell leukemia cell line (HMC-1.2) harboring the *KIT D816V* mutation. We first documented the absence of mutations (except for one annotated SNP) in the coding sequence of *TET2* in the HMC-1.2 cell line (data not shown). In absence of a reliable commercially available antibody for TET2, we determined the efficiency of five individual KD vectors by qPCR (Figure S1, panel A). We chose two vectors (sh-1 and sh-3) that achieved an average KD of TET2 of 45% and 34%, respectively (Table S1). As expected, KD of TET2 in HMC-1.2 cells caused a reduction in the total content of 5-hmC, an intermediate in the DNA demethylation reaction catalyzed by TET2 (Figure S1, panel B). In this cell line, silencing of TET2 also caused a significant increase in cellular growth over time (Fig. 1A) ($P=.05$ TET2 sh-1 vs. control shRNA [ctr sh], $P=.02$ TET2 sh-3 vs. ctr sh, at day 12 after transduction). The increase in cell numbers was associated with increased proliferation upon silencing of TET2, as assessed by BrdU incorporation (Fig. 1B and 1C) (% cells in S phase = 5.8±0.5 ctr sh vs. 12.4±3.3 TET2 sh-1 and 16.63±0.9 TET2 sh-3, P=.09 TET2 sh-1 vs. ctr sh, P=.0007 TET2 sh-3 vs. ctr). To address whether loss of TET2 would modify migratory properties of HMC-1.2 cells, we compared cells transduced with two shRNAs against TET2 (sh-1 and sh-3) to a ctr sh. There was no difference in the number of migrated cells in response to human SCF under all conditions analyzed (Figure S1, panel C). These data indicate that loss of function of TET2 cooperates with KIT D816V to increase the proliferative capacity of human malignant mast cells, without modifying their migratory properties.

Tet2$^{-/-}$;Kit D814V mice develop a more aggressive type of systemic mastocytosis compared to Tet2$^{+/+}$;Kit D814V animals

Next, we examined the *in vivo* phenotype caused by simultaneous expression of Kit D814V (the mouse homologue of *KIT D816V*) and deletion of Tet2 in the hematopoietic compartment of compound mice. In all genotypes expressing the *Kit D814V* allele there was a significant increase in mast cell infiltration of several organs. In the skin, the average number of mast cells per scored section was 56.9±4 in Tet2$^{+/+}$;Kit D814V vs. 96.3±18.9 in Tet2$^{-/-}$;Kit D814V (n = 80 from 4 independent animals/genotype, P=.04, Fig 2A). In the esophagus/stomach, the average number of mast cells per scored section was 23.1±3.6 in Tet2$^{+/}$

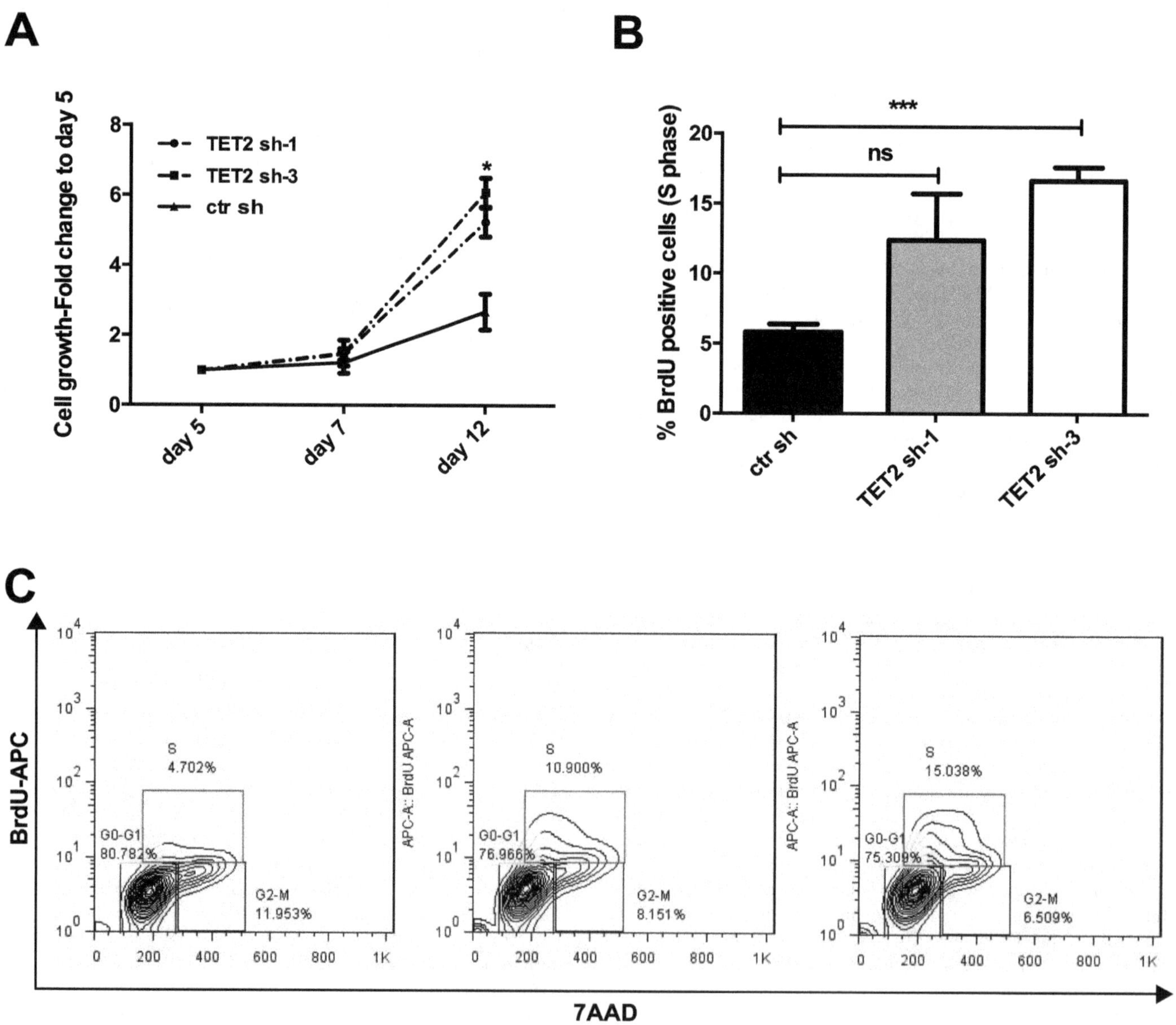

Figure 1. Increased proliferation of HMC-1.2 cells after knock down of TET2. A) HMC-1.2 cells were treated with two hairpins against TET2 (TET2 sh-1 and TET2 sh-3) or a control shRNA (ctr sh). Cell growth was calculated using the CellTiter-Glo assay from Promega. Data are presented as fold change relative to day 5 after transduction. Values represent mean ±SEM, n = 3 independent experiments. *P<.05. **B**) Percentage of cells in S-phase determined by BrdU incorporation in HMC-1.2 cells treated with TET2 sh-1 and sh-3 compared to a control hairpin. Values are mean ±SEM. n = 3 independent experiments, ***P<.001, ns = not significant. **C**) Representative FACS plots showing BrdU incorporation in relation to cell cycle stages in HMC-1.2 cells infected with control hairpin (ctr sh) compared with TET2 sh-1 and TET2 sh-3.

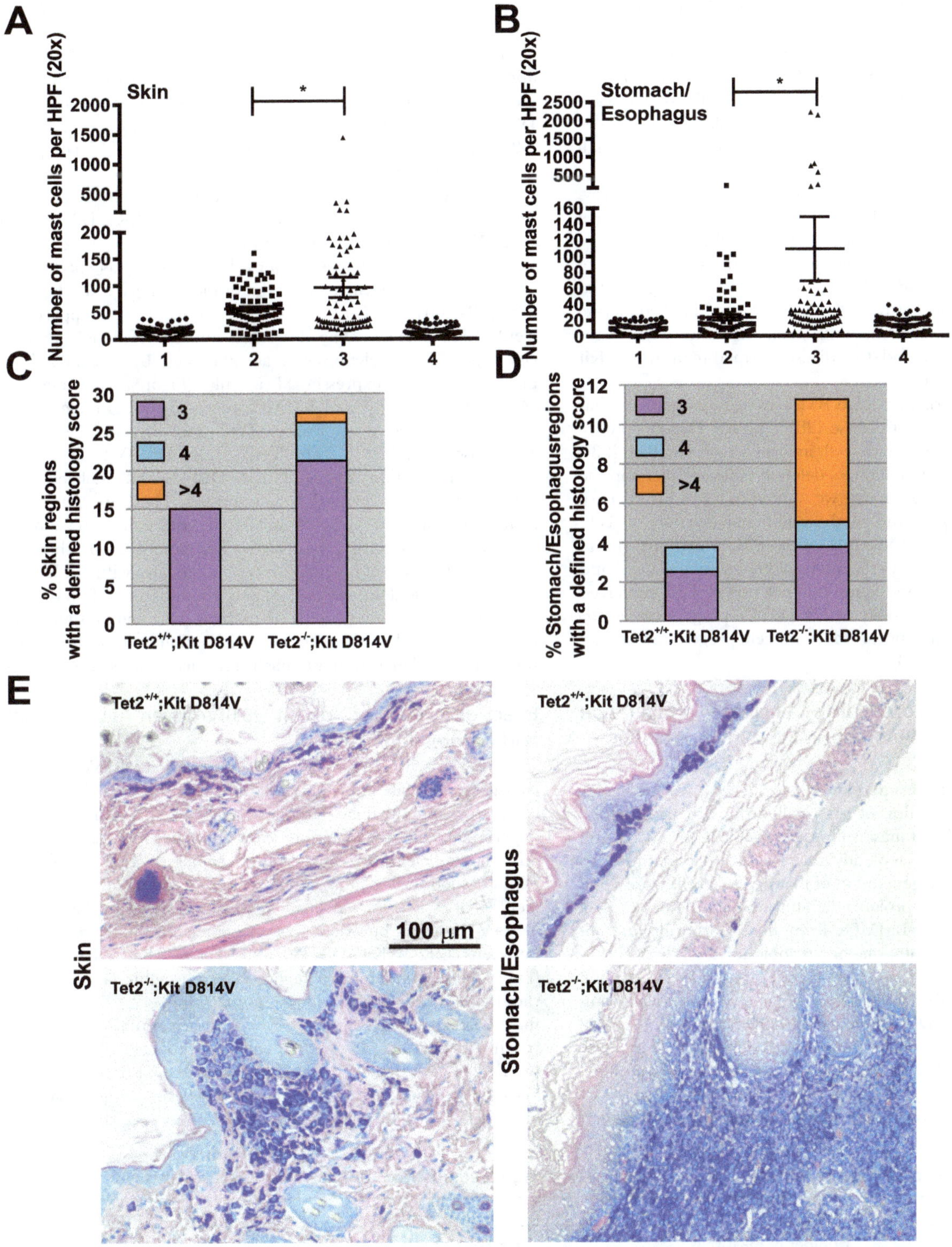

Figure 2. Loss of Tet2 accentuates a Kit D814V driven mast cell phenotype. A) Average number of mast cells per skin section across genotypes. N = 60–80 sections from 3–4 independent animals/genotype. $^*P<.05$. **B**) Average number of mast cells per stomach/esophagus section across genotypes. N = 60–80 sections from 3–4 independent animals/genotype. $^*P<.05$. For Figure 2A and 2B, numbers 1–4 indicate the following genotypes: 1 = WT ctr, 2 = Tet2$^{+/+}$;Kit D814, 3 = Tet2$^{-/-}$;Kit D814, 4 = Tet2$^{-/-}$;Kit WT. **C**) Percentage of skin sections with a defined histology score from Tet2$^{+/+}$;Kit D814V and Tet2$^{-/-}$;Kit D814V. **D**) Percentage of stomach/esophagus sections with a defined histology score in Tet2$^{+/+}$;Kit D814V and Tet2$^{-/-}$;Kit D814V animals. For Fig 2A–2D, twenty randomly chosen and independent regions of equal thickness per animal were counted in a blinded fashion at 20× magnification, and scored according to the classification reported in Table 1. Mice were all harvested between 8 and 20 weeks after the last pI:C injection. n = 4 per genotype. **E**) Representative pictures of Giemsa staining performed on skin (left panels) or stomach/esophagus sections (right panels) prepared from Tet2$^{+/+}$;Kit D814V and Tet2$^{-/-}$;Kit D814V animals. Mast cells stain dark blue in these sections. Scale bar represents 100 μm.

$^{+}$;Kit D814V vs. 108.4±40 in Tet2$^{-/-}$;Kit D814V (n = 80 from 4 independent animals/genotype, P = .03, Fig 2B). The deletion of Tet2 alone was not sufficient to cause disease in absence of Kit D814V (WT ctr vs Tet2$^{-/-}$; Kit WT P = .5 in the skin and P = .2, n = 60–80 sections) underscoring the role of Tet2 as a disease modifier, rather than a disease-initiating molecular lesion.

Given that mast cell aggregates ranged in dimension from small infiltrates to mast cell tumors, we defined a histology score (Table 1) to classify and compare disease aggressiveness across areas of affected genotypes. Loss of Tet2 in Kit D814V positive animals was associated with a more aggressive disease phenotype, as evidenced by the presence of histological sections with a score of 4 or greater in target organs (Fig. 2C–2E). These data suggest that simultaneous expression of Kit D814V and loss of Tet2 cooperate in the mast cell compartment and result in a more aggressive phenotype in the skin and the digestive tract than when Kit D814V is present alone.

SM is thought to originate from BM stem cells/progenitors that then colonize other sites of disease [28]. The Kit D814V-MxCre model does not develop mast cell infiltration of the BM [23]. However, because Mx-Cre induces deletion of floxed alleles in the BM hematopoietic compartment, we wanted to assess the effect of the Kit mutation alone and of the additional deletion of Tet2 specifically in stem/progenitor cells of the BM, which give rise to mast cells. We therefore performed colony-forming assays and competitive transplants, and found that deletion of Tet2 conferred both increased replating ability to Kit D814V progenitors *in vitro* and a competitive advantage to stem cell/progenitors *in vivo* (Figure S2, panel A and B).

Loss of one or both copies of Tet2 increases proliferation and impairs differentiation of BMMC carrying the *Kit D184V* mutation

Next, we analyzed the interplay between these two molecular hits during the specification of mast cells from BM progenitors. Given that the identity of mast cell progenitors in adult mice is still controversial [29,30], we took advantage of an established *in vitro* system that leads to the generation of mature mast cells from bone marrow (BMMCs) upon prolonged culture in the presence of IL-3 [31,32]. We compared BMMCs from mice harboring the *Kit D814V* mutation, and both, one or no copies of *Tet2* (Tet2$^{+/+}$;Kit D814V, Tet2$^{+/-}$;Kit D814V and Tet2$^{-/-}$;Kit D814V) in the hematopoietic compartment. Excision of the stop cassette allowing expression of the *Kit D814V* transgene and deletion of the *Tet2* floxed allele at the genomic level were verified in BMMCs by PCR (Figure S3, panel A–C). Tet2 mRNA was appropriately reduced according to the genotype (Fig. 3A). Loss of one or both copies of Tet2 did not alter the constitutive phosphorylation of c-Kit caused by the presence of the activating mutation *Kit D814V* in BMMCs (Fig. 3B, lanes 2–4). BMMCs carrying one or no copies of *Tet2* in addition to the *Kit D814V* mutation displayed increased proliferation compared to Tet2$^{+/+}$;Kit D814V cells as measured by BrdU incorporation (Fig. 3C) (% cells in S phase = 6.7% Tet2$^{+/+}$;Kit D814V vs. 13.2 Tet2$^{+/-}$;Kit D814V vs. 12.8 Tet2$^{-/-}$;Kit D814V, n = 3, P = .1 for Tet2$^{+/-}$ and .01 for Tet2$^{-/-}$ compared to Tet2$^{+/+}$;Kit D814V,).

Loss of Tet2 also impaired the differentiation of BMMCs. After four weeks in culture with IL-3, 92% of Tet2$^{+/+}$;Kit D814V, but only 75% of Tet2$^{+/-}$;Kit D814V and 64% of Tet2$^{-/-}$;Kit D814V stained double positive for c-Kit and Fcε (co-expression of both markers is indicative of full maturation of mast cells) (Fig. 3D, n = 3, P = .001 for Tet2$^{+/-}$ and .02 for Tet2$^{-/-}$ compared to Tet2$^{+/+}$;Kit D814V). The decreased number of double positive cells upon Tet2 deletion was accompanied by a concomitant increase in cells expressing Fcε only (Figure S3, panel D). Morphological analysis of BMMCs revealed that granule formation was reduced upon loss of Tet2 (Fig. 3E, see Tet2$^{+/+}$ in comparison with Tet2$^{+/-}$ and Tet2$^{-/-}$;Kit D814V), suggesting a delayed maturation stage of Kit D814V-Tet2 deleted cells compared to their Tet2 WT counterpart. These morphological changes did not correlate with an altered pattern of expression of a set of mast cell-specific genes (Figure S3, panel E). Together, our data show that loss of function of Tet2 cooperates with Kit D814V to enhance proliferation and alter differentiation of mast cells derived *in vitro* from murine bone marrow progenitors, supporting the hypothesis that the two hits exerts their effect during the specification of mature mast cells from uncommitted progenitors.

Effect of loss of Tet2 on Kit D814V-driven ALL initiation and progression

As previously reported [23], we noted that Kit D814V;Mx1-Cre transgenic animals induced with pI:C succumb to a disease that resembles human acute lymphoblastic leukemia (ALL). In our experiments, there was no significant difference in the incidence of ALL upon deletion of one or both copies of Tet2 (Table S2). White blood cell counts (WBCs) were significantly higher in Tet2$^{-/-}$;Kit D814V leukemic mice compared with Tet2$^{+/+}$;Kit D814V (Fig. 4A), but there was no significant difference in WBC between Tet2$^{+/+}$;Kit D814V and Tet2$^{+/-}$;Kit D814V mice (Fig. 4B). A trend toward higher spleen weights (a measure of the disease burden in moribund animals) in Tet2$^{-/-}$;Kit D814V mice correlated with higher WBC in these animals, but did not reach statistical difference when compared to Tet2$^{+/+}$;Kit D814V or Tet2$^{+/-}$;Kit D814V animals. There was also no difference across genotypes in disease latency, based on the average time after pI:C when mice were found moribund (Fig. 4C). All mice

Table 1. Histology score used to classify skin and stomach/esophagus regions from animals with mastocytosis.

Histology Score	Number of mast cells	Description
0	0–30 mast cells	
1	31–50 mast cells	Increased diffuse infiltrate
2	51–100 mast cells	Mast cell accumulation
3	101–200 mast cells	Mast cell tumor<500 μm
4	201–500 mast cells	Mast cell tumor (500–100 μm)
5	501–1000 mast cells	Mast cell tumor (1000–1500 μm)
6	>1000 mast cells	Large tumor>1500 μm

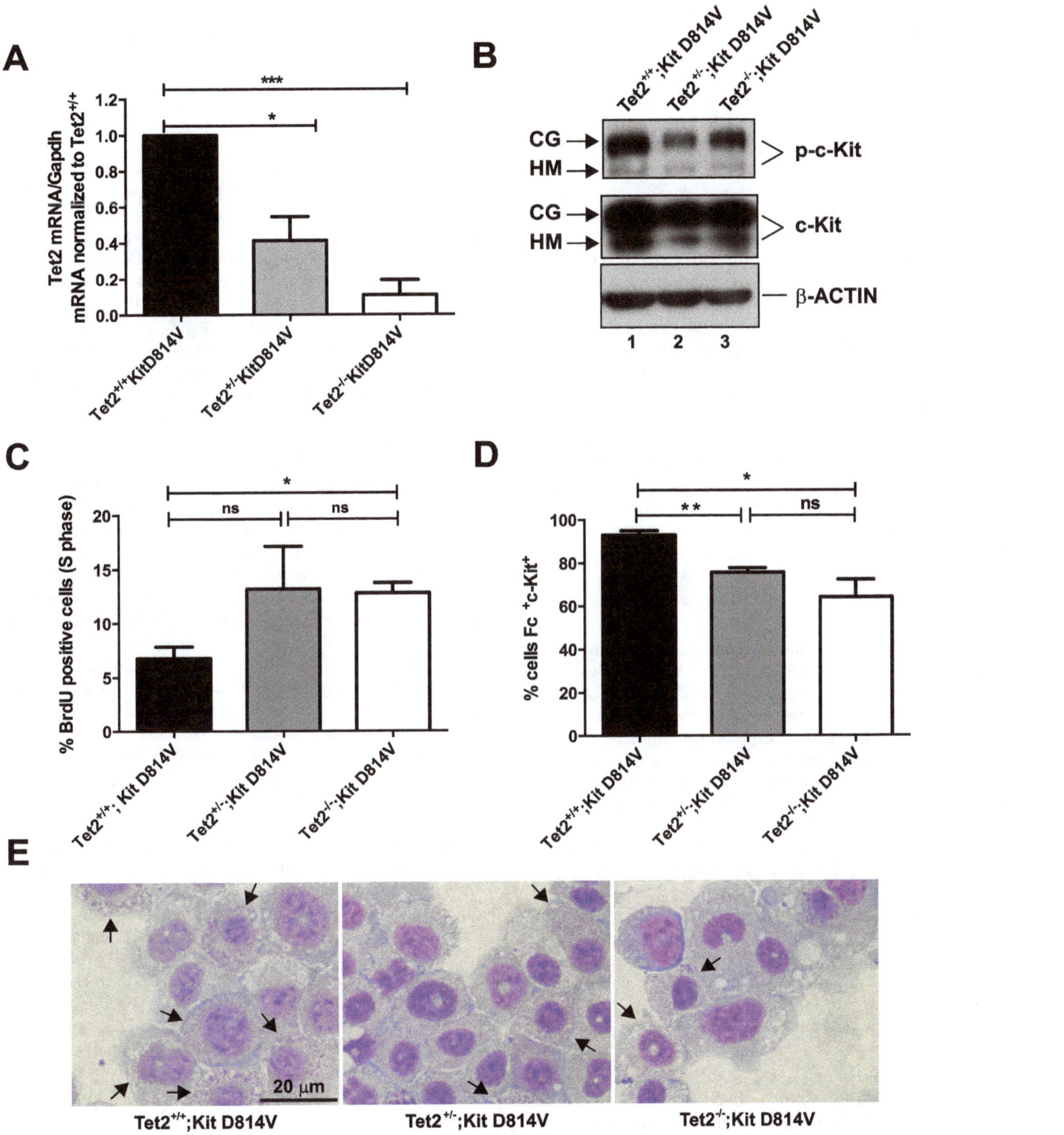

Figure 3. Effects of loss of Tet2 on BMMCs derived from Kit D814V-MxCre mice. A) Tet2 mRNA levels measured in BMMCs upon Mx1-Cre-mediated deletion of Tet2. Data are presented as fold change of Tet2 mRNA/Gapdh mRNA levels relative to Tet2$^{+/+}$;Kit D814V. Data represent mean ±SEM, n = 3, *P = <05, ***P<.001. **B**) Phosphorylation of the Kit receptor in the absence of its ligand SCF due to the presence of a Kit activating mutation in BMMCs from Tet2$^{+/+}$;Kit D814V, Tet2$^{+/-}$;Kit D814V and Tet2$^{-/-}$;Kit D814V animals. The western blot shown is representative of two independent experiments with similar results. Two different glycosylated forms of the Kit receptor are indicated. CG = complex glycosylation form; HM = high-mannose form. Total levels of c-KIT and β-actin are shown as loading controls. **C**) Proliferation of BMMCs carrying the *Kit D814V* mutation upon loss of Tet2. Data show average percentage ±SEM of BrdU-positive BMMCs across genotypes, n = 3, *P<.05, ns = not significant. **D**) Differentiation of *Kit D814V* positive BMMCs in the absence of Tet2. Data show average percentage ±SEM of double positive (Fcε^{+}c-Kit^{+}) BMMCs from Tet2$^{+/+}$;Kit D814V, Tet2$^{+/-}$;Kit D814V and Tet2$^{-/-}$;Kit D814V (64.1±8.2) after 4 weeks in culture with mIL-3. n = 3, *P = <05, **P<.01, ns = not significant **E**) Representative images of Tet2$^{+/+}$;Kit D814V,Tet2$^{+/-}$;Kit D814V and Tet2$^{-/-}$;Kit D814V BMMCs. Scale bar = 20 μm. Arrows indicate cells containing granules, which is indicative of a more differentiated phenotype.

sacrificed due to ALL had a diffuse generalized increase in cutaneous mast cells (data not shown). Leukemic blasts from all genotypes infiltrated the bone marrow, spleen and liver of diseased animals (Figure S4, panel A). Blast cells in the peripheral blood, marrow and spleen expressed B220 and CD19, suggesting that the leukemia had an immature B cell origin (Figure S4, panel B). Sorted blast cells expressed the *Kit D814V* allele (Figure S4, panel D) and displayed reduction of Tet2 expression consistent with their genotype (Figure S4, panel C), confirming that the leukemic clone harbored both genetic lesions. Upon transplantation into sublethally irradiated recipients, an equal number of blast cells from primary $Tet2^{+/+}$;Kit D814V, $Tet2^{+/-}$;Kit D814V and $Tet2^{-/-}$;Kit D814V mice generated ALL in secondary mice with the same characteristics of the primary disease. There was no difference in the penetrance of disease across the three genotypes in recipient animals, but the median survival was slightly but significantly reduced for recipients of the $Tet2^{-/-}$;Kit D814V group compare with the other two genotypes (median survival for $Tet2^{+/+}$;Kit D814V and $Tet2^{+/-}$;Kit D814V was 13 days, 11 days for $Tet2^{-/-}$;Kit D814V; $P=.009$; Fig. 4D). WBC and spleen weight were comparable across groups of secondary transplanted recipients (Fig. 4E–F). From these data, we conclude that Tet2 is not required for the initiation of Kit D814V-driven acute lymphoblastic leukemia, but may play a role in disease progression in this model.

Cooperation between the two lesions in a mast cell-specific context

Given the high percentage of mice succumbing to ALL in our Mx-Cre model, we hypothesized that using a mast cell-specific Cre would obviate lymphoid leukemias and allow full penetrance of the mast cell phenotype. Because the Mcpt5 promoter is active selectively in mature mast cells [25], expression of the *Kit D814V* allele driven by this lineage-specific Cre recombinase causes a slow onset (9 months) mastocytosis confined to the skin [23]. In our experiments, the average number of mast cells per skin section was 42.5 in $Tet2^{+/+}$;Kit D814V;Mcpt5-Cre, 77.3 in $Tet2^{+/-}$;Kit D814V;Mcpt5-Cre and 56.5 in $Tet2^{-/-}$;Kit D814V;Mcpt5-Cre (n = 56–96, n = 3–5 animals per genotype). Although there was a trend towards an increased number of mast cells in the skin of $Tet2^{+/-}$;Kit D814V;Mcpt5-Cre and $Tet2^{-/-}$;Kit D814V;Mcpt5-Cre compared to $Tet2^{+/+}$;Kit D814V;Mcpt5-Cre, the difference didn't reach statistical significance ($P=.1$ and .2, respectively). Importantly, the number of mast cells per skin section in $Tet2^{+/-}$;Kit WT;Mcpt5-Cre and $Tet2^{-/-}$;Kit WT;Mcpt5-Cre was not significantly different from the WT control group (Fig 5A), suggesting that in the absence of the Kit D814V lesion, deletion of Tet2 cannot initiate disease in mature mast cells. We also observed that only $Tet2^{+/-}$;Kit D814V;Mcpt5-Cre and $Tet2^{-/-}$;Kit D814V;Mcpt5-Cre animals had aggressive disease as assessed by sections with histology scores >4, according to the classification reported in Table 1 (Fig. 5B and 5C), although the severity of disease varied considerably across skin sections from individual mice. Thus, our data strongly suggest that the cell of origin of the transformed and more aggressive phenotype of mast cell disease likely is a more primitive hematopoietic progenitor and that loss of Tet2 restricted to mature mast cells only modestly accentuates the Kit D814V-driven mast cell skin phenotype.

Combination therapy with dasatinib and low-dose decitabine in TET2 mutated SM

Next, we exploited the cooperation between loss of function of TET2 and KIT D816V in the HMC-1.2 cell line to validate possible combinatorial approaches to treatment for ASM and MCL [8,33]. Loss of TET2 is believed to cause an aberrant methylation of promoter regions in AML [34]. We reasoned that if the same hypermethylator phenotype was caused by loss of TET2 in the *KIT D816V*-positive HMC-1.2 cell line, resulting silencing of gene expression in these cells could potentially be reversed by treatment with epigenetic modifiers, providing an enhanced effect to dasatinib (DASA). We therefore pre-treated HMC-1.2 cells transduced with a control sh or with two independent shRNAs against TET2 with low doses (0.5 μM) of decitabine (DAC) followed by treatment with DASA and performed Annexin V staining. The number of apoptotic ($7\text{-}AAD^-$/Annexin V^+) and dead cells ($7\text{-}AAD^+$/Annexin V^+) in TET2 KD cells treated with the drug combination was higher than in TET2 KD HMC-1.2 treated with either of the drugs alone (Fig. 6A). In HMC-1.2 cells treated with a ctr sh (TET2 WT), the drug combination induced only a modest effect compared to the TKI alone, due to a lower efficacy of DAC alone in TET2 WT compared to TET2 KD cells ($P=.02$ and $P=.03$ for sh-1 and sh-3 compared to ctr sh treated with DAC alone). Importantly, in the experiments reported here, the number of apoptotic and dead cells was significantly higher in TET2 sh-1 HMC-1.2 cells treated with low doses of DAC followed by DASA than in the control sh group ($P=.02$). Although not reaching statistical significance, there was also a trend towards higher numbers of apoptotic cells in TET2 sh-3 HMC-1.2 cells treated with the drug combination than in the control group ($P=.09$). Treatment with both drugs induced cleavage of CASPASE 3 to a larger extent in TET2 KD sh-1 and sh-3 than in control cells (Fig. 6B, densitometric quantitation of the ratio between cleaved CASPASE 3 and β-Actin expressed as fold change to DMSO treated sample in each condition was: 1 vs. 19.1 in TET2 sh-1, 1 vs. 26.6 in TET2 sh-3 and 1 vs. 14.7 in ctr sh). Furthermore, we observed that, as expected, loss of TET2 did not appear to alter the mechanism of action of DASA, which caused comparable inhibition of phosphorylation of its target SRC kinase and its downstream effector STAT5 in the three conditions (Fig. 6C). We also tested the feasibility of adding DAC to a novel promising TKI, midostaurin (PKC412). Addition of DAC to PKC412 caused only a modest, non-significant increase in the percentage of dead and apoptotic cells compared to the TKI alone ($P=.07$, $P=.1$ and $P=3$ for TET2 sh-1, sh-3 and ctr sh, respectively), but the number of apoptotic and dead cells was significantly higher in TET2 sh-1 and sh-3 HMC-1.2 cells treated with the two drug-combination than in the control sh group ($P=.005$ and $P=.01$, respectively)(Figure S5). Together, our data suggest that SM with activating mutations in KIT and loss of TET2 is more susceptible to treatment with DAC and DASA than either compound alone, and pretreatment with DAC might also enhance the effect of PKC412 in this setting.

Discussion

Aggressive forms of systemic mastocytosis (SM) are rare, but difficult to treat. Identifying new molecular targets in aggressive forms of SM may allow for a better stratification of patients and a more effective therapeutic approach. Recent data from primary human samples reported a high frequency of *TET2* mutations in SM and a potential role for loss of function of this gene in modifying the disease phenotype [11,12,22]. In this study, we used a combination of *in vitro* and *in vivo* models to investigate a role for TET2 in the pathogenesis of *KIT D816V*-positive systemic mastocytosis.

First, using a model where Kit D814V is expressed in all hematopoietic cells and Tet2 is deleted under the control of an

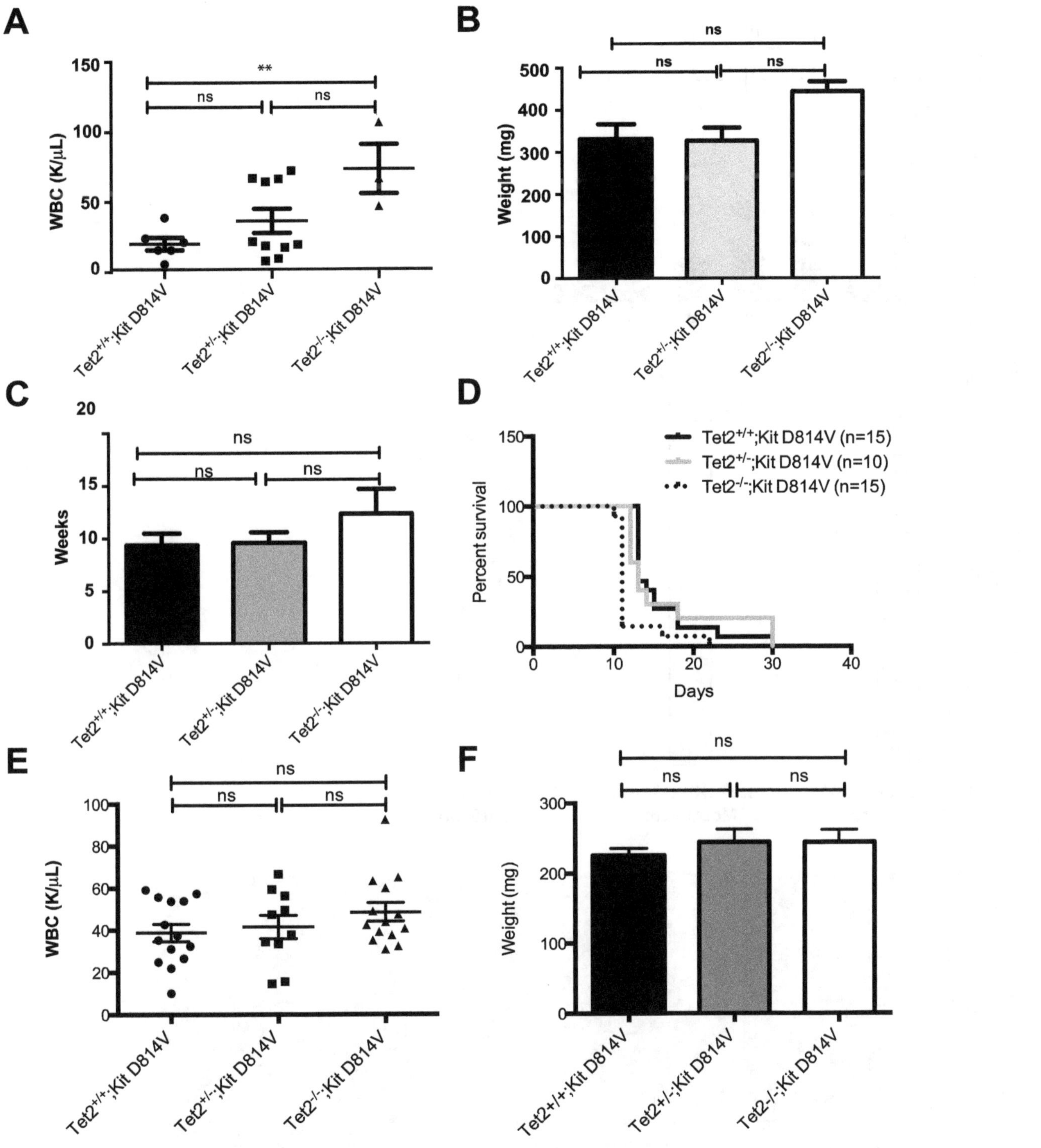

Figure 4. Tet2 deletion affects progression but not initiation of Kit D814V-driven ALL. A) Leukocyte counts in moribund leukemic animals according to genotype. Each data point represents an individual animal. $^{**}P<.01$. **B)** Leukemic infiltration of the spleen expressed as weight (in mg) across genotypes. **C)** Latency of disease (expressed as weeks after the last pI:C injection when mice were found moribund) across genotypes. Data in A B, C is presented as mean ±SEM (n = 3–12 per group). **D)** Kaplan-Meier plot demonstrating survival of recipients transplanted with Tet2$^{+/+}$;Kit D814V (black line),Tet2$^{+/-}$;Kit D814V (grey line) and Tet2$^{-/-}$;Kit D814V (black dotted line) lymphoid leukemic blasts (median survival, 13, 13 and 11 days respectively, n = 10–15 per group, $P = .009$). **E)** Leukocyte counts in secondary moribund leukemic animals according to genotype. Each data point represents an individual animal. **F)** Leukemic infiltration of the spleen expressed as weight (in mg) across genotypes of secondary animals. ns = not significant.

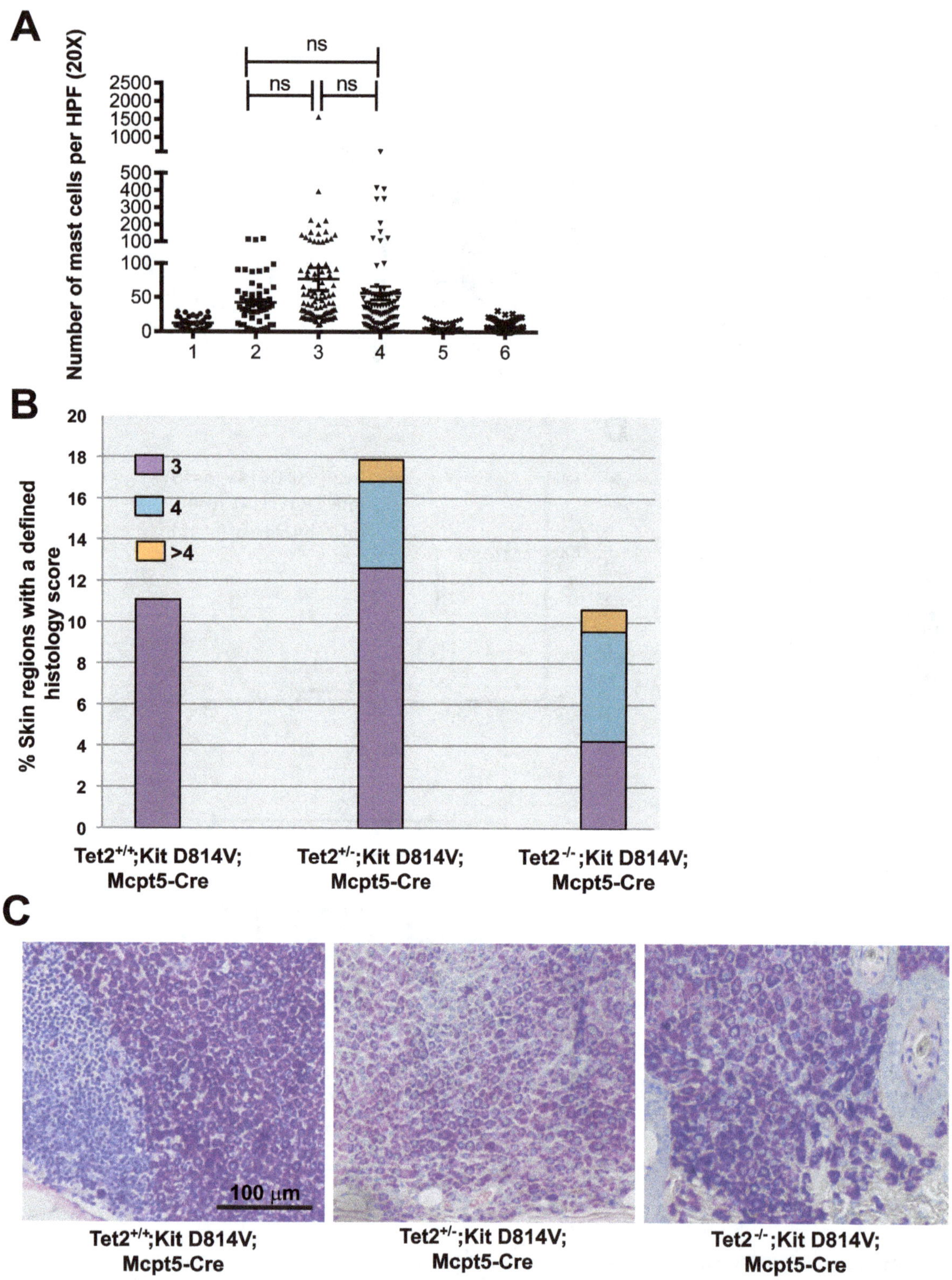

Figure 5. Expression of Kit D814V and loss of Tet2 in MC partially recapitulates the Mx1-Cre-mediated phenotype. A) Cutaneous mastocytosis in mice expressing Kit D814V under the control of a mast cell-specific Cre (Mcpt5-Cre) promoter. Graph represents the average number of mast cells/skin section across listed genotypes. N = 56–96 from 3–4 independent animals per genotype. ns = not significant. Numbers 1–6 indicate the following genotypes: 1 = WT ctr, 2 = Tet2$^{+/+}$;Kit D814;Mcpt5-Cre, 3 = Tet2$^{+/-}$;Kit D814;Mcpt5-Cre, 4 = Tet2$^{-/-}$;Kit D814V;Mcpt5-Cre, 5 = Tet2$^{+/-}$;Kit WT;Mcpt5-Cre,6 = Tet2$^{-/-}$;Kit WT;Mcpt5-Cre, **B**) Histological score of disease in affected Mcpt5-Cre animals. Each skin region was scored according to the criteria reported in Table 1. Bar graph represents the percentage of sections per genotype with a defined histology score (from 3 to >4). Mice analyzed were 9-month-old (n = 3–4 per genotype). **C**) Representative microphotographs showing mast cell infiltration in Tet2$^{+/+}$; Kit D814V;Mcpt5-Cre (dermal lymph node), Tet2$^{+/-}$;Kit D814V;Mcpt5-Cre and Tet2$^{-/-}$;Kit D814V;Mcpt5-Cre animals (skin sections). Mast cells stain dark blue in these sections. Scale = 100 μm.

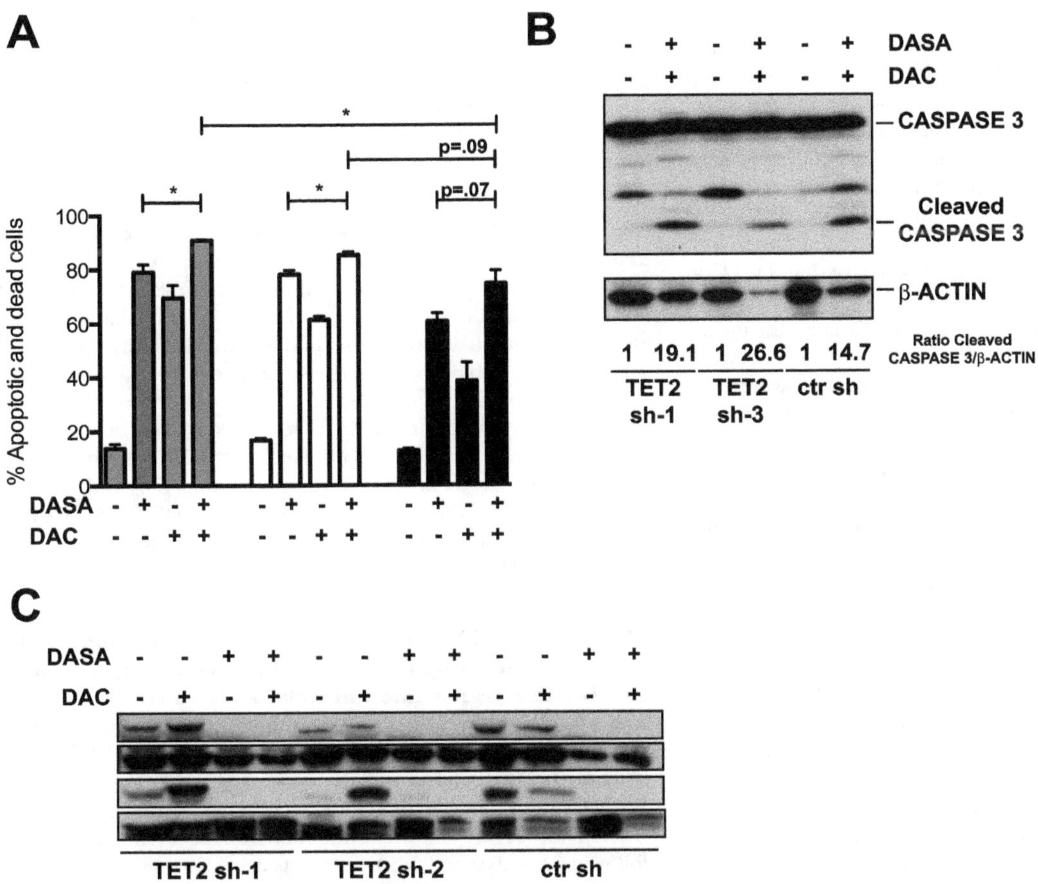

Figure 6. Knock down of TET2 enhances the response of HMC-1.2 to epigenetic modifiers. A) HMC-1.2 transduced with two hairpins against TET2 (TET2 sh-1 and TET2 sh-3) or a control shRNA (ctr sh) were treated for 72 hs with low doses of DAC (0.5 μM) or DMSO. After 72 hs, cells were washed and resuspended in media containing DMSO or DASA at a concentration of 1 μM. Annexin V staining was performed 24 hs after the addition of DASA. Bar graph shows percentage of apoptotic cells (Annexin V^+ 7-AAD^-) and dead cells (Annexin V^+ 7-AAD^+) for each treatment condition. (n = 3; data are expressed as mean ±SEM, *$P<.05$. **B**) Western blot showing cleavage of CASPASE 3 in HMC-1.2 with or without TET2 shRNA, treated with DAC and DASA or vehicle control. β-actin levels were used as a loading control. Numbers below the β-actin blot indicate the fold change to untreated of the ratio between the cleaved CASPASE 3 band and the loading control, as quantified by densitometry. One of two independent experiments with similar results is shown. **C**) Phosphorylation of SRC and STAT5 after treatment with DASA, with and without pretreatment with DAC. Total SRC and total STAT5 levels were determined to confirm equal loading. One of two or three independent experiments is shown.

Mx1-Cre promoter, we could conclusively demonstrate that the two mutations cooperate at the level of hematopoietic stem and progenitor cells in the bone marrow. This was evident in functional assays of these cells, including in vitro CFUs assays and in vivo competitive transplants, as wells as during the *in vitro* specification of mast cells from bone marrow progenitors (BMMCs).

In our experiments, loss of Tet2 led to increased proliferation and a block in differentiation of *KIT D814V* positive BMMCs. We found that the coexistence of Tet2 deletion and the *Kit D814V* mutation was insufficient to confer IL-3 independency to BMMCs (data not shown), suggesting that additional genetic alterations are required for transformation of these cells *in vitro*, or that the transforming requirement for these cells *in vitro* might differ from those required to generate a mast cell disease *in vivo*.

The interplay between loss of function of Tet2 and Kit D814V also had specific consequences on the mast cell lineage *in vivo*. We found that loss of Tet2 conferred more aggressive histological features to the SM phenotype in KitD814V transgenic mice, including increased mast cell accumulation in the skin and digestive tract. This observation contributes a possible new mechanism to the variability in clinical phenotypes of mast cell diseases.

In our *in vivo* model, expression of Kit D814V and simultaneous deletion of Tet2 in mature mast cells in the skin using the Mcpt5-Cre driver appeared to cause a more aggressive disease phenotype, but the difference between genotypes did not reach statistical significance. We conclude that the two lesions together have only modest transforming ability when expressed in the mature mast cell compartment compared with BM stem cells/progenitors. Therefore, data presented here validate loss of Tet2 as a molecular event specifically associated with more aggressive types of SM, which originate from the BM progenitor compartment and cause infiltration of various organs. Importantly, we also demonstrate here that the presence of Tet2 mutations alone is not sufficient to initiate mastocytosis, nether in the bone marrow compartment, nor in mature mast cells in the skin.

In this study, we found that all mice that succumbed to an ALL-like malignancy demonstrated an increase in cutaneous mast cells, suggesting that the Kit D814V transgenic model could serve as a model for ALL associated with SM. In humans, systemic mastocytosis with associated clonal hematological non-mast cell lineage diseases (SM-AHNMD) is a heterogeneous clinical entity [35,36,37], with a variable presence of *KIT D816V* in the malignant non-mast cell clone. Although ALL associated with SM has been reported only in sporadic cases [38,39], the presence of the *KIT D816V* mutation has been documented in lymphocytes from patients with aggressive type of disease or MCL [5], and previous retroviral and transgenic models have demonstrated that *Kit D814V* has a preferential transforming potential on B cell precursors [40,41].

Deletion of Tet2 did not influence initiation of Kit D814V-driven ALL-like disease in our experiments. This may be explained by the very short latency of the malignant disease in our model. On the other hand, *TET2* mutations have not been reported so far in human B-ALL at diagnosis [42]. However, in our experiments loss of both copies of Tet2 shortened survival of secondary recipients, suggesting that loss of Tet2 plays a role in progression of B-ALL initiated by Kit D814V. It will be interesting to analyze a larger cohort of adult patients with B-ALL (where samples at diagnosis and relapse are available), to examine the role of TET2 in this disease.

DASA has partial efficacy in patients with *KIT D816V* positive SM, and its tolerability profile frequently limits dose escalations in the clinical setting [9]. DAC and 5-azacytidine (5-AZA), which are effective for MDS and AML [43], have been shown as single agents to induce apoptosis in a human *KIT D816V* positive cell line (HMC-1.2) at high doses [44]. Recent evidence from both hematological and solid tumors has demonstrated that treatment of malignant cell lines with low doses of demethylating agents such as DAC and 5-AZA induces stable epigenetic remodeling of the treated cell genomes and induces apoptosis [45,46]. These data suggest that low doses of these epigenetic drugs could be more effective than high doses. We found that low doses of DAC in combination with DASA are effective in inducing apoptosis and cell death in HMC-1.2 cells, and that the two-drug combination is more effective upon TET2 depletion. We also provide data suggesting that the combination of midostaurin (PKC412) and DAC works well *in vitro* on cell lines carrying the Kit activating mutation *D816V* and loss of TET2. As more clinical data become available on the efficacy and toxicity profile of midostaurin as a single agent in the treatment of ASM (10), our data provide an *in vitro* rationale to exploit the cooperation between this TKI and epigenetic modifiers. Additional studies are warranted to explore how TKIs and DAC act in combination and to investigate the effect of DAC on the epigenome of malignant mast cells. We believe that our findings may lead to new approaches to the treatment of patients with ASM harboring both *KIT D816V* and mutations in *TET2*.

Supporting Information

Figure S1 shRNA-mediated knock down of TET2 in HMC-1.2 A) Reduction in the level of TET2 mRNA was quantified using qRT-PCR and normalized to the housekeeping gene GAPDH. RNA was isolated from HMC-1.2 seven days after transduction. TET2 sh-1 and TET2 sh-3 were used for experiments described in the results section. Values are presented as fold change to ctr sh and represent means ±SEM (n = 3). The Ctr sh used for this and all subsequent experiments was the Luciferase G4 construct from Sigma-Aldrich (St. Louis, MO). **B**) Histogram plot demonstrating total 5-hmC content (quantified by intracellular flow staining) in HMC-1.2 cells upon KD of TET2. The grey filled curve represents the secondary Ab control, solid and dotted black lines indicate TET2 sh-1 and sh-3 and the dashed black line represents ctr sh. Shown is one of two independent experiments with similar results. **C**) Number of HMC-1.2 cells migrated in response to hSCF in an *in vitro* transwell migration assay. Bar graph represents average fold change in number of migrated HMC-1.2 transduced with TET2 sh-1 and sh-3 relative to ctr sh (n = 3, error bars represent SEM). No significant difference was observed among experimental groups.

Figure S2 BM immunophenotype and competitive transplants in Mx1-Cre transgenic mice. A) Total number of colonies formed in methylcellulose from $Tet2^{+/+}$;Kit D814V, $Tet2^{+/-}$;Kit D814V and $Tet2^{-/-}$;Kit D814V animal at the initial density (1st round) and after a second and third round of replating. **B**) Peripheral blood chimerism data on recipient animals transplanted with equal doses of whole bone marrow test cells (45.2) and supporting cells (45.1/45.2). Data show a significant repopulation advantage for both $Tet2^{+/+}$;Kit D814V and $Tet2^{+/-}$;Kit D814V at 16 and 20 weeks over competitor cells, with a more pronounced competitive advantage for $Tet2^{+/-}$;Kit D814V 20 weeks after transplantation (*P<.05 $Tet2^{+/+}$;Kit D814V vs. $Tet2^{+/-}$;Kit D814V 45.2 donor derived cells at 20 weeks).

Figure S3 Validation of pI:C-mediated deletion of the Kit D814V flox Stop cassette and the Tet2 targeted allele in Mx1-Cre transgenic animals. A) Schematic view of the target allele in Kit D814V floxed animals. **B**) Schematic view of the target allele in Tet2 floxed animals. **C**) Kit D814V Stop deletion and Tet2 deletion PCR on genomic DNA extracted from BMMCs from induced animals. Position and size of wt, floxed and deleted alleles are shown. Numbers from 1 to 5 indicate the following genotypes: 1)Mx1-Cre, 2)$Tet2^{+/+}$;Kit D814V, 3)$Tet2^{+/-}$;Kit D814V, 4)$Tet2^{+/-}$;Kit D814V, 5)$Tet2^{Fl/WT}$;Kit $D814V^{Fl}$. **D**) Percentage of BMMCs positive for Fcε but negative for c-Kit after 4 weeks in culture with IL-3. Single positive cells were 2.6±1.2 for the $Tet2^{+/+}$;Kit D814V, 11.27±2.1 for the $Tet2^{+/-}$;Kit D814V and 19.57±9.5 for the $Tet^{-/-}$;Kit D814V group.*P<.05. **E**) qRT-PCR analysis of bone-marrow specific transcripts across genotypes. There was no significant difference in the level of carboxypeptidase 3 (Cpa-3), Il-4 and Tnfa mRNA/Gapdh across genotypes. Values are expressed as fold change to $Tet2^{+/+}$;Kit D814V, and they all represent mean ±SEM (n = 3). Ns = not significant.

Figure S4 Characterization of the ALL phenotype in diseased animals. A) Representative H&E staining of peripheral blood smear, liver, spleen and bone marrow sections from a diseased animal. Scale bars represent 25 µm and 200 µm, respectively. **B**) Expression of B220 and CD19 on ALL blasts **C**) mRNA levels of Tet2 normalized to Gapdh mRNA in sorted blasts (data are expressed as fold changes relative to $Tet2^{+/+}$;Kit D814V animals and represent means ± SEM (n = 3–4 animals/genotype)). **D**) Sequence analysis of cDNA from sorted blasts to verify the presence of the Kit D814V mutant allele in diseased animals. Data presented in A, B, D were based on one $Tet2^{+/-}$;Kit D814V animal, but were reproduced in multiple animals across different genotypes.

Figure S5 Knock-down of Tet2 enhances response of HMC-1.2 to midostaurin and decitabine. HMC-1.2 cells were infected with two sh targeting TET2 (sh-1 and sh-3) and a control sh. Transduced cells were treated with decitabine or DMSO for 72 hours, then washed and treated with midostaurin (PKC412). Annexin V staining was performed 24 hours after PKC412 treatment was started. Bar graph indicates percentage of apoptotic (Annexin V^{+}/7 AAD^{-}) and dead cells (Annexin V^{+}/7 AAD^{+}) per treatment condition according to genotype. Pretreatment of cells with decitabine did not significantly increase the percentage of dead and apoptotic cells compared to treatment with PKC412 alone ($P=.07$, $P=.1$ and $P=.3$ for TET2 sh-1, TET2 sh-3 and ctr sh). However, the combination therapy worked significantly better in TET2 KD than in ctr sh cells (**$P<.01$ for TET2 sh-1 vs ctr sh, *$P<.05$ for TET2 sh-3 vs ctr sh). All values represent mean ±SEM (n = 3).

Table S1 Sequence of the short hairpins used to target TET2.

Table S2 Incidence of ALL in primary Mx1-Cre transgenic mice. A cohort of 6–12 mice per genotype was observed for 20 weeks after the last pI:C injection, and the number of mice with ALL was recorded. There was no significant difference in the incidence of ALL across genotypes.

Methods S1 Supporting methods and references.

Acknowledgments

The authors acknowledge the helpful discussions and comments from Dr. Peter M. Gordon and other members of the Williams laboratory, and wish to thank Chad Harris and Meaghan McGuinness for expert animal husbandry and technical support. They also thank the Rodent Histopathology and Specialized Histopathology Services from the Longwood Core of the Dana-Farber/Harvard Cancer Center and the Flow Lab HSCI Core at Boston Children's Hospital, in particular Ronald Mathieu. S.D.V. is grateful to Aron B. Jaffe for critical reading of the manuscript.

Author Contributions

Conceived and designed the experiments: SDV DAW. Performed the experiments: SDV RKS M. Garcia JW M. Gavillet. Analyzed the data: SDV DAW. Contributed reagents/materials/analysis tools: BLE AG AR RLL AM. Wrote the paper: SDV DAW.

References

1. Longley BJ, Tyrrell L, Lu SZ, Ma YS, Langley K, et al. (1996) Somatic c-KIT activating mutation in urticaria pigmentosa and aggressive mastocytosis: establishment of clonality in a human mast cell neoplasm. Nat Genet 12: 312–314.
2. Horny HP, Valent P (2001) Diagnosis of mastocytosis: general histopathological aspects, morphological criteria, and immunohistochemical findings. Leuk Res 25: 543–551.
3. Valent P, Horny HP, Escribano L, Longley BJ, Li CY, et al. (2001) Diagnostic criteria and classification of mastocytosis: a consensus proposal. Leuk Res 25: 603–625.
4. Nagata H, Worobec AS, Oh CK, Chowdhury BA, Tannenbaum S, et al. (1995) Identification of a point mutation in the catalytic domain of the protooncogene c-kit in peripheral blood mononuclear cells of patients who have mastocytosis with an associated hematologic disorder. Proc Natl Acad Sci U S A 92: 10560–10564.
5. Garcia-Montero AC, Jara-Acevedo M, Teodosio C, Sanchez ML, Nunez R, et al. (2006) KIT mutation in mast cells and other bone marrow hematopoietic cell lineages in systemic mast cell disorders: a prospective study of the Spanish Network on Mastocytosis (REMA) in a series of 113 patients. Blood 108: 2366–2372.
6. Ma Y, Zeng S, Metcalfe DD, Akin C, Dimitrijevic S, et al. (2002) The c-KIT mutation causing human mastocytosis is resistant to STI571 and other KIT kinase inhibitors; kinases with enzymatic site mutations show different inhibitor sensitivity profiles than wild-type kinases and those with regulatory-type mutations. Blood 99: 1741–1744.
7. Akin C, Brockow K, D'Ambrosio C, Kirshenbaum AS, Ma Y, et al. (2003) Effects of tyrosine kinase inhibitor STI571 on human mast cells bearing wild-type or mutated c-kit. Exp Hematol 31: 686–692.
8. Shah NP, Lee FY, Luo R, Jiang Y, Donker M, et al. (2006) Dasatinib (BMS-354825) inhibits KITD816V, an imatinib-resistant activating mutation that triggers neoplastic growth in most patients with systemic mastocytosis. Blood 108: 286–291.
9. Verstovsek S, Tefferi A, Cortes J, O'Brien S, Garcia-Manero G, et al. (2008) Phase II study of dasatinib in Philadelphia chromosome-negative acute and chronic myeloid diseases, including systemic mastocytosis. Clin Cancer Res 14: 3906–3915.
10. Gotlib J, Kluin-Nelemans HC, George TI, Akin C, Sotlar K, et alKIT Inhibitor Midostaurin in Patients with Advanced Systemic Mastocytosis: Results of a Planned Interim Analysis of the Global CPKC412D2201 Trial. Blood (Annual Meeting Abstracts). November 2012 (120: 799.).
11. Tefferi A, Levine RL, Lim KH, Abdel-Wahab O, Lasho TL, et al. (2009) Frequent TET2 mutations in systemic mastocytosis: clinical, KITD816V and FIP1L1-PDGFRA correlates. Leukemia 23: 900–904.
12. Traina F, Visconte V, Jankowska AM, Makishima H, O'Keefe CL, et al. (2012) Single nucleotide polymorphism array lesions, TET2, DNMT3A, ASXL1 and CBL mutations are present in systemic mastocytosis. PLoS One 7: e43090.
13. Wilson TM, Maric I, Simakova O, Bai Y, Chan EC, et al. (2011) Clonal analysis of NRAS activating mutations in KIT-D816V systemic mastocytosis. Haematologica 96: 459–463.
14. Ito S, Shen L, Dai Q, Wu SC, Collins LB, et al. (2011) Tet proteins can convert 5-methylcytosine to 5-formylcytosine and 5-carboxylcytosine. Science 333: 1300–1303.
15. He YF, Li BZ, Li Z, Liu P, Wang Y, et al. (2011) Tet-mediated formation of 5-carboxylcytosine and its excision by TDG in mammalian DNA. Science 333: 1303–1307.
16. Delhommeau F, Dupont S, Della Valle V, James C, Trannoy S, et al. (2009) Mutation in TET2 in myeloid cancers. N Engl J Med 360: 2289–2301.
17. Tefferi A, Pardanani A, Lim KH, Abdel-Wahab O, Lasho TL, et al. (2009) TET2 mutations and their clinical correlates in polycythemia vera, essential thrombocythemia and myelofibrosis. Leukemia 23: 905–911.
18. Langemeijer SM, Kuiper RP, Berends M, Knops R, Aslanyan MG, et al. (2009) Acquired mutations in TET2 are common in myelodysplastic syndromes. Nat Genet 41: 838–842.
19. Moran-Crusio K, Reavie L, Shih A, Abdel-Wahab O, Ndiaye-Lobry D, et al. (2011) Tet2 loss leads to increased hematopoietic stem cell self-renewal and myeloid transformation. Cancer Cell 20: 11–24.
20. Quivoron C, Couronne L, Della Valle V, Lopez CK, Plo I, et al. (2011) TET2 inactivation results in pleiotropic hematopoietic abnormalities in mouse and is a recurrent event during human lymphomagenesis. Cancer Cell 20: 25–38.
21. Li Z, Cai X, Cai CL, Wang J, Zhang W, et al. (2011) Deletion of Tet2 in mice leads to dysregulated hematopoietic stem cells and subsequent development of myeloid malignancies. Blood 118: 4509–4518.
22. Soucie E, Hanssens K, Mercher T, Georgin-Lavialle S, Damaj G, et al. (2012) In aggressive forms of mastocytosis, TET2 loss cooperates with c-KITD816V to transform mast cells. Blood 120: 4846–4849.
23. Gerbaulet A, Wickenhauser C, Scholten J, Peschke K, Drube S, et al. (2011) Mast cell hyperplasia, B-cell malignancy, and intestinal inflammation in mice with conditional expression of a constitutively active kit. Blood 117: 2012–2021.
24. Kuhn R, Schwenk F, Aguet M, Rajewsky K (1995) Inducible gene targeting in mice. Science 269: 1427–1429.
25. Scholten J, Hartmann K, Gerbaulet A, Krieg T, Muller W, et al. (2008) Mast cell-specific Cre/loxP-mediated recombination in vivo. Transgenic Res 17: 307–315.
26. Butterfield JH, Marcoux JP, Weiler D, Harner SG (1988) Mast cell pharyngitis as a cause of supraglottic edema. Arch Otorhinolaryngol 245: 88–91.
27. Aichberger KJ, Gleixner KV, Mirkina I, Cerny-Reiterer S, Peter B, et al. (2009) Identification of proapoptotic Bim as a tumor suppressor in neoplastic mast cells: role of KIT D816V and effects of various targeted drugs. Blood 114: 5342–5351.
28. Yavuz AS, Lipsky PE, Yavuz S, Metcalfe DD, Akin C (2002) Evidence for the involvement of a hematopoietic progenitor cell in systemic mastocytosis from single-cell analysis of mutations in the c-kit gene. Blood 100: 661–665.
29. Chen CC, Grimbaldeston MA, Tsai M, Weissman IL, Galli SJ (2005) Identification of mast cell progenitors in adult mice. Proc Natl Acad Sci U S A 102: 11408–11413.
30. Arinobu Y, Iwasaki H, Gurish MF, Mizuno S, Shigematsu H, et al. (2005) Developmental checkpoints of the basophil/mast cell lineages in adult murine hematopoiesis. Proc Natl Acad Sci U S A 102: 18105–18110.
31. Ihle JN, Keller J, Oroszlan S, Henderson LE, Copeland TD, et al. (1983) Biologic properties of homogeneous interleukin 3. I. Demonstration of WEHI-3 growth factor activity, mast cell growth factor activity, p cell-stimulating factor activity, colony-stimulating factor activity, and histamine-producing cell-stimulating factor activity. J Immunol 131: 282–287.
32. Razin E, Ihle JN, Seldin D, Mencia-Huerta JM, Katz HR, et al. (1984) Interleukin 3: A differentiation and growth factor for the mouse mast cell that contains chondroitin sulfate E proteoglycan. J Immunol 132: 1479–1486.

33. Schittenhelm MM, Shiraga S, Schroeder A, Corbin AS, Griffith D, et al. (2006) Dasatinib (BMS-354825), a dual SRC/ABL kinase inhibitor, inhibits the kinase activity of wild-type, juxtamembrane, and activation loop mutant KIT isoforms associated with human malignancies. Cancer Res 66: 473–481.
34. Figueroa ME, Abdel-Wahab O, Lu C, Ward PS, Patel J, et al. (2010) Leukemic IDH1 and IDH2 mutations result in a hypermethylation phenotype, disrupt TET2 function, and impair hematopoietic differentiation. Cancer Cell 18: 553–567.
35. Travis WD, Li CY, Yam LT, Bergstralh EJ, Swee RG (1988) Significance of systemic mast cell disease with associated hematologic disorders. Cancer 62: 965–972.
36. Pardanani A, Lim KH, Lasho TL, Finke C, McClure RF, et al. (2009) Prognostically relevant breakdown of 123 patients with systemic mastocytosis associated with other myeloid malignancies. Blood 114: 3769–3772.
37. Horny HP, Sotlar K, Sperr WR, Valent P (2004) Systemic mastocytosis with associated clonal haematological non-mast cell lineage diseases: a histopathological challenge. J Clin Pathol 57: 604–608.
38. Masserot C, Adjaoud D, Haouy S, Deswarte C, Ballerini P, et al. (2008) Acute lymphoblastic leukemia and cutaneous mastocytosis in two children. Pediatr Blood Cancer 51: 444–445.
39. Lewis HM, Winter E, Darbyshire P, Yoong A, Marsden JR, et al. (1995) Urticaria pigmentosa and acute lymphoblastic leukaemia. J R Soc Med 88: 530P–531P.
40. Kitayama H, Tsujimura T, Matsumura I, Oritani K, Ikeda H, et al. (1996) Neoplastic transformation of normal hematopoietic cells by constitutively activating mutations of c-kit receptor tyrosine kinase. Blood 88: 995–1004.
41. Xiang Z, Kreisel F, Cain J, Colson A, Tomasson MH (2007) Neoplasia driven by mutant c-KIT is mediated by intracellular, not plasma membrane, receptor signaling. Mol Cell Biol 27: 267–282.
42. Langemeijer SM, Jansen JH, Hooijer J, van Hoogen P, Stevens-Linders E, et al. (2011) TET2 mutations in childhood leukemia. Leukemia 25: 189–192.
43. Estey EH (2013) Epigenetics in clinical practice: the examples of azacitidine and decitabine in myelodysplasia and acute myeloid leukemia. Leukemia.
44. Ghanim V, Herrmann H, Heller G, Peter B, Hadzijusufovic E, et al. (2012) 5-azacytidine and decitabine exert proapoptotic effects on neoplastic mast cells: role of FAS-demethylation and FAS re-expression, and synergism with FAS-ligand. Blood 119: 4242–4252.
45. Tsai HC, Li H, Van Neste L, Cai Y, Robert C, et al. (2012) Transient low doses of DNA-demethylating agents exert durable antitumor effects on hematological and epithelial tumor cells. Cancer Cell 21: 430–446.
46. Klco JM, Spencer DH, Lamprecht TL, Sarkaria SM, Wylie T, et al. (2013) Genomic impact of transient low-dose decitabine treatment on primary AML cells. Blood 121: 1633–1643.

14

Serum Thymidine Kinase Activity: Analytical Performance, Age-Related Reference Ranges and Validation in Chronic Lymphocytic Leukemia

Eszter Szánthó, Harjit Pal Bhattoa, Mária Csobán, Péter Antal-Szalmás, Anikó Újfalusi, János Kappelmayer, Zsuzsanna Hevessy*

Department of Laboratory Medicine, Medical and Health Science Center, University of Debrecen, Debrecen, Hungary

Abstract

Background: To date no age-related reference ranges are available for serum thymidine kinase (TK1) activity. Being a proliferation marker, it may be used as a prognostic marker in malignant diseases, including chronic lymphocytic leukemia (CLL). Our aim was to establish age-specific reference ranges for TK1 and examine its utility as a screening marker in CLL, a disease of the elderly.

Methods: Serum TK1 activity was measured by a competitive chemiluminescent immunoassay in 369 healthy adults and 115 de novo CLL patients.

Results: We observed a statistically significant decline in TK1 activity from young (18–35 years) to middle-aged (36–60 years) and further on to elderly (60–86 years) healthy individuals. Age-related reference range was: <30 U/L for young, <25 U/L for middle-aged and <19 U/L for elderly. There was no difference in TK1 activity between the studied healthy men and women. In CLL patients, TK1 activity was the highest in the advanced Rai stages. The area under the receiver operating characteristic curve (ROC-AUC) for TK1 was 0.840 (95% CI: 0.787–0.892), for differentiating CLL patients from age and sex matched healthy controls, with a cut-off value of 10.5 U/L (sensitivity: 80.9%, specificity: 73.4%). TK1 was significantly elevated in CD38+/Zap70+ CLL patients, and showed significant correlation with WBC and absolute B-cell count.

Conclusion: In the healthy, serum TK1 activity does not differ in the two sexes but declines significantly with age. As such, use of age-related reference ranges is warranted, especially when evaluating CLL patients who generally belong to the elderly age group.

Editor: Ferenc Gallyas Jr., University of Pecs Medical School, Hungary

Funding: The work is supported by the TÁMOP-4.2.2.A-11/1/KONV-2012-0025 project. The project is co-financed by the European Union and the European Social Fund. This work is supported by the OTKA 105073 research grant (HPB) and by the National Office for Research and Technology (presently National Development Agency) of Hungary (TECH-09-A1-2009-0113; mAB-CHIC) (PAS). The funders had no role in study design, data collection and analysis, decision to publish, or preparation of the manuscript.

Competing Interests: The authors have declared that no competing interests exist.

* E-mail: hevessy@med.unideb.hu

These authors contributed equally to this work.

Introduction

Distinguishing from a few tumor specific biomarkers (PSA, AFP, HCG etc) [1–3], thymidine kinase 1 (TK1, ATP; thymidine 5′-phosphotransferase; EC.2.7.1.21) is one of the non-specific tumor markers that can be measured in continuously dividing cells [4]. TK1 is a key cellular enzyme in the so-called salvage pathway of DNA synthesis. It phosphorylates thymidine into thymidine-monophosphate. The enzyme has two isoforms, TK1 is found in the cytoplasm, while TK2 remains in the mitochondria. The activity of TK1 is cell cycle-dependent, its level begins to rise in G1/S phase and reaches its peak in the G2/M phase [5–9].

TK1 can be isolated from many different cell and tissue types, and elevated serum TK1 activity is documented in many types of cancer, nonetheless, the mechanism of TK entering the systemic circulation is not well understood [10–13]. Furthermore, TK has been reported as a prognostic marker in chronic lymphocytic leukemia (CLL) and in non-Hodgkin's lymphoma [14–17]. In the last decade several studies showed the prognostic value of CD38 and Zap70 expression in CLL [18–22]. Elevated serum TK1 level was found in patients with unmutated IGHV gene, and in those with higher expression levels of Zap70 and CD38, as well as advanced disease stage [23–24]. Konoplev et al showed that high serum TK1 levels predict poorer overall survival and higher risk of developing large B-cell lymphoma (Richter syndrome) [16]. The first TK measurement method was a radio-enzymatic assay using ^{125}I-deoxyuridine [25]; later a non-radiometric, competitive, enzyme-linked, immunosorbent assay (ELISA) was developed [26]. Wu et al developed a method for measuring not the activity but the concentration of TK in serum [27]. Most recently, a liquid chromatography – tandem mass spectrometry method was described by Faria et al [28]. Nisman et al compared two commercially available immunoassays in breast cancer patients, and despite reporting differences between the two assays, concluded that both assays were adequate for tumor recurrence prediction [29].

Hallek et al found that a serum TK level of 7.1 U/L was the cutoff value that could differentiate shorter (high TK levels) and longer (low TK levels) progression-free survival subgroups in Binet A stage disease [15]. In the French-German CLL7 trial, one of the adverse risk factors to identify high-risk Binet A patients was a serum TK level >10 U/L [30,34]. Magnac et al examined the relationship between serum TK levels and IGHV mutational status and found that TK levels above 15 U/L correlated well with the IGHV unmutated status of the patients [31]. A thorough review on prognostic markers of CLL was published by Sagatys & Zhang in 2012, encouraging the establishment of a universal algorithm to improve prognostic accuracy [32]. Molica et al carried out a comparative validation analysis of the MD Anderson Cancer Center (MDACC) [33] and the modified German [34] CLL score. They found that for any novel prognostic scheme, these two scores should be the benchmark for comparison [35]. In a recent paper, Molica suggested building an international, comprehensive CLL prognostic index [36].

The primary aim of this study was to establish age-related reference ranges for serum TK. Our hypothesis was that healthy older individuals might have lower TK activity as compared to younger adults. In addition, in a cross-sectional, case-control study, we measured serum TK activity in *de novo* CLL patients who were still therapy naïve, and in an equal number of age- and sex-matched healthy volunteers. Knowing that CLL is a disease prevalent in the elderly, the utility of the age-specific reference range was examined in the studied CLL cohort.

In the CLL patients, we compared the serum TK activity with other laboratory parameters, such as white blood cell count, absolute B cell count, CD38 and Zap70 expression.

Patients and Methods

Study population, healthy cohort for establishing reference ranges

Healthy volunteers (n = 369) between 18 and 86 years of age (median: 45 years, men: 157, women: 212) were recruited from blood donors and staff of the faculty with values ≤2× upper limit of normal for all measured laboratory parameters. Exclusion criteria were cancer, metabolic and inflammatory diseases. Due to non-confirmation with selection criteria data from 24 individuals was excluded from the final statistical analysis. To examine the influence of age, the reference population was subgrouped into the following age groups: 18–35 years (young), 35–60 years (middle-aged) and 60–86 years (elderly) (Figure 1).

Study population, CLL cohort

Patients presenting with *de novo* CLL between December, 2010 and November, 2012 were included in this cross-sectional, analyst-blinded, age and sex matched case-control study (n = 115). The mean age (range) of the individuals in both groups was 65.6 (46–86) years, and the male:female ratio was ~ 1:1 (61:54). As per Rai staging, 43 were in stage Rai 0, 27 were in Rai 1, 19 were in Rai 2, 15 were in Rai 3 and 11 were in Rai 4 (Figure 1). In this cohort, 29 and 86 patients belonged to the middle-aged and elderly age-groups, respectively.

This study was approved by the Ethics Committee of the University of Debrecen in accordance with the Declaration of Helsinki. All participants gave written informed consents.

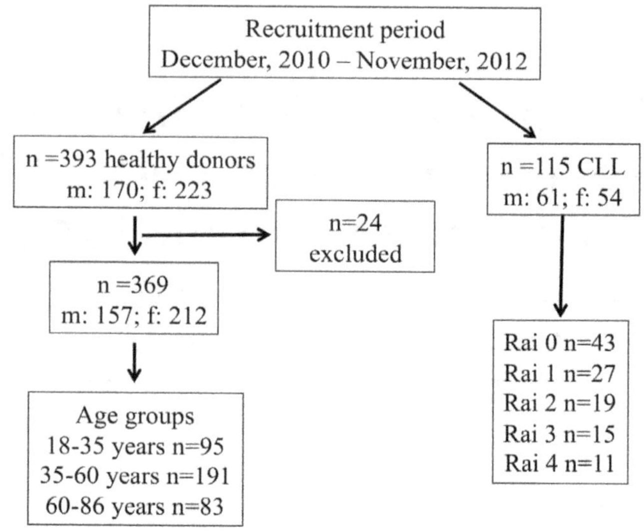

Figure 1. Flow diagram of study population.

Laboratory methods

Measurement of thymidine kinase activity. TK1 activity was measured by an indirect, modified, two-step competitive chemiluminescent immunoassay on a Liaison immunochemistry analyzer (DiaSorin S.p.A., Saluggia, Italy). The calibration curve is defined mathematically by the manufacturer (master curve), which includes the pathologic values as well. For quality control the reagent kit includes two QC samples (low and high). In order to evaluate assay performance, accuracy and precision were determined from QC samples in low and high range (QC1 and QC2, respectively). Precision was expressed in CV% and accuracy was assessed as percent deviation from the nominal activity. Intra-assay precision and accuracy were determined from 9 replicates of each QC sample on a single occasion while inter-assay precision and accuracy were determined by analyzing 18 different operating days. The results were analyzed as a linear regression of the nominal vs. observed values. Linearity was evaluated by serial dilution of a patient sample with markedly elevated TK activity.

Determination of CD38 and Zap70 positivity of CLL cells by flow cytometry

White blood cell counts were measured by an Advia 120 hematology analyzer (Siemens AG, Erlangen, Germany). Absolute B-cell count was calculated from the percentage of CD19+ cells and white blood cell count.

Flow cytometric measurements were carried out on FACS-Canto II flow cytometer, the results were evaluated by FACSDiva software (BD Biosciences, San José, CA, USA). The antibodies used were: CD19-PE-Cy7 (clone: J3-119, Beckman-Coulter, Brea, CA, USA); CD38-APC (clone: HB7, BD Biosciences) and Zap70 (unlabeled, clone: 2F3.2, Merck-Millipore (Upstate), Billerica, MA, USA). The patient was considered CD38 and/or Zap70 positive if ≥20% of the CLL cells expressed the respective markers.

Fluorescence *in situ* hybridization (FISH). Interphase fluorescence *in situ* hybridization (FISH) was performed on cell suspension originated from peripheral blood according to standard protocol. Cells were obtained by 72 hour culture in the presence of 12-O-tetradecanoylphorbol-13-acetate (TPA) (Sigma-Aldrich, Munich, Germany) or by direct preparation from uncultured peripheral blood. The probes used for FISH analysis included LSI Rb1(13q14)/13q34, LSI p53, LSI ATM (Abbott Molecular Inc, Des Plaines, USA). Cells were counterstained with DAPI

(4,6-diamidino-2-phenylindole). At least 200 interphase cells were analysed for each probe in each case. The images were captured by Zeiss Axioplan2 (Carl Zeiss, Zaventem, Brussels) fluorescence microscope and analysed by ISIS software (MetaSystems, Altlussheim, Germany).

Statistical Analyses

Kolmogorov-Smirnov test was used for the evaluation of the normality of the data. Most parameters were non-normally distributed; therefore analyses were performed by Mann-Whitney U test. The Spearman's rho was calculated for correlation analysis. P<0.05 was regarded as statistically significant. All analyses, including drawing of receiver operating characteristic (ROC) curves and estimation of the area under the ROC curve (AUC), were performed using the SPSS Statistics software, version 19.0 (IBM Corps., Armonk, NY, USA).

Results

Reproducibility and accuracy tests gave excellent results. The nominal mean TK1 activity of QC1 was 14.8 U/L. Intra-assay measured mean was 15.0±1.58 U/L, precision CV of QC1 was 10.54%, accuracy was 101%. Inter-assay measured mean of QC1 was 14.8±2.23 U/L, precision CV was 15.03% and accuracy was 100%. The nominal mean activity of QC2 was 53.7 U/L, intra-assay measured mean was 62.4±6.34 U/L, precision CV was 10.16% and accuracy was 116%. Inter-assay measured mean of QC2 was 49.15±6.27 U/L, precision CV was 12.76% and accuracy was 92% (Table 1). The test was linear from 0.5 U/L to 100 U/L.

In the healthy cohort, there was no significant difference in TK1 activity between the men and women studied, as such gender was not taken into consideration when defining age groups. TK1 activities of 3 age groups are shown on Figure 2A-C. There was a significant difference between the TK1 activity of the young (n = 95) and the elderly (n = 83), (11.85±5.7 U/L vs. 8.65±3.9 U/L; p<0.001) and between the young and the middle-aged (n = 191) (11.85±5.7 U/L vs. 9.79±5.2 U/L; p<0.001). The difference was at the limit of statistical significance between the middle-aged and the elderly (9.79±5.2 U/L vs. 8.65±3.9 U/L; p = 0.050). Overall, the lowest observed TK1 level was 0.5 U/L and the highest was 35.6 U/L. The 97.5 percentiles in the 3 age groups were 29.8 U/L (young), 25.4 U/L (middle-aged) and 19 U/L (elderly) (Figure 2D).

Table 1. Inter-assay and Intra-assay precision and accuracy for serum thymidine kinase activity of QC1 and QC2 samples.

	Nominal concentration (U/L)	
	14.8 (QC1)	53.7 (QC2)
Observed concentration (U/L)		
Intra-assay mean ± SD	15.0±1.58	62.4±6.34
Intra-assay precision (%CV)	10.54	10.16
Intra-assay accuracy (%DFN)	1.35	16
Inter-assay mean ± SD	14.8±2.23	49.15±6.27
Inter-assay precision (%CV)	15.03	12.76
Inter-assay accuracy (%DFN)	0	-8.5

SD, standard deviation; %CV, percent coefficient of variation; %DFN, percent deviation from nominal value.

Results of 115 CLL patients on presentation were compared with an equal number of age- and sex-matched controls (n = 115). This age- and sex-matched control group was derived from the over-all healthy cohort (n = 393), that was used to define the reference ranges of TK1 in the different age groups. Patient characteristics are given in Table 2. We found significant difference in TK1 activity between the healthy control group and all Rai stages of CLL. As we had few individuals in Rai 2, Rai 3 and Rai 4 stages, we grouped them as being in a more advanced stage of the disease. The observed mean TK1 activity in the age and sex matched healthy group (n = 115) was 9.18±5.0 U/L, which was significantly lower than that in Rai 0 (n = 43; mean: 18.58±15.6 U/L; p<0.001), Rai 1 (n = 27; mean: 28.16±32.9 U/L; p<0.001) and Rai 2-3-4 (n = 45; mean: 72.88±101.1 U/L; p<0.001). We also noticed significant difference in TK1 activity between Rai 0 and Rai 2-3-4 stages (p<0.001) and Rai 1 and Rai 2-3-4 stages (p = 0.002) (Figure 3).

CLL patients were on average 65.6 years old (range: 46–86). There was no difference in TK1 levels upon comparing those below and equal to 60 years (middle aged, n = 29) and those over 60 years (elderly, n = 86) of age belonging to the different Rai stages (Table 3).

The area under the receiver operating characteristic curve (ROC-AUC) for TK1 was 0.840 (95% CI: 0.787–0.892) for differentiating CLL patients from age and sex matched healthy controls, with a cut-off value of 10.5 U/L (sensitivity: 80.9%, specificity: 73.4%) (Figure 4A.). Furthermore, at the same cut-off value, the ROC-AUC for TK1 was 0.760 (95% CI: 0.671–0.849) for differentiating Rai 0 stage CLL patients from healthy controls (sensitivity: 73.9%, specificity: 72.1%) (Figure 4B.).

We also compared the TK1 results of the CLL patients with other known prognostic factors, i.e., CD38 and Zap70 expression. The mean TK1 activity in the CD38–/Zap70– group (n = 52) was significantly lower than that in the CD38+/Zap70+ group (n = 31) (22.3±17.8 U/L vs. 109±130.3 U/L; p<0.001). The difference was also significant between the CD38–/Zap70+ group (n = 17) and the CD38+/Zap70+ group (26.25±33 U/L vs. 109±130.3 U/L; p = 0.002); and between the CD38+/Zap70– group (n = 15) and the CD38–/Zap70– group (40.87±38 U/L vs. 22.3±17.8 U/L; p = 0.022); and the CD38–/Zap70+ group and the CD38+/Zap70– group (26.25±33 U/L vs. 40.87±38 U/L; p = 0.021) (Figure 5.).

With ROC analysis, the TK1 cut-off value to distinguish CD38–/Zap70– patients from those with either or both positivity was 30 U/L (ROC-AUC: 0.710, 95%CI: 0.601–0.819, Specificity:76.6%, Sensitivity: 54.3%).

Out of 115 CLL patients, 95 had FISH data. Upon comparing those with no chromosomal alterations, del(13q), 12 trisomy (n = 76) with the group with del(17p13), del(11q22) (n = 19) no statistically significant difference was found in the TK1 values (38.7±65.7 U/L vs. 55.5±96.5 U/L, p = 0.347). The non-significance did not change when patients with 12 trisomy were excluded from the statistical analysis (33.0±44.5 vs. 55.5±96.5, p = 0.211).

We observed a statistically significant correlation between TK1 activity and WBC (Spearman's rho: 0.367, p<0.001) and absolute B cell count (Spearman's rho: 0.369, p<0.001).

Discussion

According to the 2008 guideline of the Clinical Laboratory Standards Institute, it may be necessary to carry out a minor reference value study to validate a reference interval given by the test manufacturer or a donor laboratory [37]. Soon after we

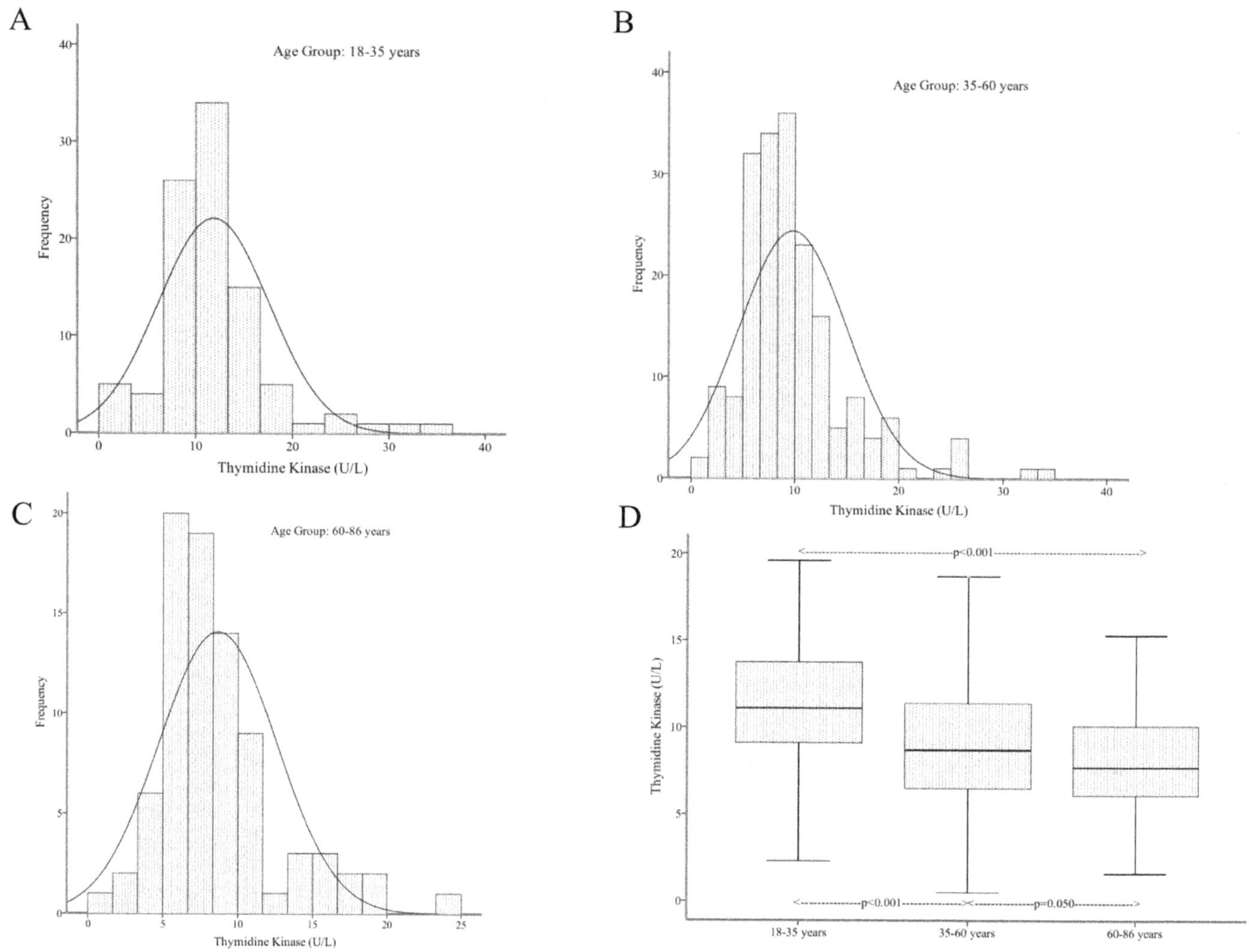

Figure 2. Age-related frequency distributions of serum thymidine kinase activity in age groups 18–35 years (A), 35–60 years (B) and 60–86 years (C). Box and whisker plots showing significant difference of serum TK activity in the studied age groups (D).

Table 2. CLL patient characteristics.

	CLL patients (n = 115)
Age, years (mean, range)	65.6 (46–86)
Males (n, %)	61 (53)
Females (n, %)	54 (47)
Rai 0 (n, %)	43 (37)
Rai 1 (n, %)	27 (23)
Rai 2 (n, %)	19 (17)
Rai 3 (n, %)	15 (13)
Rai 4 (n, %)	11 (10)
CD38–/Zap70– (n, %)	52 (45)
CD38–/Zap70+ (n,%)	17 (15)
CD38+/Zap70– (n, %)	15 (13)
CD38+/Zap70+ (n, %)	31 (27)
White blood cell count, G/L (mean, range)	50.6 (12.4–447)
Absolute B cell count, G/L (mean, range)	39.9 (5.2–392)

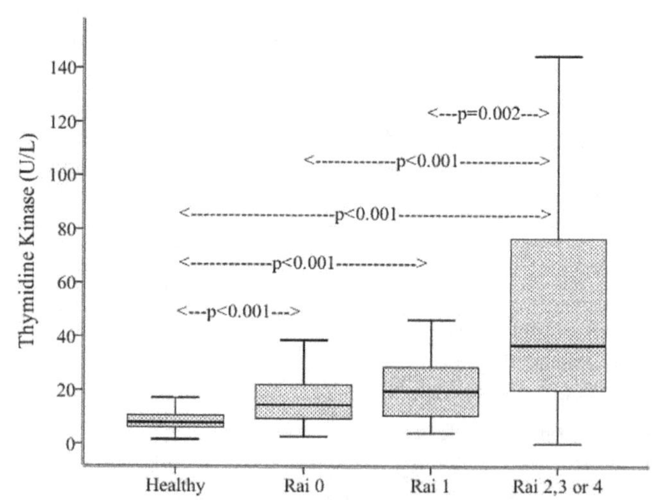

Figure 3. Comparison of serum thymidine kinase activity in de novo CLL patients in Rai 0, Rai 1 and Rai 2-3-4 clinical stages with the age and sex matched healthy cohort.

Table 3. Comparison of thymidine kinase activity between middle-aged and elderly CLL patients belonging to different Rai stages.

Rai stages	Age		p values
	46–60 years	60.1–86 years	
	Thymidine kinase activity, mean ± SD (U/L)		
Rai 0 (n = 43)	15.5±8.9 (n = 15)	20.2±18.2 (n = 28)	0.558
Rai 1 (n = 27)	59.7±67.7 (n = 5)	21.0±13.3 (n = 22)	0.524
Rai 2, 3 or 4 (n = 45)	89.0±151.6 (n = 9)	68.8±86.7 (n = 36)	0.645

started our TK1 measurements with the test manufacturer's reference range (2 – 7.5 U/L) it turned out that it was not applicable to our population, as we often observed higher TK1 activity than the suggested upper reference limit even in healthy individuals. The interpretation of these results was not always convincing and caused some unnecessary anxiety for physicians and patients. The observed elevated TK1 activity in our healthy population and the significant differences in TK1 activity between the age groups encouraged us to define our own reference ranges for TK1. Although TK1 measurements are widely used in malignant diseases for prognostic purposes and even in routine health screening [38], to our knowledge no age-related reference ranges have been published so far for TK1 activity.

In each age group we had sufficient numbers of reference subjects to determine the 97.5 percentiles. Based on our 97.5 percentile results, the suggested reference values are <30 U/L for young (18–35 years), <25 U/L for middle-aged (36–60 years) and <19 U/L for elderly (60–86 years) adults. The age-specific reference ranges may be crucial in the context of chronic lymphocytic leukemia, where most of the affected are older individuals. We also identified a cutoff point of 10.5 U/L distinguishing CLL patients in the RAI 0 stage from healthy individuals. This result correlates well with the finding of Letestu et al, who found a serum TK1 activity of 10 U/L to be an independent predictor of progression-free survival with a hazard ratio of 2.98, p<0.0001 [39].

As TK1 is a general proliferation marker, several non-malignant conditions like infection, inflammation, autoimmune disorders and benign tissue proliferations might also cause mildly elevated TK1 levels [40]. Hagberg et al showed that severe vitamin B12 deficiency caused elevated serum TK1 levels, as the proliferating tissues became unstable in the absence of the vitamin [41]. Chen et al also showed that serum TK1 concentration was useful in health screening as their patients with elevated TK1 concentration had a significantly increased risk of developing malignancies [42]. The above study also showed that a significantly larger proportion of oilfield workers had elevated serum TK1 concentrations than city dwellers [42]. As such, in routine medical practice, non-malignant medical conditions and environmental factors need to be considered when using TK1 as a health screening marker.

It is also known that CD38+ CLL has a more adverse prognosis [43]. Hus et al showed that CD38 combined with Zap70 expression amplified the prognostic power of both markers. They found that Zap70+/CD38+ patients had shorter event-free survival than CD38–/Zap70– patients [44]. In our study, we found significantly higher TK1 activity in CD38+/Zap70+ as compared to CD38–/Zap70– patients and there was no significant difference between CD38–/Zap70– and CD38–/Zap70+ patients. Higher serum TK1 activities of CD38+ CLL patients can be

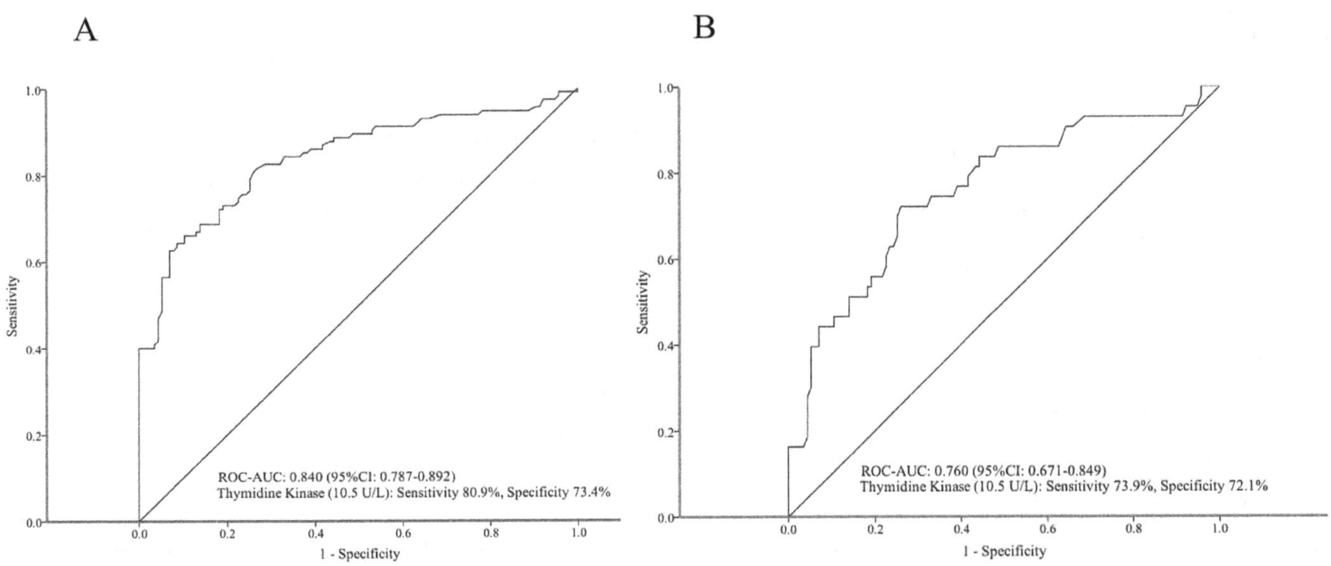

Figure 4. Receiver operating characteristic (ROC) analysis of serum thymidine kinase activity for differentiating all CLL patients (A) and Rai 0 CLL patients (B) from age and sex matched healthy controls. AUC, area under the receiver operating characteristic curve.

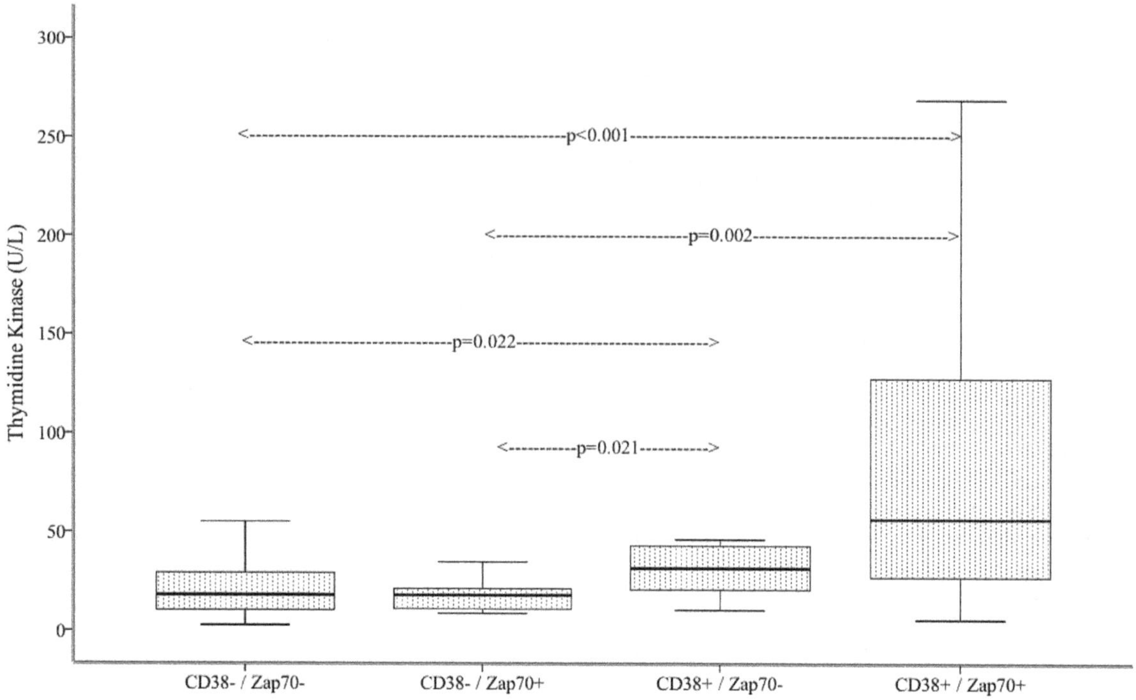

Figure 5. Serum thymidine kinase activity of CLL patients upon presentation in different prognostic groups.

explained by the intense proliferation of cells, as both TK1 and CD38 are proliferation markers [45,35].

Furthermore, in line with published data, del(13q), 12 trisomy, del(17p13) and del(11q22) FISH aberrations did not influence TK1 values in our patients [16].

TK1 activity correlated with WBC and absolute B cell count in our study, this finding supports the data reported previously by Hallek et al [15].

Each laboratory should establish its own age-related reference ranges as even minor ethnical or lifestyle differences in a particular region may have a significant impact on reference ranges, not disregarding the influence of age and sex. These differences make it difficult to obtain universally applicable reference intervals, even though the applied methodology is traceable to reference measurement systems [46,47]. As producing reference ranges is an expensive task for an individual laboratory, one possible solution is to establish reference ranges for a homogeneous population by involving all the laboratories measuring the certain analyte with the same method [47]. Siest et al emphasized that the boundaries between healthy and pathological conditions are not clear-cut, and reference intervals or cut-off values should be established to expedite clinical decision making [48].

Limitations of the present results include the cross-sectional nature of the CLL study, a prospective design would have enabled us to examine the utility of TK1 as a prognostic marker. Although the CLL population was represented by a cohort of 115 de novo patients, the non-similar number of patients in the different Rai stages, and as per their CD38 and Zap70 characteristics may have distorted the statistical findings. Furthermore, our age-specific reference ranges need to be validated in other healthy populations as well.

In conclusion, serum TK1 levels decline significantly with age in the healthy, and this finding warrants the use of age-related reference ranges. Furthermore, it may distinguish CLL patients in the RAI 0 stage from healthy individuals in the diagnostic work-up of CLL suspect cases.

Author Contributions

Conceived and designed the experiments: ES HPB JK ZH. Performed the experiments: ES PAS MC AU. Analyzed the data: HPB ZH. Contributed reagents/materials/analysis tools: JK MC AU. Wrote the paper: ES HPB ZH.

References

1. O'Neill KL, Buckwalter MR, Murray BK (2001) Thymidine kinase: diagnostic and prognostic potential. Expert Rev Mol Diagn 1: 428–433.
2. Stenman UH, Leinonen J, Zhang WM, Finne P (1999) Prostate-specific antigen. Semin Cancer Biol 9: 83–93.
3. Houstek J, Masopust J, Kithier K, Rádl J (1968) Hepatocellular carcinoma in association with a specific fetal alpha-1-globulin, fetoprotein. J Pediatr 72: 186–193.
4. Vaitukaitis JL (1974) Human chorionic gonadotropin as a tumor marker. Ann Clin Lab Sci 4(4): 276–280.
5. Reichard P, Estborn B (1951) Utilization of deoxyribosides in the synthesis of polynucleotides. J Biol Chem 188: 839–846.
6. Kornberg A, Lehman IR, Bessman MJ, Simms ES (1989) Enzymic synthesis of deoxyribonucleic acid. 1956. Biochim Biophys Acta 1000: 57–8.
7. Weissman SM, Smellie RM, Paul J (1960) Studies on the biosynthesis of deoxyribonucleic acid by extracts of mammalian cells IV. The phosphorylation of thymidine. Biochim Biophys Acta 45: 101–110
8. Berk AJ, Clayton DA (1973) A genetically distinct thymidine kinase in mammalian mitochondria. Exclusive labeling of mitochondrial deoxyribonucleid acid. J Biol Chem 248: 2722–2729
9. Sherley JL, Kelly TJ (1988) Regulation of human thymidine kinase during the cell cycle. J Biol Chem 263: 8350–8358.
10. Hallek M, Wanders L, Strohmeyer S, Emmerich B (1992) Thymidine kinase: a tumor marker with prognostic value for non-Hodgkin's lymphoma and a broad range for potential clinical applications. Ann Hematol 65: 1–5.

11. Thomas WM, Robertson JF, McKenna PG, O'Neill KL, Robinson MH, et al. (1995) Serum thymidine kinase in colorectal neoplasia. Eur J Surg Oncol 21: 632–634.
12. Foekens JA, Romain S, Look MP, Martin PM, Klijn JG (2001) Thymidine kinase and thymidilate synthase in advanced breast cancer: response to tamoxifen and chemotherapy. Cancer Res 61: 1421–1425.
13. Fujiwaki R, Hata K, Moriyama M, Iwanari O, Katabuchi H, et al. (2001) Clinical value of thymidine kinase in patients with cervical carcinoma. Oncology 61: 47–51.
14. Källander CFR, Simonsson B, Hagberg H, Gronowitz JS (1984) Serum deoxythymidine kinase gives prognostic information in chronic lymphocytic leukemia. Cancer 54: 2450–5.
15. Hallek M, Langenmayer I, Nerl C, Knauf W, Dietzfelbinger H, et al. (1999) Elevated serum thymidine kinase levels identify a subgroup at high risk of disease progression in early, nonsmoldering chronic lymphocytic leukemia. Blood 93: 1732–1737.
16. Konoplev SN, Fritsche HA, O'Brien S, Wierda WG, Keating MJ, et al. (2010) High serum thymidine kinase 1 level predicts poorer survival in patients with chronic lymphocytic leukemia. Am J Clin Pathol 134: 472–477.
17. Gronowitz JS, Hagberg H, Källander CFR, Simonsson B (1983) The use of serum deoxythymidine kinase as a prognostic marker, and in the monitoring of patients with non-Hodgkin's lymphoma. Br J Cancer 47: 487–495.
18. Damle RN, Ghiotto F, Valetto A, Albesiano E, Fais F et al. (2002) B-cell chronic lymphocytic leukemia cells express a surface membrane phenotype of activated, antigen-experienced B lymphocytes. Blood 99: 4087–4093.
19. Damle RN, Wasil T, Fais F, Ghiotto F, Valetto A, Allen SL, et al. (1999) Ig V gene mutation status and CD38 expression as novel prognostic indicators in chronic lymphocytic leukemia. Blood 94: 1840–1847.
20. Wiestner A, Rosenwald A, Barry TS, Wright G, Davis RE, et al. (2003) ZAP-70 expression identifies a chronic lymphocytic leukemia subtype with unmutated immunoglobulin genes, inferior clinical outcome, and distinct gene expression profile. Blood 101: 4944–4951.
21. D'Arena G, Tarnani M, Rumi C, Vaisitti T, Aydin S, et al. (2007) Prognostic significance of combined analysis of Zap70 and CD38 in chronic lymphocytic leukemia. Am J Hematol 82: 787–791.
22. Malavasi F, Deaglio S, Rajendra D, Cutrona G, Ferrarini M, et al. (2011) CD38 and chronic lymphocytic leukemia: a decade later. Blood 118: 3470–3478.
23. Xu W, Cao X, Miao KR, Qiao C, Wu YJ, et al. (2009) Serum thymidine kinase 1 concentration in Chinese patients with chronic lymphocytic leukemia and its correlation with other prognostic factors. Int J Hematol 90: 205–211.
24. Rivkina A, Vitols G, Murovska M, Lejniece S (2011) Identifying the stage of new CLL patients using TK, ZAP-70, CD38 levels. Exp Oncol 33: 99–103.
25. Gronowitz JS, Källander CFR (1980) Optimized assay for thymidine kinase and its application to the detection of antibodies against herpes simplex virus type 1 and 2-induced thymidine kinase. Infect Immun 29: 425–434.
26. Öhrvik A, Lindh M, Einarsson R, Grassi J, Eriksson S (2004) Sensitive nonradiometric method for determining thymidine kinase 1 activity. Clin Chem 50: 1597–1606.
27. Wu C, Yang R, Zhou J, Bao S, Zou L, et al. (2003) Production and characterisation of a novel chicken IgY antibody raised against C-terminal peptide from human thymidine kinase 1. J Immunol Methods 277: 157–169.
28. Faria M, Halquist MS, Kindt E, Li W, Karnes HT, et al. (2012) Liquid chromatography-tandem mass spectrometry method for quantification of thymidine kinase activity in human serum by monitoring the conversion of 3'-deoxy-3'-fluorothymidine to 3'-deoxy-3'-fluorothymidine monophosphate. J of Chromatogr B 907: 13–20.
29. Nisman B, Allweis T, Kadouri L, Mali B, Hamburger T, et al. (2013) Comparison of diagnostic and prognostic performance of two assays measuring thymidine kinase 1 activity in serum of breast cancer patients. Clin Chem Lab Med 51: 439–447.
30. Furman RR (2010) Prognostic markers and stratification of chronic lymphocytic leukemia. Hematology Am Soc Hematol Educ Program. 1: 77–81.
31. Magnac C, Porcher R, Davi F, Nataf J, Payelle-Brogard B, et al. (2003) Predictive value of serum thymidine kinase level for Ig-V mutational status in B-CLL. Leukemia 17: 133–137.
32. Sagatys EM, Zhang L (2012) Clinical and laboratory prognostic indicators in chronic lymphocytic leukemia. Cancer Control 19: 18–25.
33. Wierda WG, O'Brien S, Wang X, Faderl S, Ferrajoli A, et al. (2011) Multivariate model for time to first treatment in patients with chronic lymphocytic leukemia. J Clin Oncol 29: 4088–4095.
34. Bahlo J, Pflug N, Elter T, Bauer K, Eichhorst B, et al. (2011) Proposal of a prognostic score for previously untreated patients with chronic lymphocytic leukemia based on an overall survival analysis of three German CLL Study Group Phase III trials. Blood 118(Suppl. 1), abstr. 2831.
35. Molica S, Giannarelli D, Gentile M, Cutrona G, Di Renzo N, et al. (2013) The utility of two prognostic models for predicting time to first treatment in early chronic lymphocytic leukemia patients: Results of a comparative analysis. Leuk Res 37: 943–947.
36. Molica S (2013) Is it perhaps time for a comprehensive international prognostic index in chronic lymphocytic leukemia? Leuk Lymphoma DOI: 10.3109/10428194.2013.825908
37. Clinical and Laboratory Standards Institute (2008) Defining, establishing and verifying reference intervals in the clinical laboratory: approved guideline, 3rd ed. CLSI document C28-A3: Wayne PA, Clinical and Laboratory Standards Institute 28(30):61
38. Zhou J, He E, Skog S (2013) The proliferation marker thymidine kinase 1 in clinical use. Mol Clin Onc 1: 18–28.
39. Letestu R, Lévy V, Eclache V, Baran-Marszak F, Vaur D, et al. (2010) Prognosis of Binet stage A chronic lymphocytic leukemia patients: the strength of routine parameters. Blood 116: 4588–4590.
40. Chen ZH, Zhou H, Li S, He E, Hu J, et al. (2008) Serological thymidine kinase indicates an elevated risk for the development of malignant tumors. Anticancer Res 28: 3897–3908.
41. Hagberg H, Gronowitz S, Killander A, Källander C (1984) Serum thymidine kinase in vitamin B12 deficiency. Scand J Haematol 32: 41–45.
42. Chen ZH, Huang SQ, Wang Y, Yang AZ, Wen J, et al. (2011) Serological thymidine kinase 1 is a biomarker for early detection of tumours: a health screening study on 35 365 people, using a sensitive chemiluminescent dot blot assay. Sensors 11: 11064–11080.
43. Dürig J, Naschar M, Schmücker U, Renzig-Köhler K, Hölter T (2002) CD38 expression is an important prognostic marker in chronic lymphocytic leukemia. Leukemia 16: 30–35.
44. Hus I, Podhorecka M, Bojarska-Junak A, Rolinski J, Schmitt M, et al. (2006) The clinical significance of ZAP-70 and CD38 expression in B-cell chronic lymphocytic leukaemia. Ann Oncol 17: 683–690.
45. Funaro A, Morra M, Calosso L, Zini MG, Ausiello CM, et al. (1997) Role of the human CD38 molecule in B cell activation and proliferation. Tissue Antigens 49: 7–15.
46. Panteghini M, Ceriotti F (2012) Obtaining reference intervals traceable to reference measurement systems: is it possible, who is responsible, what is the strategy? Clin Chem Lab Med 50: 813–817.
47. Henny J (2013) Multicenter reference intervals studies: a promising perspective for the future? Clin Chem Lab Med 51: 1335–1338.
48. Siest G, Henny J, Gräsbeck R, Wilding P, Petitclerk C, et al. (2013) The theory of reference values: an unfinished symphony. Clin Chem Lab Med 51: 47–64.

FTY720 Induces Apoptosis of M2 Subtype Acute Myeloid Leukemia Cells by Targeting Sphingolipid Metabolism and Increasing Endogenous Ceramide Levels

Limin Chen[1,2], Liu-Fei Luo[1], Junyan Lu[2], Lianchun Li[2], Yuan-Fang Liu[1], Jiang Wang[2], Hong Liu[2], Heng Song[3], Hualiang Jiang[2], Sai-Juan Chen[1], Cheng Luo[2*¶], Keqin Kathy Li[1*¶]

1 State Key Laboratory of Medical Genomics, Shanghai Institute of Hematology, Rui Jin Hospital Affiliated to Shanghai Jiao Tong University School of Medicine, Shanghai, China, **2** Drug Discovery and Design Center, State Key Laboratory of Drug Research, Shanghai Institute of Materia Medica, Chinese Academy of Sciences, Shanghai, China, **3** Department of Chemistry, East China University of Science and Technology, Shanghai, China

Abstract

The M2 subtype Acute Myeloid Leukemia (AML-M2) with t(8;21) represents an unmet challenge because of poor clinical outcomes in a sizable portion of patients. In this study,we report that FTY720 (Fingolimod), a sphingosine analogue and an FDA approved drug for treating of multiple sclerosis, shows antitumorigenic activity against the Kasumi-1 cell line, xenograft mouse models and leukemic blasts isolated from AML-M2 patients with t(8;21) translocation. Primary investigation indicated that FTY720 caused cell apoptosis through caspases and protein phosphatase 2A (PP2A) activation. Transcriptomic profiling further revealed that FTY720 treatment could upregulate AML1 target genes and interfere with genes involved in ceramide synthesis. Treatment with FTY720 led to the elimination of AML1-ETO oncoprotein and caused cell cycle arrest. More importantly, FTY720 treatment resulted in rapid and significant increase of pro-apoptotic ceramide levels, determined by high-performance liquid chromatography-electrospray ionization tandem mass spectrometry based lipidomic approaches. Structural simulation model had also indicated that the direct binding of ceramide to inhibitor 2 of PP2A (I2PP2A) could reactivate PP2A and cause cell death. This study demonstrates, for the first time, that accumulation of ceramide plays a central role in FTY720 induced cell death of AML-M2 with t(8;21). Targeting sphingolipid metabolism by using FTY720 may provide novel insight for the drug development of treatment for AML-M2 leukemia.

Editor: Leah J. Siskind, University of Louisville, United States of America

Funding: This work was supported by China 973 Program (2013CB733700, 2011CB510102, and 2009CB918502), the National Natural Science Foundation of China grants (81270622, 91029704, 91229204, 21210003, 81230076, 21021063 and 81200373), the National High Technology Research and Development Program of China (2012AA020302), and the National Science and Technology Major Project "Key New Drug Creation and Manufacturing Program" (2013ZX09507-004). The funders had no role in study design, data collection and analysis, decision to publish, or preparation of the manuscript.

Competing Interests: The authors have declared that no competing interests exist.

* Email: cluo@simm.ac.cn (CL); kli@epigenetic.us (KKL)

These authors contributed equally to this work.

¶ These authors are co-senior authors on this work.

Introduction

Acute myeloid leukemia (AML)is a heterogeneous clonal disorder of the myeloid line of blood cells and is characterized by the accumulation of immature myeloid progenitors in the bone marrow and peripheral blood. Clinical outcomes are particularly poor for AML subtypes with contain chromosomal abnormalities, such as t(8;21) translocation, which accounts for 40% to 80% of M2 type AML (AML-M2) [1].AML1-ETO fusion proteinis generated by t(8:21) translocation [2], which is thought to be a transcriptional repressor of AML1 target genes. The median survival time of these patients is no more than two years and the five-year survival rate is less than 40% [3]. Currently, cytosine arabinoside (Ara-C) based chemotherapy is one of the standard induction therapies for AML patients. However, since Ara-C is a nucleoside analog, high dosages cause a number of undesirable side effects. Thus, despite the conventional chemotherapeutic approaches, there is an urgent need to identify novel anti-tumor agents for treating AML-M2 with new mechanisms and low toxicity.

As an immunosuppressive agent, FTY720 (2-amino-2-[2-(4-*n*-octylphenyl)ethyl]-1, 3-propanediol hydrochloride) is synthetically derived from myriocin (ISP-1), a metabolite isolated from fungus *Isaria Sinclairii*, and was approved by the US Food and Drug Administration (FDA) for treatment of multiple sclerosis in 2010 [4]. FTY720 has previously shown activity in several hematologic malignancies [5–10]. In another study,FTY720demonstrated the potential toincrease the radio therapeutic sensitivity of prostate cancer cells and reduce tumor growth and metastasis without toxic side effects [11].Despite the extensive investigations intothe anti-cancer effects of FTY720, the mechanism of FTY720 induced cell death is disputed, asFTY720 shows an apparent heterogeneous effectsacross different hematologic malignancies. FTY720 could induce apoptosis or non-apoptotic cell death through either caspase dependent or independent pathways [5,6,12–14]. Meanwhile, activation of PP2A has been considered to be a common event in FTY720 induced cell death [5,6,12,14]. Other distinct mechanisms for FTY720 induced cell death, such as down regulating nutrient transporter proteins [15],inducing reactive oxygen species (ROS) [16], and activating sterol regulatory element-binding protein (SREBP) [17] have also been proposed.

Herein, we report that FTY720 has potent *in vitro* and *in vivo* antitumorigenic activity against AML-M2 with t (8;21). FTY720 mediates apoptosis of Kasumi-1 cells in a caspase-dependent manner. In accordance with previous studies [5], we found that FTY720 treatment activated PP2A, butisonly partially responsible for the apoptosis. In order to explore the mechanism of FTY720's antitumorigenic activity in AML-M2 leukemia, a combination of microarray based bioinformatic and high-performance liquid chromatography–electrospray ionization tandem mass spectrometry (HPLC-ESI-MS/MS) lipidomic studies were carried out. It was revealed that FTY720 treatment could upregulateAML1 targeted genes, interfere with genes involved in ceramide synthesis and rapidly increase the intracellular levels of ceramide. Using small molecule inhibitors to block ceramide generation effectively reduced the pro-apoptic effect of FTY720, indicating that ceramide accumulation is a crucial event in FTY720 induced apoptosis. Furthermore, mass spectrum measurements of mitochondrial sphingolipid metabolites and simulated structural model of the ceramide and inhibitor 2 of protein phosphatase 2A (I2PP2A) complex imply that ceramide initiates caspase-dependent apoptosis machinery through directly activating mitochondria, and binding to and inhibiting I2PP2A, which results in PP2A activation and cell death. Since novel agents with new anti-tumor mechanisms for AML-M2 are in urgent demand, targeting sphingolipid metabolism by using FTY720 or FTY720 mimics may provide newinsights into the development of anti-AML drugs.

Materials and Methods

Cells and Chemical reagents

AML cell lines Kasumi-1 and SKNO-1 were obtained from American Type Culture Collection (ATCC, Manassas, VA). Peripheral blood mononuclear cells (PBMCs) enriched by Ficoll separation were obtained from leukemia patients and healthy donor. The protocols used in this study were approved by Rui Jin Hospital Ethics Review Boards. Written informed consents were obtained from all the patients and healthy donors in accordance with the Declaration of Helsinki. Animals were used according to the protocols approved by Rui Jin Hospital Animal Care and Use Committee. Kasumi-1 cells and PBMC were incubated in RPMI 1640 media (Gibco/Life Technologies, Carlsbad, CA) supplemented with 10% heat-inactivated fetal bovine serum and 1% antibiotic/antimycotic (FBS; Hyclone Laboratories, Logan, UT) at 37°C in an atmosphere of 5% CO_2. FTY720 was purchased from Selleck. Caspase-3 specific inhibitor N-acetyl-Asp-Glu-Val-Asp-aldehyde (Ac-DEVD-cho), neutral sphingomyelinase (nSMase) inhibitor GW4869, and protein phosphatase 2A (PP2A) inhibitor okadaic acid (OA) were purchased from Sigma-Aldrich. N-benzyloxycabonyl-Val-Ala-Asp-fluoromethylketone (z-VAD-fmk) was purchase from R&D System. Sphingolipid standards such as C14, C16, C18, C20, and C22 ceramides were available from Toronto Research Chemicals Inc and sphingosine, S1P were purchased from Sigma.

Cell viability analysis

Cell growth was assessed using the cell counting kit-8 (CCK8; Dojindo) assay. The cells (2×10^4) were plated in 100 µL of media with FTY720 (ranging from 0 to 10 µM) in each well of a 96-well flat-bottomed microtiter plates in triplicate cultures and incubated at 37°C in an incubators at 5% CO_2 atmosphere. 10 µL CCK8 solution was added to each well after46 hours treatment. The cell was culturedfor another 2 hours at 37°C. The absorbance was measured at a 450 nm wavelength with 600 nm wavelength as reference using a micro plate reader (Nanoquant; Tecan). The cell viability was expressed as a percentage of absorbance in cells with indicated treatments to that in cells of control.

Colony formation assay

Kasumi-1 cells were plated in 24-well plates at the concentration of 4000 cells/ml with 0.5 ml IMDM medium containing 0.56% methylcellulose, 30% fetal calf serum, 1% penicillin-streptomycin, and DMSO or FTY720. Fourteen days later, colonies were counted.

Flow cytometry assays

The cell apoptosis was determined by dual staining with annexin V conjugated to phycoerythrin (PE) and 7-amino-actinomycin (7AAD). Kasumi-1 cells or PBMCs were treated with 0, 2.5, 5, 7.5, and 10 µM FTY720 for 24 hours.Then according to the protocol, 1×10^6 cells were stained with annexin V-PE and 7AAD (BD Pharmingen) for 15 minutes in the dark and analyzed by flow cytometry using a LSR II cytometer (BD Pharmingen). Apoptotic cells were identified as annexin V^+ and/or $7AAD^+$ cells. Cells excluding both annexin V-PE and 7AAD were considered viable. The annexin V^-/PI^- cells normalized to untreated controls are represented as a percentage oflive cells.

To evaluate effects of indicated inhibitor in FTY720-induced apoptosis, Kasumi-1 cells were incubated with indicated inhibitor for 3 h prior to treat with 7.5 µM FTY720 for 24 h. After treatment, Kasumi-1 cells were collected, and cell viability analysis was performed as described above.

Invivo therapeutic efficacy evaluation in Xenograft model

The *in vivo* therapeutic efficacy evaluation of FTY720 was performed in nude mice (*nu/nu*) Xenograft model. This model was generated by subcutaneous inoculation of 3×10^7 Kasumi-1 cells with more than 95% viability into the right flank of female nude mice 5- to 6-weeks-old. The nude mice were divided into four treatment groups when tumorsreached 100 mm^3 approximately 10 days after inoculation. The four groups (7 or 8 mice per group) were treated with control (received placebo: 5% glucose), 5 mg/kg Ara-C (positive control), 1 mg/kg FTY720 or 5 mg/kg FTY720 per day for 3 weeks intraperitoneally. Body weight was measured every three days. The longest perpendicular tumor diameters were measured every three days, and the tumor volume was calculated by using the following formula: $0.5\times(\text{width})^2\times(\text{length})$. Animals were euthanized at day 21.

Tumors excised from animals were formalin-fixed, paraffin-embedded, then the paraffin-embedded tumor sections (control, Ara-C (5 mg/kg), and FTY720 (5 mg/kg)) were used in TUNEL assay. TUNEL assay was performed to detect in situ apoptosis on tissue section using an *in situ* cell death detection kit (Roche) according to the manufacturer's protocol.

Western blot analysis

Kasumi-1 cells were treated with FTY720, then cells were lysed with RIPA buffer (50 mM TrisHCl PH 8.0; 150 mM NaCl; 1% NP-40; 0.5% sodium deoxycholate; 0.1% SDS). Lysate with 50 µg of total protein were separated with SDS-PAGE, and transferred to PVDF membrane (GE healthcare). The blots were probed with indicated primary antibodies followed by horseradish peroxidase (HRP)-conjugated goat anti-rabbit or goat anti-mouse IgG.

Detection was performed with chemi-luminescent HRP substrate (Millipore). The caspase-3, caspase-8, and caspase-9 antibodies were purchased from Cell Signaling Technology (CST). ETO antibody was purchased from Santa Cruz Biotechnology (Santa Cruz).

PP2A activity assay

The protein phosphatase 2A activity in Kasumi-1 cells treated with or without FTY720 was determined according to PP2A immuno-precipitation phosphatase assay kit (Millipore). Kasumi-1 cells were treated with indicated concentrations of FTY720 for 24 h and thencells were pelleted and washed with ice-cold PBS. Cell pellets were incubated with phosphatase extraction buffer (20 mM imidazole-HCl, 2 mM EDTA, 2 mM EGTA, PH 7.0 with protease inhibitor cocktail and 1 mM PMSF), and then cells were subjected to sonication for 10 seconds and centrifuged at 13000 rpm for 5 min at 4°C. The protein concentration in supernatantwas quantified by BCA method. Supernatants with 100 μg protein were used to check the PP2A activity.

Molecular Docking

The PP2A/SET protein structure was derived from the SET/TAF-1beta/INHAT complex structure (PDB: 2E50) with waters and small molecules deleted. C22-ceramide was docked to the PP2A/SET protein using Autodock Vina [18].The final docking poses were chosen based on binding free energy calculated by docking program and referring to reported studies [19,20].

Microarray and bioinformatics analysis

The quality of total RNA was tested by denaturing agarose gel electrophoresis. The total RNA from each sample was quantified by Nanodrop ND-1000 (GE)and RNA integrity was assessed by standard denaturing agarose gel electrophoresis. Amplification of RNA was performed with the Invitrogen Superscript ds-cDNA synthesis kit. The ds-cDNA was labeled by using NimbleGen one-color DNA labeling kit. After array hybridization using the NimbleGen Hybridization System followed by washing with the NimbleGen wash buffer kit, the array scanning was finally performed using the Axon GenePix 4000B microarray scanner (Molecular Devices Corporation). Scanned images (TIFF format) were then imported into NimbleScan software (version 2.5) for grid alignment and expression data analysis. Expression data were normalized through quantile normalization and the Robust Multichip Average (RMA) algorithm included in the NimbleScan software. All gene expression level files were imported into Agilent GeneSpring GX software (version 11.5.1) for further analysis. Genes that have values greater than or equal to lower cut-off: 100.0 in 4 out of 6 samples ("All Targets Value") were chosen for data analysis. The microarray data was submitted to Gene Expression Omnibus (accession number: GSE55772).

Differentially expressed genes with statistical significance were identified through Volcano Plot filtering. Functional enrichment analysis of the differentially expressed genes was performed using Database for Annotation, Visualization and Integrated Discovery (DAVID) [21]. Gene set enrichment analysis (GSEA) was performed as described previously on gene lists ranked by expression level after treatment of FTY720 [22].

Quantitative real-time PCR

For microarray analysis, total cellular RNA of Kasumi-1 cells treated or untreated with 5 μM FTY720 for 6 hours was extracted. For quantitative real-time PCR (qRT -PCR), total RNA was extracted and reverse transcribed into cDNA. qRT-PCR was performed on ABI PRISM 7900HT using SYBR Green PCR Master mix (Takara). The fold change was calculated and normalized to the transcript level of GAPDH, and the results were presented as fold change of copy number of mRNA of indicated genes. The primers used were shown in Table S1.

Preparation of cytosol and mitochondria

Kasumi-1 cells (1×10^7) treated or untreated with FTY720 were collected and washed with ice-cold PBS. The cell pelletswerere-suspended in 100 μl buffer (20 mM HEPES (PH 7.4), 250 mM sucrose, 5 mM $MgCl_2$, 10 mMKCl, 1 mM EDTA, 1 mM EGTA, and 0.025% digitonin) and incubated on ice for 20 min. After incubation, cytosol and mitochondria fractions were prepared according to previous report [23].

Quantization of sphingolipids by HPLC-ESI-MS/MS

Calibration curves for ceramide (C14-, C16-, C18-, C20-, and C22-ceramide), sphingosine, and sphingosine-1-phosphated were prepared by using indicated standards with concentrations ranging from 0, 10, 50, 100, 500, 1000, 5000, 10000 ng/ml. No internal standard was used in the experimental system, but all samples were prepared in the same protocol.

Kasumi-1 cell pellets (5×10^6 cells) treated with or without FTY720 were collected and washed with ice-cold PBS. The cell pellets were sonicated 3 times periodically for 30 s after the addition of 100 μl of water. Protein content was quantified by the bicinchoninic acid (BCA) method (Beyotime Institute of Biotechnology). Lysates with 1 mg of total protein were used for sphingolipids extraction. Samples were added 1 ml of chloroform/methanol 2:1 (v/v) and were mixed for 20 min on a rotator at room temperature, 400 μl of 0.5 M KH_2PO_4 was added, and samples were mixed for another 20 min on a rotator at room temperature. Samples were centrifuged at 13000 rpm for 5 min, the lower phase containing sphingolipids was collected. 1 ml chloroform was added to the remnant sample for re-extraction, the sample was mixed by vortex and centrifugated at 13000 rpm for 5 min. The lower phase was collected; the two fractions were combined and dried under a steady nitrogen stream at 40°C.

The dried residue was reconstituted with 200 μl of chloroform/methanol 1:1 (v/v) and centrifuged for 5 min at 13000 rpm, transferred supernatant to an auto-sampler HPLC vial, injected 1 μl on Agilent HPLC system to analyze ceramide, sphingosine, and sphingosine-1-phosphate. For the ESI-MS/MS analysis, 1 mM ammonium formate in methanol containing 0.2% formic acid was served as mobile phase.

Ceramides with different carbon chain length, sphingosine, and S1P content of Kasumi-1 treated or untreated with FTY720 were calculated according to indicated calibration curves.

Statistical analysis

All results were obtained from three separate experiments and expressed as the mean ± S.D. of data. SPSS software (version 16.0) was used for all statistical analysis. Significance was tested based on two-side P values, and all statistical analyses were performed by using paired *t*-test. $P<0.05$ level was considered significant.

Results

FTY720 induces apoptosisof leukemic cells from cultured Kasumi-1 cell line, Xenograft nude mouse model and AML patients

Various studies showed that FTY720 had significant anti-tumorigenic activities against hematologic malignancies including

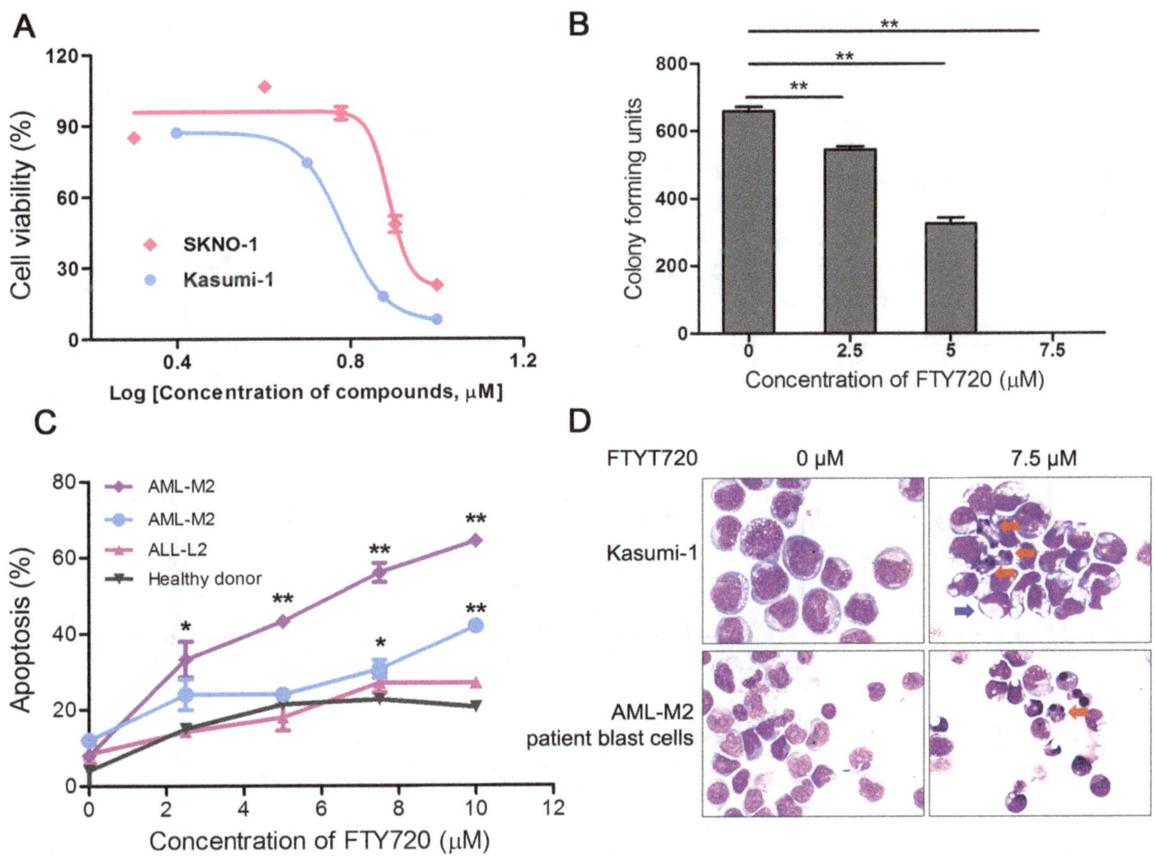

Figure 1. ***In vitro*** **efficacy of FTY720 on Kasumi-1 cells and fresh leukemic cells.** (A) Kasumi-1 and SKNO-1 cells were treated with indicated concentration of FTY720 for 48 h, and the cell viability was determined with a CCK-8 kit. (B) Kasumi-1 cells were grown in methylcellulose for 14 d in presence of FTY720. **P<0.01, student's *t* test compared with untreated. (C) PBMCs from leukemia patients or healthy donor were treated with or without FTY720 for 24 h, and then subjected to apoptosis analysis by flow cytometry. *P<0.05, **P<0.01. (D) Kasumi-1 (top panel) and fresh leukemic cells (bottom panel) from AML-M2 patient were treated or untreated with FTY720 (7.5 μM), and analyzed by wright staining. Partial apoptotic cells were indicated by red arrows, and blue arrow presented cells might undergo differentiation.

acute lymphoblastic leukemia (ALL), chronic lymphocytic leukemia (CLL) [5], NK-cell leukemia [6], T-cell large granular lymphocyte (LGL) leukemia(T-LGL) [7], Blast crisis of chronic myelogenous leukemia (CML-BC) [8] and AML with c-kit mutation [9]. However, fewstudies reported the activity and mechanisms of FTY720 in M2 subtype acute myeloid leukemia (AML-M2), which is associated with t(8;21) chromosomal translocation and the resultant AML1-ETO fusion gene. Kasumi-1 cell line,which wasestablished from an AML-M2 patient harbors AML1-ETO fusion protein and Asn822Lys mutation of C-KIT protein [24]. Our initial experiments demonstrated that FTY720 inhibited proliferation and mediated apoptosis of Kasumi-1 cell line in a dose-dependent manner(IC_{50} = 5.9 μM) (Fig. 1A), and FTY720 significantly inhibited colony formation of Kasumi-1 cells *in vitro* (Fig. 1B).Kasumi-1 cells subjected to FTY720 treatment largelypresented apoptotic morphological changes with condensation and fragmentation of nuclei and cells, but only a few showed morphologic characteristics of differentiation (Fig. 1D). FTY720 also significantly inhibited proliferation of another AML1-ETO containing cell line SKNO-1 with IC_{50} of 6.2 μM (Fig. 1A). In order to evaluate the*in vivo* effect of FTY720 on AML1-ETO harbored cells, we used Kasumi-1 cell-inoculated Xenograft mouse model by subcutaneous injection of Kasumi-1 cells in nude mice. Compared to the control mice of Ara-C treatment, treatment with FTY720 at 1 mg/kg and 5 mg/kg significantly inhibited tumor growth, exerted more antitumorigenic activity than Ara-C and induced in situ apoptosis (Fig. 2A–D). In addition, we incubated blast cells from AML-M2, ALL-L2 (acute lymphoblastic leukemia) patients and healthy donors with increasing concentration of FTY720, and observed a dose-dependent increase in the percentage of the cells that underwent apoptosis identified as annexin V^+ and/or $7AAD^+$ cells by flow cytometry (Fig. 1C). Blast cells from AML-M2 with t(8;21) patients were more sensitive to FTY720 induced apoptosis, while mononuclear cells from healthy donors were resistant to FTY720 induced apoptosis (Fig.1C–D). Taken together, FTY720 has significant anti-leukemia efficacy for AML-M2 with t(8;21).Due to the limited material available from patients, and FTY720 induced similar dose-dependent apoptotic cell death in SKNO-1 and Kasumi-1 cell lines, we used Kasumi-1 cell line throughout the remainder experiments for further mechanistic studies.

FTY720-mediated apoptosis in Kasumi-1 cells is dependent on activation of caspases

To study the mechanism of FTY720 induced apoptosis, we firstly sought to determine whether caspase activation was involved, since FTY720 has been reported to induce either caspase dependent or caspase independent cell death in leukemic cells [5,6,12–14]. We foundthat FTY720 treatment activated caspase-3, 8, 9simultaneously (Fig.3A–B). Kasumi-1 cells were

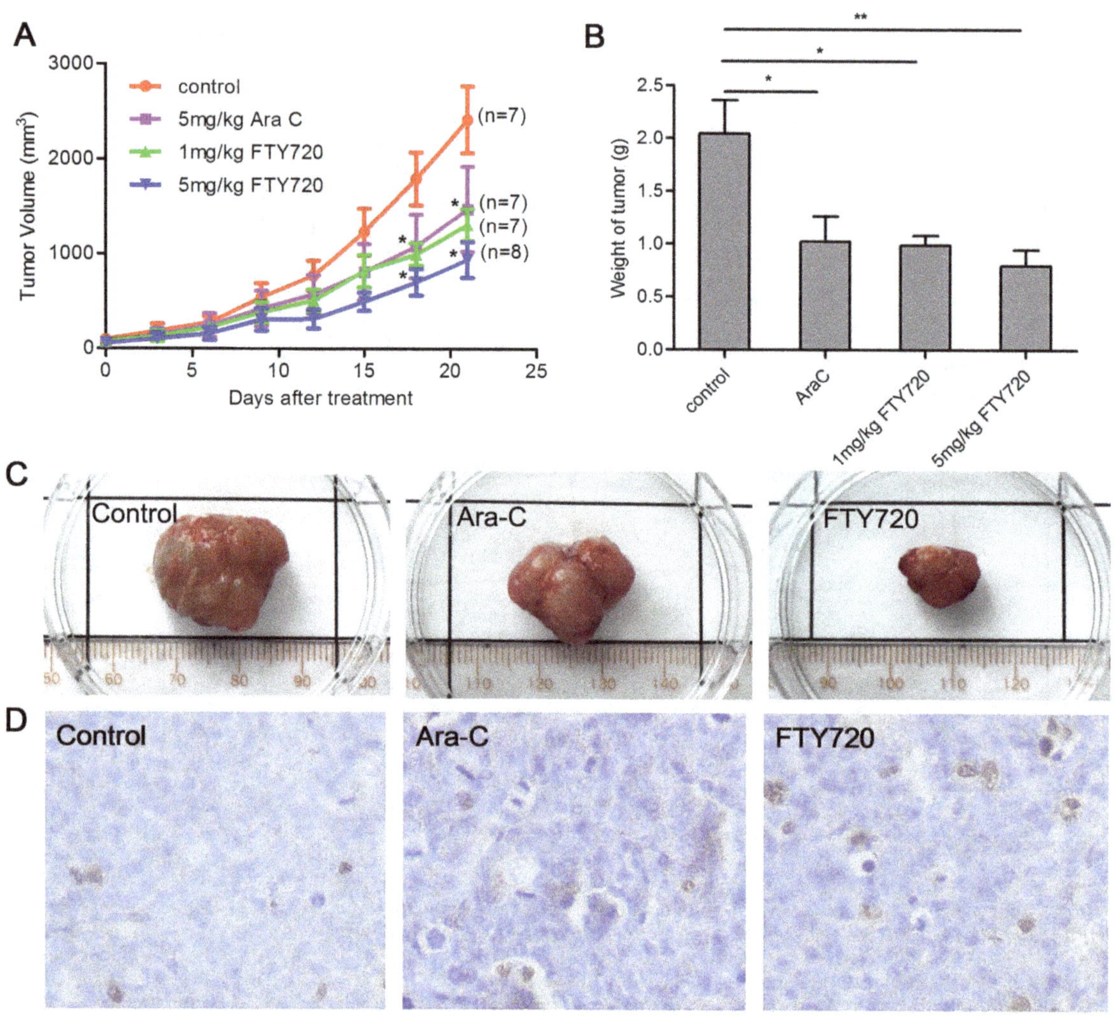

Figure 2. FTY720 suppresses Kasumi-1 xenograft tumor growth. Nude mice (7 or 8 mice per group) with Kasumi-1 tumor were injected intraperitoneally with vehicle (5% glucose), Ara C (5 mg/kg, positive control) or FTY720 (1 mg/kg, 5 mg/kg) for 21days. (A) Tumor volumes were measured every three days. Data are expressed as mean volumes. *$P<0.05$. (B, C) Animals were sacrificed at day 21, and tumors were excised and weighed. Average (B) and representative (C) results are shown. *$P<0.05$. **$P<0.01$ (D) TUNEL assay was used to detect apoptotic cells in tumors of Kasumi-1 Xenograft models treated with vehicle, Ara-C (5 mg/kg), or FTY720 (5 mg/kg).

pretreated with or without 40 μM Caspase-3 specific inhibitor N-acetyl-Asp-Glu-Val-Asp-aldehyde (Ac-DEVD-cho, DEVD) or a broad-spectrum caspases inhibitor, N-benzyloxycabonyl-Val-Ala-Asp-fluoromethylketone (z-VAD-fmk, VAD)for 3 hours, and then treated with 7.5 μM FTY720 for another 21 hours. DEVD partially rescued FTY720-induced apoptosis while VAD effectively blocked FTY720-mediated apoptosis (Fig. 3C). Then, we checked the time dependent manner of FTY720 (7.5 μM)-induced activation of various caspases. It was shown that all tested caspases (caspase-3, 8, 9) needed more than 12 hours of treatment to be activated. Caspase-8,caspase-3 and caspase-9 were activated in Kasumi-1 cells treated with FTY720 after12 hours, 18 hours and 24 hours, respectively (Fig. 3D).

FTY720-mediated apoptosis partially depends on PP2A activation

Previous studies have shown that FTY720 could induce caspase activation and apoptosis by activating protein phosphatase 2A (PP2A) [5,8,9,25]. We then tested whether FTY720 induced apoptosis through activating PP2A in Kasumi-1 cells. We treated Kasumi-1 cells with different dosages of FTY720 for 24 hours, and determinedthe PP2A activity in cell lysates. The results showedFTY720 activated PP2A in a dose-dependent manner (Fig. 4A). However, 3 hours pretreatment of Kasumi-1 cells with okadaic acid (OA), a small molecule inhibitor ofPP2A,only partially inhibited FTY720-mediated apoptosis (Fig. 4B), whilethe increased activity of PP2A in Kausmi-1 cellsupon FTY720 treatment was inhibited by OA (Fig. 4C).The results suggested thatother factors and mechanisms may play more important roles in the FTY720 induced apoptosis in Kasumi-1 cells.

Gene expression profile analysis reveals FTY720 treatment interferes with sphingolipid metabolism and upregulates AML1 target genes.

The molecular basis of FTY720 induced apoptosis in different type of cells was not clear and even controversial [26]. Therefore,we performed gene expression microarray profiling analysis of Kasumi-1 cells treated with 5 μM FTY720 for 6 hours, when the

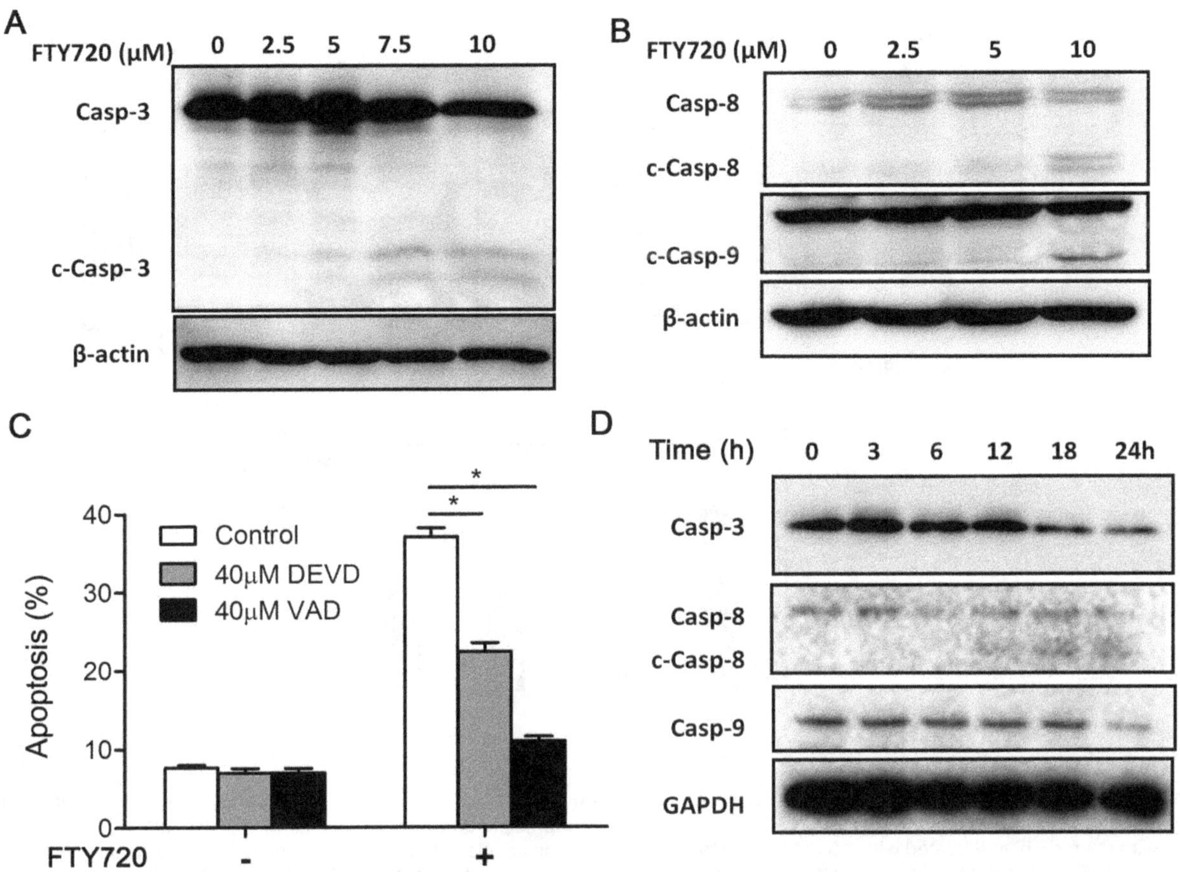

Figure 3. FTY720 results in caspase-dependent cell apoptosis. Western blotting assay was used to analyze the activation of caspases in Kasumi-1 cells treated with FTY720. Kasumi-1 cells were treated with indicated concentrations of FTY720 for 24 h. Caspase-3 (casp-3) and activated caspase-3 (c-casp-3) were shown by the same antibody blotting (A), caspase-8 (casp-8), active caspase-8 (c-casp-8), caspase-9 (casp-9) and active caspase-9 (c-casp-9) were analyzed by indicated antibodies blotting (B). (C) Kasumi-1 cells were pretreated with DEVD or VAD for 3 h, and subjected to 7.5 μM FTY720 for another 21 h. The effects of DEVD and VAD on FTY720-induced apoptosis were evaluated by flow cytometry. *$P<0.05$. (D) Kasumi-1 cells were treated with 7.5 μM FTY720 for indicated times, and then western blotting assay was carried out to analysis casp-3, casp-8, and casp-9 activation in Kasumi-1 cells treated with FTY720 for different time.

cells were on the early stage of reacting to the drug, to find out thedirect factors initiating FTY720 induced apoptosis. Volcano plot filtering was used to identify differentially expressed genes between control group and FTY720 treated group (Fig. 5A). According to the results, 687 genes were significantly upregulated and 277 genes were significantly downregulated after treatment of FTY720 (fold change≥1.5, *P*value≤0.05). Functional annotation clustering of these differentially expressed genes using the DAVID annotation database [21] indicatedthat the set of up-regulated genes were highly enriched in functional groups that related to cellular metabolism such as sterol biosynthetic process (*P* value = 3.2E-7) and lipid biosynthesis (*P* value = 5.7E-5). This effect may be a protective reaction of AML cells when treated with apoptosis-inducing agents [27]. Further, results from Gene Set Enrichment Analysis (GSEA) suggested thatsome genes involved in sphingolipid metabolism were upregulated upon treatment of FTY720 (Fig. 5B). Among them, the genes involved in *de novo* salvage pathways of ceramide synthesis, such as acid sphingomyelinase (aSmase, SMPD1) [28], acid beta-glucosidase (GBA) [29]and delta (4)-desaturase sphingolipid 1 (DEGS1) [30], were shown to be upregulated by treatment of FTY720 (Fig. 5C). Ceramide is a sphingosine-based lipid signaling molecule and has been considered to be tightly correlated with programmed cell death [31].Thus, the upregulation of genes encoding enzymes involved in ceramide synthesis may be a new mechanism of FTY720 induced Kasumi-1 apoptosis.

In addition, the upregulated genesofFTY720 treatment were shown to be highly enriched in the set of downstream targets of AML1 transcription factor (*P* value = 3.68E-10) (Table S2). In accordance, GSEA using the transcription factor target sets(c3.tft.v3.1.symbols.gmt) also indicated the upregulated genes were enriched in the set of target genes of AML1 (Fig. 5D).

The qRT-PCR experiments proved that treatment with FTY720 upregulated multiple genes belonging to ceramide biosynthesis pathway such as DEGS1, SMPD1 and GBA (Figure 5E). qRT-PCR assays also revealed that neutral sphingomyelinase2 (nSmase2, SMPD3), another key enzyme in the salvage pathway of ceramide synthesis [32], was up-regulated following FTY720 treatment (Fig. 5E). The qRT-PCR assay also validated that a well-defined target gene of AML1, NFE2 [33], was upregulated after treatment of FTY720. Other genespreviouslysuggested as AML1 target genes by Chip-Seq experiment [34,35], such as Erbb2 Interacting Protein (ERBB2IP), Lymphocyte Antigen 9 (LY9) and Modulator of Apoptosis 1 (MOAP1), were also shown to be upregulated upon treatment of FTY720 (Fig. 5F). The upregulation of AML1 target genes indicated that the function of AML1, which was blocked by the AML1-ETO fusion protein [1,36], was partially rescued upon treatment of FTY720. Restoration of AML1 function may further

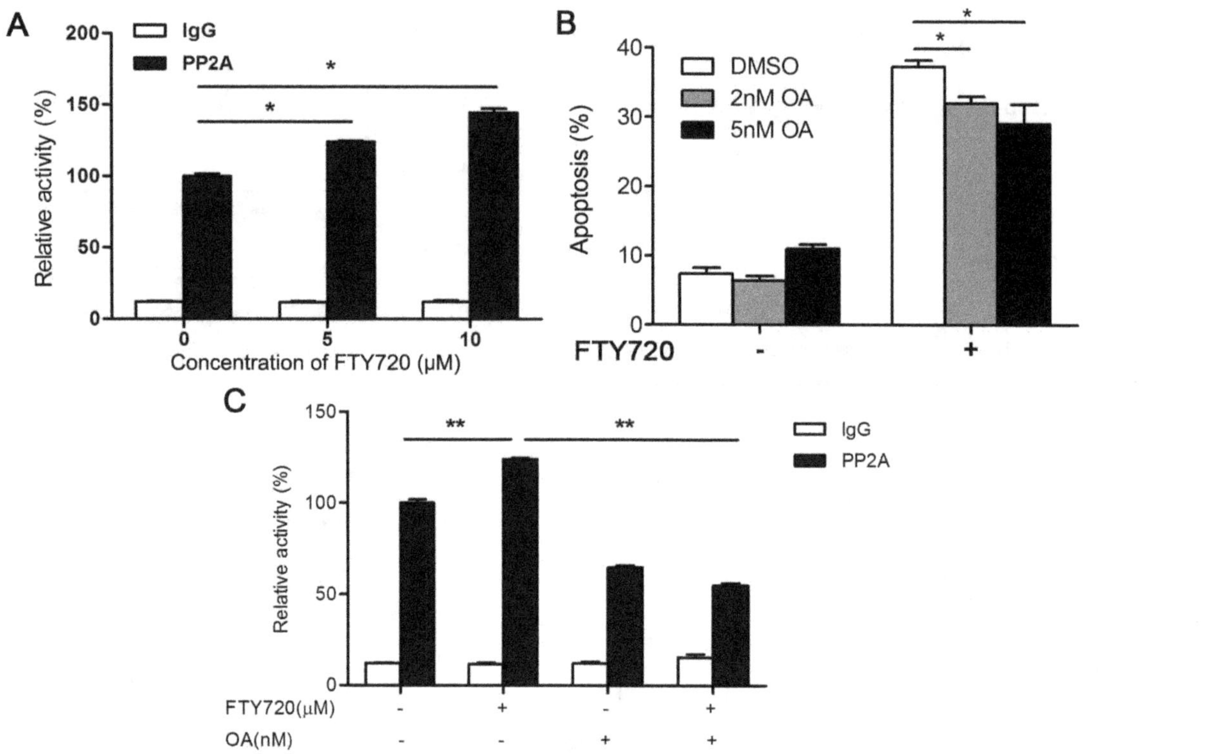

Figure 4. FTY720 induces Kasumi-1 apoptosis is partially dependent on PP2A. (A) Kasumi-1 cells were treated with FTY720 for 24 h, then the cell lysate was used to determine the activity of PP2A by PP2A immunoprecipitation phosphatase assay kit. *P<0.05. (B) Kasumi-1 cells were pretreated with OA for 3 h, and treated with 7.5 μM FTY720 for further 21 h. The effects of OA on FTY720-induced apoptosis were evaluated by flow cytometry. *P<0.05. (C) Kasumi-1 cells were pretreated with OA or DMSO for 3 h, and treated with 7.5 μM FTY720 for further 21 h. Then the cell lysate was used to determine the activity of PP2A according to the protocol of PP2A immunoprecipitation phosphatase assay kit. **P<0.01.

reduce tumor growth and contribute to enhancing potency of FTY720 in Kasumi-1 cells.

FTY720 causes AML1-ETO oncoprotein elimination and G_0/G_1 cell cycle arrest

As gene expression profiling results indicated FTY720 could reverse AML1-ETO mediated transcriptional repression, we performed western blot assays to investigate whether the expression of AML1-ETO oncoprotein was affected by FTY720. We saw a dramatic elimination of AML1-ETO fusion protein in Kasumi-1 treated with 7.5 μM or higher dosage of FTY720 for 24 hours (Fig. 6A). AML1-ETO could repress AML1 target genes and block the differentiation of hematopoietic stem cells [34,36]. Studies have shown that siRNA-mediated depletion of AML1-ETO in Kasumi-1 cells led to a sensitization towards myeloid differentiation and increase of the G_1/G_0 fraction [1]. As mentioned above, a few of FTY720 treated Kasumi-1 cells presented morphological characteristics of differentiation. We then further evaluated the differentiation of Kasumi-1 cells treated with FTY720 by following criteria: cell cycle arrest in G_1 phase, and expression of differentiation markers. DNA content showed an increment of the percentage of cells in G_0/G_1 phase after incubation with FTY720 for 48 hours (Fig. 6B–C). However, we failed to detect any expression changes of CD117, CD11b and CD11c, three differentiation markers for hematopoietic stem cells, after FTY720 treatment for 72 hours (Fig. 6E–F), while signs of apoptosis were significant (Fig. 6D). The cell cycle results were similar to previous report that FTY720 could induce G_0/G_1 cell cycle arrest of human lymphoma cell lines [37].Taken together, these results suggested that FTY720 could eliminate AML1-ETO fusion protein and induce cell cycle arrest. However, the cells underwent apoptosis before showing detectable sign of differentiation. Therefore, another dominant mechanism forFTY720's effect on Kasumi-1 cells may exist.

FTY720 induces the accumulation of ceramide in Kasumi-1 cells

Since the upregulation of AML1 target genes may not be the major effects of FTY720 induced apoptosis and our gene expression profiling demonstrated that FTY720 disturbed the sphingolipid metabolism and could activate ceramide synthesis pathway, we used HPLC-ESI-MS/MS analysis to monitor the changes of three functional sphingolipid metabolites - ceramide, sphingosine, and sphingosine-1-phosphate (S1P) in Kasumi-1 cells treated with or without FTY720 for 24 hours. The contents of ceramide C18, C20 and C22 were increased in Kasumi-1 cells treated with FTY720 in a concentration-dependent manner (Fig. 7A, G). Significant accumulation of ceramide was detected as early as 6 hours after treatment, when cells showed normal morphology and were negative for 7AAD and Annexin V staining (Fig. 7B). However, 7.5 μM of Ara-C treatment did not alter the cellular level of sphingolipids in Kasumi-1 cells (Fig. 7D). On the

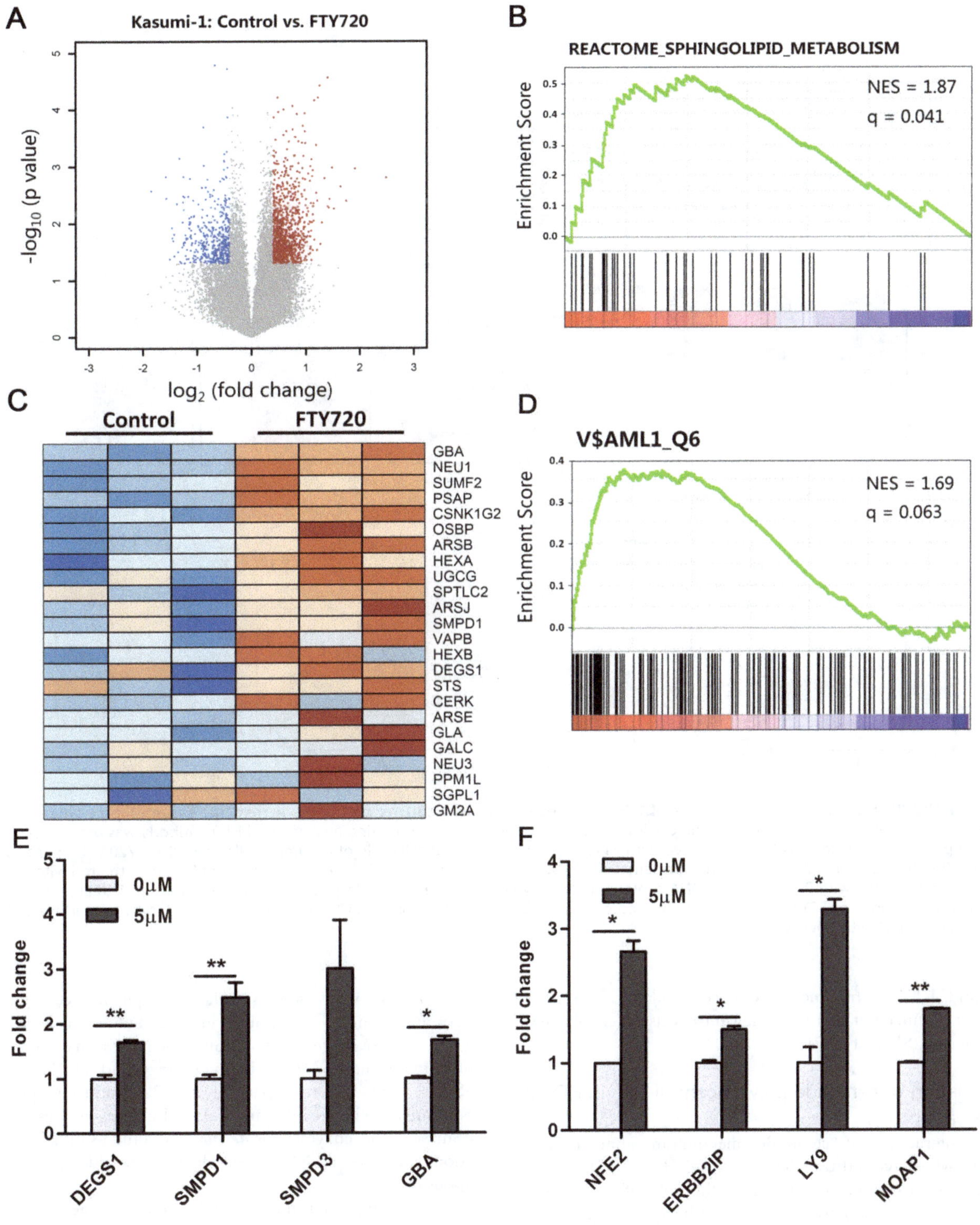

Figure 5. Gene expression profile analysis of FTY720 treated Kasumi-1 cells. (A) Volcano plots of gene expression differences for Kasumi-1 cells treated with FTY720 for 6 hours. Blue dots represent gene probes with *P* value <0.05 by t test and down-regulated fold change >1.5 ($log_2FC < -0.58$). Red dots represent gene probes with *P*<0.05 and fold change >1.5 ($log_2FC > 0.58$). Gray dots represent gene probes with *P*>0.05 or fold change <1.5 (B) Gene Set Enrichment Analysis of sphingolipid metabolism signature. The enrichment is depicted by FDR q value and NES. (C) Heat map of the core enrichment genes (subset of genes that contributes the most to the enrichment result) in sphingolipid metabolism. (D) Gene set enrichment analysis of AML1 transcription factor signature. The enrichment is depicted by FDR q value and NES. (E, F) Kasumi-1 cells were treated with 5 μM FTY720 for 6 h, and RNA was extracted from cells. qRT-PCR was used to analyzetranscription of genes of ceramide synthesis pathway (E) and AML1 targets (F). *P<0.05, **P<0.01.

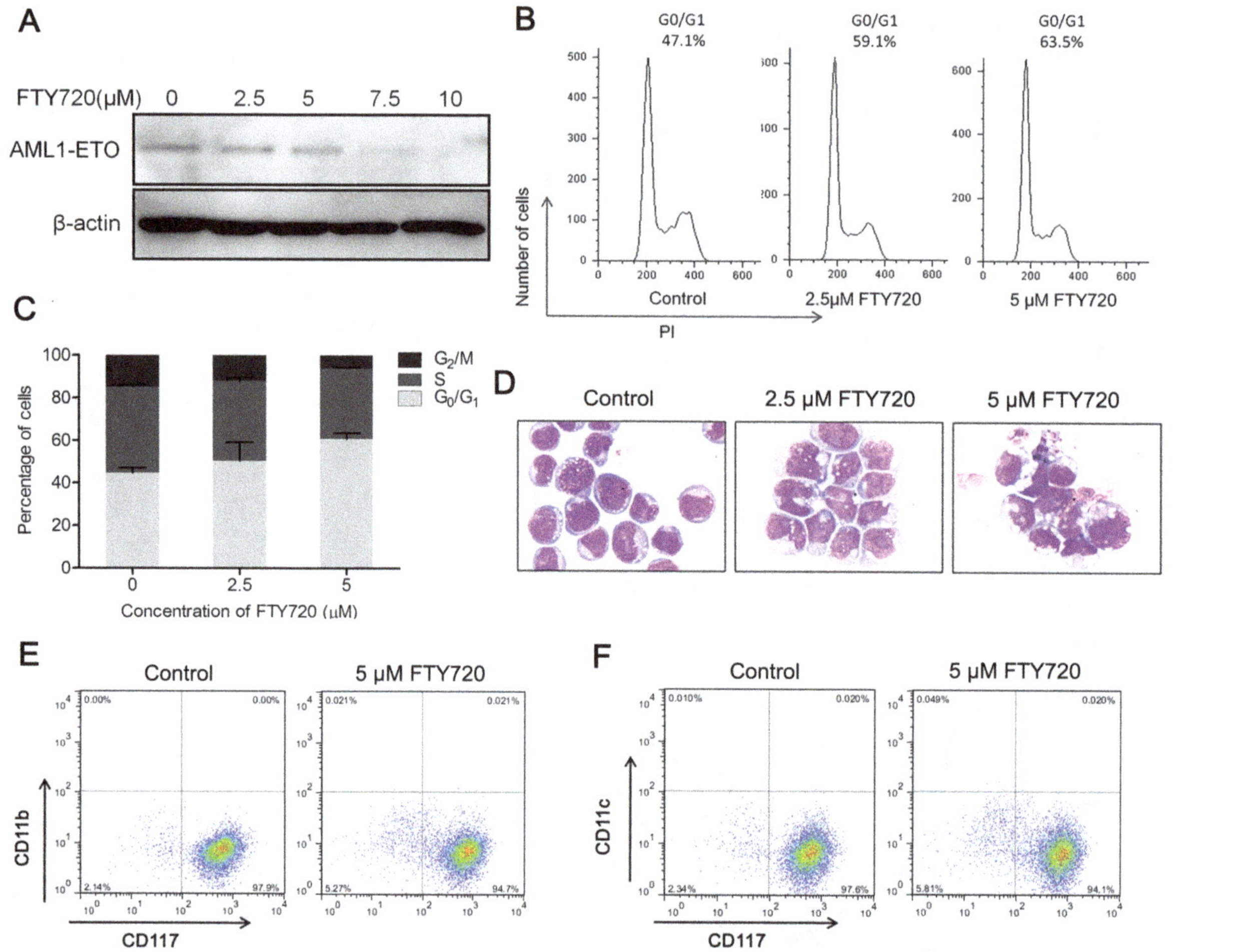

Figure 6. FTY720 induces elimination of AML1-ETO oncoprotein and causes cell cycle arrest. (A) Kasumi-1 cells were treated with indicated concentrations of FTY720 for 24 h, and cell lysate was subjected to western blotting analysis. Anti-ETO antibody was used to detect AML1-ETO fusion protein. (B) Kasumi-1 cells were treated with FTY720 for 72 hours, and cell cycle of Kasumi-1 cells treated FTY720 was analyzed by flow cytometry after propidium iodide (PI) staining, representative histograms were shown. (C) Cell cycle progression of Kasumi-1 treated with FTY720 was evaluated, nuclei stained with PI was used to DNA content analysis by flow cytometry. (D) Morphologic changes in Kasumi-1 treated for 3 days with indicated concentrations of FTY720. (E, F) Quantification of CD11b (E), CD11c (F), and CD117 expression in Kaumi-1 cells treated for 3 days with FTY720 was detected with flow cytometry.

other hand, FTY720 treatment decreased cellular S1P in a dose dependent manner but had no significant effects on cellular level of sphingosine (SPH) (Fig. 7E–F).

Accumulation of ceramide plays a central role in FTY720 induced apoptosis

Since alterations of ceramide metabolism after FTY720 treatment were revealed by microarray and HPLC-ESI-MS/MS assay, it was necessary to investigate the role of ceramide in FTY720 induced apoptosis signaling pathway. We pretreated Kasumi-1 cells with 20 μM GW4869, a neutral sphingomyelinase (nSMase) inhibitor [38] for blocking the salvage pathway of ceramide generation, prior to FTY720 treatment. As expected, GW4869 significantly reduced FTY720-mediated apoptosis (Fig. 7H). In addition, using a ceramide synthases inhibitor Fumonisin B1 (FB1, 20 μM), which could block the *de novo* pathway of ceramide synthesis [39], also partly rescued Kasumi-1 cells from FTY720 induced apoptosis. However, pretreatment with amitriptyline, an acid sphingomyelinase (aSmase) inhibitor, failed to protect Kasumi-1 cells from FTY720-mediated apoptosis (Fig. 7I). Previous studies indicated that the contribution of lysosomal aSmase was limited in stress-induced cell death [40]. Therefore, we suggest that, although we have seen an upregulation of aSmase gene *SMPD1* in microarray and qRT-PCR assays, aSmase may not take part in FTY720 induced apoptosis in Kasumi-1 cells, while neutral sphingomyelinases, such as nSmase2, and enzymes for *de novo* ceramide synthesis may play adominant role in FTY720-mediated ceramide generation and apoptosis.

Studies suggested that ceramide could target mitochondria directly and lead to mitochondria outer membrane permeabilization (MOMP), resulting in caspase activation and apoptosis, and mitochondrial ceramide levels increasing prior to the mitochondrial stage of apoptosis [41]. Thus, we extractedthe mitochondria of Kasumi-1 cells treated or untreated with FTY720, and used HPLC-ESI-MS/MS to detect ceramide levels on mitochondria. Same as the total cellular ceramide accumulation, HPLC-ESI-MS/MS analysis revealed a significant increase of mitochondrial ceramide, especially C22-ceramide, as early as 4 hours after FTY720 treatment (Fig. 7C).

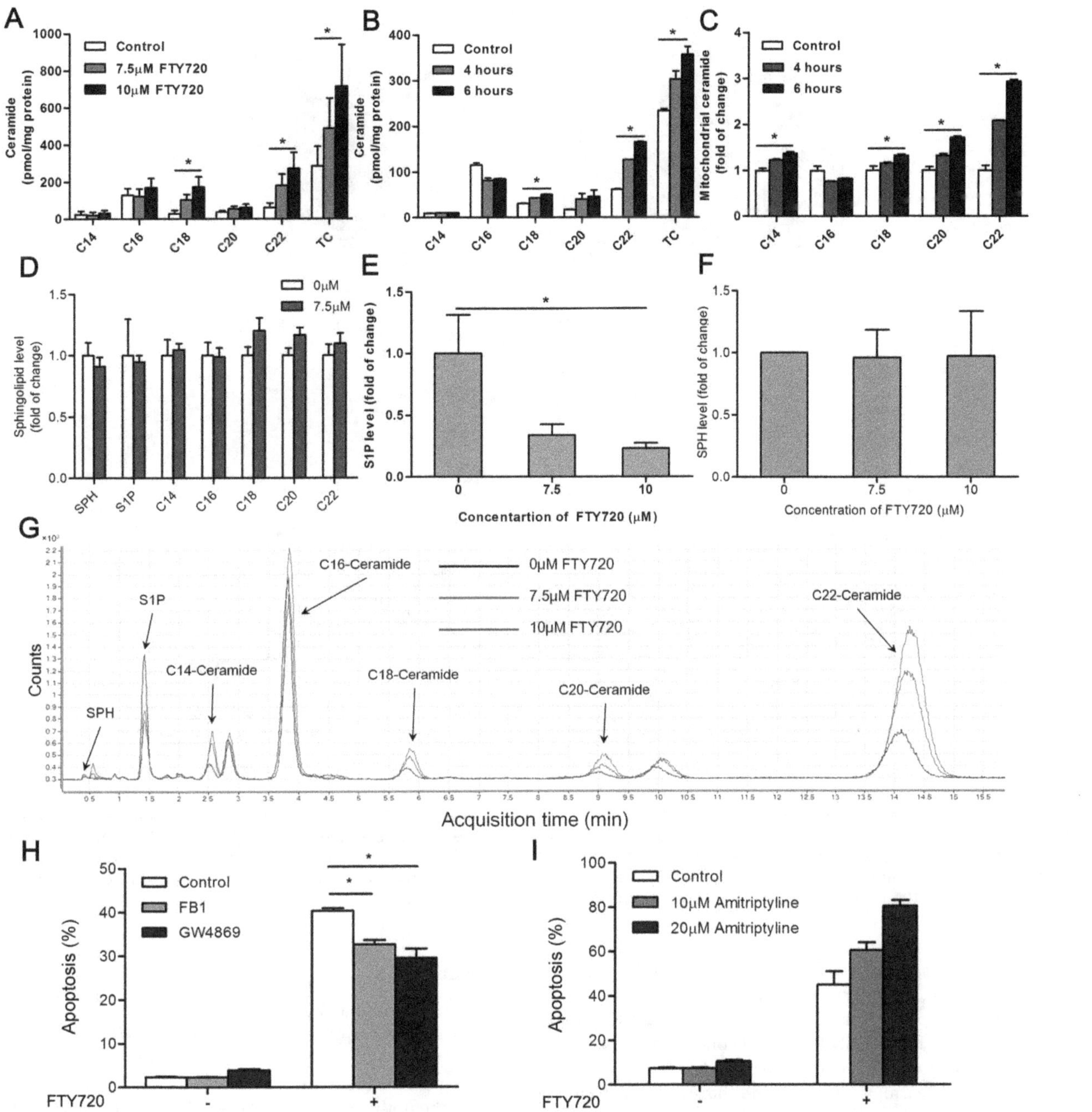

Figure 7. FTY720 induces Kasumi-1 cell apoptosis primarily through elevating ceramide levels. (A, B) Ceramide levels in Kasumi-1 cells treated FTY720 with indicated concentrations (A) and different times (B) were determined by HPLC-ESI-MS/MS assay, TC means total ceramide (C14-, C16-, C18-, C20-, and C22-Ceramide). *$P<0.05$. (C) Kasumi-1 cells were treated with FTY720 for indicated times, and mitochondria was separated. The contents of ceramide in mitochondria of FTY720 treated Kasumi-1 cells were determined by HPLC-ESI-MS/MS assay. * $P<0.05$. (D) Kasumi-1 cells treated with or without Ara-C (7.5 μM) for 24 h, the contents of sphingolipid were determined by HPLC-ESI-MS/MS assay. (E, F) Kasumi-1 cells treated with indicated concentrations of FTY720 for 24 h, the contents of S1P (E) or SPH (F) were determined by HPLC-ESI-MS/MS assay. *$P<0.05$. (G) Kasumi-1 cells treated with indicated concentrations of FTY720 for 24 h, the signals of sphingolipids detected by HPLC-ESI-MS/MS assay were shown. (H) Kasumi-1 cells were pretreated with 20 μM FB1 or GW4869 for 3 h, and treated with 7.5 μM FTY720 for further 21 h. The effects of FB1 or GW4869 on FTY720-induced apoptosis were evaluated by flow cytometry. *$P<0.05$. (I) Kasumi-1 cells were pretreated with amitriptyline for 3 h, and treated with 7.5 μM FTY720 for further 21 h. The effects of amitriptyline on FTY720-mediated apoptosis were determined by flow cytometry.

Since our experiment indicated that FTY720 induced apoptosis only partially depended on the PP2A activation, we thought to seek the direct factors responsible in Kasumi-1 cells. We noticed a newly released study in A549 human lung cancer cells identified the inhibitor 2 of PP2A (I2PP2A/SET) as a ceramide-binding protein [25,42]. FTY720 and ceramide both directly bind to I2PP2A/SET with a high affinity (K_d ~10 nM). As I2PP2A/SET is an endogenous inhibitor of PP2A, I2PP2A/SET inhibition by ceramide binding could lead to PP2A activation and cell death [25,42]. During our current studies in AML leukemia cells, we observed PP2A activation and a significant accumulation of cellular ceramide following FTY720 treatment. Therefore, we

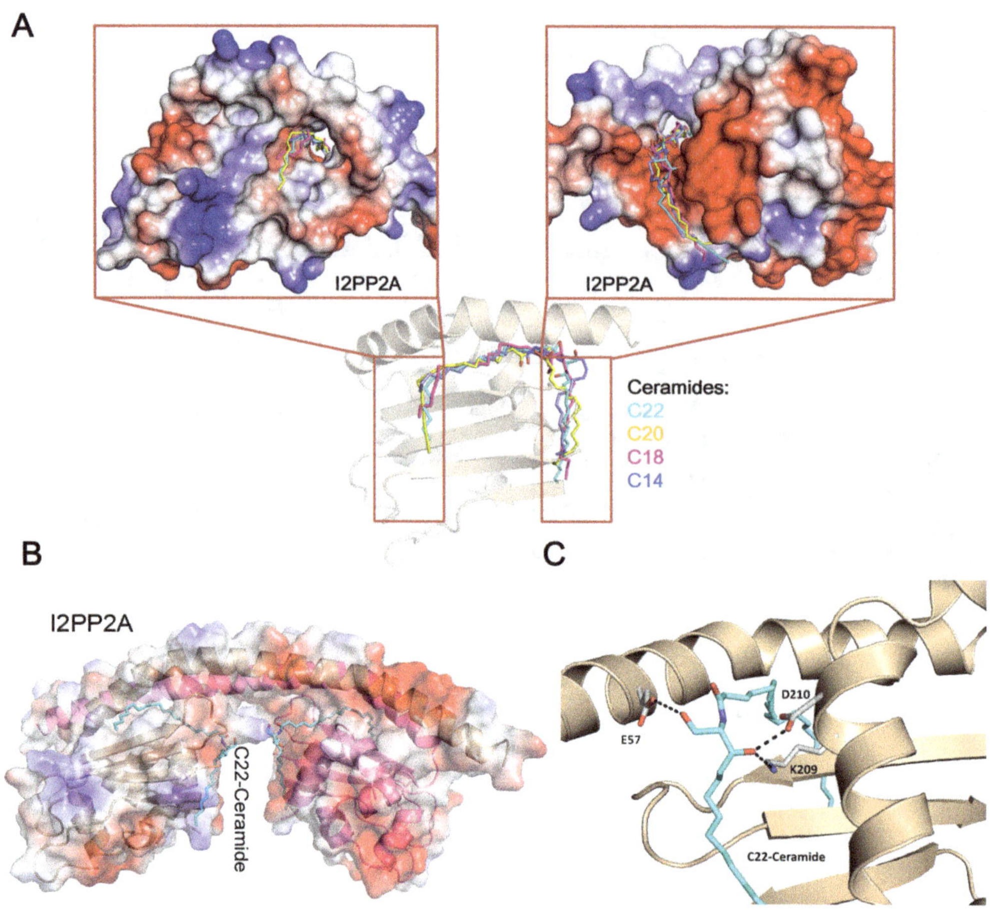

Figure 8. Binding of ceramides to I2PP2A/SET. (A) Docking of C22-ceramide to I2PP2A/SET. The surface contour was colored by electrostatic potential. The atoms of C22-ceramide were shown as sticks. (B) The binding mode of C22-ceramide with I2PP2A/SET. C22-ceramide and the residues involved in the interactions with C22-ceramide are shown as sticks. The hydrogen bonds formed between C22-ceramide and I2PP2A/SET were shown as black dashes. (C) Binding modes between I2PP2A/SET and ceramide with various chain lengths predicted by molecular docking. Front and rear direction views show the bond ceramide composed sphingosine and fatty acid chains.

docked ceramide species that increased significantly following FTY720 treatment, i.e. C18-, C20- and C22-ceramide, to the dimmerized "headphone"-like structure of I2PP2A/SET (PDB: 2E50), which is the biologically functional conformation inside the cell. It is interesting that the ceramide lies on the bottom surface of the I2PP2A/SET "earmuff" domain, and thisregion is engaged in histone chaperone activity for binding to core histones and double-stranded DNA [43]. All ceramides adopted similar docking poses and bound to the hydrophobic concave, whichcould accommodate thevarious chain lengths of ceramide (Fig. 8A) [25,42]. Figure 8B and Figure 8C showedthe detailed binding pose between C22-ceramide and I2PP2A/SET. The simulated binding mode between C22-ceramide and I2PP2A/SET suggested that E57, K209, D210 form three hydrogen bonds with two hydroxyl groups of C22-ceramide (Fig. 8C). The role of K209 in I2PP2A/SET-ceramide interaction has been validated by reported mutational studies [25,42].

Taken together, these results indicate that FTY720 induces apoptosis of Kasumi-1 cells mainly through accumulation of ceramide, and that ceramide may initiate apoptosis machinery through directly activating mitochondria and binding to I2PP2A/SET, resulting in PP2A activation and apoptosis.

Discussion

We showed that FTY720, an FDA approved oral drug, could induce apoptosis of Kasumi-1 cells, an AML cell line possessing both t(8;21)(q22:q22) and c-kit mutations, *in vitro* and in Xenograft model. FTY720 showed higher efficacy than currently used chemotherapy agent, Ara-C. In addition, FTY720 induced apoptosis of blast cells from AML patients in a dose dependent manner and showed selectivity for blast cells from AML-M2 patients. Given the high potency of inducing apoptosis of AML cells and low toxicity towards normal cells, FTY720 or FTY720 mimic may provide novel insight into drug development for AML-M2 treatment. Considering that our initial findings of the caspase activation is a terminal event in programmed cell death, and thatPP2A activation is only partially responsible for FTY720 induced apoptosis, we sought to discover the dominant factors controlling the mechanism of FTY720 induced apoptosis. Through a combined bioinformatic and lipidomic study, we identified a perturbation of sphingolipid metabolism pathway by FTY720 treatment, which ledto the accumulation of ceramide- a pro-apoptotic second messenger. Microarray and qRT-PCR studies indicated that enzymes encoded by some of the upregulated genes, such as DEGS1, SMPD1, SMPD3, and GBA, were involved in the ceramide synthesis pathway, which indicated that FTY720 treatment might elevate the endogenous ceramide levels. In accordance with microarray and qRT-PCR results, HPLC-ESI-MS/MS analysis revealed a significant accumulation of ceramide in Kasumi-1 cells following FTY720 treatment.On the other hand, FTY720 could upregulate AML1 target genes and result in an increase of G_1/G_0 fraction in Kasumi-1 cell.Thecellstreated with FTY720 might partially undergo differentiation; however, the endogenous ceramide accumulation ultimately dictates cell death by apoptosis. Our current study revealed that ceramide related molecular events might be the upstream and dominant effect behindthe mechanism of FTY720 induced apoptosis in Kasumi-1 cell.

Although FTY720, which is a sphingosine mimic, is structurally similar to ceramide, the role of ceramide in FTY720 induced apoptosis has rarely been studied. However, the role of ceramide as a second messenger in cellular apoptosis has been well characterized [31]. In the present study, we have shown that FTY720 treatment significantly and rapidly increased endogenous ceramide of various chain lengths. Ceramide levels in FTY720-treated Kasumi-1 cells were elevated as early as 4 hours, when caspases were inactive and apoptotic markers were negative.Ithas been known that ceramide is played greater potency than FTY720 in PP2A activation [44,45], and ceramide could also increase the permeability of the mitochondrial outer membrane directly, releasing pro-apoptotic proteins such as cytochrom C and eventually led to caspase activation and apoptosis [41]. Although the mitochondrial preparation may contain endoplasmic reticulum(ER), we observed a significant accumulation of ceramide on mitochondrial membrane after FTY720 treatment. Therefore, we suggest that apoptosis induced by FTY720 largely owes to ceramide accumulation after FTY720 treatment.

The precise mechanism of how FTY720 perturbs the sphingolipid metabolism and leads to ceramide accumulation remains elusive. A study on prostate cancer cells has shown that FTY720 could moderately elevate cellular ceramide levels by directly inhibiting SPHK1 [11]. In addition, Steven et al. have shown that a SPHK1 specific inhibitor named SKI-1 could induce apoptosis of U937 cells [46]. In their study, SKI-1 inhibited SPHK1 and caused ceramide increasing and S1P decreasing. Although decrement slight decrease of cellular S1P after FTY720 treatment was observed, we would exclude the possibility that the accumulation of ceramide in Kasumi-1 cells resulted from the direct inhibition of SPHK1 by FTY720, asthe amount of increased ceramide far exceeded the amount of decreased S1P and we did not observe increase of sphingosine after FTY720 treatment, as reported in prostate cancer cells [11] and NK-cell leukemia [6]. Thus, the majority of increased ceramide must come from other sources such as salvage or *de novo* ceramide synthesis (Figure S1). Furthermore, it was reported that FTY720 could increase the generation of long chain ceramide in part through the salvage pathway and fumonisin B1 treatment also partially rescued cells from FTY720-induced death [15]. However, as a multi-target drug, it's difficultto rule out the ability of FTY720 inhibition to SPHK1 contributes to its cytotoxicity on Kasumi-1 cells, because reducing the cellular level of anti-apoptotic S1P could further sensitize tumor cells to FTY720 and ceramide induced apoptosis [47]. In addition, the role of nSmase2 in stress-induced ceramide generation has been well recognized [32] and nSmase2 gene is frequently mutated or downregulated in acute leukemia [48,49]. Therefore, combining our qRT-PCR assays and chemical inhibitor experiment, we suggest nSmase2 might be crucial for the ceramide accumulation and cell death induced by FTY720.

In conclusion, our studies demonstrated that FTY720 exerted potent antitumorigenic effects on Kasumi-1 cells, both in animal models, as well as in blast cells derived from AML-M2 patients. Our data indicated FTY720 treatment could activate ceramide synthesis pathway, which in turn leads to the increase of ceramide in Kasumi-1 cells, particularly on mitochondria membrane. Endogenous ceramide activates PP2A or targets mitochondria to induce MOMP, which eventually activates caspase cascade and initiates apoptosis machinery. In addition, the elimination of AML1-ETO may still facilitate FTY720 induced apoptosis of Kasumi-1 cells by mediating cell cycle arrest, although it failed to induce cell differentiation. Collectively, these data demonstrate that FTY720 may provide a novel insight into drug development for AML-M2 treatment and targeting sphingolipid metabolism may also be a promising way to treat AML-M2.

Supporting Information

Figure S1 Metabolic pathways of sphingolipids.

Table S1 Primers of indicated genes used in RT-PCR.

Table S2 Top 10 enriched transcription factors identified by functional annotation clustering using DAVID database.

Acknowledgments

The authors give special thanks to Professor Zhu Chen, Professor Samuel Waxman and the Waxman Cancer Research Foundation Co-PI Program. The authors also thank the medicinal chemistry advices from Professor Binghe Wang and Peng George Wang at Georgia State University. The authors are grateful for the valuable help from Dr. Ping Liu and Dr. Jian-Xiang Liu in the Medical Genomics State Key Lab. We give special thanks for the carefully proofreading of this article, provided by Kenneth Huang from Georgia State University. Computational bioinformatics analyses were partially supported by the Computer Network Information Center, Chinese Academy of Sciences and Shanghai Supercomputing Center.

Author Contributions

Conceived and designed the experiments: KKL CL. Performed the experiments: LC LFL JL KKL. Analyzed the data: YFL JL CL KKL LFL. Contributed reagents/materials/analysis tools: LL HS JW HJ HL. Wrote the paper: KKL JL CL SJC.

References

1. Martinez N, Drescher B, Riehle H, Cullmann C, Vornlocher HP, et al. (2004) The oncogenic fusion protein RUNX1-CBFA2T1 supports proliferation and inhibits senescence in t(8;21)-positive leukaemic cells. BMC Cancer 4: 44.
2. Miyoshi H, Kozu T, Shimizu K, Enomoto K, Maseki N, et al. (1993) The t(8;21) translocation in acute myeloid leukemia results in production of an AML1-MTG8 fusion transcript. The EMBO journal 12: 2715–2721.
3. Billstrom R, Johansson B, Fioretos T, Garwicz S, Malm C, et al. (1997) Poor survival in t(8;21) (q22;q22)-associated acute myeloid leukaemia with leukocytosis. Eur J Haematol 59: 47–52.
4. Cohen JA, Barkhof F, Comi G, Hartung HP, Khatri BO, et al. (2010) Oral fingolimod or intramuscular interferon for relapsing multiple sclerosis. N Engl J Med 362: 402–415.
5. Liu Q, Zhao X, Frissora F, Ma Y, Santhanam R, et al. (2008) FTY720 demonstrates promising preclinical activity for chronic lymphocytic leukemia and lymphoblastic leukemia/lymphoma. Blood 111: 275–284.
6. Liao A, Broeg K, Fox T, Tan SF, Watters R, et al. (2011) Therapeutic efficacy of FTY720 in a rat model of NK-cell leukemia. Blood 118: 2793–2800.

7. Shah MV, Zhang R, Irby R, Kothapalli R, Liu X, et al. (2008) Molecular profiling of LGL leukemia reveals role of sphingolipid signaling in survival of cytotoxic lymphocytes. Blood 112: 770–781.
8. Neviani P, Santhanam R, Oaks JJ, Eiring AM, Notari M, et al. (2007) FTY720, a new alternative for treating blast crisis chronic myelogenous leukemia and Philadelphia chromosome-positive acute lymphocytic leukemia. J Clin Invest 117: 2408–2421.
9. Yang Y, Huang Q, Lu Y, Li X, Huang S (2012) Reactivating PP2A by FTY720 as a novel therapy for AML with C-KIT tyrosine kinase domain mutation. J Cell Biochem 113: 1314–1322.
10. Payne SG, Oskeritzian CA, Griffiths R, Subramanian P, Barbour SE, et al. (2007) The immunosuppressant drug FTY720 inhibits cytosolic phospholipase A2 independently of sphingosine-1-phosphate receptors. Blood 109: 1077–1085.
11. Pchejetski D, Bohler T, Brizuela L, Sauer L, Doumerc N, et al. (2010) FTY720 (fingolimod) sensitizes prostate cancer cells to radiotherapy by inhibition of sphingosine kinase-1. Cancer Res 70: 8651–8661.
12. Matsuda S, Minowa A, Suzuki S, Koyasu S (1999) Differential activation of c-Jun NH2-terminal kinase and p38 pathways during FTY720-induced apoptosis of T lymphocytes that is suppressed by the extracellular signal-regulated kinase pathway. Journal of Immunology 162: 3321–3326.
13. Wallington-Beddoe CT, Hewson J, Bradstock KF, Bendall LJ (2011) FTY720 produces caspase-independent cell death of acute lymphoblastic leukemia cells. Autophagy 7: 707–715.
14. Nagahara Y, Ikekita M, Shinomiya T (2000) Immunosuppressant FTY720 induces apoptosis by direct induction of permeability transition and release of cytochrome c from mitochondria. Journal of Immunology 165: 3250–3259.
15. Romero Rosales K, Singh G, Wu K, Chen J, Janes MR, et al. (2011) Sphingolipid-based drugs selectively kill cancer cells by down-regulating nutrient transporter proteins. Biochem J 439: 299–311.
16. Liao A, Hu R, Zhao Q, Li J, Li Y, et al. (2012) Autophagy induced by FTY720 promotes apoptosis in U266 cells. Eur J Pharm Sci 45: 600–605.
17. Yoshino T, Tabunoki H, Sugiyama S, Ishii K, Kim SU, et al. (2011) Non-phosphorylated FTY720 induces apoptosis of human microglia by activating SREBP2. Cell Mol Neurobiol 31: 1009–1020.
18. Trott O, Olson AJ (2010) AutoDock Vina: improving the speed and accuracy of docking with a new scoring function, efficient optimization, and multithreading. J Comput Chem 31: 455–461.
19. Mukhopadhyay A, Saddoughi SA, Song P, Sultan I, Ponnusamy S, et al. (2009) Direct interaction between the inhibitor 2 and ceramide via sphingolipid-protein binding is involved in the regulation of protein phosphatase 2A activity and signaling. The FASEB Journal 23: 751–763.
20. Saddoughi SA, Gencer S, Peterson YK, Ward KE, Mukhopadhyay A, et al. (2013) Sphingosine analogue drug FTY720 targets I2PP2A/SET and mediates lung tumour suppression via activation of PP2A-RIPK1-dependent necroptosis. EMBO Molecular Medicine 5: 105–121.
21. Huang DW, Sherman BT, Lempicki RA (2009) Systematic and integrative analysis of large gene lists using DAVID bioinformatics resources. Nature Protocols 4: 44–57.
22. Subramanian A, Tamayo P, Mootha VK, Mukherjee S, Ebert BL, et al. (2005) Gene set enrichment analysis: a knowledge-based approach for interpreting genome-wide expression profiles. Proc Natl Acad Sci U S A 102: 15545–15550.
23. Dewson G, Snowden RT, Almond JB, Dyer MJ, Cohen GM (2003) Conformational change and mitochondrial translocation of Bax accompany proteasome inhibitor-induced apoptosis of chronic lymphocytic leukemic cells. Oncogene 22: 2643–2654.
24. Larizza L, Magnani I, Beghini A (2005) The Kasumi-1 cell line: a t(8;21)-kit mutant model for acute myeloid leukemia. Leuk Lymphoma 46: 247–255.
25. Saddoughi SA, Gencer S, Peterson YK, Ward KE, Mukhopadhyay A, et al. (2013) Sphingosine analogue drug FTY720 targets I2PP2A/SET and mediates lung tumour suppression via activation of PP2A-RIPK1-dependent necroptosis. EMBO Mol Med 5: 105–121.
26. Pitman MR, Woodcock JM, Lopez AF, Pitson SM (2012) Molecular Targets of FTY720 (Fingolimod). Current Molecular Medicine 12: 1207–1219.
27. Banker DE, Mayer SJ, Li HY, Willman CL, Appelbaum FR, et al. (2004) Cholesterol synthesis and import contribute to protective cholesterol increments in acute myeloid leukemia cells. Blood 104: 1816–1824.
28. Takahashi T, Suchi M, Desnick RJ, Takada G, Schuchman EH (1992) Identification and expression of five mutations in the human acid sphingomyelinase gene causing types A and B Niemann-Pick disease. Molecular evidence for genetic heterogeneity in the neuronopathic and non-neuronopathic forms. J Biol Chem 267: 12552–12558.
29. Kitatani K, Sheldon K, Rajagopalan V, Anelli V, Jenkins RW, et al. (2009) Involvement of acid beta-glucosidase 1 in the salvage pathway of ceramide formation. J Biol Chem 284: 12972–12978.
30. Ternes P, Franke S, Zahringer U, Sperling P, Heinz E (2002) Identification and characterization of a sphingolipid delta 4-desaturase family. J Biol Chem 277: 25512–25518.
31. Hannun YA, Obeid LM (1995) Ceramide: an intracellular signal for apoptosis. Trends Biochem Sci 20: 73–77.
32. Marchesini N, Luberto C, Hannun YA (2003) Biochemical properties of mammalian neutral sphingomyelinase 2 and its role in sphingolipid metabolism. J Biol Chem 278: 13775–13783.
33. Wang W, Schwemmers S, Hexner EO, Pahl HL (2010) AML1 is overexpressed in patients with myeloproliferative neoplasms and mediates JAK2V617F-independent overexpression of NF-E2. Blood 116: 254–266.
34. Gardini A, Cesaroni M, Luzi L, Okumura AJ, Biggs JR, et al. (2008) AML1/ETO oncoprotein is directed to AML1 binding regions and co-localizes with AML1 and HEB on its targets. PLoS Genet 4: e1000275.
35. Ptasinska A, Assi SA, Mannari D, James SR, Williamson D, et al. (2012) Depletion of RUNX1/ETO in t(8;21) AML cells leads to genome-wide changes in chromatin structure and transcription factor binding. Leukemia 26: 1829–1841.
36. Petrie K, Zelent A (2007) AML1/ETO, a promiscuous fusion oncoprotein. Blood 109: 4109–4110.
37. Nagahara Y, Matsuoka Y, Saito K, Ikekita M, Higuchi S, et al. (2001) Coordinate involvement of cell cycle arrest and apoptosis strengthen the effect of FTY720. Jpn J Cancer Res 92: 680–687.
38. Luberto C, Hassler DF, Signorelli P, Okamoto Y, Sawai H, et al. (2002) Inhibition of tumor necrosis factor-induced cell death in MCF7 by a novel inhibitor of neutral sphingomyelinase. J Biol Chem 277: 41128–41139.
39. Merrill AH, Jr., van Echten G, Wang E, Sandhoff K (1993) Fumonisin B1 inhibits sphingosine (sphinganine) N-acyltransferase and de novo sphingolipid biosynthesis in cultured neurons in situ. J Biol Chem 268: 27299–27306.
40. Bezombes C, Segui B, Cuvillier O, Bruno AP, Uro-Coste E, et al. (2001) Lysosomal sphingomyelinase is not solicited for apoptosis signaling. FASEB J 15: 297–299.
41. Perera MN, Ganesan V, Siskind LJ, Szulc ZM, Bielawski J, et al. (2012) Ceramide channels: Influence of molecular structure on channel formation in membranes. Biochim Biophys Acta 1818: 1291–1301.
42. Mukhopadhyay A, Saddoughi SA, Song P, Sultan I, Ponnusamy S, et al. (2009) Direct interaction between the inhibitor 2 and ceramide via sphingolipid-protein binding is involved in the regulation of protein phosphatase 2A activity and signaling. FASEB J 23: 751–763.
43. Muto S, Senda M, Akai Y, Sato L, Suzuki T, et al. (2007) Relationship between the structure of SET/TAF-Ibeta/INHAT and its histone chaperone activity. Proc Natl Acad Sci U S A 104: 4285–4290.
44. Ruvolo PP, Deng XM, Ito T, Carr BK, May WS (1999) Ceramide induces Bcl2 dephosphorylation via a mechanism involving mitochondrial PP2A. Journal of Biological Chemistry 274: 20296–20300.
45. Dobrowsky RT, Kamibayashi C, Mumby MC, Hannun YA (1993) Ceramide Activates Heterotrimeric Protein Phosphatase-2a. Journal of Biological Chemistry 268: 15523–15530.
46. Paugh SW, Paugh BS, Rahmani M, Kapitonov D, Almenara JA, et al. (2008) A selective sphingosine kinase 1 inhibitor integrates multiple molecular therapeutic targets in human leukemia. Blood 112: 1382–1391.
47. Cuvillier O, Pirianov G, Kleuser B, Vanek PG, Coso OA, et al. (1996) Suppression of ceramide-mediated programmed cell death by sphingosine-1-phosphate. Nature 381: 800–803.
48. Kim WJ, Okimoto RA, Purton LE, Goodwin M, Haserlat SM, et al. (2008) Mutations in the neutral sphingomyelinase gene SMPD3 implicate the ceramide pathway in human leukemias. Blood 111: 4716–4722.
49. Sobue S, Iwasaki T, Sugisaki C, Nagata K, Kikuchi R, et al. (2006) Quantitative RT-PCR analysis of sphingolipid metabolic enzymes in acute leukemia and myelodysplastic syndromes. Leukemia 20: 2042–2046.

16

Phenotypic, Genomic and Functional Characterization Reveals no Differences between CD138^{++} and CD138^{low} Subpopulations in Multiple Myeloma Cell Lines

Teresa Paíno[1,3], María E. Sarasquete[2,3], Bruno Paiva[4], Patryk Krzeminski[1,3], Laura San-Segundo[1,3], Luis A. Corchete[2], Alba Redondo[2], Mercedes Garayoa[1,3], Ramón García-Sanz[2,3], Norma C. Gutiérrez[2,3], Enrique M. Ocio[1,2,3]*, Jesús F. San-Miguel[4]

1 Centro de Investigación del Cáncer, Instituto de Biología Molecular y Celular del Cáncer/Consejo Superior de Investigaciones Científicas-Universidad de Salamanca, Salamanca, Spain, **2** Hospital Universitario de Salamanca, Salamanca, Spain, **3** Instituto de Investigación Biomédica de Salamanca (IBSAL), Salamanca, Spain, **4** Clínica Universidad de Navarra; Centro de Investigaciones Médicas Aplicadas (CIMA), Pamplona, Spain

Abstract

Despite recent advances in the treatment of multiple myeloma (MM), it remains an incurable disease potentially due to the presence of resistant myeloma cancer stem cells (MM-CSC). Although the presence of clonogenic cells in MM was described three decades ago, the phenotype of MM-CSC is still controversial, especially with respect to the expression of syndecan-1 (CD138). Here, we demonstrate the presence of two subpopulations - CD138^{++} (95–99%) and CD138^{low} (1–5%) - in eight MM cell lines. To find out possible stem-cell-like features, we have phenotypically, genomic and functionally characterized the two subpopulations. Our results show that the minor CD138^{low} subpopulation is morphologically identical to the CD138^{++} fraction and does not represent a more immature B-cell compartment (with lack of CD19, CD20 and CD27 expression). Moreover, both subpopulations have similar gene expression and genomic profiles. Importantly, both CD138^{++} and CD138^{low} subpopulations have similar sensitivity to bortezomib, melphalan and doxorubicin. Finally, serial engraftment in CB17-SCID mice shows that CD138^{++} as well as CD138^{low} cells have self-renewal potential and they are phenotypically interconvertible. Overall, our results differ from previously published data in MM cell lines which attribute a B-cell phenotype to MM-CSC. Future characterization of clonal plasma cell subpopulations in MM patients' samples will guarantee the discovery of more reliable markers able to discriminate true clonogenic myeloma cells.

Editor: Evren Alici, Karolinska Institutet, Sweden

Funding: This work was supported by the Cooperative Research Thematic Network (RTICs; RD06/0020/0006), the "Junta de Castilla y León. Consejería de Sanidad" (GRS 391/B/09), the "Ministerio de Ciencia e Innovación" (PS09/01897), the "Fundación Memoria D. Samuel Solórzano Barruso" (FS/2-2010) and Asociación Española Contra el Cáncer (AECC)(GCB120981SAN). The funders had no role in study design, data collection and analysis, decision to publish, or preparation of the manuscript.

Competing Interests: The authors have declared that no competing interests exist.

* E-mail: emocio@usal.es

Introduction

Multiple myeloma (MM) is characterized by the accumulation of malignant plasma cells (PCs) in the bone marrow. Despite recent advances in therapy that contributed to double patients' survival [1], MM remains an incurable disease which may potentially be explained, at least in part, to the persistence of resistant MM cancer stem cells (MM-CSC) with clonogenic potential. The presence of clonogenic cells in MM was described more than 30 years ago [2], but the phenotype of this population is still a matter of debate. It is well known that syndecan-1 (CD138), a heparan sulfate proteoglycan, is expressed by both normal and malignant PCs in most of MM patient samples and cell lines [3,4,5], while absent on all earlier B-cells [5,6,7,8]. Interestingly, some authors have described the presence of potential MM-CSC that lacked expression of CD138 both in MM cell lines and patient samples [9,10,11]. However, other studies have also demonstrated that CD138^{+} PCs are clonogenic and can engraft in different mice models [12,13,14]. It has also been reported that the tumor microenvironment enhances the clonogenicity of human myeloma cells and promotes their de-differentiation towards a more CD138 negative phenotype [15,16]. Therefore, whether MM-CSCs are CD138^{+} or CD138^{-} is still controversial and multiple factors could be implicated in this particular phenotype. Moreover, it has been recently suggested that the CD138^{-} MM subpopulation seems to represent an apoptotic artifact due to sample handling and procedures [17]. In the present study, we have analyzed eight MM cell lines and we have observed that all of them contain a minor subpopulation of CD138^{low} cells. Overall, our results show that the subpopulation of CD138^{low} cells does not differ from the major CD138^{++} subpopulation regarding phenotypic, genomic and functional features.

Materials and Methods

Ethics statement

All animal experiments were conducted according to Institutional Guidelines for the Use of Laboratory Animals of the

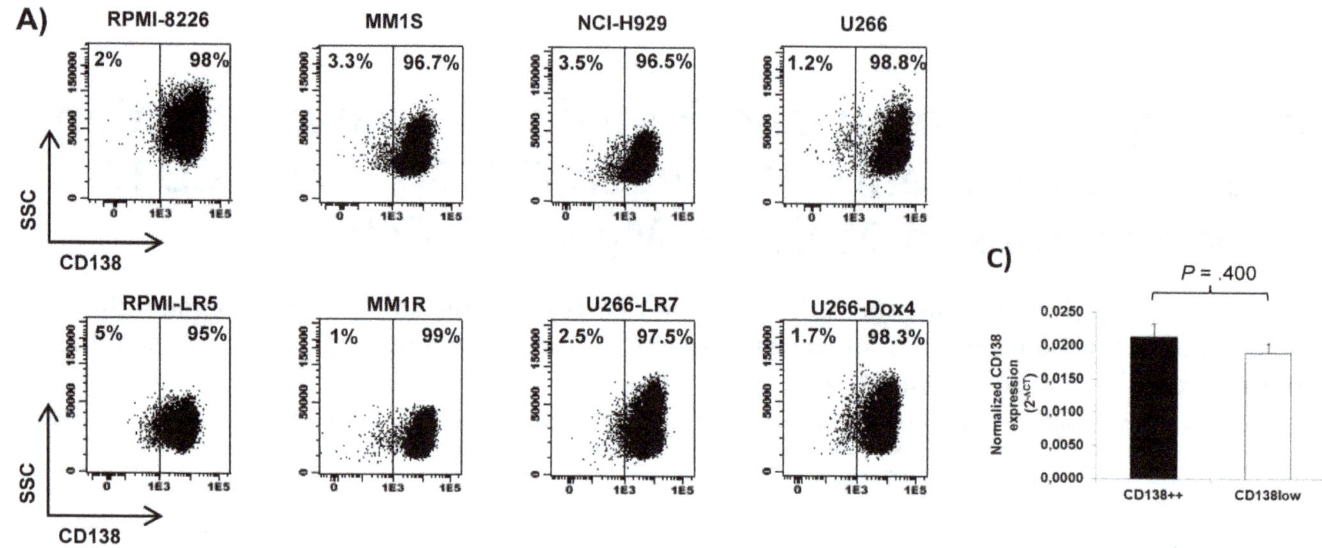

B)

	RPMI-8226	MM1S	NCI-H929	U266	RPMI-LR5	MM1R	U266-LR7	U266-Dox4
CD138⁺⁺	CD19- CD20- CD27- CD38++ CD45- CD56++	CD19- CD20- CD27- CD38-/+ CD45- CD56+	CD19- CD20- CD27- CD38++ CD45- CD56++	CD19- CD20- CD27- CD38- CD45-/+ CD56-/+	CD19- CD20- CD27- CD38++ CD45- CD56-	CD19- CD20- CD27- CD38+ CD45- CD56dim	CD19- CD20- CD27- CD38+ CD45- CD56-/+	CD19- CD20- CD27- CD38-/+ CD45- CD56-
CD138^low	CD19- CD20- CD27- CD38++ CD45- CD56++	CD19- CD20- CD27- CD38-/+ CD45- CD56+	CD19- CD20- CD27- CD38++ CD45- CD56+	CD19- CD20- CD27- CD38- CD45-/+ CD56-/+	CD19- CD20- CD27- CD38++ CD45- CD56-	CD19- CD20- CD27- CD38+ CD45- CD56dim	CD19- CD20- CD27- CD38+ CD45- CD56-/+	CD19- CD20- CD27- CD38-/+ CD45- CD56-

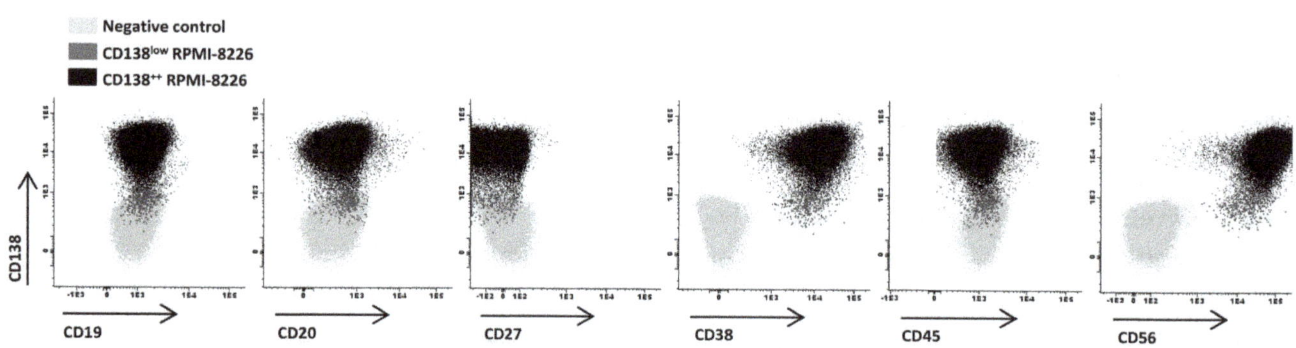

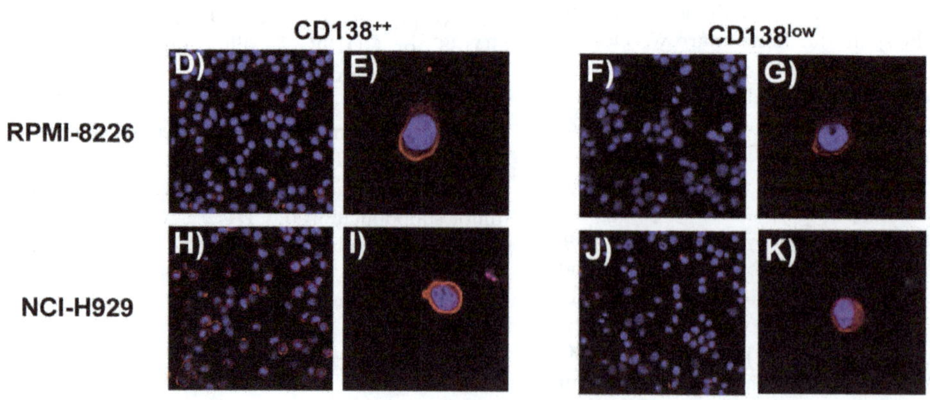

Figure 1. CD138 expression in MM cell lines. (A) Dot plots showing the percentage of $CD138^{++}$ and $CD138^{low}$ cells in MM cell lines. (B) Top: summary of the expression of CD19, CD20, CD27, CD38, CD45 and CD56 in $CD138^{++}$ and $CD138^{low}$ subpopulations in MM cell lines. Code: – (negative); −/+ (heterogeneity); dim (weak positive); + (positive); ++ (high positive). Bottom: representative dot plots corresponding to non-stained RPMI-8226 cells (negative control; light grey) and stained $CD138^{++}$ (black) and $CD138^{low}$ (dark grey) RPMI-8226 cells. (C) Expression of CD138 by real-time quantitative PCR in $CD138^{++}$ and $CD138^{low}$ RPMI-8226 subpopulations. Relative values were calculated by the $2^{-\Delta Ct}$ method ($\Delta Ct = Ct_{(Gene)} - Ct_{(GAPDH)}$). The *GAPDH* gene was used as a control gene. Results are expressed as the means ± SEM (n = 3). (D–K) Confocal images corresponding to the immunocytochemistry for CD138 (red) in $CD138^{++}$ and $CD138^{low}$ RPMI-8226 and NCI-H929 cells. Nuclear DNA was stained with DAPI (blue). Magnification of the lens, 63x. Specific "4× zoom" was made in E, G, I, K.

University of Salamanca (Spain), after acquiring permission from the Bioethics Committee of the University of Salamanca, Spain (Reg. N° 201100030128) and in accordance with current Spanish laws on animal experimentation (RD53/2013).

Reagents and immunochemicals

Cell-culture media, serum, and penicillin-streptomycin were purchased from Invitrogen (Carlsbad, CA). Bortezomib was provided by Millennium Pharmaceuticals (Cambridge, MA) and melphalan and doxorubicin were obtained from Sigma-Aldrich (St Louis, MO). Annexin-V–FITC was purchased from Immunostep (Salamanca, Spain). May-Grünwald and Giemsa stains were obtained from Merck (Darmstadt, Germany). The origin of the antibodies used in immunocytochemistry and flow cytometry was as follows: anti-CD138-APC (clone B-B4), used for immunocytochemistry and flow cytometry, from Miltenyi Biotec (Auburn, CA); anti-CD20-FITC (clone L27), anti-CD138-PerCP-Cy5 (clone MI15), anti-CD56-APC (clone NCAM16.2), anti-CD45-AmCyan (clone 2D1) and anti-CD38-PE (clone HB7) from BD Biosciences (San Jose, CA, USA); anti-CD19-PacificBlue (clone HIB19) and anti-CD27-PE-Cy7 (clone O323) antibodies from eBioscience (San Diego CA, USA); anti-CD38-AlexaFluor700 antibody (clone HIT2) from Exbio (Vestec, Czech Republic) and anti-CD138-FITC (clone B-A38) from Cytognos S.L. (Salamanca, Spain). The FITC anti-Ki-67 Set was purchased from BD Biosciences (San Diego, CA) and DRAQ5® was obtained from Biostatus (Leicestershire, UK).

Cell lines, cell culture and morphological characterization

The multiple myeloma cell lines used were: MM1S and MM1R (from Dr. S. T. Rosen, Northwestern University, Chicago, IL) [18]; NCI-H929 (from Dr. J. Teixidó, Centro de Investigaciones Biológicas, Madrid, Spain) [19] and RPMI-8226, U266, RPMI-LR5, U266-LR7 and U266-Dox4 (from Dr. W.S. Dalton, Moffitt Cancer Center, Tampa, FL) [20,21]. Briefly, cells were cultured in RPMI-1640 medium supplemented with 2 mM L-glutamine, 100 U/mL penicillin, 100 mg/mL streptomycin and 10% fetal bovine serum at 37°C and 5% CO_2/95% air. Morphological characterization of $CD138^{++}$ and $CD138^{low}$ myeloma cells was performed with May-Grünwald-Giemsa staining.

Fluorescence-activated cell sorting and flow cytometry

MM cell lines were immunophenotyped on a FACSCanto II cytometer (Becton Dickison Biosciences) using a 7-color immunofluorescence technique [22] with the following combination of monoclonal antibodies (Pacific Blue (PB)/anemonia majano cyan (AmCyan)/fluorescein isothiocyanate (FITC)/peridinin chlorophyllprotein-cyanin 5.5 (PerCP-Cy5.5)/PE-cyanin 7 (PE-Cy7)/ allophycocyanin (APC)/alexafluor 700 (AF700)): CD19/CD45/ CD20/CD138/CD27/CD56/CD38. Data analysis was performed using the Infinicyt software (Cytognos S.L.). $CD138^{++}$ and $CD138^{low}$ cells were sorted on a FACSAria cytometer (BD Biosciences) after incubation with CD138-APC plus 7AAD. Sorting was performed exclusively on viable cells ($7AAD^{-}$), excluding debris by scatter properties and gating on the lowest and highest 5% CD138-expressing cells. The $CD138^{++}$ and $CD138^{low}$ sorted cells had a final purity >95% (Figure S1). In

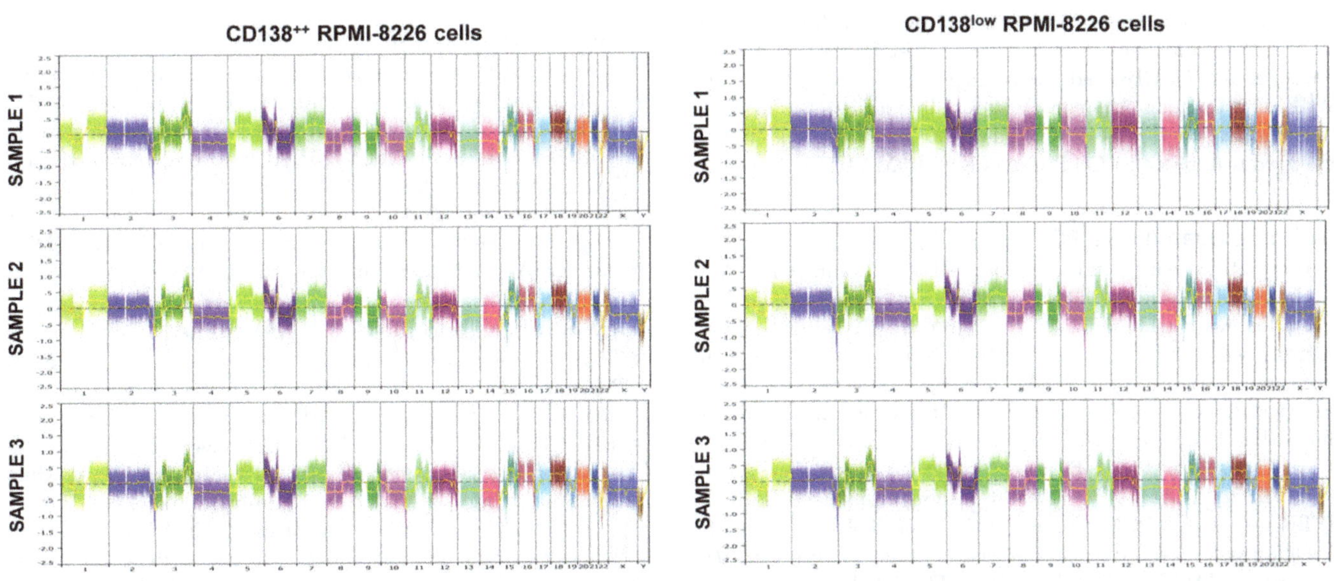

Figure 2. Copy number abnormalities analysis of $CD138^{++}$ and $CD138^{low}$ cells. Log ratio plot of all chromosomes corresponding to $CD138^{++}$ RPMI-8266 cells (n = 3; left panel) and $CD138^{low}$ RPMI-8266 cells (n = 3; right panel) on the basis of Cytoscan HD array generated with Nexus.

Table 1. Genes differentially expressed in CD138^{low} RPMI-8226 *versus* CD138^{++} RPMI-8226 cells.

Probe set	Fold change	Gene Title	Gene Symbol
8118548	2,25	major histocompatibility complex, class II, DR alpha	HLA-DRA
7952335	2,29	small nucleolar RNA, C/D box 14E	SNORD14E
8179481	2,37	major histocompatibility complex, class II, DR alpha	HLA-DRA
8178193	2,96	major histocompatibility complex, class II, DR alpha	HLA-DRA
8101126	4,14	chemokine (C-X-C motif) ligand 10	CXCL10

some experiments the phenotype of the sorted populations was re-analyzed after their expansion *in vitro*. Thus, either CD138^{++} or CD138^{low} RPMI-8226 cells were single-sorted into 96 multiwell plates (1 cell/well) and serially expanded into 48, 24 and 12 multiwell plates for 25 up to 37 days. Afterwards, the phenotype of each clone was analyzed by flow cytometry using CD138-APC plus 7AAD. Apoptosis was determined by double staining with CD38-PE plus CD138-APC followed by incubation with Annexin-V-FITC/7AAD. To analyze the expression of Ki-67 in CD138^{++} and CD138^{low} populations, cells were first surface-stained with CD138-APC. Afterwards, they were fixed and permeabilized with the Cytofix/Cytoperm^{TM} Fixation/Permeabilization Solution Kit (BD Biosciences) and then stained either with Ki-67-FITC or isotype control. To analyze the cell cycle, cells were first incubated with CD138-FITC followed by DRAQ5® and measured on a FACSCanto II cytometer. The expression of aldehyde dehydrogenase (ALDH) was assessed using the Aldefluor Kit (StemCell Technologies, Grenoble, France) following the manufacturer's instructions with further staining with CD138-PerCP-Cy5.

Immunocytochemistry

After FACS sorting, cells were collected, washed with PBS, centrifuged at 800 g for 3 minutes and then resuspended in 200 µl of PBS. An aliquot was taken from each sample and placed on glass slides coated with poly-L-lysine followed by 15 minutes incubation in a cell culture incubator. Then, cells were fixed with 4% paraformaldehyde for 30 minutes, blocked with BSA 100 µg/ml for 1 h at room temperature and incubated with anti-CD138-APC (1:100) overnight at 4°C. Glass slides were then mounted using VECTASHIELD Mounting Medium (Vector Laboratories, Burlingame, CA). Finally, images were collected under Zeiss confocal microscope equipped with 63×/1.4 Oil Plan-APOCRHOMAT DIC.

Real time quantitative PCR (qRT-PCR)

Total RNA was extracted from CD138^{++} and CD138^{low} myeloma cells using an RNeasy Mini Kit (Qiagen, Valencia, USA) following the manufacturer's protocol. RNA quality and quantity were assessed with the RNA Nano LabChip (Agilent Tech. Inc., Palo Alto, CA, USA). The retrotranscription reaction was performed using SuperScript^{TM} III First-Strand Synthesis SuperMix (Invitrogen) according to the manufacturer's recommendations. Finally, qRT-PCR was performed to detect the target gene (*SDC1*) using iQ^{TM} SYBR GreenSupermix kit (BioRad). SYBR green qRT-PCR was performed using Bio-Rad iQ5 PCR detection system with the following gene-specific primers: *GAPDH*, forward 5′-CAGGGCTGCTTTTAACTCTGGTAA-3′ and reverse 5′-GGGTGGAATCATATTGGAACATGTA-3′; *SDC1*, forward 5′-GGCTGTAGTCCTGCCAGAAG-3′ and reverse 5′-GTTGAGGCCTGATGAGTGGT-3′. Relative gene expression was calculated by the $2^{-\Delta Ct}$ method, $\Delta Ct = Ct\ (gene) - Ct\ (GAPDH)$.

Cell viability assay

Viability of multiple myeloma cells was assessed using 3-(4,5-dimethylthiazol-2-yl)-2,5-diphenyltetrazolium bromide (MTT) colorimetric assay as previously described [23]. Briefly, CD138^{++} or CD138^{low} RPMI-8226 sorted cells were plated into 96-well culture dishes (20000 cells/well) in the absence (control) or presence of 10 nM bortezomib, 10 µM melphalan or 250 nM doxorubicin and incubated for 24 and 48 hours.

Microarray RNA analyses

RNA was isolated from CD138^{++} (n = 3) and CD138^{low} (n = 3) RPMI-8226 cells using an RNeasy Mini Kit (Qiagen, Valencia, USA) following the manufacturer's protocol. RNA was hybridized to Human Gene 1.0 ST array (Affymetrix) according to Affymetrix protocols [24]. Microarray data were normalized using the Robust Multichip Analysis (RMA) algorithm implemented in the Affymetrix Expression Console. Data analysis was carried out using DNA-Chip Analyzer software (DChip). The comparison criteria used in DChip analysis were fold change E/B≥2 or B/E≥2, mean difference E-B>100 or B-E>100 and the lower 90% confidence bound of fold-change was used. All microarray data have been deposited with the Gene Expression Omnibus (http://www.ncbi.nlm.nih.gov/geo/; accession number GSE49482).

Identification of IGH rearrangements

Complete VDJH rearrangements were amplified using two multiplexed tubes containing VH-family specific primers for FR1 and FR3 regions with a JH consensus primer according to the BIOMED-2 Concerted Action [25]. All reactions were carried out in 25 µL containing 100 ng of DNA samples and 10 pm of each primer. Then the clonal nature of the PCR fragments was confirmed by Gene-Scanning analysis in an ABI 3130 DNA Sequencer (Applied Biosystems, Foster City, CA, USA).

Copy number abnormalities (CNA) studies

DNA was isolated from CD138^{++} (n = 3) and CD138^{low} (n = 3) RPMI-8226 cells using GenElute Mammalian Genomic DNA Miniprep Kit (Sigma-Aldrich) following the manufacturer's protocol. The detection of CNA was investigated using the CytoScan HD array (Affymetrix, Santa Clara, CA, USA) which includes more than 2.6 million copy number markers and 750.000 SNPs. Briefly, genomic DNA was digested with Nsp I restriction endonuclease, ligated to adaptors that recognize the cohesive four base pair overhangs and amplified by PCR. PCR product was purified and fragmented with DNAse I and then end-labeled using terminal deoxynucleotidyl transferase and hybridized to the CytoScan HD array. The arrays were processed using the Fluidics

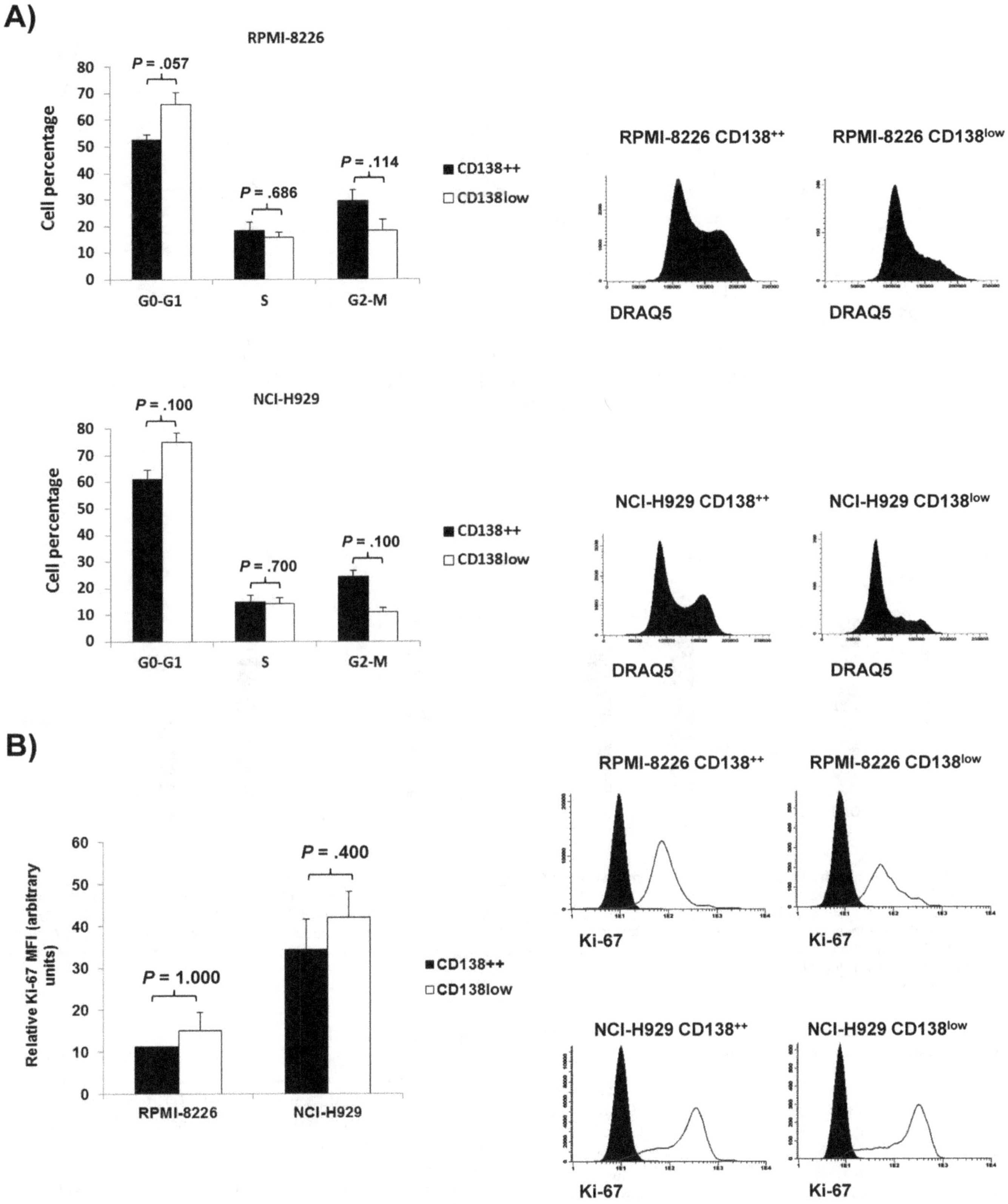

Figure 3. Proliferation of CD138^{++} and CD138^{low} subpopulations. (A) Left: Cell percentage of CD138^{++} and CD138^{low} RPMI-8226 or NCI-H929 cells in G0-G1, S and G2-M phases. The results are expressed as the means ± SEM of at least three independent experiments. Right: Representative DRAQ5 histograms for each indicated population. (B) Left: Relative Ki-67 MFI of CD138^{++} and CD138^{low} RPMI-8226 and NCI-H929 cells with respect to isotype control. Results are expressed as the means ± SEM of three independent experiments. Right: Representative Ki-67 histograms for each indicated population. Filled histograms (isotype control); open histograms (Ki-67).

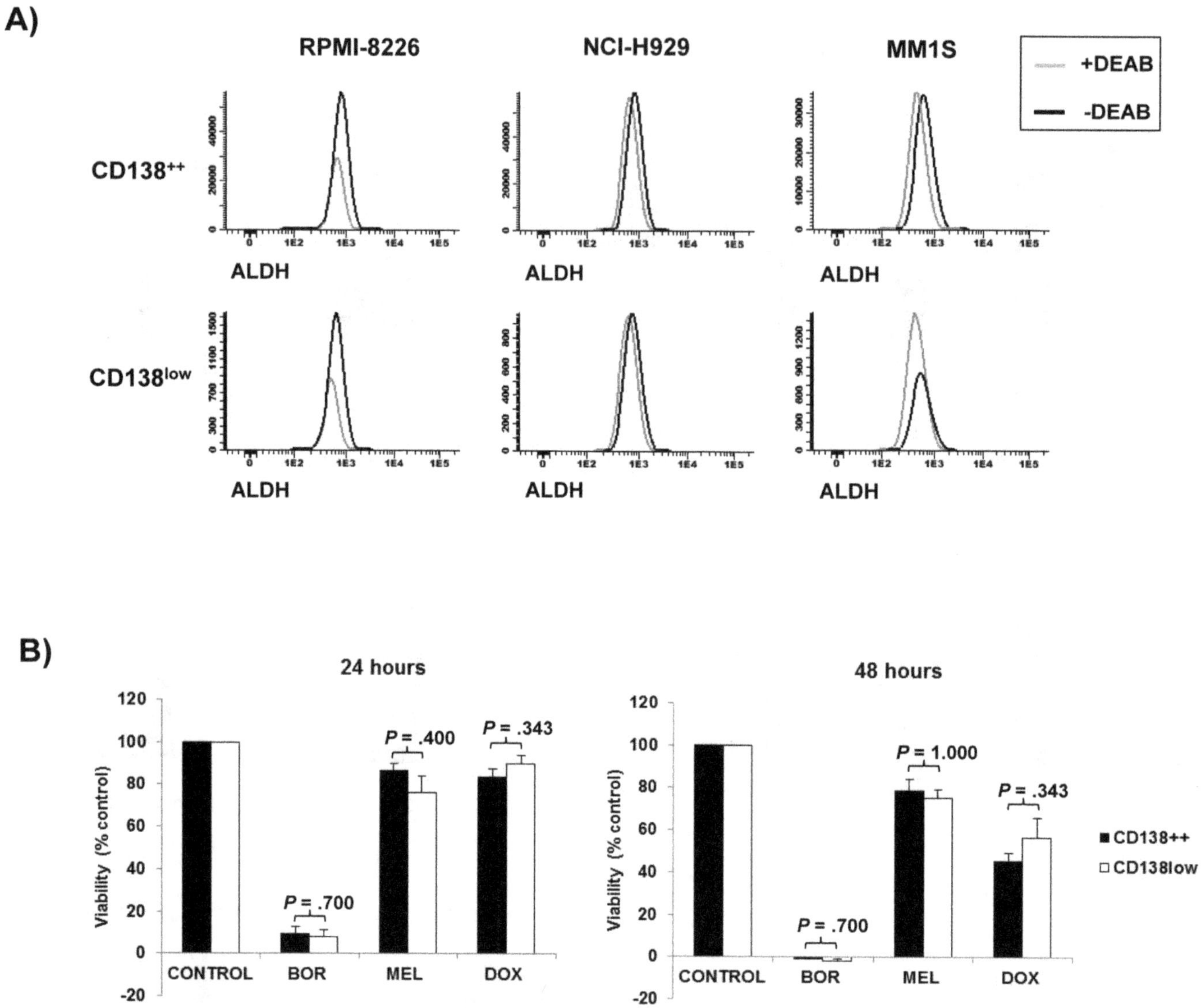

Figure 4. Study of aldehyde dehydrogenase expression and drug sensitivity in CD138^{++} and CD138^{low} subpopulations. (A) Single parameter histograms illustrating the expression of ALDH in the presence or absence of the ALDH inhibitor DEAB (diethylaminobenzaldehyde) in CD138^{++} and CD138^{low} subpopulations of the cell lines RPMI-8226, NCI-H929 and MM1S (B) Sorted CD138^{++} or CD138^{low} RPMI-8226 cells were incubated in the absence (control) or presence of bortezomib (10 nM), melphalan (10 μM) or doxorubicin (250 nM) for 24 and 48 hours. After the incubation time, cell viability was measured by MTT assay and the percentage of cell viability was calculated considering control as 100%. Results are the means ± SEM of at least three independent experiments.

Station 450, GeneChip Scanner 3000 7 G and AGCC (AffymetrixGeneChip Command Console Software).

For the analysis we employed the Affymetrix Chromosome Analysis Suite (ChAS) Software v2.0 and Nexus Copy Number Software Version 7.0 (BioDiscovery, El Segundo, CA, USA). The complete data set was analyzed by visual inspection using ChAS software. CNA were reported when the three following criteria were achieved: minimum of 50 markers per segment, 200 Kb minimum genomic sizes and 50% overlap with known copy number variants (Database of Genomic Variants). Nexus software was employed to obtain the presented Figures. All microarray data have been deposited with the Gene Expression Omnibus (accession number GSE49483).

Myeloma xenografts

For serial engrafting assays, either sorted CD138^{++} or CD138^{low} RPMI-8266 cells were subcutaneously inoculated into the right flank of 6–7 week old female CB17-SCID mice (Charles River, Spain) as previously described [26] to generate primary tumors (5 mice were inoculated per group with 3×10^4 cells) and subsequently cells isolated from primary tumors were serially transplanted into new mice to generate secondary tumors (6 mice were inoculated per group with 3×10^6 cells). Caliper measurement of the tumor diameters were performed three times per week and the tumor volume was estimated as the volume of an ellipse using the following formula: $V = 4/3\ \pi \times (a/2) \times (b/2)^2$, where "a" and "b" correspond to the longest and shortest diameter, respectively. Animals were sacrificed when their tumor diameter was ≤2 cm. To investigate the phenotype of the generated tumors, we mechanically

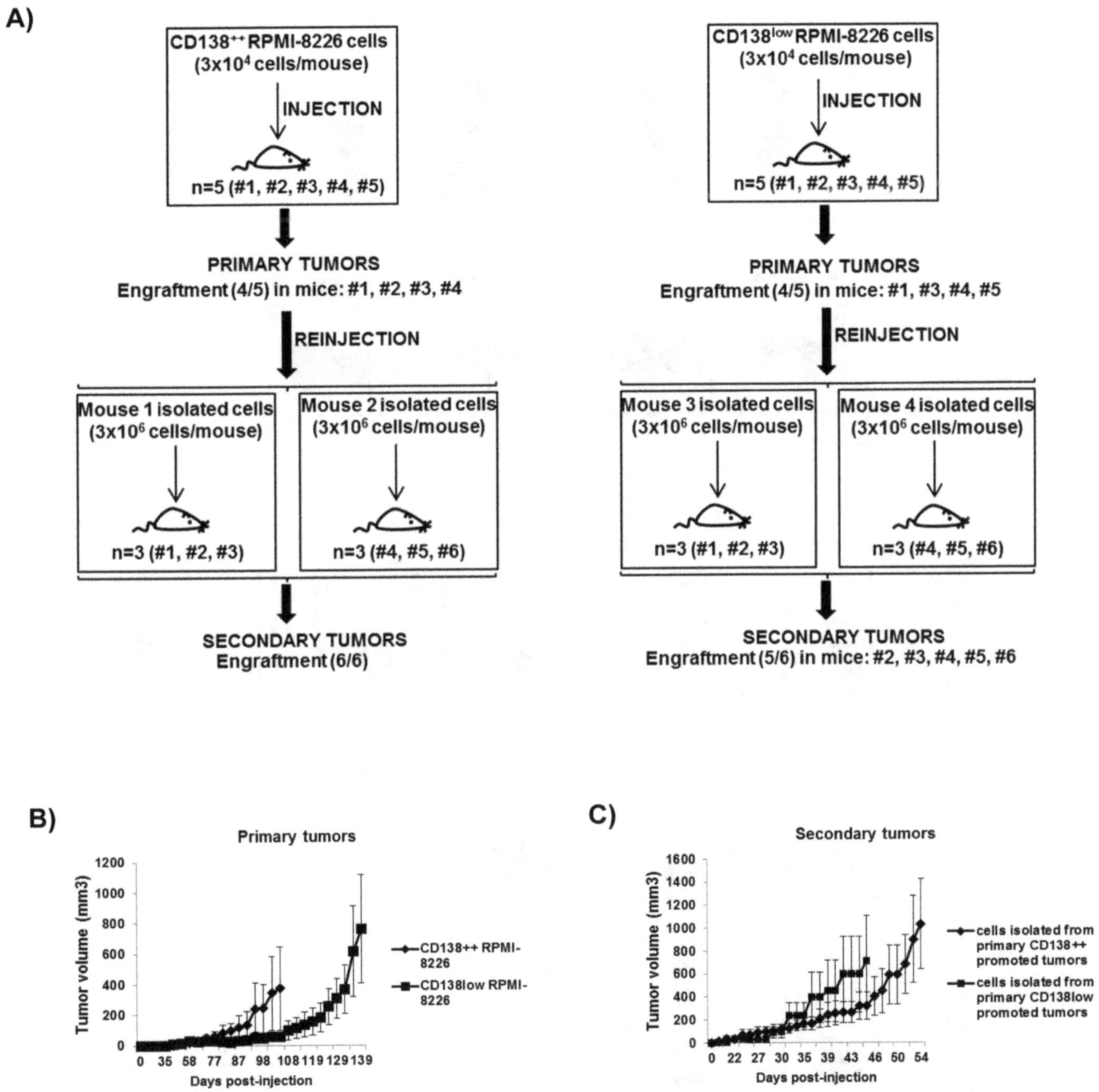

Figure 5. Tumorigenic potential of CD138^{++} and CD138^{low} subpopulations. (A) 3×10^4 sorted CD138^{++} RPMI-8226 or CD138^{low} RPMI-8226 cells were subcutaneously injected into CB17-SCID mice to generate primary tumors. Subsequently, 3×10^6 cells isolated from selected primary tumors were serially transplanted into new CB17-SCID mice to generate secondary tumors. The engraftment efficacy is indicated in each case. (B, C) Tumor growth curves for CB17-SCID mice that developed measurable primary and secondary tumors. Growth curves represent tumor volumes (means ± SEM; n = 4–6) until the time point in which the first mouse in every group is sacrificed.

minced and filtered the tumors through 40 μm cell-strainers and stained the obtained cell suspension with CD38-FITC plus CD138-APC. 7AAD was used also to exclude dead cells.

Statistical analysis

Statistical analysis was performed using the SPSS-20.0 software (SPSS, Chicago, IL, USA). Significant differences between groups were assessed by Mann-Whitney U tests.

Results

CD138 expression in MM cell lines

We analyzed the phenotypic profile of eight MM cell lines (RPMI-8226, MM1S, NCI-H929, U266, RPMI-LR5, MM1R, U266-LR7 and U266-Dox4) to investigate the presence of CD138^{-} or CD138^{low} MM cells. All eight MM cell lines contained two populations with different intensity of CD138 expression: one with bright staining (CD138^{++}) that represented

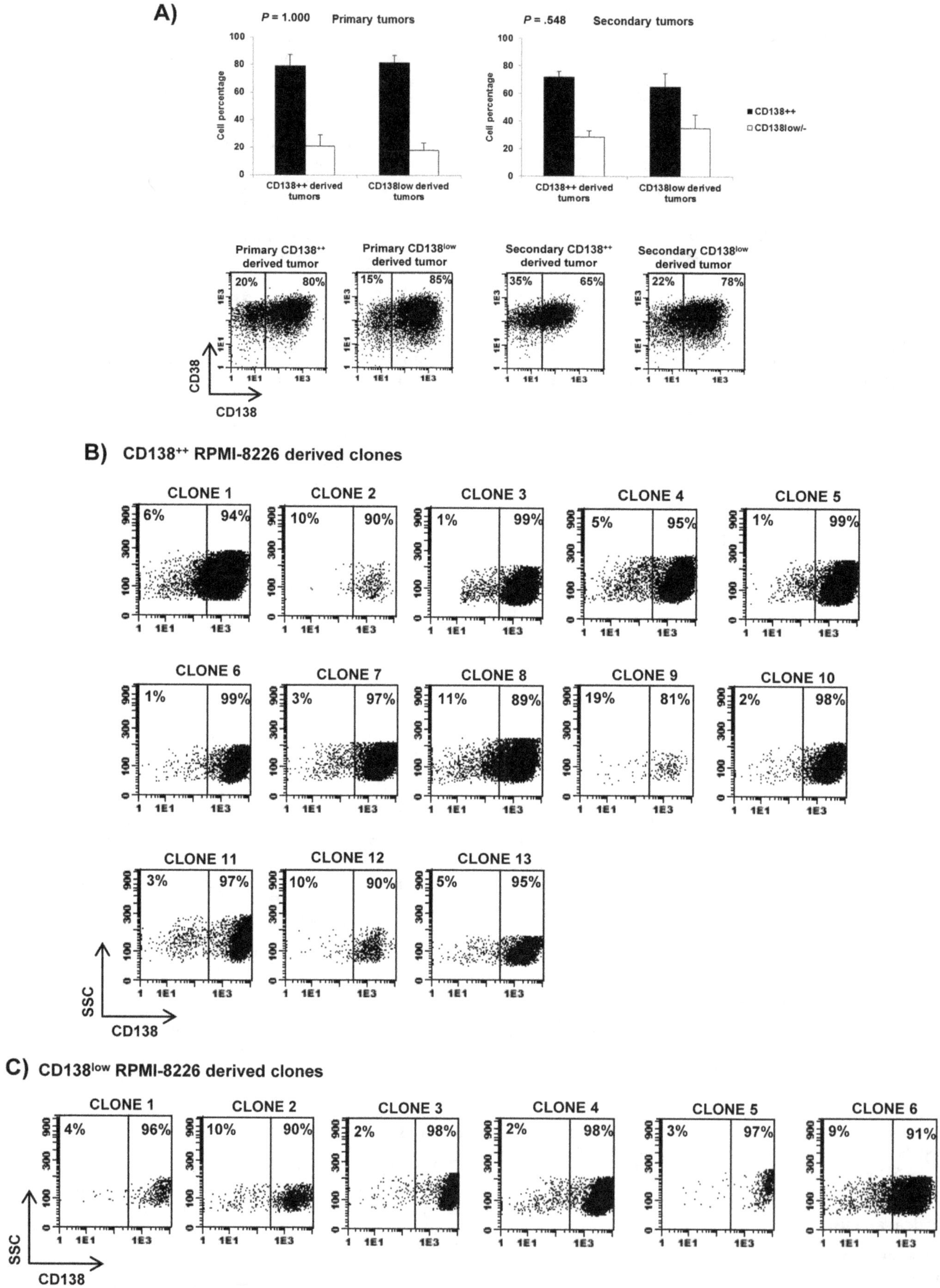
A)
P = 1.000 Primary tumors
P = .548 Secondary tumors
Cell percentage
CD138++ derived tumors
CD138low derived tumors
■ CD138++
□ CD138low/-
Primary CD138++ derived tumor
Primary CD138low derived tumor
Secondary CD138++ derived tumor
Secondary CD138low derived tumor
20% 80%
15% 85%
35% 65%
22% 78%
CD38
CD138
B) CD138++ RPMI-8226 derived clones
CLONE 1 6% 94%
CLONE 2 10% 90%
CLONE 3 1% 99%
CLONE 4 5% 95%
CLONE 5 1% 99%
CLONE 6 1% 99%
CLONE 7 3% 97%
CLONE 8 11% 89%
CLONE 9 19% 81%
CLONE 10 2% 98%
CLONE 11 3% 97%
CLONE 12 10% 90%
CLONE 13 5% 95%
SSC
CD138
C) CD138low RPMI-8226 derived clones
CLONE 1 4% 96%
CLONE 2 10% 90%
CLONE 3 2% 98%
CLONE 4 2% 98%
CLONE 5 3% 97%
CLONE 6 9% 91%
SSC
CD138

Figure 6. CD138^{++} cells give rise to CD138^{low} cells and *vice versa*. (A) The graphs represent the percentage of CD38^{++}CD138^{++} and CD38^{++}CD138$^{low/-}$ cells of primary and secondary CD138^{++} RPMI-8226 and CD138^{low} RPMI-8226 derived tumors. Results are expressed as the means ± SEM (n = 4-6). A representative dot plot for every group of tumors is shown and the percentage of CD38^{++}CD138^{++} and CD38^{++}CD138$^{low/-}$ is indicated in each case (B, C) Phenotype of each individual clone derived from CD138^{++} RPMI-8226 or CD138^{low} RPMI-8226 cells. The percentage of CD138^{++} and CD138^{low} cells is indicated in each dot plot.

around 95–99% of all MM cells and a minor fraction showing dim intensity (CD138^{low}) that represented 1–5% (Figure 1A). No differences were observed between these two populations regarding other myeloma-related markers (CD38, CD45, CD56) and both subpopulations were negative for the B-cell markers CD19, CD20 and CD27 (Figure 1B). Moreover, in one cell line (RPMI-8226) we analyzed the morphology of both subpopulations and CD138^{low} cells did not display different morphological characteristics as compared to CD138^{++} cells (Figure S2). The expression of CD138 was also explored by alternative techniques in two cell lines (RPMI-8226 and NCI-H929). By qRT-PCR, no differences were noted in CD138 mRNA levels between CD138^{++} and CD138^{low} RPMI-8226 cells (Figure 1C). However, by immunocytochemistry a clear higher surface staining for CD138 in the CD138^{++} subpopulation from both RPMI-8226 and NCI-H929 cells was found (Figures 1D–K) in accordance with the results observed by flow cytometry. It should be noted that neither CD138^{++} nor CD138^{low} subpopulations contained apoptotic nuclei (Figures 1D–K) and in fact both were negative for annexin-V and 7AAD (Figure S3).

Genomic characterization of CD138^{++} and CD138^{low} subpopulations

To confirm the clonal relationship among CD138^{++} and CD138^{low} subpopulations, we analyzed the *IGH* rearrangements of CD138^{++} RPMI-8226 cells (n = 2) and CD138^{low} RPMI-8226 cells (n = 2). The monoclonal VDJH rearrangement was present in all samples with the same pattern and size in the GeneScan analysis (340 bp for FR1 and 131 bp for FR3), demonstrating a common clonal origin of CD138^{++} and CD138^{low} subpopulations. To explore if phenotypically distinct CD138^{++} and CD138^{low} subpopulations had different genomic changes, we comparatively studied CNA of CD138^{++} RPMI-8226 (n = 3) and CD138^{low} RPMI-8226 (n = 3) subpopulations, but no relevant differences were observed (Figure 2). Finally, we compared the gene expression profile of CD138^{++} and CD138^{low} RPMI-8226 cells. As shown in Table 1, only three genes (*HLA-DRA*, SNORD14E and *CXCL10*) were differentially expressed between the two populations, and specifically overexpressed in the CD138^{low} cells.

Proliferation of CD138^{++} and CD138^{low} subpopulations

We analyzed the cell cycle of CD138^{++} and CD138^{low} subpopulations in two cell lines (RPMI-8226 and NCI-H929) and we observed that none of them is truly quiescent, although the CD138^{low} subpopulation shows a numerically -not significantly- lower percentage of cells in G2-M phase as compared to the CD138^{++} subpopulation (Figure 3A). These results were further confirmed by Ki-67 staining. Both CD138^{++} and CD138^{low} subpopulations in RPMI-8226 and NCI-H929 cell lines showed considerable and similar levels of Ki-67 (Figure 3B).

Study of ALDH expression and drug sensitivity in CD138^{++} and CD138^{low} subpopulations

Since drug resistance is a hallmark of stem cells [27,28] we next studied the expression of the drug resistance and stem cell-associated marker ALDH [29] in CD138^{++} and CD138^{low} cells. In three different cell lines (RPMI-8226, NCI-H929 and MM1S) the expression of ALDH was barely noted in both CD138^{++} and CD138^{low} subpopulations with no differences between them (Figure 4A). To compare the sensitivity of CD138^{++} and CD138^{low} cells to different anti-myeloma drugs we sorted both subpopulations from the RPMI-8226 cell line and incubated the two subpopulations in the absence (control) or presence of bortezomib, melphalan or doxorubicin. No differences in the sensitivity of CD138^{++} and CD138^{low} cells to any of the tested drugs was found (Figure 4B).

Tumorigenic potential of CD138^{++} and CD138^{low} subpopulations

We compared the engrafting potential of CD138^{++} and CD138^{low} RPMI-8226 cells in a serial transplantation assay in CB17-SCID mice. Initially, the same number (3×10^4) of sorted CD138^{++} and CD138^{low} cells were subcutaneously injected into CB17-SCID mice to generate primary tumors, and subsequently the cells isolated from primary tumors were serially transplanted into new mice (3×10^6 cells/mouse) to generate secondary tumors (Figure 5A). No significant differences were found for primary and secondary tumors neither in the growth curves (Figures 5B–C) nor in the engrafting capacity (Figure 5A).

CD138^{++} cells give rise to CD138^{low} cells and vice versa

Since differentiation potential is a characteristic of stem cells [30], we wanted to know if CD138^{++} cells give rise to CD138^{low} cells or *vice versa*. To this aim, we analyzed the phenotype of the tumors derived from purified CD138^{++} RPMI-8226 or CD138^{low} RPMI-8226 cells. As shown in Figure 6A, primary and secondary tumors derived from both populations contained similar percentages of CD138^{++} and CD138$^{low/-}$ cells, indicating that, *in vivo*, each population is able to give rise to the other. To confirm these results and to dismiss that they are due to contamination of the sorted populations injected into the mice, we performed an *in vitro* experiment of single-cell sorting. Thus, we single-sorted either CD138^{++} or CD138^{low} RPMI-8226 cells into 96 multiwell plates (1 cell/well) and allowed them to expand for a period of time between 25–37 days. We found a higher number of clones derived from CD138^{++} subpopulation (13 clones out of 96) as compared to CD138^{low} subpopulation (6 clones out of 96). The phenotypic analysis of all clones showed that, independently of the initiating cell (CD138^{++} or CD138^{low}), every clone contained CD138^{++} and CD138^{low} cells (Figures 6B and 6C). Overall, these results indicate that CD138^{++} cells give rise to CD138^{low} cells and *vice versa*.

Discussion

Although the presence of clonogenic cells in MM was described more than 30 years ago [2] the phenotype of the resistant putative MM-CSC is still a matter of debate. In this work, we have focused on myeloma cells with low expression of the maturation associated surface marker CD138. Our results show that the minor subpopulation of CD138^{low} cells contained in MM cell lines does not differ from the major CD138^{++} subpopulation regarding phenotypic, genomic and functional features.

An immature phenotype is a typical hallmark of cancer stem cells [31]. However, in MM there is still an ongoing controversy with respect to the phenotype of MM-CSC. Thus, some authors have suggested that MM-CSC are CD138 negative [9,10,11], whereas others have demonstrated the existence of CD138 positive plasma cells with stem cell properties [12,13,14,32]. Traditionally, a better understanding of cancer stem cell properties has been possible, in part, by analyzing cell lines obtained from different types of tumors [33,34,35]. Here, we investigated in a panel of eight MM cell lines for the presence of a $CD138^{low/-}$ population and we analyzed its biological characteristics. As previously suggested by other authors [9,16,36,37] we confirmed that all cell lines contain a minor subpopulation of $CD138^{low}$ cells. However, it has been recently described that infraexpression of CD138 in MM cells may be an artifact due to apoptotic induction [17]. Our results show that the $CD138^{low}$ subpopulation is viable as demonstrated by DAPI-nuclear as well as Annexin-V/7ADD staining.

The presence of $CD138^{low/-}$ cells in myeloma is intriguing because it could imply a less differentiated state. In fact, it has been previously reported that the interaction of myeloma cells with different types of cells of the bone marrow microenvironment promotes a reduction of CD138 expression, a less differentiated morphology and an increase of the B-cell associated transcription factor, Bcl6 [15,16,38]. Here, we have detected the presence of myeloma cells with low expression of CD138 in the absence of bone marrow microenvironment cells and under these circumstances, the population of $CD138^{low}$ cells does not seem to represent a more immature compartment since it does not express the B-cell associated markers CD19, CD20 and CD27 and it does not show a less differentiated morphology. Moreover, VDJH rearrangement analysis, CNA analysis and gene expression profiling did not show relevant differences between $CD138^{++}$ and $CD138^{low}$ cells. In fact, the absence of substantial differences in the gene expression profiling of both populations has also been revealed using single molecule microarray in a recent study [39]. Furthermore, the higher or lower surface expression of CD138 in MM cells seems to be regulated at the protein rather than transcriptional level, as demonstrated by similar CD138 mRNA levels found in the two subpopulations. It should be noted that our *in vitro* and *in vivo* results demonstrate the bidirectional origin of the two populations since $CD138^{++}$ cells give rise to $CD138^{low}$ cells and *vice versa*. These data suggest a dynamic between the two phenotypic subpopulations that tend to equilibrium, and could be responsible of the heterogeneity typically found in MM cells, as previously demonstrated through statistical modeling in breast cancer cell lines [33]. In fact, it has been demonstrated in myeloma patient samples the presence of interconvertible phenotypic and functional states responsible of myeloma-propagating activity and drug resistance [40].

Apart from the immature phenotype, other hallmarks of normal and cancer stem cells are quiescence, chemoresistance and potential to self-renew [41,42]. Here, we have compared the cell cycle of $CD138^{++}$ and $CD138^{low}$ cells and found that none of them is quiescent as demonstrated by a considerable percentage of cells ($\geq$25%) in the proliferative phases (S and G2-M) of the cell cycle. This was further confirmed by substantial expression of the proliferation-associated marker Ki-67. Nevertheless, we observed a numerically -not significantly- lower percentage of cells in G2-M phase in $CD138^{low}$ cells as compared to the $CD138^{++}$ fraction that could be the cause of the lower number of clones expanded *in vitro* from the $CD138^{low}$ subpopulation. These results are in line with previous data by Fuhler and col. in RPMI-8226 cells [16], but differ from those by Matsui and col. who found that the CD138 negative subpopulation within RPMI-8226 and NCI-H929 cell lines is mainly quiescent (>98% cells in G0–G1) [10], but paradoxically express higher levels of Ki-67 than CD138 positive cells [9]. The proliferation rate of $CD138^{+}$ and $CD138^{-}$ myeloma cells has also been described in primary patient samples with discordant results. Reid and col. observed a higher proliferation rate of $CD38^{++}CD138^{-}$ myeloma cells as compared with $CD38^{++}CD138^{+}$ myeloma cells [43], whereas Chaidos and col. identified a so-called pre-plasma cell compartment ($CD38^{++}CD138^{-}$) that is relatively quiescent [40].

The chemoresistance of cancer stem cells is mainly associated to their specific properties such as quiescence [28], expression of multidrug resistance efflux pumps [44] and expression of detoxifying enzymes [45]. Here, we investigated the expression of the detoxifying enzyme ALDH and, in contrast to previous observations [10], we have not found higher ALDH expression in $CD138^{low}$ cells as compared to $CD138^{++}$ cells. Moreover, $CD138^{++}$ and $CD138^{low}$ RPMI-8226 cells displayed similar sensitivity to different antimyeloma drugs. Overall, these results indicate that the $CD138^{low}$ subpopulation within myeloma cell lines does not represent a specific chemoresistant compartment. In fact, our results support recent data by Jakubikova and col. who found a lack of correlation between the drug resistant "side population" and $CD138^{-/low}$ subpopulations in MM cell lines [37].

As previously mentioned, the potential to self-renew is another hallmark of stem cells [41,42]. This specific property is linked to the potential of stem cells to serially engraft into immunocompromised mice [46]. In MM, the first evidence of self-renewal pointed to the capacity of circulating cells to engraft into NOD-SCID mice [47]. Nevertheless, later studies have been controversial, with some authors demonstrating the tumorigenic potential of post-germinal center memory B-cells [9,10] while others of MM plasma cells [12,14,32,40,48,49,50]. Here, we demonstrated in a serial transplantation assay in SCID mice that both $CD138^{++}$ and $CD138^{low}$ RPMI-8226 cells have tumorigenic and self-renewal potential. These results are in line with previous studies in which the tumorigenic potential of $CD19^{-}CD38^{+}CD138^{+}$ and $CD19^{-}CD38^{+}CD138^{-}$ primary plasma cells was compared and both populations were able to engraft into immunocompromised mice [32,40].

In conclusion, our results show that the minor $CD138^{low}$ subpopulation in MM cell lines does not represent an immature B-cell compartment and has similar genomic and functional profile as compared to the major $CD138^{++}$ fraction. Both $CD138^{++}$ and $CD138^{low}$ subpopulations have self-renewal potential, similar drug sensitivity and are phenotypically interconvertible. Therefore, these results highlight the need to explore new and more reliable markers able to discriminate true clonogenic myeloma cells.

Supporting Information

Figure S1 Gating strategy for sorting $CD138^{++}$ and $CD138^{low}$ subpopulations in RPMI-8226 cells. Top panel: viable cells were gated as $7AAD^{-ve}$ (R1) and subsequently debris were eliminated by scatter properties (R2). Finally, the lowest and highest 5% CD138-expressing cells were gated on R2. Bottom panel: $CD138^{++}$ and $CD138^{low}$ sorted cells had a final purity >95% in the post-sort analysis.

Figure S2 Morphology of $CD138^{++}$ and $CD138^{low}$ RPMI-8226 cells. May-Grünwald-Giemsa staining of sorted $CD138^{++}$ and $CD138^{low}$ RPMI-8226 cells. Scale bar = 10 μm.

Figure S3 Analysis of apoptosis in $CD138^{++}$ and $CD138^{low}$ subpopulations in RPMI-8226, NCI-H929,

MM1S and U266 cell lines. Non-apoptotic cells were gated as annexin-V^{-ve}/7AAD^{-ve} (R1) and subsequently debris were eliminated by scatter properties (R2). The third dot plot for every MM cell line corresponding to R2 shows the percentage of CD138^{low} cells.

Acknowledgments

We are grateful to Dr. W. S. Dalton (Moffitt Cancer Center, Tampa, FL) for providing the RPMI-8226, U266, RPMI-LR5, U266-LR7 and U266-Dox4 cell lines, to Dr. S. T. Rosen (Northwestern University, Chicago, IL) for providing the MM1S and MM1R cell lines and to Dr. J. Teixidó (Centro de Investigaciones Biológicas, Madrid, Spain) for providing the NCI-H929 cell line.

Author Contributions

Conceived and designed the experiments: TP EMO JFSM. Performed the experiments: TP MES BP PK LSS AR MG. Analyzed the data: TP MES BP PK LAC AR RGS NCG EMO. Contributed reagents/materials/analysis tools: TP MES BP LAC RGS NCG EMO JFSM. Wrote the paper: TP MES BP PK RGS NCG EMO JFSM.

References

1. San-Miguel JF, Mateos MV (2011) Can multiple myeloma become a curable disease? Haematologica 96: 1246–1248.
2. Hamburger A, Salmon SE (1977) Primary bioassay of human myeloma stem cells. J Clin Invest 60: 846–854.
3. Chilosi M, Adami F, Lestani M, Montagna L, Cimarosto L, et al. (1999) CD138/syndecan-1: a useful immunohistochemical marker of normal and neoplastic plasma cells on routine trephine bone marrow biopsies. Mod Pathol 12: 1101–1106.
4. Wei A, Juneja S (2003) Bone marrow immunohistology of plasma cell neoplasms. J Clin Pathol 56: 406–411.
5. Wijdenes J, Vooijs WC, Clement C, Post J, Morard F, et al. (1996) A plasmocyte selective monoclonal antibody (B-B4) recognizes syndecan-1. Br J Haematol 94: 318–323.
6. Jego G, Robillard N, Puthier D, Amiot M, Accard F, et al. (1999) Reactive plasmacytoses are expansions of plasmablasts retaining the capacity to differentiate into plasma cells. Blood 94: 701–712.
7. Jego G, Bataille R, Pellat-Deceunynck C (2001) Interleukin-6 is a growth factor for nonmalignant human plasmablasts. Blood 97: 1817–1822.
8. Calame KL (2001) Plasma cells: finding new light at the end of B cell development. Nat Immunol 2: 1103–1108.
9. Matsui W, Huff CA, Wang Q, Malehorn MT, Barber J, et al. (2004) Characterization of clonogenic multiple myeloma cells. Blood 103: 2332–2336.
10. Matsui W, Wang Q, Barber JP, Brennan S, Smith BD, et al. (2008) Clonogenic multiple myeloma progenitors, stem cell properties, and drug resistance. Cancer Res 68: 190–197.
11. Boucher K, Parquet N, Widen R, Shain K, Baz R, et al. (2012) Stemness of B-cell progenitors in multiple myeloma bone marrow. Clin Cancer Res 18: 6155–6168.
12. Yata K, Yaccoby S (2004) The SCID-rab model: a novel in vivo system for primary human myeloma demonstrating growth of CD138-expressing malignant cells. Leukemia 18: 1891–1897.
13. Chiron D, Surget S, Maiga S, Bataille R, Moreau P, et al. (2012) The peripheral CD138+ population but not the CD138- population contains myeloma clonogenic cells in plasma cell leukaemia patients. Br J Haematol 156: 679–683.
14. Kim D, Park CY, Medeiros BC, Weissman IL (2012) CD19-CD45 low/- CD38 high/CD138+ plasma cells enrich for human tumorigenic myeloma cells. Leukemia 26: 2530–2537.
15. Kukreja A, Hutchinson A, Dhodapkar K, Mazumder A, Vesole D, et al. (2006) Enhancement of clonogenicity of human multiple myeloma by dendritic cells. J Exp Med 203: 1859–1865.
16. Fuhler GM, Baanstra M, Chesik D, Somasundaram R, Seckinger A, et al. (2010) Bone marrow stromal cell interaction reduces syndecan-1 expression and induces kinomic changes in myeloma cells. Exp Cell Res 316: 1816–1828.
17. Christensen JH, Jensen PV, Kristensen IB, Abildgaard N, Lodahl M, et al. (2012) Characterization of potential CD138 negative myeloma "stem cells". Haematologica 97: e18–20.
18. Greenstein S, Krett NL, Kurosawa Y, Ma C, Chauhan D, et al. (2003) Characterization of the MM.1 human multiple myeloma (MM) cell lines: a model system to elucidate the characteristics, behavior, and signaling of steroid-sensitive and -resistant MM cells. Exp Hematol 31: 271–282.
19. Sanz-Rodriguez F, Ruiz-Velasco N, Pascual-Salcedo D, Teixido J (1999) Characterization of VLA-4-dependent myeloma cell adhesion to fibronectin and VCAM-1. Br J Haematol 107: 825–834.
20. Chen Q, Van der Sluis PC, Boulware D, Hazlehurst LA, Dalton WS (2005) The FA/BRCA pathway is involved in melphalan-induced DNA interstrand cross-link repair and accounts for melphalan resistance in multiple myeloma cells. Blood 106: 698–705.
21. Ma MH, Yang HH, Parker K, Manyak S, Friedman JM, et al. (2003) The proteasome inhibitor PS-341 markedly enhances sensitivity of multiple myeloma tumor cells to chemotherapeutic agents. Clin Cancer Res 9: 1136–1144.
22. Paiva B, Perez-Andres M, Vidriales MB, Almeida J, de las Heras N, et al. (2011) Competition between clonal plasma cells and normal cells for potentially overlapping bone marrow niches is associated with a progressively altered cellular distribution in MGUS vs myeloma. Leukemia 25: 697–706.
23. Carvajal-Vergara X, Tabera S, Montero JC, Esparis-Ogando A, Lopez-Perez R, et al. (2005) Multifunctional role of Erk5 in multiple myeloma. Blood 105: 4492–4499.
24. Gutierrez NC, Lopez-Perez R, Hernandez JM, Isidro I, Gonzalez B, et al. (2005) Gene expression profile reveals deregulation of genes with relevant functions in the different subclasses of acute myeloid leukemia. Leukemia 19: 402–409.
25. van Dongen JJ, Langerak AW, Bruggemann M, Evans PA, Hummel M, et al. (2003) Design and standardization of PCR primers and protocols for detection of clonal immunoglobulin and T-cell receptor gene recombinations in suspect lymphoproliferations: report of the BIOMED-2 Concerted Action BMH4-CT98-3936. Leukemia 17: 2257–2317.
26. Ocio EM, Maiso P, Chen X, Garayoa M, Alvarez-Fernandez S, et al. (2009) Zalypsis: a novel marine-derived compound with potent antimyeloma activity that reveals high sensitivity of malignant plasma cells to DNA double-strand breaks. Blood 113: 3781–3791.
27. Zhou S, Schuetz JD, Bunting KD, Colapietro AM, Sampath J, et al. (2001) The ABC transporter Bcrp1/ABCG2 is expressed in a wide variety of stem cells and is a molecular determinant of the side-population phenotype. Nat Med 7: 1028–1034.
28. Li L, Bhatia R (2011) Stem cell quiescence. Clin Cancer Res 17: 4936–4941.
29. Charafe-Jauffret E, Ginestier C, Iovino F, Wicinski J, Cervera N, et al. (2009) Breast cancer cell lines contain functional cancer stem cells with metastatic capacity and a distinct molecular signature. Cancer Res 69: 1302–1313.
30. Bharadwaj S, Liu G, Shi Y, Wu R, Yang B, et al. (2013) Multi-Potential Differentiation of Human Urine-Derived Stem Cells: Potential for Therapeutic Applications in Urology. Stem Cells 31:1840–56
31. Bonnet D, Dick JE (1997) Human acute myeloid leukemia is organized as a hierarchy that originates from a primitive hematopoietic cell. Nat Med 3: 730–737.
32. Hosen N, Matsuoka Y, Kishida S, Nakata J, Mizutani Y, et al. (2012) CD138-negative clonogenic cells are plasma cells but not B cells in some multiple myeloma patients. Leukemia 26: 2135–2141.
33. Gupta PB, Fillmore CM, Jiang G, Shapira SD, Tao K, et al. (2011) Stochastic state transitions give rise to phenotypic equilibrium in populations of cancer cells. Cell 146: 633–644.
34. Li H, Chen X, Calhoun-Davis T, Claypool K, Tang DG (2008) PC3 human prostate carcinoma cell holoclones contain self-renewing tumor-initiating cells. Cancer Res 68: 1820–1825.
35. Roesch A, Fukunaga-Kalabis M, Schmidt EC, Zabierowski SE, Brafford PA, et al. (2010) A temporarily distinct subpopulation of slow-cycling melanoma cells is required for continuous tumor growth. Cell 141: 583–594.
36. Spisek R, Kukreja A, Chen LC, Matthews P, Mazumder A, et al. (2007) Frequent and specific immunity to the embryonal stem cell-associated antigen SOX2 in patients with monoclonal gammopathy. J Exp Med 204: 831–840.
37. Jakubikova J, Adamia S, Kost-Alimova M, Klippel S, Cervi D, et al. (2011) Lenalidomide targets clonogenic side population in multiple myeloma: pathophysiologic and clinical implications. Blood 117: 4409–4419.
38. Yaccoby S (2005) The phenotypic plasticity of myeloma plasma cells as expressed by dedifferentiation into an immature, resilient, and apoptosis-resistant phenotype. Clin Cancer Res 11: 7599–7606.
39. Jacak J, Schnidar H, Muresan L, Regl G, Frischauf A, et al. (2013) Expression analysis of multiple myeloma CD138 negative progenitor cells using single molecule microarray readout. J Biotechnol 164: 525–530.
40. Chaidos A, Barnes CP, Cowan G, May PC, Melo V, et al. (2013) Clinical drug resistance linked to interconvertible phenotypic and functional states of tumor-propagating cells in multiple myeloma. Blood 121: 318–328.
41. Reya T, Morrison SJ, Clarke MF, Weissman IL (2001) Stem cells, cancer, and cancer stem cells. Nature 414: 105–111.
42. Nguyen LV, Vanner R, Dirks P, Eaves CJ (2012) Cancer stem cells: an evolving concept. Nat Rev Cancer 12: 133–143.
43. Reid S, Yang S, Brown R, Kabani K, Aklilu E, et al. (2010) Characterisation and relevance of CD138-negative plasma cells in plasma cell myeloma. Int J Lab Hematol 32: e190–196.
44. Wulf GG, Wang RY, Kuehnle I, Weidner D, Marini F, et al. (2001) A leukemic stem cell with intrinsic drug efflux capacity in acute myeloid leukemia. Blood 98: 1166–1173.

45. Luo Y, Dallaglio K, Chen Y, Robinson WA, Robinson SE, et al. (2012) ALDH1A isozymes are markers of human melanoma stem cells and potential therapeutic targets. Stem Cells 30: 2100–2113.
46. Dick JE (1996) Human stem cell assays in immune-deficient mice. Curr Opin Hematol 3: 405–409.
47. Pilarski LM, Hipperson G, Seeberger K, Pruski E, Coupland RW, et al. (2000) Myeloma progenitors in the blood of patients with aggressive or minimal disease: engraftment and self-renewal of primary human myeloma in the bone marrow of NOD SCID mice. Blood 95: 1056–1065.
48. Van Valckenborgh E, Matsui W, Agarwal P, Lub S, Dehui X, et al. (2012) Tumor-initiating capacity of CD138- and CD138+ tumor cells in the 5T33 multiple myeloma model. Leukemia 26: 1436–1439.
49. Paino T, Ocio EM, Paiva B, San-Segundo L, Garayoa M, et al. (2012) CD20 positive cells are undetectable in the majority of multiple myeloma cell lines and are not associated with a cancer stem cell phenotype. Haematologica 97: 1110–1114.
50. Paino T, Paiva B, San Miguel J (2013) Reply to "Response to"CD20 positive cells are undetectable in the majority of multiple myeloma cell lines and are not associated with a cancer stem cell phenotype". Haematologica 2012;97(7):1110–1114. Haematologica 98: e10.

17

Dissecting the Regulatory Microenvironment of a Large Animal Model of Non-Hodgkin Lymphoma: Evidence of a Negative Prognostic Impact of FOXP3$^+$ T Cells in Canine B Cell Lymphoma

Dammy Pinheiro[1], Yu-Mei Chang[2], Hannah Bryant[1], Balazs Szladovits[3], Tim Dalessandri[1¤], Lucy J. Davison[4,5], Elizabeth Yallop[6], Emily Mills[6], Chiara Leo[7], Ana Lara[7], Anneliese Stell[7], Gerry Polton[8], Oliver A. Garden[1,7*]

1 Department of Clinical Sciences and Services, Immune Regulation Laboratory, The Royal Veterinary College, London, United Kingdom, **2** Research Office, The Royal Veterinary College, London, United Kingdom, **3** Department of Pathology and Pathogen Biology, The Royal Veterinary College, Hatfield, Hertfordshire, United Kingdom, **4** Henry Wellcome Building, Centre for Cellular and Molecular Physiology, University of Oxford, Oxford, United Kingdom, **5** Department of Veterinary Medicine, University of Cambridge, Cambridge, United Kingdom, **6** Clinical Investigation Centre, The Royal Veterinary College, Hatfield, Hertfordshire, United Kingdom, **7** Department of Clinical Sciences and Services, Queen Mother Hospital for Animals, The Royal Veterinary College, Hatfield, Hertfordshire, United Kingdom, **8** Oncology Service, North Downs Specialist Referrals, Bletchingley, Surrey, United Kingdom

Abstract

The cancer microenvironment plays a pivotal role in oncogenesis, containing a number of regulatory cells that attenuate the anti-neoplastic immune response. While the negative prognostic impact of regulatory T cells (Tregs) in the context of most solid tissue tumors is well established, their role in lymphoid malignancies remains unclear. T cells expressing FOXP3 and Helios were documented in the fine needle aspirates of affected lymph nodes of dogs with spontaneous multicentric B cell lymphoma (BCL), proposed to be a model for human non-Hodgkin lymphoma. Multivariable analysis revealed that the frequency of lymph node FOXP3$^+$ T cells was an independent negative prognostic factor, impacting both progression-free survival (hazard ratio 1.10; $p = 0.01$) and overall survival (hazard ratio 1.61; $p = 0.01$) when comparing dogs showing higher than the median FOXP3 expression with those showing the median value of FOXP3 expression or less. Taken together, these data suggest the existence of a population of Tregs operational in canine multicentric BCL that resembles thymic Tregs, which we speculate are co-opted by the tumor from the periphery. We suggest that canine multicentric BCL represents a robust large animal model of human diffuse large BCL, showing clinical, cytological and immunophenotypic similarities with the disease in man, allowing comparative studies of immunoregulatory mechanisms.

Editor: Kristy L. Richards, University of North Carolina at Chapel Hill, United States of America

Funding: This work was generously funded by the Petplan Charitable Trust, grant number 10–19, URL: http://www.petplantrust.org/. LJD is supported by a Wellcome Trust Veterinary Postdoctoral Fellowship (WT/096398/Z/11/Z). The funders had no role in the study design, data collection and analysis, decision to publish, or preparation of the manuscript.

Competing Interests: GP is affiliated with a private practice (North Downs Specialist Referrals).

* Email: ogarden@rvc.ac.uk

¤ Current address: Department of Medicine, Imperial College London, London, United Kingdom

Introduction

Non-Hodgkin lymphoma (NHL), a heterogeneous group of lymphoid malignancies [1,2], is the eleventh most common cause of death from cancer in humans worldwide, estimated to be responsible for approximately 192,000 deaths in 2008 alone [3]. Despite advances in therapy in recent years, five-year survival rates are as low as 25% for the more aggressive subtypes of NHL [3]. There is thus an urgent need to develop novel, targeted therapies for this group of diseases, driven by advances in our understanding of their pathogenesis and specific prognosis. Current rodent models of lymphoma are far from predictive of the natural course of the human disease, relying either on the subcutaneous implantation of xenogeneic lymphoma cells into immune-compromised mice, or on genetic manipulations that artificially increase the likelihood of lymphoma in a monogenic fashion [4]. Key to advancing the field will be the development of natural, polygenic animal models of NHL, allowing the further interrogation of molecular and cellular pathogenesis, as well as trials of novel anti-cancer agents. The dog has gained traction in recent years as a model for a number of human diseases, including various malignancies [5–8]. Its spontaneous development of mesenchymal, epithelial and round cell tumors, relatively short lifespan, and cohabitation of our environment, as well as the availability of advanced diagnostic and therapeutic modalities that are similar to those available in human oncology clinics, all make this species attractive as a model for cancer research [7,9,10].

Furthermore, the most prevalent subtype of canine lymphoma, diffuse large (DL) BCL, mirrors the most common form of NHL [11], and various studies suggest that the molecular pathogenesis of DLBCL in the two species is fundamentally similar [12–15].

One of the key pathogenic determinants in oncogenesis is the cancer microenvironment [16–20]. Interactions with stromal and immune cells and extracellular matrix components conspire to inhibit anti-neoplastic immune responses, allowing the cancer to grow and metastasize. Central among such cellular interactions are those occurring with Tregs, of which the thymic subset is generally identified by its expression of the Forkhead box transcription factor FOXP3 in addition to the classical markers CD4 and CD25^{high} [21]. While the negative prognostic impact of FOXP3^{+} Tregs in various solid tumors of both mesenchymal and epithelial origin has been well documented [22,23], these cells have also been associated with a favorable outcome in certain solid tumors [24,25] and their role in the pathogenesis of lymphoid malignancies is much less clear [26]. Some papers suggest that intra-tumoral Tregs predict a negative outcome in human lymphoma [27–31], while others suggest that they may have a beneficial effect [32–40]; yet others propose that they have neither a positive nor a negative prognostic impact [41]. The situation is further complicated by the presence of more than one subset of Treg – including both thymic and peripheral IL-10-secreting (Tr1) phenotypes – and interactions with other cells with suppressive properties, including myeloid-derived suppressor cells, natural killer T (NKT) cells and tolerogenic dendritic cells [42–45].

While a number of recent studies have added weight to the suggestion that lymphoma in the dog closely resembles human NHL [12–15], very little is known about the role of Tregs in canine BCL. We and others have recently characterised FOXP3^{+} Tregs in the dog [46], demonstrating that they have similar properties to those of human Tregs; we were thus optimally poised to interrogate their role in various canine diseases, including lymphoma. The aim of the present study was therefore to document the presence of FOXP3^{+} Tregs in the resident T cell population of affected lymph nodes of dogs with B cell lymphoma (BCL) and to test the hypothesis that intra-tumoral CD4^{+}FOXP3^{+} Tregs have a negative impact on treatment outcome, making comparisons with dogs with T cell lymphoma (TCL), non-neoplastic causes of lymphadenomegaly, and metastatic mast cell tumors (MCTs). Our goal was to advance our understanding of the pathogenesis of canine BCL, thus further validating this spontaneous, naturally occurring disease as a large animal model of NHL in which to study the role of immunoregulatory pathways.

Materials and Methods

Case accession

Dogs were recruited to this study from four different veterinary practices, three located in the UK and one in Sweden. Complete clinical histories were obtained from every dog. Diagnostic investigations appropriate to the presenting complaints were undertaken in all dogs, including cytological and, or histopathological review of enlarged lymph nodes by a board-certified veterinary pathologist. Standard clinical staging was undertaken by means of thoracic radiographs or computed tomography; abdominal ultrasound examination; fine needle aspirates (FNAs) of the liver and spleen when sonographic lesions of these organs were identified; and bone marrow aspirates when prompted by peripheral cytopenias. Stages IV and V were thus assigned with the caveat that aspirates of the liver, spleen and bone marrow were not undertaken in every dog. Study samples comprised blood collected by venepuncture of a peripheral vein into EDTA and serum gel tubes, and three to four fine needle aspirates (FNAs) of a representative, enlarged lymph node deposited into neat fetal bovine serum (PAA Laboratories Ltd, Yeovil, UK) for flow cytometry. Staining of cells for flow cytometry was performed within 48 hours of sample collection, followed by acquisition of the fixed cells within a further 72 hours. (Pilot studies had established that the immunophenotype of samples remained stable up to 48 hours after sample collection.) Serum was harvested within two hours of sample collection and was stored at a temperature of − 20°C until analysis.

Twenty-two of the dogs recruited were diagnosed with BCL, whilst the remaining cases were recruited to three different control groups. The first comprised 14 dogs with TCL; the second comprised 14 dogs with reactive hyperplasia (RH) associated with cutaneous inflammation/dermatitis, immune-mediated disease, distant neoplasia (i.e. non-draining lymph nodes were sampled) or systemic infection; while the third comprised six dogs with metastatic MCTs, the samples in these cases having been collected from draining lymph nodes. Flow cytometric analyses of peripheral blood were undertaken in these dogs and a group of 25 healthy control (HC) dogs, which also contributed serum samples. (C-reactive protein and cytokine assays, reported elsewhere, were undertaken on all of the serum samples.) For ethical and legal reasons, lymph node samples could not be obtained from HC dogs. All patient samples were collected by licensed veterinarians in routine diagnostic fashion following written informed consent and all study protocols were approved by the Royal Veterinary College Ethics and Welfare Committee (Permit Number: URN-20101005). None of the dogs suffered any adverse consequences of sample procurement.

Cytomorphological classification

When available, slides of diagnostic specimens were retrieved from the receiving diagnostic laboratories for review by a board-certified clinical pathologist involved in the study (BS) for cytomorphological classification. Cytological features that were recorded in the study are presented in Table S1. Based on these observations and the immunophenotype of the lymphoma, the most likely subtype was deduced – for example, DLBCL – though histopathological review would have been required to confirm such tissue diagnoses.

Flow cytometry

A panel of canine-specific or cross-reactive fluorochrome-conjugated monoclonal antibodies (mAbs) against both extra- and intra-cellular antigens was applied (Table 1). The manufacturer's protocol for FOXP3 staining was applied. Briefly, lymphocytes were washed and stained with mAbs for 20 minutes on ice. Lymphocytes were then washed and incubated overnight in a 1:4 (concentrate:diluent) fixation/permeabilization solution. Following incubation, the lymphocytes were washed twice and then stained with mAbs against intracellular antigens for 30 minutes on ice. All incubations were carried out in the dark. Upon completion, lymphocytes were washed twice and re-suspended in 200 μl phosphate buffered saline (PBS) solution. Isotype control antibodies were used to define gates in all experiments. Three-colour staining was used throughout the study, T cells identified in a panel comprising mAbs against CD5 and FOXP3 with CD4, CD8 or Helios. Data were acquired using a FACS Canto II flow cytometer (BD Biosciences) and were analyzed using Flowjo (Tree Star Inc) software.

Table 1. Staining antibodies, isotype controls and fluorochromes.

Antigen	Clone	Isotype	Fluorochrome	Supplier
CD5	YKIX322.3	Rat IgG2a	FITC/PE	AbD Serotec, UK
CD4	YKIX302.9	Rat IgG2a	FITC/PE	AbD Serotec, UK
CD8	YCATE55.9	Rat IgG1	FITC/PE	AbD Serotec, UK
CD79b	AT107-2	Rat IgG1	FITC	AbD Serotec, UK
CD21	CA2.1D6	Mouse IgG1	PE	AbD Serotec, UK
CD34	1H6	Mouse IgG1	PE	AbD Serotec, UK
FOXP3	FJK-16s	Rat IgG2a	APC	eBioscience, UK
Helios	22F6	Armenian hamster IgG	PE	Biolegend, UK

Abbreviations: FITC, fluorescein isothiocyanate; PE, phycoerythrin; APC, allophycocyanin.

Immunophenotypic determination

A threshold of 60% marker expression was used to classify patient samples as being of either a B or T cell phenotype, adopting a previously validated diagnostic protocol [47]. This threshold was applied to the 30% of largest events following removal of dead cells and debris by appropriate gating, as determined by forward and side scatter characteristics (Figure 1). Where at least 60% of cells expressed CD21 or CD79b, a classification of BCL was made. Conversely, when at least 60% of cells expressed CD5, CD4 or CD8 a classification of TCL was made. To further interrogate the composition of cell populations in FNAs, an 'All' gate was applied, which again excluded dead events. Non-neoplastic and neoplastic populations of cells within the BCL FNAs were then evaluated on the basis of CD5 expression, which was limited to the resident (non-neoplastic) T cells in the majority of such cases. An equivalent strategy was applied to both the RH and MCT groups; however, TCL samples were excluded from this analysis owing to CD5 expression by both neoplastic and non-neoplastic cells, which precluded distinction of the two populations within the aspirated cells. In all cases, the expression of CD34 in peripheral blood was negligible, ruling out leukemia.

Clinical definitions and statistical analysis

The following outcome metrics were derived from patient records and communications with the clinicians involved in this study: time to remission (TTR), progression-free survival (PFS) and overall survival (OS). These parameters were determined following assessment of the response to therapy using Veterinary Cooperative Oncology Group-approved definitions of complete response (CR), partial response (PR), stable disease (SD) and progressive disease (PD) applied to peripheral lymph nodes measured by the attending clinicians [48].

Comparisons between two groups of continuous data were undertaken using Mann-Whitney U tests and for three or more groups using Kruskal-Wallis tests. Summary data are presented in the text in the following format: median, range [lowest to highest value], number of cases or experimental repeats (n); p value. Summary data are presented in the form of box plots, in which the boxes show the respective 25th and 75th percentiles, the horizontal lines median values, and the whiskers, the lowest and highest data points still within 1.5 times the interquartile range of the respective lower and upper quartiles. Dots represent the data from individual dogs. Red symbols correspond to data from dogs 'pre-treated' with corticosteroids or any chemotherapeutic drug within three weeks of sampling. In the case of RH cases, square symbols represent data from dogs with *dermatitis*; diamonds represent data from dogs with *distant neoplasia*; triangles represent data from dogs with *immune-mediated disease*; and inverted triangles represent data from dogs with *systemic infection*.

Survival analysis of the dogs with lymphoma was performed using Cox's proportional hazards regression and presented in the form of Kaplan-Meier curves. Continuous variables were categorised to produce the Kaplan-Meier curves using the median value as a threshold. Both univariable and multivariable analyses were undertaken. Criteria for inclusion of variables into the multivariable model included significance at the level of univariable analysis, lack of overlap of the respective survival curves, and constancy of the risk (hazard) with time. Only the BCL cases were analyzed as a separate group for the prognostic impact of phenotypic variables; there were too few TCL cases to make survival analysis of phenotypic variables of this group meaningful. Dogs that failed to go into complete remission were censored for TTR analysis; those that did not show progression, including death, at the last known follow-up time point were censored for PFS analysis; and those that were still alive at the last known follow-up time point were censored for OS analysis. Rescue therapy was not a criterion for censorship in the OS analysis.

Results

Clinical and immunophenotypic details of cases and controls

A total of 22 BCL, 14 TCL, 14 RH, six MCT and 25 HC dogs were recruited into the study. A summary of the signalment and clinical details of the BCL, TCL, RH, MCT and HC cases is presented in Table 2; further details are presented in Tables S2 to S5.

Comparing the BCL, TCL, RH and MCT dogs, there was no significant difference in age ($p = 0.51$), sex ($p = 0.14$), neutering status ($p = 0.27$), bodyweight ($p = 0.09$) or body condition ($p = 0.86$) between the groups. The BCL dogs tended to be of higher stage (III 41%, IV 32%, V 27%) than the TCL (II 7%, III 79%, IV 14%; $p = 0.02$), but there was no difference in sub-stage between the groups ($p = 1.00$). In common with the prevailing literature, TCL dogs were more commonly hypercalcemic (4/13; 31%) than BCL (1/22, 4.5%; $p = 0.05$). Among the lymphoma dogs, the cytomorphological characteristics when considered alongside immunophenotype were most commonly consistent with DLBCL (11/22; 50%) and peripheral TCL (8/14, 57%; Table 2, Figure S1). The most common chemotherapy protocol in both BCL and TCL dogs was CHOP, comprising cyclophospha-

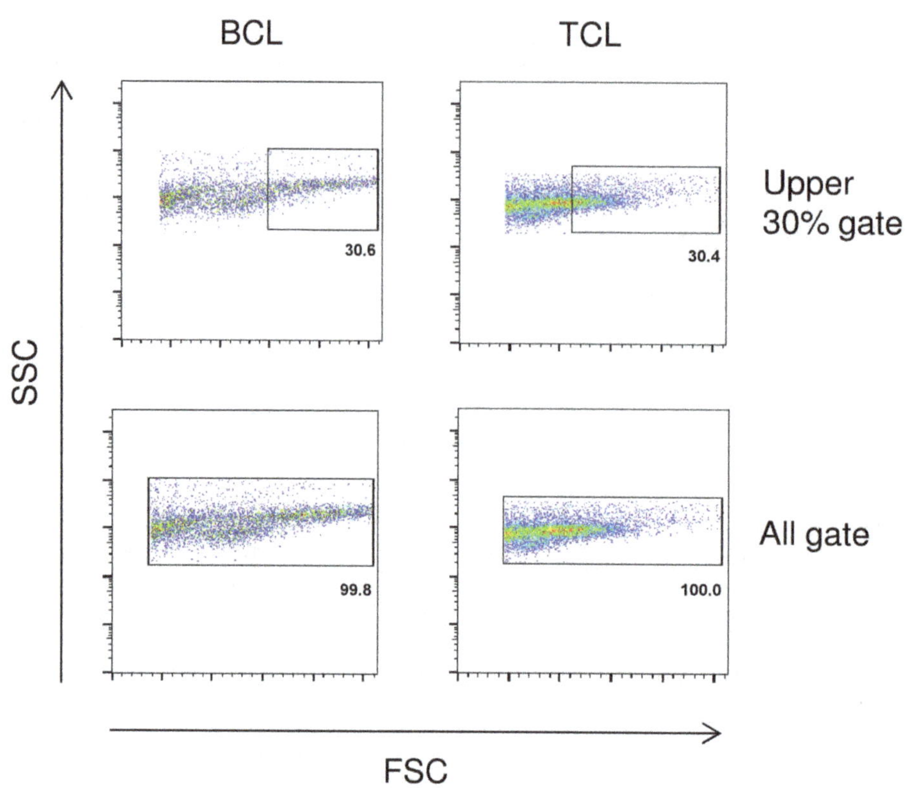

Figure 1. Gating strategies used to interrogate the neoplastic and non-neoplastic cell populations. Following exclusion of dead cells and debris, two different gating strategies were employed to evaluate the cells isolated from lymph node aspirates. For the purposes of generating an immunophenotyping profile, an upper 30% gate was applied to identify the population of largest events, enriched in neoplastic cells. The immunophenotype was then determined using a 60% expression threshold within this population. For the purposes of evaluating frequencies of T cells within fine needle aspirates of B cell lymphoma (BCL), reactive hyperplasia (RH) and mast cell tumour (MCT) cases, an 'All' gate was applied and then the populations subsequently delineated by means of CD5 expression. Non-neoplastic cells were identified as $CD5^+$ and neoplastic populations $CD5^-$ in the context of BCL; TCL cases were excluded from such comparisons on account of their CD5 expression by both neoplastic and non-neoplastic cells.

mide, doxorubicin, vincristine and prednisolone (Tables 1, S2 and S3).

Treatment of the BCL and TCL dogs with a corticosteroid or any cytotoxic chemotherapeutic drugs within three weeks of sampling was considered a confounding factor, since such drugs may theoretically alter the frequency of peripheral Tregs. Of the BCL cases, 9/21 (43%) dogs had been 'pre-treated' in this way, compared to 5/13 (38%) of the TCL cases. (In each respective BCL and TCL group, one dog received no treatment at all.) Phenotypic characteristics of the pre-treated dogs were no different from those that had not received such drugs prior to sampling (BCL, $p>0.05$; TCL, $p>0.05$) and pre-treatment had no impact on outcome variables (TTR: BCL, $p=0.58$; TCL, $p=0.46$; PFS: BCL, $p=0.30$; TCL, $p=0.11$; OS: BCL, $p=0.28$; TCL, $p=0.91$). The pre-treated and treatment-naïve groups were therefore considered as a single group in respective BCL and TCL cases. A complete response to chemotherapy was achieved in 17/21 (81%) of the BCL cases and in 8/13 (62%) of the TCL cases. Thus, four of the BCL and five of the TCL dogs were censored from TTR analysis. One dog in each lymphoma group was censored from PFS analysis, while five BCL and two TCL dogs were censored from OS analysis. Comparing the BCL with TCL groups, there was no difference in TTR (BCL: median 20 days *versus* TCL: median 27 days; $p=0.09$), PFS (BCL: median 117 days *versus* TCL: median 63 days; $p=0.47$) or OS (BCL: median 294 days *versus* TCL: median 151 days; $p=0.21$). In the case of the BCL group, older dogs had shorter PFS (median 74 days) than younger dogs (median 174 days; $p=0.006$) and dogs treated with CHOP had longer PFS (median 175 days) than those treated with the other protocols (median 45 days; $p=0.01$) (Figure S2). Rescue therapy, which was unstandardized, was administered to 10 of the BCL dogs and nine of the TCL dogs (Tables S2 and S3). In the case of both the BCL and TCL groups, dogs receiving rescue therapy had longer OS than those not receiving it (BCL: median OS 322 days *versus* 174 days respectively, $p=0.049$; TCL: median OS 230 days *versus* 9.5 days respectively, $p=0.008$; combined BCL+TCL: 294 days *versus* 102 days respectively, $p=0.013$). There was no association with prognosis in either the BCL or the TCL groups for sex, neutering status, body weight, body condition, stage, substage or presence of hypercalcemia (in all cases $p>0.05$).

Neoplastic effacement of normal lymphoid tissue impacts FOXP3, Helios and CD8 expression, but the ratio of cytotoxic to regulatory T cells is not decreased in canine B cell lymphoma

The median frequency of $FOXP3^+$ cells within the whole population of cells harvested by fine needle aspiration, identified by the 'All' gate, was significantly lower in BCL (1.1% [0.16%–

Table 2. Clinical, cytological and treatment details of dogs in the study.

		B cell lymphoma	T cell lymphoma	Reactive hyperplasia	Mast cell tumor	Healthy control dogs
Age (months)[1]	Median (range)	113 (33–171)	93 (58–163)	108 (15–156)	138 (84–176)	55 (19–324)
Sex	Me	6	4	1	0	2
	Mn	7	3	6	0	11
	Fe	4	1	1	1	2
	Fn	5	6	6	5	10
Breed		Labrador retriever (n = 2); Afghan hound, Australian silky, Bernese mountain dog, Border collie, bullmastiff, cocker spaniel, Doberman, English springer spaniel, flat-coated retriever, German shepherd dog, golden retriever, Jack Russell terrier, Shar pei, Shetland sheepdog, shih tzu, spaniel cross, Staffordshire bull terrier, Tibetan terrier, undefined cross breed, West Highland white terrier (all n = 1)	Boxer (n = 4); Labrador retriever (n = 3); cocker spaniel (n = 2); Border collie, Dogue de Bordeaux, English springer spaniel, golden retriever, Shetland sheepdog (all n = 1)	Fox terrier (n = 2); Labrador retriever (n = 2); Border collie, cocker spaniel, French bulldog, German shepherd dog, Irish terrier, Jack Russell terrier, Labrador cross, Patterdale terrier, Rottweiler, undefined cross breed (all n = 1)	Golden retriever (n = 2); Labrador retriever (n = 2); Rottweiler, undefined cross breed (all n = 1)	Rhodesian ridgeback (n = 3); Border terrier (n = 2); Jack Russell terrier (n = 2); Labrador retriever (n = 2); whippet (n = 2); greyhound, lurcher, standard poodle, boxer cross, Dogue de Bordeaux, Hungarian vizsla, English springer spaniel, Japanese akita, Labrador/English springer spaniel cross, Staffordshire bull terrier (all n = 1); undefined cross breed (n = 4)
Body condition[2]	Under	4	1	2	0	0
	Optimal	13	9	10	4	24
	Over	5	4	2	2	1
WHO stage	II	0	1	N/A	N/A	N/A
	III	9	11	N/A	N/A	N/A
	IV	7	2	N/A	N/A	N/A
	V	6	0	N/A	N/A	N/A
Sub-stage	a	11	6	N/A	N/A	N/A
	b	11	8	N/A	N/A	N/A
Hyper-calcemic?[3]	No	21	9	N/A	N/A	N/A
	Yes	1	4	N/A	N/A	N/A
Cytological appearance		DLBCL: n = 11; DLBCL or Burkitt-type: n = 2; Undefined: n = 1; Slides not available for review: n = 8	PTCL: n = 8; Small cell: n = 1; T zone: n = 1; Undefined: n = 1; Slides not available for review: n = 3	Reactive lymphoid hyperplasia confirmed in every case	Metastatic mast cell tumor confirmed in every case	N/A
Chemotherapy protocol[4]	CHOP	14	8	Various drugs administered, including antimicrobials, NSAIDs and prednisolone	Various drugs administered, including vinblastine, prednisolone, lomustine, masitinib and toceranib	N/A
	COP	3	1	N/A	N/A	N/A
	Other	3	4	N/A	N/A	N/A
	Pred	1	0	N/A	N/A	N/A
	None	1	1	N/A	N/A	N/A

Abbreviations: Me, entire male; Mn, neutered male; Fe, entire female; Fn, neutered female; WHO, World Health Organization; N/A, not applicable; DLBCL, diffuse large B cell lymphoma; PTCL, peripheral T cell lymphoma; CHOP, cyclophosphamide, doxorubicin, vincristine, prednisolone protocol; COP, cyclophosphamide, vincristine, prednisolone protocol; Pred, prednisolone alone; NSAIDS, non-steroidal anti-inflammatory drugs.

Notes: [1]: Age when presenting signs were first observed. [2]: Body condition score was assessed by different clinicians on either a 5 or 9 point scale: 'under-conditioned' was defined by a score of 1–2/5 or 1–3/9; 'optimal' was defined by a score of 2.5–3/5 or 4–5/9; while 'over-conditioned' was defined by a score of 3.5–5/5 or 6–9/9. [3]: Serum or plasma calcium concentration was not measured in one of the T cell lymphoma cases prior to initiation of therapy. [4]: The initial treatment protocol is listed. 'Other' treatments included cytarabine, L-asparaginase and lomustine (B cell lymphoma) and L-asparaginase, lomustine, prednisolone, masitinib and chlorambucil (T cell lymphoma).

6.01%]; n = 22) and TCL (0.86% [0.01%–5.15%]; n = 14) cases than in both RH (6.06% [0.93%–9.50%]; n = 13) and MCT (5.36% [2.52%–9.57%]; n = 4) cases (p = 0.00005; Figure 2A,B). This was attributed to effacement and thus 'dilution' of normal lymphoid tissue by tumor cells, prompting further examination of FOXP3 expression specifically within the T cell population of BCL, RH and MCT cases. A similarly defined sub-population of non-neoplastic cells could not be delineated in TCLs owing to CD5 expression by the neoplastic cells themselves, precluding such analysis in the TCL cases.

A variable pattern of FOXP3 expression was observed in BCL lymph node aspirates, but there was no overall difference between groups when FOXP3 was examined in either the $CD5^+$ population (BCL: 8.56% [0.77%–18.1%], n = 22; RH: 10.8% [0.37%–18.1%], n = 14; MCT: 9.43% [0.96%–11.7%], n = 4; p = 0.41) or the specific $CD4^+CD5^+$ T cells (BCL: 6.21% [0.57%–17.1%], n = 22; RH: 6.79% [0.38%–13.4%], n = 14; MCT: 9.51% [5.64%–10.6%], n = 4; p = 0.74) within the lymph nodes (Figure 2C,D). Furthermore, there was no overall difference in expression of FOXP3 by PBMCs between groups (BCL: 0.57% [0.05%–5.07%], n = 10; TCL: 0.31% [0.05%–1.96%], n = 9; RH: 0.67% [0.07%–6.67%], n = 5; MCT: 12.04%, n = 1; p = 0.21) (Figure 2E). A similar lack of difference in FOXP3 expression between groups was also apparent when its expression within the $CD5^+$ (BCL: 2.03% [0.25%–9.91%], n = 11; TCL: 4.31% [0.18%–6.48%], n = 8; RH: 4.74% [2.43%–10.30%], n = 6; MCT: 5.9%, n = 1; p = 0.53) or specific $CD4^+CD5^+$ T cell fractions of PBMCs was examined (BCL: 5.29% [0.21%–13.85%], n = 10; TCL: 5.41% [0.258%–16.02%], n = 9; RH: 8.36% [5.23%–10.96%], n = 6; MCT: 16.13%, n = 1; p = 0.15) (Figure 2F,G).

The median frequency of expression of Helios within the whole population of aspirated cells was markedly higher in TCL cases (33.1% [0.6%–94.0%]; n = 13) than in the other three groups of dogs (BCL: 3.0% [0.1%–52.3%], n = 22; RH: 6.65% [0.60%–8.90%], n = 12; MCT: 6.38% [0.50%–9.13%], n = 5; p = 0.00003), compatible with neoplastic T cell Helios expression rather than localization of Helios to the thymic Tregs alone (Figure 3A,B).

Expression of Helios was therefore of limited use in the identification of thymic Tregs in TCL.

The median frequency of $CD8^+$ cells within the whole population of harvested cells was significantly lower in the BCL cases (2.68% [0.89%–10.7%]; n = 20) than in RH cases (11.1% [1.17%–17.1%], n = 20; p = 0.0005), again attributed to effacement of the normal lymphoid population by neoplastic cells (Figure 4A,B). In the case of this marker, median expression was also low in the MCT cases (2.24% [0.82%–6.9%]; n = 4). The median expression of CD8 specifically by T cells was also lower in the neoplastic groups than in the RH group (BCL: 11.3% [0.57%–30.4%], n = 20; MCT: 7.06% [5.35%–9.76%], n = 3; RH: 18.4% [0.6%–37.1%], n = 11; p = 0.04) (Figure 4C). Rationalizing that the balance of cytotoxic to regulatory T cells may be perturbed in BCL, we then examined the ratio of $CD8^+$ to $FOXP3^+$ T cells within the whole population of harvested cells. Rather than being lower in BCL cases, the median $CD8^+$:$FOXP3^+$ ratio showed a trend towards being higher in this group of dogs when compared to RH (or MCT) cases (BCL: 2.09 [0–27.7], n = 22; RH: 1.63 [0–5.89], n = 13; MCT: 0.35 [0–1.07]; n = 4; p = 0.06), which became significant when thymic Tregs were specifically examined by means of co-expression of FOXP3 and Helios within the overall population (BCL: 15.6 [2.11–36.1], n = 11; RH: 4.26 [0–12.0], n = 13; p = 0.04) (Figure 4D,E).

FOXP3, Helios and MHC class II expression all have prognostic significance in canine B cell lymphoma

The impact of FOXP3, Helios and MHC class II expression on BCL prognosis was then interrogated using both univariable and multivariable analysis. FOXP3 expression was a negative prognostic factor in the context of OS and PFS. Patients with total FOXP3 expression less than or equal to the median value (1.23%) survived longer than those with expression above the median value (≤1.23%, median OS = 322 days, >1.23%, median OS = 169 days; median ratio 0.52; p = 0.018) (Figure 5A). A similar phenomenon was observed for PFS: patients with lower FOXP3 expression in the $CD5^+CD4^+$ population had a longer PFS than those with higher FOXP3 expression (≤10.2%, median PFS = 211 days, >10.2%, median PFS = 61 days; median ratio 0.29; p = 0.012) (Figure 5B). The proportional expression of Helios was also a negative prognostic factor, as patients with expression lower than the median value had longer PFS (≤3.00%, median PFS = 175 days, >3.00%, median PFS = 62 days; median ratio 0.35; p = 0.014) (Figure 5C). The intensity of MHC class II expression by the lymphoma cells, expressed as the ratio of geometric mean fluorescence intensity of MHC II^+:MHC II^- cells within the $CD5^-$ subset of the 'All' gate, was also of prognostic significance (Figure 5D): TTR was longer in those cases with expression ratios less than or equal to the median value (≤4.40, median 22 days, >4.40, median 10 days; p = 0.017).

Multivariable analysis yielded two independent factors impacting PFS, age and frequency of FOXP3 expression by lymph node $CD5^+CD4^+$ T cells, and two independent factors impacting OS, the administration of rescue therapy and the frequency of FOXP3 expression within the total harvested population (Table 3). In the case of OS analysis, a similar proportion of dogs in the $FOXP3^{low}$ (≤1.23%: 6/11) and $FOXP3^{high}$ (>1.23%: 4/10) group had received rescue therapy (p = 0.67). Univariable analysis identified only a single factor impacting TTR (MHC class II expression), obviating the need for multivariable analysis for this outcome variable.

Discussion

To the authors' knowledge, this study represents the first attempt to define the prognostic impact of Tregs in a well-characterized cohort of canine cases of multicentric BCL. Despite the relatively small size of the cohort and heterogeneity of treatment protocols, the expression of FOXP3 emerged as an independent prognostic factor, alongside the expression of MHC class II, age at presentation and the administration of rescue therapy. This observation raises the intriguing possibility that the dog, in common with other species, harbors thymic Tregs within the neoplastic microenvironment of BCL, which are likely to interact with the neoplastic B cells, stromal cells, and other regulatory populations such as tolerogenic dendritic cells, tumor-associated macrophages, myeloid-derived suppressor cells and $\gamma\delta$ T cells.

Control dogs included those with TCL, non-neoplastic lymphadenomegaly (RH) and metastatic MCTs, the latter as an example of an alternative round cell tumor. In common with previous literature, boxers appeared to be over-represented in the TCL group (4/14, 29%) [49–52] and dogs with TCL were more commonly hypercalcemic than those with BCL [53,54]. Cytological reviews were possible in 14 of 22 BCL and 11 of 14 TCL cases, suggesting a predominance of DLBCL and peripheral TCL. This observation accords with both previous veterinary literature, in which these cytological classifications were the most commonly recognized among multicentric BCL and TCL cases [51,55,56],

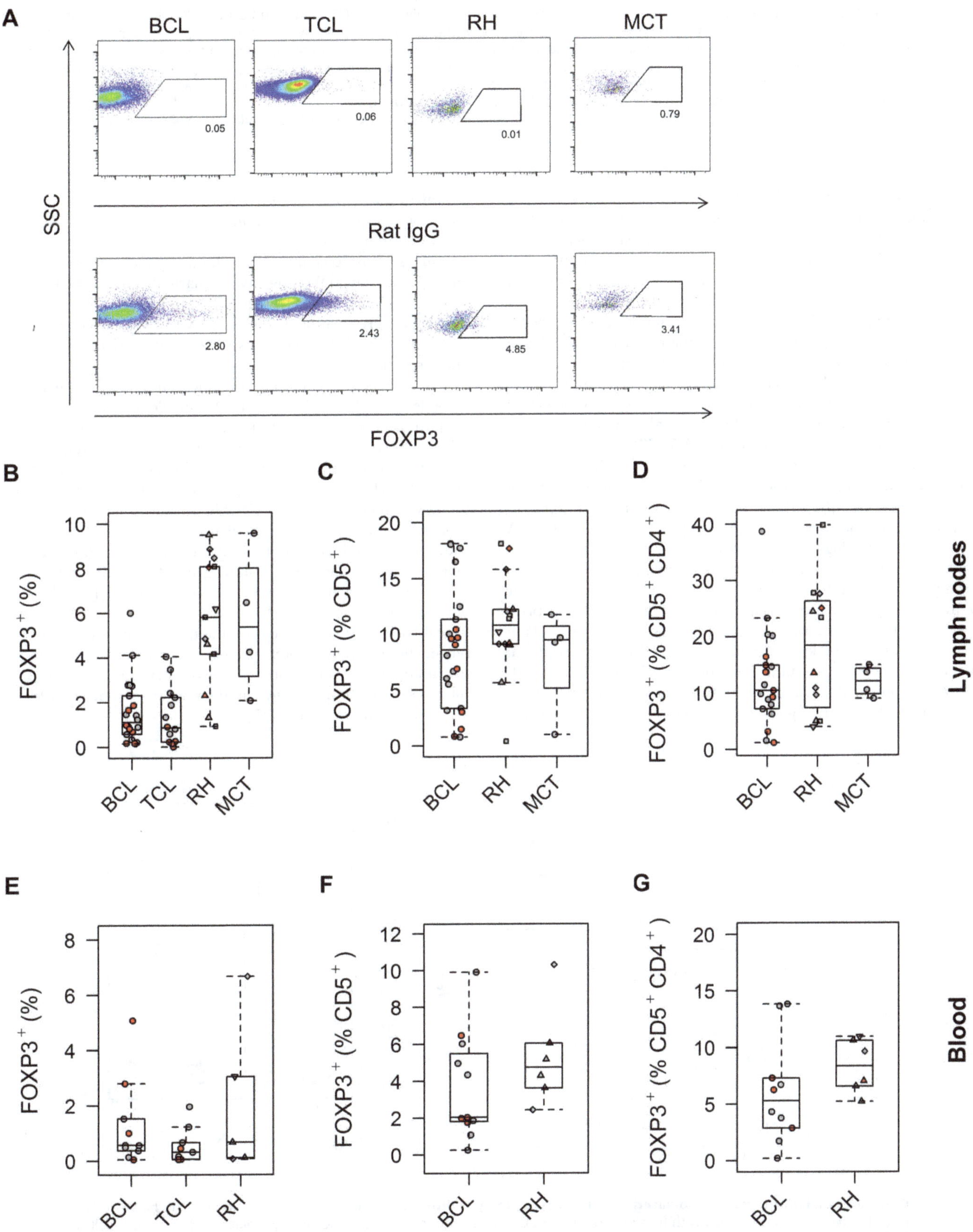

Figure 2. FOXP3$^+$ Treg frequency is no higher in canine B cell lymphoma than control samples. The frequency of FOXP3$^+$ cells in fine needle aspirates harvested from the lymph nodes of dogs with B cell lymphoma (BCL), T cell lymphoma (TCL), reactive hyperplasia (RH) and mast cell tumors (MCT) is shown, expressed as a proportion of all cells (A, B, showing the effect of neoplastic effacement of normal lymphoid tissue;

p = 0.00005), gated CD5$^+$ cells (C, showing the resident T cells; p = 0.41), or sequentially gated CD5$^+$ and then CD4$^+$ T cells (D, showing specifically the resident CD4$^+$ T cells; p = 0.74). Representative dot plots are shown for each of the groups, followed by box-and-whisker plots summarising the data. In each of the dot plots, the respective isotype control stain is shown above the specific stain. In this and subsequent figures, red symbols correspond to data from dogs 'pre-treated' with corticosteroids or any chemotherapeutic drug within three weeks of sampling. In the case of RH cases, square symbols (□) represent data from dogs with dermatitis; diamonds (◇) represent data from dogs with distant neoplasia; triangles (Δ) represent data from dogs with immune-mediated disease; and inverted triangles (▼) represent data from dogs with systemic infection. The expression of FOXP3 by PBMCs (E; p = 0.21) or by the CD5$^+$ (F; p = 0.53) or specific CD5$^+$CD4$^+$ (G; p = 0.15) T cells within PBMCs similarly showed no differences between groups.

and reviews of human NHL [2,57]. The similar cytological appearance of the most common types of canine and human BCL adds weight to the notion that the canine disease could model NHL [11]. However, although FNAs are still the cornerstone of lymphoma diagnosis in canine patients and serve an important triaging role in people with lymphadenomegaly by virtue of their ease of procurement [58–60], solid tissue biopsies are considered the gold standard for diagnosis of human patients, allowing a detailed tissue architectural classification of lymphoma subtypes [1,2]. Recent years have seen an increasing recognition of the diagnostic and prognostic value of histopathological subtypes of lymphoma in dogs [56,61,62], which generally show remarkable similarity to those of human patients [51,55,63].

Most of the dogs in this study were treated with a CHOP protocol, considered to be the standard of care in the treatment of canine lymphoma [64,65]; anti-canine CD20 mAbs similar to rituximab are not currently available, precluding R-CHOP. A proportion of the dogs had received at least one of the drugs on at least one occasion within three weeks of sampling for this study, prompting concern that such 'pre-treatment' might influence their immune cell profile. In particular, we were concerned that prior use of corticosteroids or cyclophosphamide would alter Treg frequencies, given the known impact of these drugs on peripheral T cells in rodents [66–68], humans [69–71] and dogs [72]. However, neither the cellular phenotype nor the prognosis of the pre-treated dogs was significantly different from that of the treatment-naïve patients, presumably because such drugs were administered on a limited number of occasions prior to sampling and would thus have had only minimal opportunity to impact the immune system. Recent studies of human patients receiving short-term glucocorticoid therapy have similarly shown no change in the frequency of peripheral Tregs [73,74]. In view of the lack of impact of pre-treatment on these variables, all dogs of the respective B and T cell groups were considered together in our final analysis.

The impact of a number of clinical and immunophenotypic variables on TTR, PFS and OS of dogs with multicentric lymphoma was examined in the current study, including B or T cell phenotype, age, sex, neutering status, bodyweight, body condition, stage, substage, presence of hypercalcemia, treatment protocol (CHOP *versus* 'Other') and the administration of rescue therapy. Other than the predictable impact of rescue therapy on OS, multivariable analysis revealed that age was the only factor with an independent impact on prognosis, younger dogs enjoying longer PFS. This has been a finding in other canine studies [62] and also reflects the situation in human NHL, for which the prognosis is worse in elderly patients [75,76]. The pathophysiological basis of this observation remains unclear, but is thought to reflect the generally poorer cellular repair mechanisms, progressive immunosenescence, propensity for chemoresistant molecular subtypes of DLBCL, and increased spectrum of comorbidities that occur with advancing age [77].

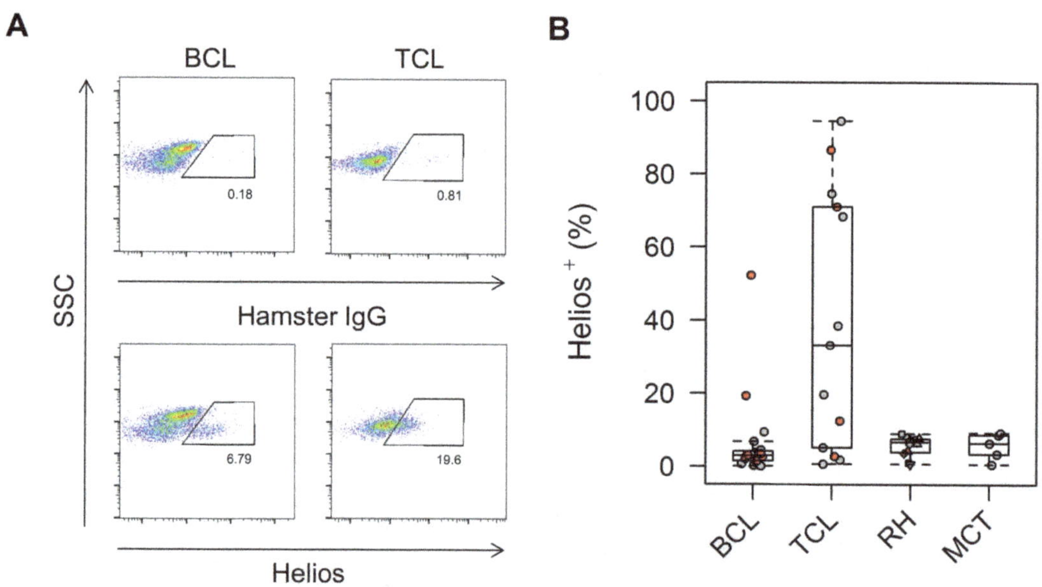

Figure 3. Canine T cell lymphoma is associated with high-frequency Helios expression. Helios expression by cells harvested by fine needle aspiration from the lymph nodes of dogs with B cell lymphoma (BCL), T cell lymphoma (TCL), reactive hyperplasia (RH) and mast cell tumors (MCT) was examined as a marker for thymic Tregs, but the unexpectedly high frequency of Helios$^+$ events in a few B cell and several T cell lymphoma cases suggested neoplastic expression of this marker. Median frequency of Helios expression was significantly different between the groups (p = 0.00003). Representative dot plots for BCL and TCL cases, with their respective isotype control stains, is shown (A), followed by box-and-whisker plots summarising the data (B). (For key to symbols, refer to Figure 2).

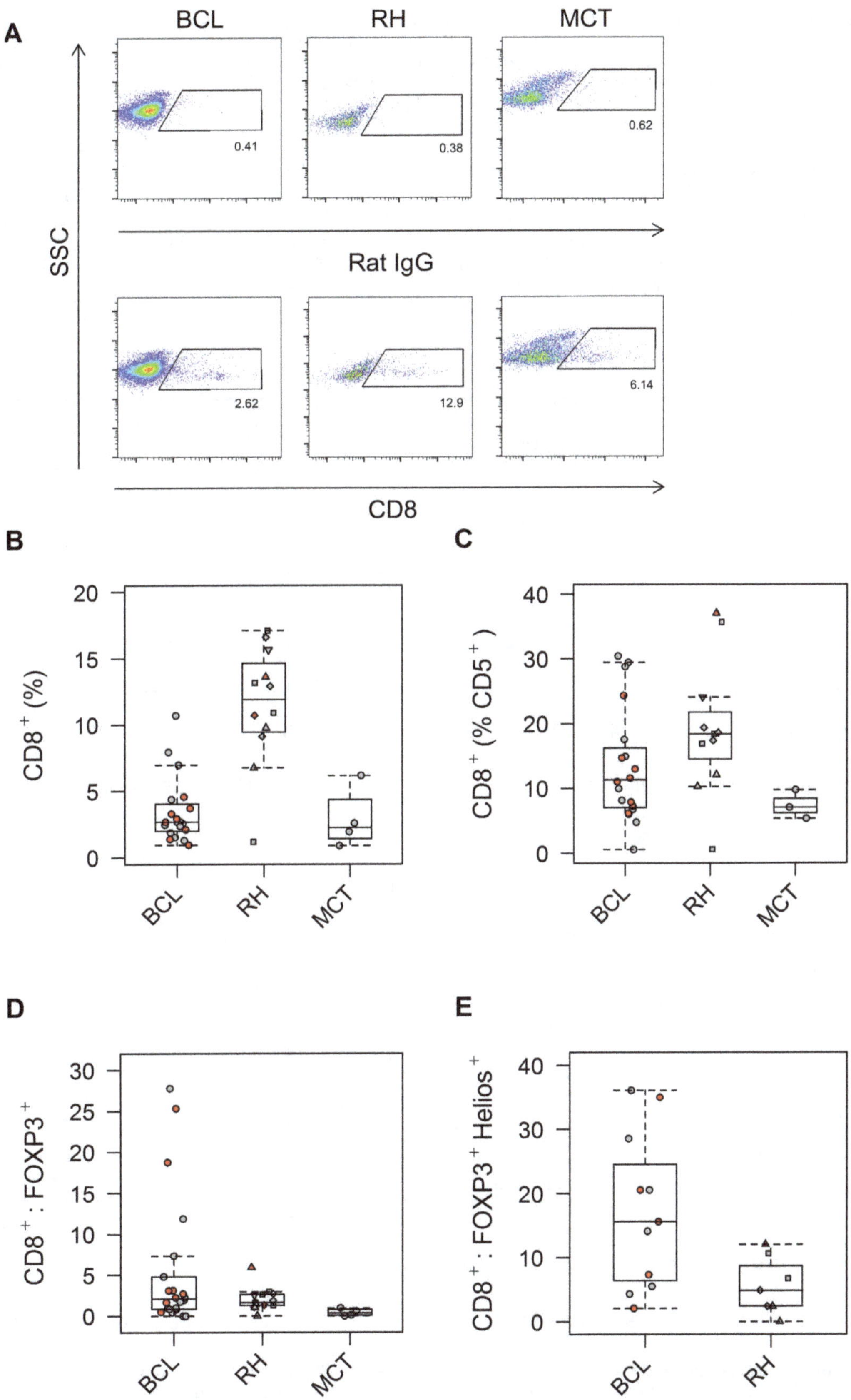

Figure 4. Canine B cell lymphoma shows no deficit of cytotoxic T cells relative to thymic Tregs. When expressed as a proportion of all cells aspirated from the lymph node, the frequency of $CD8^+$ T cells (A,B) was decreased in BCL (and MCT), again attributed to neoplastic effacement ($p = 0.0005$). The frequency of $CD8^+$ cells within the $CD5^+$ T cell population also showed differences between groups (C; $p = 0.04$). The ratio of

CD8⁺:FOXP3⁺ cells (D) was not significantly different between groups (p = 0.06), though dogs with BCL showed the six highest ratios of the cohort, and a trend for higher values in the BCL group was observed. Indeed, the ratio of $CD8^+$:$FOXP3^+Helios^+$ cells (E) was higher in the BCL than RH cases (p = 0.04); only two data points for the MCT (3.48; 3.95) were available for this variable and were not therefore represented. Representative dot plots for all the groups are shown alongside their respective isotype controls, followed by box-and-whisker plots summarising the data. (For key to symbols, refer to Figure 2).

Prognostic factors in other canine studies of multicentric lymphoma have included sex [78,79], B or T immunophenotype [53,80–82], stage [81,83–85], substage [79,83], serum calcium concentration [86], packed cell volume [87], monocyte concentration [88], prior administration of corticosteroids [89,90], treatment protocol [62,91], coagulation profile [92], presence of minimal residual disease after treatment [93], and cytomorphological and histopathological characteristics [56,61,62,81]. However, in common with our own observations, different studies have yielded different conclusions and have not all been able to demonstrate a prognostic impact of every one of the examined variables: factors such as the number and clinical heterogeneity of recruited patients and the nature of the specific end points examined influence the results of such outcome analyses [94].

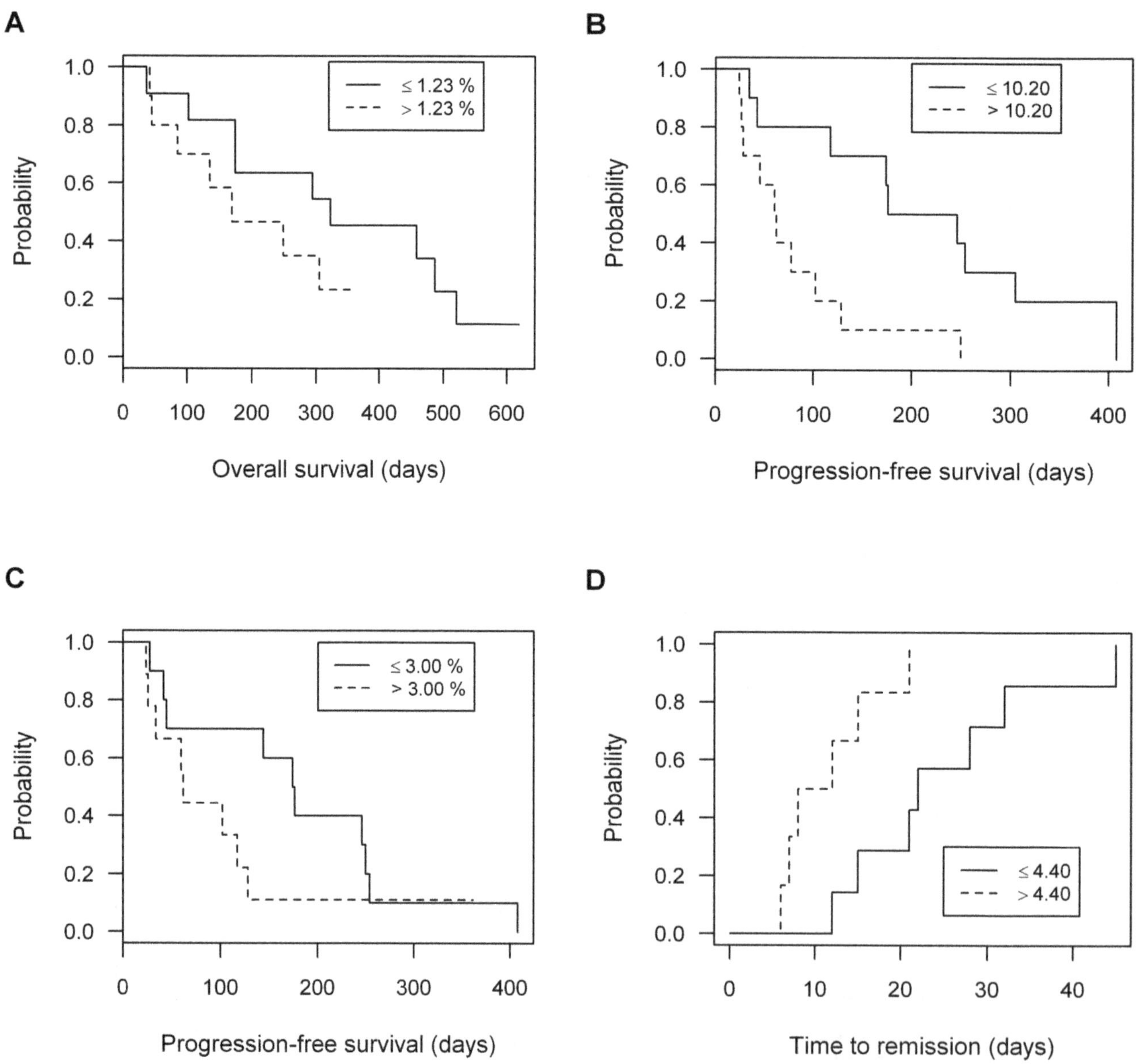

Figure 5. Expression of T cell FOXP3 and Helios, and tumor cell MHC class II, all impact prognosis in dogs with B cell lymphoma. The frequency of $FOXP3^+$ cells within the 'All' gate (A), or within a cascaded All→$CD5^+$→$CD4^+$ gate (B), influenced survival times. Overall survival times were shorter in those dogs with frequencies of $FOXP3^+$ T cells higher than the median value (A: p = 0.02); a similar pattern in progression-free survival (PFS) was observed (B: p = 0.01). The frequency of $Helios^+$ cells within the 'All' gate also influenced PFS (C: p = 0.01). The intensity of MHC class II expression by the lymphoma cells, expressed as the ratio of geometric mean fluorescence intensity of MHC II^+:MHC II^- cells within the $CD5^-$ subset of the 'All' gate, was also of prognostic significance: time to remission was longer in those cases with less MHC class II expression per cell (D: p = 0.02).

Table 3. FOXP3, MHC class II, age at presentation and rescue therapy are independent prognostic factors in canine B cell lymphoma.

Outcome metric	Variable	Median ratio	Hazard ratio (95% CI)	p value
TTR	MHC class II	0.45	2.44 (1.36–4.35)	0.003
PFS	Age	0.43	1.02 (1.01–1.04)	0.007
	$FOXP3^+$ (% $CD5^+CD4^+$)	0.29	1.10 (1.02–1.18)	0.01
OS	Rescue therapy	0.54	0.29 (0.09–0.90)	0.03
	$FOXP3^+$ (%)	0.52	1.61 (1.11–2.32)	0.01

Abbreviations: TTR, time to remission; PFS, progression-free survival; OS, overall survival; CI, confidence interval; $FOXP3^+$ (% $CD5^+CD4^+$), frequency of $FOXP3^+$ cells within the sequential $CD5^+$ and $CD4^+$ gates; $FOXP3^+$ (%), frequency of $FOXP3^+$ cells within the total harvested population; median ratio = ratio of median remission or survival time (TTR/PFS/OS) of the sub-group of dogs with a value of the variable greater than the median of the group to that of the sub-group of dogs with a value of the variable less than or equal to the median of the group.

More recent studies have stratified canine BCL patients by gene profiling, demonstrating that in common with human DLBCL two subtypes with different survival times – the germinal center B cell-like and the activated B cell-like – can be distinguished, the latter associated with a poorer prognosis [14,15]. While the individual genes were different between the species, the general pathways characterizing these subtypes were strikingly similar [14].

We used a cross-reactive mAb against murine Foxp3, validated for use in dogs [46,95], to identify Tregs in this study. While a large number of markers for Tregs have been proposed, FOXP3 remains the single most widely applied phenotypic credential of regulatory activity in cancer and other studies [96–98], despite being transiently expressed in activated human and canine conventional T cells lacking regulatory function [46,99]. Comparisons of respective $FOXP3^+$ and $CD8^+$ cells between the study groups yielded the initially surprising observation that dogs with lymphoma had lower frequencies of these cells than those with RH and MCTs. While FNAs of lymph nodes only ever approximate the cellular content of the node, a consistent aspiration technique was applied between patients and we could not attribute these differences to trivial anomalies in the cellular harvest of lymphomatous lymph nodes, which readily exfoliate cells. Rather, we attributed this observation to cellular effacement of the normal lymphoid tissue by neoplastic B or T cells.

The expression pattern of Helios was also unanticipated. Applied as a marker of thymic Tregs in our study [100], the high frequency of its expression in a number of TCL and two BCL cases suggested that neoplastic lymphocytes may also express this transcription factor, especially those of T cell origin. This intriguing observation accords with similar findings in human TCL, in which over-expression of non-DNA-binding, dominant negative isoforms of Helios is thought to be involved in disease progression [101]. Indeed, transgenic expression of short Helios isoforms in mice promotes the development of TCL [102], while ectopic expression of full-length Helios in B cells promotes BCL [103], suggesting a potential pathogenic role in both immunophenotypes. It is tempting to speculate that deregulated expression of Helios may also be implicated in a minority of BCLs and some TCLs in dogs. Insufficient data were available to allow survival analysis of the $Helios^{high}$ group, but this could be a rewarding avenue for future research; furthermore, immunocytochemical staining could be employed to confirm expression of Helios by the malignant T cells. In the light of these observations, Helios was used as a surrogate marker for thymic Tregs only in the BCL dogs.

Review of the initial flow cytometric data prompted us to adopt a cascaded gating approach in subsequent analysis of the BCL cases, in which sequential $CD5^+$ and $CD4^+$ gates were applied to identify the resident T cells. By 'normalizing' the data in this manner, we endeavored to remove the dilutional influence of the neoplastic B cells. We found no significant difference in the frequency of $FOXP3^+$ cells between the BCL and two control groups, when expressed either as a proportion of $CD5^+$ or of $CD5^+CD4^+$ T cells. This observation contrasts with both a comparison of the cellular phenotype of lymph nodes in human patients with Hodgkin lymphoma and RH [104], and a recent study by Mitchell *et al*, who examined the cytotoxic T cell response in dogs with multicentric BCL treated with doxorubicin: the mean initial frequency of Tregs was approximately four-fold higher in Mitchell's study than in ours [105]. While this disparity is difficult to explain given the commonality of the species and disease, there were some notable differences between the studies. Thus, Mitchell *et al* harvested excisional biopsies, which represent a more accurate sampling technique than FNAs, but recruited only five dogs with BCL in total. We speculate that the five dogs included in their study represented a $Treg^{high}$ phenotype, reminiscent of the highest-expressing patients in our own work, but that the pattern of expression is generally more heterogeneous among all dogs with BCL. Furthermore, for ethical and legal reasons we were unable to sample the lymph nodes of healthy animals; our comparisons were thus restricted to dogs with non-neoplastic lymphadenomegaly and infiltration of the lymph nodes by another round cell tumor, both of which could have harbored higher frequencies of Tregs than healthy dogs. Indeed, this notion of non-malignant expansion of Tregs reconciles with the known activation of these cells in the context of inflammatory microenvironments [106].

Among the populations of cytotoxic cells within a tumor, $CD8^+$ T cells play a prominent role in the elimination of neoplastic cells [107]. Conventional wisdom places them on the other side of a balancing act with Tregs and additional regulatory cells in solid cancers [108]. We thus explored the possibility of a perturbation of the relative frequencies of $CD8^+$ and $FOXP3^+$ T cells in BCL, but found no evidence of a deficit of the former when compared to the control groups. Rather, the ratio of $CD8^+$ to regulatory T cells tended to be higher in the lymph nodes of the BCL than RH dogs, especially when thymic Tregs were identified by means of Helios expression. While Helios has been criticized as a marker for thymic Tregs [109], it is still generally regarded to be a valid surrogate for this population of regulatory cells [110]. Future studies could also examine the cross-reactivity of available mAbs against neuropilin-1, considered by some to be a superior marker [111] and implicated in Treg-mediated suppression within certain cancer microenvironments [112]. Taken together, these data provided no support for a gross numerical deficit of $CD8^+$ T cells in canine BCL, but further work will be required to explore possible functional deficits of these critical cells.

Despite the lack of a significant difference in overall T cell FOXP3 expression between the BCL and control groups, FOXP3 nevertheless emerged as an independent negative prognostic factor in this study. This apparent paradox was likely to reflect the very different microenvironments of B cell neoplasia and lymphoid hyperplasia and the role of Tregs within them: in the context of cancer, Tregs have traditionally been viewed as having a pathogenic influence [22,23,42], co-opted by the cancer to help thwart anti-neoplastic immune responses [113], while in the context of RH, Tregs are likely to serve a beneficial role by limiting over-exuberant inflammatory responses and collateral tissue damage, adapting their suppressive program to the prevailing milieu [106]. While our data reconciled with this view of Tregs as being 'bad' in the context of canine BCL, aligning with a plethora of studies of solid tissue cancers in humans and other species [22,23,42] and some studies of human NHL [27–31], it was at odds with a proportion of studies of human lymphoma that have suggested the exact opposite – that Tregs are actually part of the anti-neoplastic defenses [32–40], presumably because they are able to draw on their armamentarium of suppressive mechanisms to neutralize or kill neoplastic T and B cells, as well as a host of innate immune cells subverted by the lymphoma. The bewildering complexity of the microenvironment in both solid tissue and hemolymphatic tumors is only now beginning to be elucidated [16–20] and we speculate that Tregs may have divergent and dynamic roles in this context that are predicated on both micro-anatomical and temporal factors. Whether $FOXP3^+$ Tregs play a negative prognostic role in all canine BCL subtypes remains to be determined, but they appeared to be deleterious in the context of the cohort of dogs we examined. High Helios and low MHC II expression were also of prognostic significance in this study. We suggest that the Helios result reflects its predominant co-localization with FOXP3 in thymic Tregs, while the MHC II result reconciles with studies of both human [114–116] and canine [117] BCL patients, in which low-level expression of this molecule is thought to compromise the activation of T cell responses against the neoplastic B cells and thus shorten survival. Interestingly, the current study revealed an impact of MHC II expression on TTR alone, but differences in patients and study design were likely to account for this discrepancy from existing publications.

In common with all clinical research of an exploratory nature, this study suffered a number of limitations. Staging was not complete in every case and our end-point variables (TTR, PFS and OS) were defined by owners' and attending veterinarians' observations of clinical signs and lymph node size. While diligent follow-up of cases was undertaken, the pragmatic nature of clinical veterinary practice meant that these values were likely to be best estimates only. Furthermore, the cohort of BCL patients examined was uncontrolled and relatively small, incorporating a number of different treatment regimens. We chose not to censor dogs that had received rescue therapy, instead incorporating them in the analysis of OS to maximize power. Nevertheless, despite the heterogeneity of the cohort, we were able to demonstrate that frequency of FOXP3 expression was an independent prognostic factor. Future studies of carefully stratified canine lymphoma patients treated with the same chemotherapy protocol are planned to confirm the results of the current work, which must be considered preliminary until they are prospectively validated in this manner.

In summary, we have presented evidence suggesting that $FOXP3^+$ Tregs have a negative prognostic impact in canine multicentric BCL. We suggest that dogs with BCL, in common with human NHL patients, harbor a spectrum of interacting regulatory cells within the neoplastic lymph nodes, including thymic Tregs. We present further evidence of similarities between canine BCL and human NHL, thus helping to vindicate this large animal model of lymphoid cancer. There is an increasing need to find new ways of modulating the immune system as an integral part of multimodal veterinary cancer therapy. Regulatory T cells are an obvious candidate in such therapeutic endeavors, since this work suggests that they play a decisive role in the pathogenesis of canine BCL.

Supporting Information

Figure S1 Cytological characteristics of representative B cell lymphoma, T cell lymphoma, reactive hyperplasia and mast cell tumor cases. Smears of fine needle aspirates were stained with modified Wright's stain and examined by a board-certified clinical pathologist in each case to reach a cytological diagnosis. A representative image of each group is presented (100x oil immersion lens; bar = 10 μm). (A) Diffuse large B cell lymphoma (DLBCL), characterized by a dominance of medium-to-large lymphocytes with immature chromatin and prominent nucleoli. (B) Peripheral T cell lymphoma (PTCL), characterized by a dominance of medium-to-large lymphocytes with eccentric and occasionally indented nuclei, smooth chromatin and multiple nucleoli. (C) Reactive hyperplasia (RH), characterized by a mixed population of lymphocytes with predominance of small lymphocytes, and increased numbers of medium-to-large lymphocytes, plasma cells and Mott cells. (D) Draining lymph node of a mast cell tumor (MCT), characterized by numerous moderately-to-well granulated mast cells, occasional eosinophils and a mixed lymphocyte population, consistent with a metastatic mast cell tumor.

Figure S2 Younger dogs, those treated with CHOP and those 'rescued' show longer survival in B cell lymphoma. (A) Dogs with B cell lymphoma that were less than or equal to the median age of the group (112 months) had longer progression-free survival (PFS: median 174 *vs* 74 days; median ratio = 0.43, $p = 0.006$) but not overall survival (OS, $p = 0.11$; data not shown); time to remission (TTR) was also no different between younger and older dogs ($p = 0.57$; data not shown). The significance of age on PFS remained in the multivariable regression model, demonstrating that it was an independent prognostic factor in this cohort of dogs. (B) CHOP chemotherapy was associated with longer PFS than the other treatments in the BCL group (CHOP, median 175 days; Other [including COP (n = 3), cytarabine, L-asparaginase, lomustine (n = 3) and prednisolone alone (n = 1)], median 45 days; $p = 0.01$). However, when interrogated in multivariable analysis, the variable 'protocol' no longer remained significant after accounting for age, reflecting the younger mean age of dogs treated with CHOP than 'Other' protocols (93 *versus* 123 months; $p = 0.05$). (C) Dogs receiving rescue therapy had longer OS (median 322 days) than those not receiving rescue therapy (174 days, median ratio 0.54; $p = 0.049$).

Table S1 Cytomorphological criteria for the assessment of lymphoma cases.

Table S2 Signalment, therapy and immunophenotype of B cell lymphoma dogs. Abbreviations: mo, months; m, male; f, female; n, neutered; e, entire; ND, not determined; chemotherapy agents: CHOP, protocol in which cyclophosphamide (C), doxorubicin (H), vincristine (O) and prednisolone (P) are administered; COP, protocol in which cyclophosphamide (C), vincristine (O) and prednisolone (P) are administered; L, lomustine; Cy, cytosine arabinoside; Ap, L-asparaginase; Chl, chlorambucil; VCAA, protocol in which vincristine (V), cyclophosphamide (C), L-asparaginase (A) and doxorubicin (A) are administered; LMP, protocol in which chlorambucil (L), methotrexate (M) and prednisolone (P) are administered; DMAC, protocol in which dexamethasone (D), melphelan (M), actinomycin-D (A) and cytosine arabinoside (C) are administered; Ma, masitinib; Vb, vinblastine; Pr, procarbazine; -, no rescue therapy administered (Rescue therapy) or remission not achieved (TTR); +, no progression (PFS) or alive at conclusion of study (OS) and therefore censored from survival analysis. Notes: The immunophenotype lists the per cent positive staining for the listed antigen; [1]: these cases were classified as B cell lymphomas with aberrant CD5 expression.

Table S3 Signalment, therapy and immunophenotype of T cell lymphoma dogs. Abbreviations: mo, months; m, male; f, female; n, neutered; e, entire; ND, not determined; chemotherapy agents: see Table S2 and Dex, dexamethasone; -, no rescue therapy administered (Rescue therapy) or remission not achieved (TTR); +, no progression (PFS) or alive at conclusion of study (OS) and therefore censored from survival analysis. Notes: The immunophenotype lists the per cent positive staining for the listed antigen.

Table S4 Disease subtype and signalment of reactive hyperplasia dogs. Abbreviations: mo, months; m, male; f, female; n, neutered; e, entire.

Table S5 Signalment of mast cell tumor dogs. Abbreviations: mo, months; f, female; n, neutered; e, entire.

Acknowledgments

The authors would like to thank the following clinicians for submission of patient samples during the course of this study: Dr Francesca Fabrizio, Dr Angela Taylor, Dr Shasta Lynch, Dr Isabelle Desmas, Dr Sofia Carvalho, Mr David Walker, Dr Majbritt Larsen, Mr Graeme McKeown and Ms Lucy Gardiner. This project was undertaken as part of DP's Fellowship in Regulatory T Cell and Cancer Biology in the Immune Regulation Laboratory of OG.

Author Contributions

Conceived and designed the experiments: DP TD OAG. Performed the experiments: DP TD LJD EY EM CL AL AS GP OAG. Analyzed the data: DP YMC HB BS TD OAG. Contributed reagents/materials/analysis tools: YMC BS. Wrote the paper: OAG.

References

1. Guerard EJ, Bishop MR (2012) Overview of non-Hodgkin's lymphoma. Dis Mon 58: 208–218.
2. Shankland KR, Armitage JO, Hancock BW (2012) Non-Hodgkin lymphoma. Lancet 380: 848–857.
3. UK CR (2013) Cancer Statistics Report: Non-Hodgkin Lymphoma.
4. O'Connor OA, Toner LE, Vrhovac R, Budak-Alpdogan T, Smith EA, et al. (2005) Comparative animal models for the study of lymphohematopoietic tumors: strengths and limitations of present approaches. Leuk Lymphoma 46: 973–992.
5. Head E (2013) A canine model of human aging and Alzheimer's disease. Biochim Biophys Acta 1832: 1384–1389.
6. Potschka H, Fischer A, von Ruden EL, Hulsmeyer V, Baumgartner W (2013) Canine epilepsy as a translational model? Epilepsia 54: 571–579.
7. Ranieri G, Gadaleta CD, Patruno R, Zizzo N, Daidone MG, et al. (2013) A model of study for human cancer: Spontaneous occurring tumors in dogs. Biological features and translation for new anticancer therapies. Crit Rev Oncol Hematol 88: 187–197.
8. Tsai KL, Clark LA, Murphy KE (2007) Understanding hereditary diseases using the dog and human as companion model systems. Mamm Genome 18: 444–451.
9. Gordon I, Paoloni M, Mazcko C, Khanna C (2009) The Comparative Oncology Trials Consortium: using spontaneously occurring cancers in dogs to inform the cancer drug development pathway. PLoS Med 6: e1000161.
10. Paoloni M, Khanna C (2008) Translation of new cancer treatments from pet dogs to humans. Nat Rev Cancer 8: 147–156.
11. Marconato L, Gelain ME, Comazzi S (2013) The dog as a possible animal model for human non-Hodgkin lymphoma: a review. Hematol Oncol 31: 1–9.
12. Frantz AM, Sarver AL, Ito D, Phang TL, Karimpour-Fard A, et al. (2013) Molecular profiling reveals prognostically significant subtypes of canine lymphoma. Vet Pathol 50: 693–703.
13. Mooney M, Bond J, Monks N, Eugster E, Cherba D, et al. (2013) Comparative RNA-Seq and microarray analysis of gene expression changes in B-cell lymphomas of Canis familiaris. PLoS One 8: e61088.
14. Richards KL, Motsinger-Reif AA, Chen HW, Fedoriw Y, Fan C, et al. (2013) Gene Profiling of Canine B-Cell Lymphoma Reveals Germinal Center and Postgerminal Center Subtypes with Different Survival Times, Modeling Human DLBCL. Cancer Res 73: 5029–5039.
15. Su Y, Nielsen D, Zhu L, Richards K, Suter S, et al. (2013) Gene selection and cancer type classification of diffuse large-B-cell lymphoma using a bivariate mixture model for two-species data. Hum Genomics 7: 2.
16. Schiavoni G, Gabriele L, Mattei F (2013) The tumor microenvironment: a pitch for multiple players. Front Oncol 3: 90.
17. Becker JC, Andersen MH, Schrama D, Thor Straten P (2013) Immune-suppressive properties of the tumor microenvironment. Cancer Immunol Immunother 62: 1137–1148.
18. Gribben JG (2010) Implications of the tumor microenvironment on survival and disease response in follicular lymphoma. Curr Opin Oncol 22: 424–430.
19. Coupland SE (2011) The challenge of the microenvironment in B-cell lymphomas. Histopathology 58: 69–80.
20. Fridman WH, Dieu-Nosjean MC, Pages F, Cremer I, Damotte D, et al. (2013) The immune microenvironment of human tumors: general significance and clinical impact. Cancer Microenviron 6: 117–122.
21. Garden OA, Pinheiro D, Cunningham F (2011) All creatures great and small: regulatory T cells in mice, humans, dogs and other domestic animal species. Int Immunopharmacol 11: 576–588.
22. Gallimore A, Godkin A (2008) Regulatory T cells and tumour immunity - observations in mice and men. Immunology 123: 157–163.
23. Oleinika K, Nibbs RJ, Graham GJ, Fraser AR (2013) Suppression, subversion and escape: the role of regulatory T cells in cancer progression. Clin Exp Immunol 171: 36–45.
24. Dobrzanski MJ (2013) Expanding roles for CD4 T cells and their subpopulations in tumor immunity and therapy. Front Oncol 3: 63.
25. deLeeuw RJ, Kost SE, Kakal JA, Nelson BH (2012) The prognostic value of FoxP3+ tumor-infiltrating lymphocytes in cancer: a critical review of the literature. Clin Cancer Res 18: 3022–3029.
26. Lindqvist CA, Loskog AS (2012) T regulatory cells in B-cell malignancy - tumour support or kiss of death? Immunology 135: 255–260.
27. Marshall NA, Christie LE, Munro LR, Culligan DJ, Johnston PW, et al. (2004) Immunosuppressive regulatory T cells are abundant in the reactive lymphocytes of Hodgkin lymphoma. Blood 103: 1755–1762.
28. Yang ZZ, Novak AJ, Ziesmer SC, Witzig TE, Ansell SM (2006) Attenuation of $CD8^+$ T-cell function by $CD4^+CD25^+$ regulatory T cells in B-cell non-Hodgkin's lymphoma. Cancer Res 66: 10145–10152.
29. Yang ZZ, Novak AJ, Stenson MJ, Witzig TE, Ansell SM (2006) Intratumoral $CD4^+CD25^+$ regulatory T-cell-mediated suppression of infiltrating $CD4^+$ T cells in B-cell non-Hodgkin lymphoma. Blood 107: 3639–3646.
30. Yang ZZ, Novak AJ, Ziesmer SC, Witzig TE, Ansell SM (2009) Malignant B cells skew the balance of regulatory T cells and TH17 cells in B-cell non-Hodgkin's lymphoma. Cancer Res 69: 5522–5530.
31. Schreck S, Friebel D, Buettner M, Distel L, Grabenbauer G, et al. (2009) Prognostic impact of tumour-infiltrating Th2 and regulatory T cells in classical Hodgkin lymphoma. Hematol Oncol 27: 31–39.
32. Alvaro T, Lejeune M, Salvado MT, Bosch R, Garcia JF, et al. (2005) Outcome in Hodgkin's lymphoma can be predicted from the presence of accompanying cytotoxic and regulatory T cells. Clin Cancer Res 11: 1467–1473.

33. Carreras J, Lopez-Guillermo A, Fox BC, Colomo L, Martinez A, et al. (2006) High numbers of tumor-infiltrating FOXP3-positive regulatory T cells are associated with improved overall survival in follicular lymphoma. Blood 108: 2957–2964.
34. Kelley TW, Pohlman B, Elson P, Hsi ED (2007) The ratio of FOXP3+ regulatory T cells to granzyme B+ cytotoxic T/NK cells predicts prognosis in classical Hodgkin lymphoma and is independent of bcl-2 and MAL expression. Am J Clin Pathol 128: 958–965.
35. Lee NR, Song EK, Jang KY, Choi HN, Moon WS, et al. (2008) Prognostic impact of tumor infiltrating FOXP3 positive regulatory T cells in diffuse large B-cell lymphoma at diagnosis. Leuk Lymphoma 49: 247–256.
36. Tzankov A, Meier C, Hirschmann P, Went P, Pileri SA, et al. (2008) Correlation of high numbers of intratumoral FOXP3+ regulatory T cells with improved survival in germinal center-like diffuse large B-cell lymphoma, follicular lymphoma and classical Hodgkin's lymphoma. Haematologica 93: 193–200.
37. Wahlin BE, Aggarwal M, Montes-Moreno S, Gonzalez LF, Roncador G, et al. (2010) A unifying microenvironment model in follicular lymphoma: outcome is predicted by programmed death-1–positive, regulatory, cytotoxic, and helper T cells and macrophages. Clin Cancer Res 16: 637–650.
38. Koreishi AF, Saenz AJ, Persky DO, Cui H, Moskowitz A, et al. (2010) The role of cytotoxic and regulatory T cells in relapsed/refractory Hodgkin lymphoma. Appl Immunohistochem Mol Morphol 18: 206–211.
39. Felcht M, Heck M, Weiss C, Becker JC, Dippel E, et al. (2012) Expression of the T-cell regulatory marker FOXP3 in primary cutaneous large B-cell lymphoma tumour cells. Br J Dermatol 167: 348–358.
40. Dehghani M, Sharifpour S, Amirghofran Z, Zare HR (2012) Prognostic significance of T cell subsets in peripheral blood of B cell non-Hodgkin's lymphoma patients. Med Oncol 29: 2364–2371.
41. Koch K, Hoster E, Unterhalt M, Ott G, Rosenwald A, et al. (2012) The composition of the microenvironment in follicular lymphoma is associated with the stage of the disease. Hum Pathol 43: 2274–2281.
42. Lindau D, Gielen P, Kroesen M, Wesseling P, Adema GJ (2013) The immunosuppressive tumour network: myeloid-derived suppressor cells, regulatory T cells and natural killer T cells. Immunology 138: 105–115.
43. Whiteside TL, Schuler P, Schilling B (2012) Induced and natural regulatory T cells in human cancer. Expert Opin Biol Ther 12: 1383–1397.
44. Tanchot C, Terme M, Pere H, Tran T, Benhamouda N, et al. (2013) Tumor-infiltrating regulatory T cells: phenotype, role, mechanism of expansion in situ and clinical significance. Cancer Microenviron 6: 147–157.
45. Adeegbe DO, Nishikawa H (2013) Natural and induced T regulatory cells in cancer. Front Immunol 4: 190.
46. Pinheiro D, Singh Y, Grant CR, Appleton RC, Sacchini F, et al. (2011) Phenotypic and functional characterization of a $CD4^+CD25^{high}FOXP3^{high}$ regulatory T-cell population in the dog. Immunology 132: 111–122.
47. Wilkerson MJ, Dolce K, Koopman T, Shuman W, Chun R, et al. (2005) Lineage differentiation of canine lymphoma/leukemias and aberrant expression of CD molecules. Vet Immunol Immunopathol 106: 179–196.
48. Vail DM, Michels GM, Khanna C, Selting KA, London CA (2010) Response evaluation criteria for peripheral nodal lymphoma in dogs (v1.0)–a Veterinary Cooperative Oncology Group (VCOG) consensus document. Vet Comp Oncol 8: 28–37.
49. Modiano JF, Breen M, Burnett RC, Parker HG, Inusah S, et al. (2005) Distinct B-cell and T-cell lymphoproliferative disease prevalence among dog breeds indicates heritable risk. Cancer Res 65: 5654–5661.
50. Lurie DM, Milner RJ, Suter SE, Vernau W (2008) Immunophenotypic and cytomorphologic subclassification of T-cell lymphoma in the boxer breed. Vet Immunol Immunopathol 125: 102–110.
51. Ponce F, Marchal T, Magnol JP, Turinelli V, Ledieu D, et al. (2010) A morphological study of 608 cases of canine malignant lymphoma in France with a focus on comparative similarities between canine and human lymphoma morphology. Vet Pathol 47: 414–433.
52. Pastor M, Chalvet-Monfray K, Marchal T, Keck G, Magnol JP, et al. (2009) Genetic and environmental risk indicators in canine non-Hodgkin's lymphomas: breed associations and geographic distribution of 608 cases diagnosed throughout France over 1 year. J Vet Intern Med 23: 301–310.
53. Greenlee PG, Filippa DA, Quimby FW, Patnaik AK, Calvano SE, et al. (1990) Lymphomas in dogs. A morphologic, immunologic, and clinical study. Cancer 66: 480–490.
54. Fournel-Fleury C, Ponce F, Felman P, Blavier A, Bonnefont C, et al. (2002) Canine T-cell lymphomas: a morphological, immunological, and clinical study of 46 new cases. Vet Pathol 39: 92–109.
55. Fournel-Fleury C, Magnol JP, Bricaire P, Marchal T, Chabanne L, et al. (1997) Cytohistological and immunological classification of canine malignant lymphomas: comparison with human non-Hodgkin's lymphomas. J Comp Pathol 117: 35–59.
56. Ponce F, Magnol JP, Ledieu D, Marchal T, Turinelli V, et al. (2004) Prognostic significance of morphological subtypes in canine malignant lymphomas during chemotherapy. Vet J 167: 158–166.
57. Mey U, Hitz F, Lohri A, Pederiva S, Taverna C, et al. (2012) Diagnosis and treatment of diffuse large B-cell lymphoma. Swiss Med Wkly 142: w13511.
58. Das DK (1999) Value and limitations of fine-needle aspiration cytology in diagnosis and classification of lymphomas: A review. Diagn Cytopathol 21: 240–249.
59. Landgren O, Porwit MacDonald A, Tani E, Czader M, Grimfors G, et al. (2004) A prospective comparison of fine-needle aspiration cytology and histopathology in the diagnosis and classification of lymphomas. Hematol J 5: 69–76.
60. Vigliar E, Cipullo C, Todaro P, Giuffre G, Pepe S (2012) Fine needle cytology, infectious diseases and non-Hodgkin lymphoma. Infez Med 20 Suppl 3: 39–42.
61. Aresu L, Martini V, Rossi F, Vignoli M, Sampaolo M, et al. (2013) Canine indolent and aggressive lymphoma: clinical spectrum with histologic correlation. Vet Comp Oncol. doi: 10.1111/vco.12048.
62. Valli VE, Kass PH, Myint MS, Scott F (2013) Canine lymphomas: association of classification type, disease stage, tumor subtype, mitotic rate, and treatment with survival. Vet Pathol 50: 738–748.
63. Valli VE, San Myint M, Barthel A, Bienzle D, Caswell J, et al. (2011) Classification of canine malignant lymphomas according to the World Health Organization criteria. Vet Pathol 48: 198–211.
64. Marconato L (2011) The staging and treatment of multicentric high-grade lymphoma in dogs: a review of recent developments and future prospects. Vet J 188: 34–38.
65. Chun R (2009) Lymphoma: which chemotherapy protocol and why? Top Companion Anim Med 24: 157–162.
66. Liu P, Jaffar J, Hellstrom I, Hellstrom KE (2010) Administration of cyclophosphamide changes the immune profile of tumor-bearing mice. J Immunother 33: 53–59.
67. Rico MJ, Rozados VR, Mainetti LE, Zacarias Fluck MF, Matar P, et al. (2012) Regulatory T cells but not NKT I cells are modulated by a single low-dose cyclophosphamide in a B cell lymphoma tumor-model. Exp Oncol 34: 38–42.
68. Mao R, Xiao W, Liu H, Chen B, Yi B, et al. (2013) Systematic evaluation of 640 FDA drugs for their effect on $CD4^+Foxp3^+$ regulatory T cells using a novel cell-based high throughput screening assay. Biochem Pharmacol 85: 1513–1524.
69. Zhao J, Cao Y, Lei Z, Yang Z, Zhang B, et al. (2010) Selective depletion of $CD4^+CD25^+Foxp3^+$ regulatory T cells by low-dose cyclophosphamide is explained by reduced intracellular ATP levels. Cancer Res 70: 4850–4858.
70. Camisaschi C, Filipazzi P, Tazzari M, Casati C, Beretta V, et al. (2013) Effects of cyclophosphamide and IL-2 on regulatory $CD4^+$ T cell frequency and function in melanoma patients vaccinated with HLA-class I peptides: impact on the antigen-specific T cell response. Cancer Immunol Immunother 62: 897–908.
71. Zen M, Canova M, Campana C, Bettio S, Nalotto L, et al. (2011) The kaleidoscope of glucorticoid effects on immune system. Autoimmun Rev 10: 305–310.
72. Burton JH, Mitchell L, Thamm DH, Dow SW, Biller BJ (2011) Low-dose cyclophosphamide selectively decreases regulatory T cells and inhibits angiogenesis in dogs with soft tissue sarcoma. J Vet Intern Med 25: 920–926.
73. Moniuszko M, Bodzenta-Lukaszyk A, Dabrowska M (2010) Effects of oral glucocorticoid therapy on $CD4^+CD25^+CD127^-$ and $CD4^+CD25^{high}$ T cell levels in asthmatic patients. Inflammation 33: 415–420.
74. Sbiera S, Dexneit T, Reichardt SD, Michel KD, van den Brandt J, et al. (2011) Influence of short-term glucocorticoid therapy on regulatory T cells in vivo. PLoS One 6: e24345.
75. Armand P, Welch S, Kim HT, LaCasce AS, Jacobsen ED, et al. (2013) Prognostic factors for patients with diffuse large B cell lymphoma and transformed indolent lymphoma undergoing autologous stem cell transplantation in the positron emission tomography era. Br J Haematol 160: 608–617.
76. (1993) A predictive model for aggressive non-Hodgkin's lymphoma. The International Non-Hodgkin's Lymphoma Prognostic Factors Project. N Engl J Med 329: 987–994.
77. Fields PA, Linch DC (2012) Treatment of the elderly patient with diffuse large B cell lymphoma. Br J Haematol 157: 159–170.
78. MacEwen EG, Hayes AA, Mooney S, Patnaik A, Kurzman I, et al. (1985) Levamisole as adjuvant to chemotherapy for canine lymphosarcoma. J Biol Response Mod 4: 427–433.
79. Keller ET, MacEwen EG, Rosenthal RC, Helfand SC, Fox LE (1993) Evaluation of prognostic factors and sequential combination chemotherapy with doxorubicin for canine lymphoma. J Vet Intern Med 7: 289–295.
80. Dobson JM, Blackwood LB, McInnes EF, Bostock DE, Nicholls P, et al. (2001) Prognostic variables in canine multicentric lymphosarcoma. J Small Anim Pract 42: 377–384.
81. Teske E, van Heerde P, Rutteman GR, Kurzman ID, Moore PF, et al. (1994) Prognostic factors for treatment of malignant lymphoma in dogs. J Am Vet Med Assoc 205: 1722–1728.
82. Ruslander DA, Gebhard DH, Tompkins MB, Grindem CB, Page RL (1997) Immunophenotypic characterization of canine lymphoproliferative disorders. In Vivo 11: 169–172.
83. Jagielski D, Lechowski R, Hoffmann-Jagielska M, Winiarczyk S (2002) A retrospective study of the incidence and prognostic factors of multicentric lymphoma in dogs (1998–2000). J Vet Med A Physiol Pathol Clin Med 49: 419–424.
84. Marconato L, Martini V, Aresu L, Sampaolo M, Valentini F, et al. (2013) Assessment of bone marrow infiltration diagnosed by flow cytometry in canine large B cell lymphoma: Prognostic significance and proposal of a cut-off value. Vet J 197: 776–781.

85. Wiedemann AL, Charney SC, Barger AM, Schaeffer DJ, Kitchell BE (2005) Assessment of corticosteroid-induced alkaline phosphatase as a prognostic indicator in canine lymphoma. J Small Anim Pract 46: 185–190.
86. Weller RE, Theilen GH, Madewell BR (1982) Chemotherapeutic responses in dogs with lymphosarcoma and hypercalcemia. J Am Vet Med Assoc 181: 891–893.
87. Miller AG, Morley PS, Rao S, Avery AC, Lana SE, et al. (2009) Anemia is associated with decreased survival time in dogs with lymphoma. J Vet Intern Med 23: 116–122.
88. Perry JA, Thamm DH, Eickhoff J, Avery AC, Dow SW (2011) Increased monocyte chemotactic protein-1 concentration and monocyte count independently associate with a poor prognosis in dogs with lymphoma. Vet Comp Oncol 9: 55–64.
89. Price GS, Page RL, Fischer BM, Levine JF, Gerig TM (1991) Efficacy and toxicity of doxorubicin/cyclophosphamide maintenance therapy in dogs with multicentric lymphosarcoma. J Vet Intern Med 5: 259–262.
90. Khanna C, Lund EM, Redic KA, Hayden DW, Bell FW, et al. (1998) Randomized controlled trial of doxorubicin versus dactinomycin in a multiagent protocol for treatment of dogs with malignant lymphoma. J Am Vet Med Assoc 213: 985–990.
91. Carter RF, Harris CK, Withrow SJ, Valli VEO, Susaneck SJ (1987) Chemotherapy of canine lymphoma with histopathological correlation - doxorubicin alone compared to COP as first treatment regimen. J Am Anim Hosp Assoc 23: 587–598.
92. Kol A, Marks SL, Skorupski KA, Kass PH, Guerrero T, et al. (2013) Serial haemostatic monitoring of dogs with multicentric lymphoma. Vet Comp Oncol. doi: 10.1111/vco.12041.
93. Sato M, Yamzaki J, Goto-Koshino Y, Takahashi M, Fujino Y, et al. (2013) The prognostic significance of minimal residual disease in the early phases of chemotherapy in dogs with high-grade B-cell lymphoma. Vet J 195: 319–324.
94. Webster JD, Dennis MM, Dervisis N, Heller J, Bacon NJ, et al. (2011) Recommended guidelines for the conduct and evaluation of prognostic studies in veterinary oncology. Vet Pathol 48: 7–18.
95. Mizuno T, Suzuki R, Umeki S, Okuda M (2009) Crossreactivity of antibodies to canine CD25 and Foxp3 and identification of canine $CD4^+CD25^+Foxp3^+$ cells in canine peripheral blood. J Vet Med Sci 71: 1561–1568.
96. Flammiger A, Weisbach L, Huland H, Tennstedt P, Simon R, et al. (2013) High tissue density of $FOXP3^+$ T cells is associated with clinical outcome in prostate cancer. Eur J Cancer 49: 1273–1279.
97. Lee S, Cho EY, Park YH, Ahn JS, Im YH (2013) Prognostic impact of FOXP3 expression in triple-negative breast cancer. Acta Oncol 52: 73–81.
98. Kryczek I, Liu R, Wang G, Wu K, Shu X, et al. (2009) FOXP3 defines regulatory T cells in human tumor and autoimmune disease. Cancer Res 69: 3995–4000.
99. Wang J, Ioan-Facsinay A, van der Voort EI, Huizinga TW, Toes RE (2007) Transient expression of FOXP3 in human activated nonregulatory $CD4^+$ T cells. Eur J Immunol 37: 129–138.
100. Thornton AM, Korty PE, Tran DQ, Wohlfert EA, Murray PE, et al. (2010) Expression of Helios, an Ikaros transcription factor family member, differentiates thymic-derived from peripherally induced $Foxp3^+$ T regulatory cells. J Immunol 184: 3433–3441.
101. Fujii K, Ishimaru F, Nakase K, Tabayashi T, Kozuka T, et al. (2003) Overexpression of short isoforms of Helios in patients with adult T-cell leukaemia/lymphoma. Br J Haematol 120: 986–989.
102. Zhang Z, Swindle CS, Bates JT, Ko R, Cotta CV, et al. (2007) Expression of a non-DNA-binding isoform of Helios induces T-cell lymphoma in mice. Blood 109: 2190–2197.
103. Dovat S, Montecino-Rodriguez E, Schuman V, Teitell MA, Dorshkind K, et al. (2005) Transgenic expression of Helios in B lineage cells alters B cell properties and promotes lymphomagenesis. J Immunol 175: 3508–3515.
104. Hudnall SD, Betancourt E, Barnhart E, Patel J (2008) Comparative flow immunophenotypic features of the inflammatory infiltrates of Hodgkin lymphoma and lymphoid hyperplasia. Cytometry B Clin Cytom 74: 1–8.
105. Mitchell L, Dow SW, Slansky JE, Biller BJ (2012) Induction of remission results in spontaneous enhancement of anti-tumor cytotoxic T-lymphocyte activity in dogs with B cell lymphoma. Vet Immunol Immunopathol 145: 597–603.
106. Chaudhry A, Rudensky AY (2013) Control of inflammation by integration of environmental cues by regulatory T cells. J Clin Invest 123: 939–944.
107. Lanca T, Silva-Santos B (2012) The split nature of tumor-infiltrating leukocytes: Implications for cancer surveillance and immunotherapy. Oncoimmunology 1: 717–725.
108. Lakshmi Narendra B, Eshvendar Reddy K, Shantikumar S, Ramakrishna S (2013) Immune system: a double-edged sword in cancer. Inflamm Res 62: 823–834.
109. Akimova T, Beier UH, Wang L, Levine MH, Hancock WW (2011) Helios expression is a marker of T cell activation and proliferation. PLoS One 6: e24226.
110. Onoe T, Kalscheuer H, Danzl N, Chittenden M, Zhao G, et al. (2011) Human natural regulatory T cell development, suppressive function, and postthymic maturation in a humanized mouse model. J Immunol 187: 3895–3903.
111. Lin X, Chen M, Liu Y, Guo Z, He X, et al. (2013) Advances in distinguishing natural from induced $Foxp3^+$ regulatory T cells. Int J Clin Exp Pathol 6: 116–123.
112. Hansen W, Hutzler M, Abel S, Alter C, Stockmann C, et al. (2012) Neuropilin 1 deficiency on $CD4^+Foxp3^+$ regulatory T cells impairs mouse melanoma growth. J Exp Med 209: 2001–2016.
113. Malchow S, Leventhal DS, Nishi S, Fischer BI, Shen L, et al. (2013) Aire-dependent thymic development of tumor-associated regulatory T cells. Science 339: 1219–1224.
114. Rimsza LM, Farinha P, Fuchs DA, Masoudi H, Connors JM, et al. (2007) HLA-DR protein status predicts survival in patients with diffuse large B-cell lymphoma treated on the MACOP-B chemotherapy regimen. Leuk Lymphoma 48: 542–546.
115. Rimsza LM, Roberts RA, Miller TP, Unger JM, LeBlanc M, et al. (2004) Loss of MHC class II gene and protein expression in diffuse large B-cell lymphoma is related to decreased tumor immunosurveillance and poor patient survival regardless of other prognostic factors: a follow-up study from the Leukemia and Lymphoma Molecular Profiling Project. Blood 103: 4251–4258.
116. Veelken H, Vik Dannheim S, Schulte Moenting J, Martens UM, Finke J, et al. (2007) Immunophenotype as prognostic factor for diffuse large B-cell lymphoma in patients undergoing clinical risk-adapted therapy. Ann Oncol 18: 931–939.
117. Rao S, Lana S, Eickhoff J, Marcus E, Avery PR, et al. (2011) Class II major histocompatibility complex expression and cell size independently predict survival in canine B-cell lymphoma. J Vet Intern Med 25: 1097–1105.

18

NSFC Health Research Funding and Burden of Disease in China

Gelin Xu, Zhizhong Zhang, Qiushi Lv, Yun Li, Ruidong Ye, Yunyun Xiong, Yongjun Jiang, Xinfeng Liu*

Department of Neurology, Jinling Hospital, Nanjing University School of Medicine, Nanjing, Jiangsu Province, China

Abstract

Background: Allocation of health research funds among diseases has never been evaluated in China. This study aimed to examine the relationship between disease-specific funding levels of National Nature Science Foundation of China (NSFC), the main governmental resource for health research in China, and burden of disease.

Methods: Funding magnitudes for 53 diseases or conditions were obtained from the website of NSFC. Measures of disease burden, mortality, years of life lost (YLLs) and disability-adjusted life years (DALYs), were derived from the Global Burden of Disease Study 2010. The relationship between NSFC funding and disease burden was analyzed with univariate linear regression. For each measure associated with funding, regression-derived estimates were used to calculate the expected funds for each disease. The actual and expected funds were then compared. We also evaluated the impacts of changes of disease burden metrics since 1990, and differences from the world averages on NSFC funding.

Results: NSFC health research funding was associated with disease burden measured in mortality ($R = 0.33$, $P = 0.02$), YLLs ($R = 0.39$, $P = 0.004$), and DALYs ($R = 0.40$, $P = 0.003$). But none of the changes of mortality ($R = 0.22$, $P = 0.12$), YLLs ($R = -0.04$, $P = 0.79$) and DALYs ($R = -0.003$, $P = 0.98$) since 1990 was associated with the funding magnitudes. None of the differences of mortality ($R = -0.11$, $P = 0.45$), YLLs ($R = -0.11$, $P = 0.43$) and DALYs ($R = -0.12$, $P = 0.38$) from that of the concurrent world averages were associated with the funding magnitudes. Measured by DALY, stroke and COPD received the least funding compared to expected; while leukemia and diabetes received the most funding compared to expected.

Conclusion: Although NSFC funding were roughly associated with disease burden as measured in mortality, YLLs and DALYs. Some major diseases such as stroke were underfunded; while others such as leukaemia were overfunded. Change of disease burden during the last 20 years and country-specialized disease burden were not reflected in current allocation of NSFC funds.

Editor: Guangyuan He, Huazhong University of Science and Technology, China

Funding: This study was sponsored by Nature Science Foundation of Jiangsu (BE2013713) to GX. The funders had no role in study design, data collection and analysis, decision to publish, or preparation of the manuscript.

Competing Interests: The authors have declared that no competing interests exist.

* Email: xfliu2@vip.163.com

Introduction

In recent years, China is pouring cash into science and technology faster than its economy has expanded [1]. The total research and development (R&D) expenditure in China has increased by 23% annually on average over the past decade [2]. The central government's budget on science and technology reached 267.4 billion yuan renminbi (RMB), or US $43.6 billion, in 2014 [2]. Consistent with this trend, the governmental funding for health research is also increasing. Although still dwarfed by that of US (US $ 3.1 billion for National Natural Science Foundation of China (NSFC) against US $ 30 billion for US National Institute of Health (NIH) in 2014), China's governmental funds, principally NSFC, are becoming an important supporter for health research in the world [3].

However, the allocation of research funds among diseases, and its rationality has never been evaluated in China. The disbursement of grant money has been criticized for lack of transparency, and funding tends to go to eminent scientists and safe projects [4,5]. There are short-term (annual) and long-term (5 years) national priorities for health researches, but they are merely results of government decisions based on politic will, public opinions, extemporaneous expert comments and immediate experience from western countries, rather than on systematic analysis of China's own disease burden. Considering the limited resources, it is important for China to optimize the process for health fund allocation with disease burden as a reference, as did in USA and other countries [6–8].

NSFC is a centre goverment agency specialized in administrating basic research funds, and it is the main source for the health research funds. Utilizing the design and methods in previous studies for evaluating association of NIH funding level and disease burden in USA [6,7], this study evaluated the relationship between NSFC funding levels and measures of disease burden. We also

Table 1. Funding levels of NSFC and disease burden in China.

Condition or disease	NSFC research fund	Measure of disease burden in 2010					
		thousands (rank)					
	thousands in RMB (% of total)	Mortality	Mortality change since 1990	YLLs	YLLs change since 1990	DALYs	DALYs change since 1990
Leukaemia	327854 (12.8)	58 (17)	5 (25)	2390 (15)	−366 (40)	2418 (19)	−354 (42)
Diabetes	176635 (6.9)	160 (11)	90 (5)	3173 (13)	1251 (5)	7835 (9)	2989 (4)
Ischemic heart disease	169185 (6.6)	949 (2)	499 (1)	16084 (3)	7093 (1)	17886 (3)	7759 (1)
Dementia	115785 (4.5)	50 (20)	24 (11)	616 (30)	159 (17)	1593 (23)	636 (13)
Liver cancer	114225 (4.5)	370 (6)	131 (4)	10014 (6)	2684 (4)	10089 (7)	2718 (5)
Injury	103560 (4.0)	796 (4)	−56 (47)	31759 (1)	−12827 (51)	40804 (1)	−10386 (51)
Breast cancer	95360 (3.7)	53 (19)	23 (12)	1563 (17)	645 (8)	1671 (22)	716 (10)
Asthma	80060 (3.1)	20 (32)	−32 (45)	358 (37)	−173 (38)	1095 (30)	−143 (39)
Colorectal cancer	75990 (3.0)	150 (12)	57 (6)	3305 (11)	901 (7)	3423 (15)	975 (8)
Chronic kidney diseases	75389 (2.9)	82 (15)	28 (9)	2054 (16)	413 (11)	2782 (17)	696 (11)
Cirrhosis	68085 (2.7)	114 (13)	−61 (48)	3180 (12)	−2095 (47)	3316 (16)	−2088 (47)
Neonatal disorders	63730 (2.5)	83 (14)	−260 (52)	7173 (7)	−22334 (53)	8679 (8)	−22534 (53)
Lung cancer	63580 (2.5)	513 (5)	253 (3)	11197 (5)	4943 (2)	11318 (6)	5013 (3)
Hypertensive heart disease	61463 (2.4)	173 (10)	39 (7)	2734 (14)	458 (10)	2767 (18)	460 (15)
Stroke	55330 (2.2)	1727 (1)	387 (2)	29173 (2)	4829 (3)	30139 (2)	5262 (2)
Stomach cancer	53610 (2.1)	297 (7)	0 (38)	6523 (8)	−849 (43)	6616 (10)	−825 (43)
Hepatitis	53245 (2.1)	44 (23)	11 (16)	1319 (19)	−48 (34)	1443 (28)	−38 (37)
Brain cancers	52610 (2.1)	49 (21)	13 (14)	1473 (18)	232 (14)	1497 (26)	240 (19)
Depression	51335 (2.0)	0 (53)	0 (36)	0 (53)	0 (30)	11767 (5)	2297 (6)
Pneumonia	46600 (1.8)	195 (8)	−197 (51)	4771 (9)	−20173 (52)	5135 (11)	−20166 (52)
Schizophrenia	43260 (1.7)	9 (42)	−4 (40)	279 (39)	−171 (37)	3472 (14)	918 (9)
HIV-AIDS	40075 (1.6)	36 (24)	36 (8)	1111 (23)	1100 (6)	1752 (20)	1739 (7)
Peptic ulcer	39870 (1.6)	19 (33)	−36 (46)	382 (35)	−942 (45)	453 (41)	−958 (45)
Atrial fibrillation and flutter	39150 (1.5)	13 (37)	8 (18)	154 (47)	91 (22)	596 (39)	259 (18)
Prostate cancer	34530 (1.3)	11 (39)	7 (19)	165 (45)	97 (21)	178 (50)	109 (25)
Nasopharynx cancer	31250 (1.2)	34 (26)	12 (15)	1046 (24)	314 (13)	1060 (31)	320 (17)
Epilepsy	31240 (1.2)	12 (38)	−7 (42)	559 (32)	−424 (41)	1507 (25)	−216 (40)
Maternal disorders	30260 (1.2)	5 (49)	−16 (43)	272 (40)	−911 (44)	546 (40)	−855 (44)
COPD	29450 (1.2)	934 (3)	−493 (53)	12995 (4)	−10808 (50)	16724 (4)	−9746 (50)
Parkinson disease	29160 (1.1)	7 (47)	3 (30)	121 (49)	25 (28)	265 (44)	91 (28)
Tuberculosis	26710 (1.0)	45 (22)	−124 (50)	1172 (22)	−4059 (49)	1733 (21)	−4418 (49)
Cervical cancer	26245 (1.0)	25 (29)	5 (26)	727 (28)	180 (16)	742 (35)	185 (21)

Table 1. Cont.

Condition or disease		NSFC research fund	Measure of disease burden in 2010					
			thousands (rank)					
		thousands in RMB (% of total)	Mortality	Mortality change since 1990	YLLs	YLLs change since 1990	DALYs	DALYs change since 1990
Pancreatic cancer		24051 (0.9)	58 (16)	26 (10)	1315 (20)	551 (9)	1322 (29)	555 (14)
Ovarian cancer		22270 (0.9)	21 (31)	6 (23)	594 (31)	141 (19)	603 (38)	145 (23)
Mouth cancer		19970 (0.8)	14 (36)	7 (21)	351 (38)	150 (18)	361 (43)	156 (22)
Oesophageal cancer		19480 (0.8)	176 (9)	7 (20)	3824 (10)	−15 (32)	3858 (12)	−10 (34)
Multiple sclerosis		18085 (0.7)	2 (51)	−2 (39)	50 (51)	−60 (35)	149 (52)	−26 (36)
Lymphoma		16400 (0.6)	29 (28)	6 (22)	835 (26)	40 (26)	854 (33)	50 (31)
Malaria		15050 (0.6)	0 (52)	0 (37)	2 (52)	−6 (31)	12 (53)	−4 (33)
Schistosomiasis		14650 (0.6)	9 (43)	0 (35)	222 (42)	−34 (33)	251 (45)	−23 (35)
Bladder cancer		13280 (0.5)	23 (30)	8 (17)	399 (34)	106 (20)	411 (42)	115 (24)
Pancreatitis		13110 (0.5)	8 (44)	2 (32)	188 (44)	25 (29)	205 (48)	27 (32)
Anaemias		12860 (0.5)	15 (35	−5 (41)	420 (33)	−494 (42)	1513 (24)	−346 (41)
Cardiomyopathy and myocarditis		12710 (0.5)	35 (25)	3 (31)	985 (25)	−125 (36)	1013 (32)	−127 (38)
Alcohole Chinae disorders		10720 (0.4)	5 (50)	1 (33)	163 (46)	32 (27)	3489 (13)	688 (12)
Kidney cancer		10020 (0.4)	32 (27)	18 (13)	823 (27)	400 (12)	837 (34)	384 (16)
Melanoma		8330 (0.3)	7 (48)	4 (28)	153 (48)	75 (24)	156 (51)	77 (29)
Gallbladder cancer		7560 (0.3)	18 (34)	0 (34)	637 (29)	225 (15)	644 (37)	229 (20)
Peripheral vascular disease		6990 (0.3)	9 (41)	6 (24)	119 (50)	−346 (39)	182 (49)	100 (26)
Thyroid cancer		6660 (0.3)	8 (45)	3 (29)	201 (43)	67 (25)	213 (47)	76 (30)
Meningitis		5350 (0.2)	8 (46)	−23 (44)	358 (36)	−1488 (46)	675 (36)	−1555 (46)
Rheumatic heart disease		4470 (0.2)	57 (18)	−74 (49)	1270 (21)	−2581 (48)	1487 (27)	−2654 (48)
Multiple myeloma		1710 (0.1)	9 (40)	4 (27)	246 (41)	90 (23)	250 (46)	93 (27)
Association with NSFC research fund	R		0.33	0.22	0.39	−0.04	0.40	−0.003
	P		0.02	0.12	0.004	0.79	0.003	0.98

discussed the differences of health research system in China and USA and the possible factors influencing the health fund allocation among diseases.

Methods

The budgets for NSFC are determined at least one year before each fiscal year, and some major research plans are made even five years ago. To reflect this time lag, data of 2010 disease burden and 2012 NSFC funding were chose to evaluate the relationship between disease burden and magnitude of research funding. Diseases were included in this study if 1) they were defined in *International Classification of Diseases, 9th revision, Clinical Modification (ICD-9-CM);* 2) their funding levels of NSFC were available; and 3) their measures of the burden of disease were available in Global Burden of Disease (GBD) Study 2010 [9].

Data Sources

NSFC has eight departments responsible for funding researches in different scientific subjects: mathematics, chemistry, life science, geoscience, engineering and material science, information science, management science and health. Before 2010, health research was included in the life science department, which also involved specialties of biology, botany, ecology, zoology, forestry, microbiology, immunology, psychology, agronomy and veterinary medicine. In 2010, health research was separated from life science department as a separate department.

The health department of NSFC has a similar framework to NIH, but with fewer "institutes" (currently eight compared with 27 institutes and centers in NIH), and endued with less functions. Applicants submit their protocols to different institutes according to target disease. For example, No.1 institute is responsible for diseases in circulatory, respiratory, blood and digestive systems. No.2 institute is responsible for disease in urinary, genital and endocrine systems, and diseases of ophthalmology, otolaryngology and dentistry. No. 3 institute is responsible for diseases of neurology and psychology. No.4 institute is responsible for diseases of skin, locomotor system and injury. No. 5 institute is responsible for cancer. No. 6 institute is responsible for communicable diseases and occupational diseases. No. 7 institute is responsible for pharmacology and pharmaceutics. No. 8 institute is responsible for Traditional Chinese Medicine.

Data concerning the funding levels for specific diseases or conditions in 2012 fiscal year were obtained from the NSFC website (http://isisn.nsfc.gov.cn/egrantweb/). The funding data were updated annually by NSFC. Data concerning disease burden were derived from GBD Study 2010 [9].

Three measures were chose to reflect disease burden from the GBD Study 2010: mortality, years of life lost (YLLs), and disability-adjusted life years (DALYs). In GBD Study, YLLs are calculated by multiplying the number of deaths in each age group by a reference life expectancy at that age. YLDs are calculated from the prevalence of a sequela multiplied by the disability weight for that sequela. Disability weights are based on surveys of general population. DALYs are the sum of YLLs and YLDs [10].

Due to the rapid population ageing and widespread westernized lifestyle changing, there is a remarkable change of disease

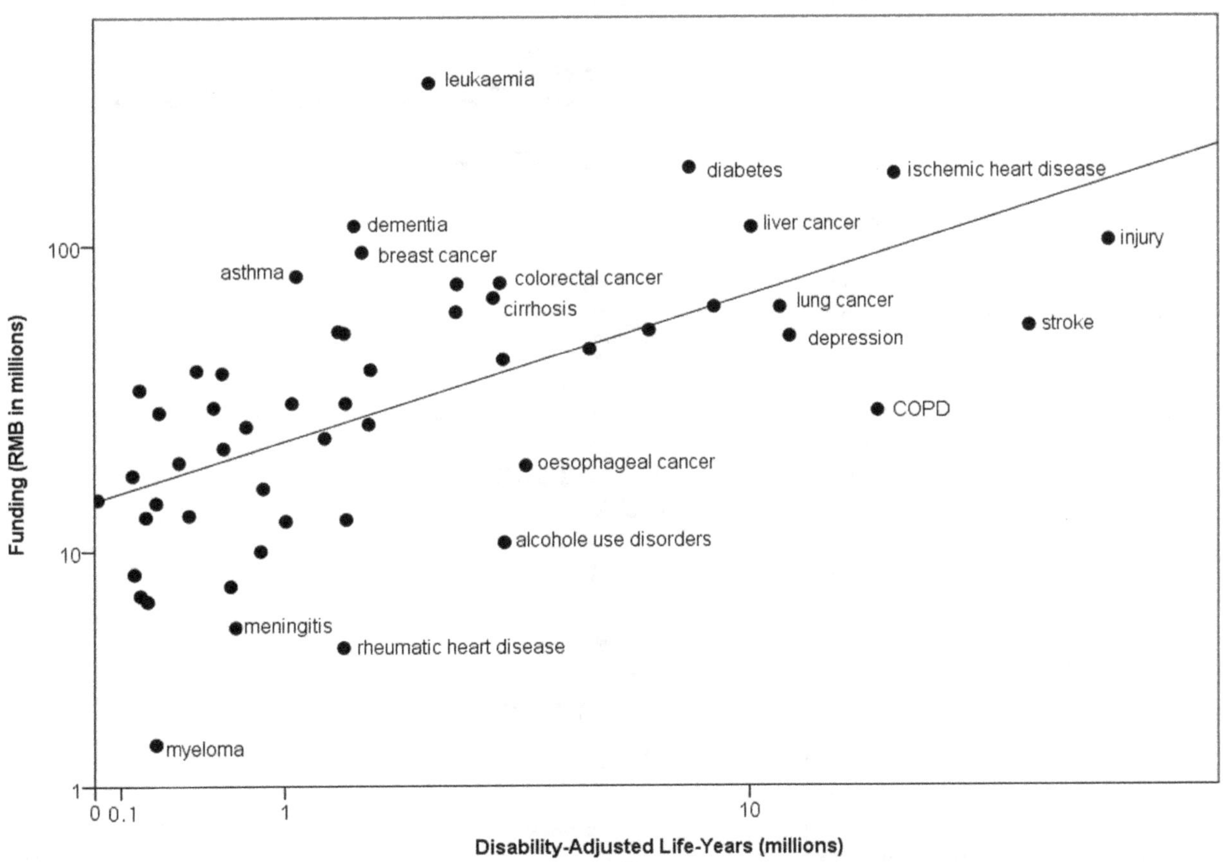

Figure 1. Relationship between NSFC disease-specific funding in 2012 and disability-adjusted life-years (DALYs) in 2012. Both X and Y axes are submitted to logarithmic scale. The line represents funding predicted on the basis of a linear regression with DALYs.

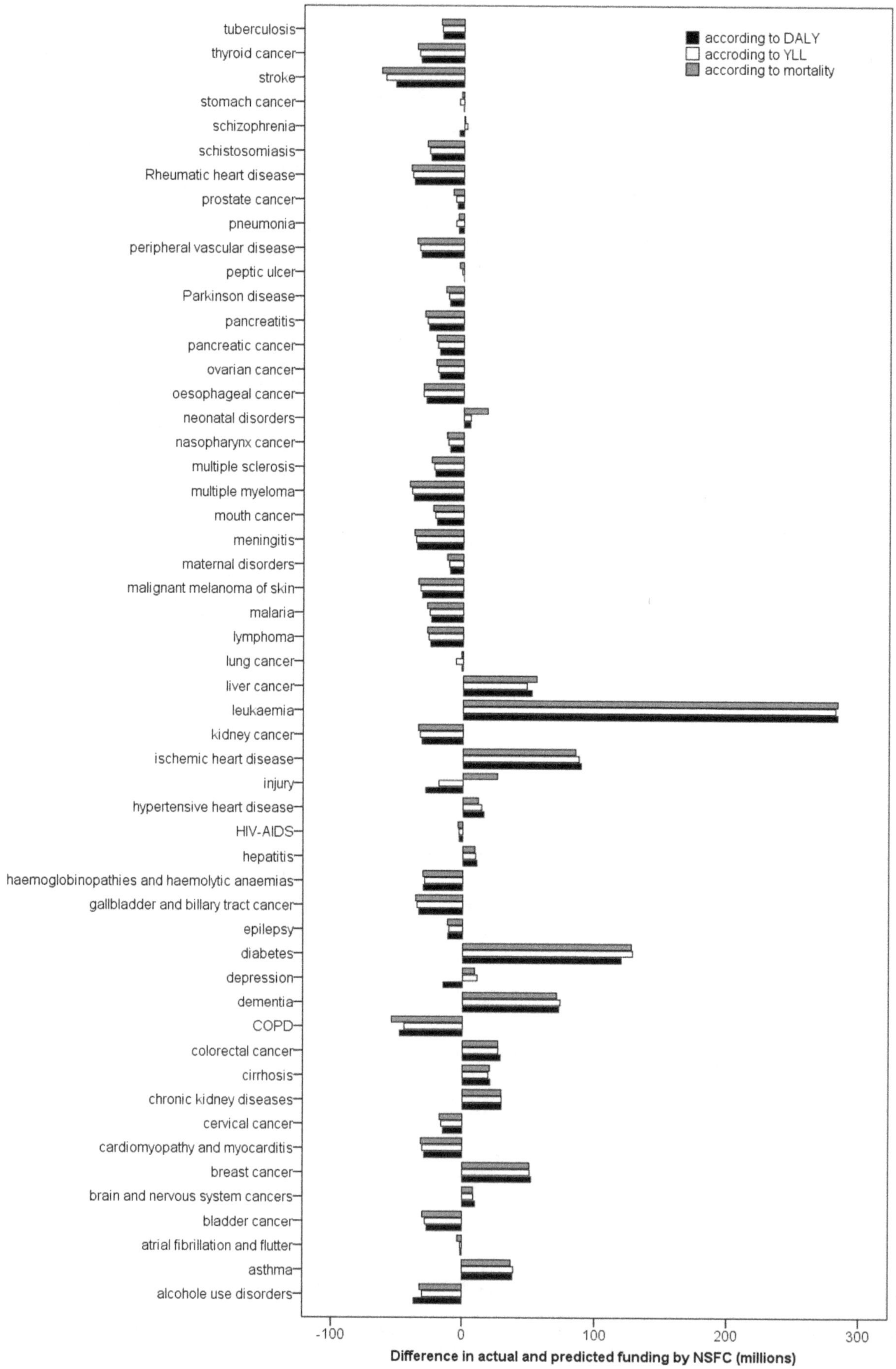
according to DALY
accroding to YLL
according to mortality
tuberculosis
thyroid cancer
stroke
stomach cancer
schizophrenia
schistosomiasis
Rheumatic heart disease
prostate cancer
pneumonia
peripheral vascular disease
peptic ulcer
Parkinson disease
pancreatitis
pancreatic cancer
ovarian cancer
oesophageal cancer
neonatal disorders
nasopharynx cancer
multiple sclerosis
multiple myeloma
mouth cancer
meningitis
maternal disorders
malignant melanoma of skin
malaria
lymphoma
lung cancer
liver cancer
leukaemia
kidney cancer
ischemic heart disease
injury
hypertensive heart disease
HIV-AIDS
hepatitis
haemoglobinopathies and haemolytic anaemias
gallbladder and biliary tract cancer
epilepsy
diabetes
depression
dementia
COPD
colorectal cancer
cirrhosis
chronic kidney diseases
cervical cancer
cardiomyopathy and myocarditis
breast cancer
brain and nervous system cancers
bladder cancer
atrial fibrillation and flutter
asthma
alcohole use disorders
-100
0
100
200
300
Difference in actual and predicted funding by NSFC (millions)

Figure 2. Differences between actual and expected disease-specific NSFC funding as predicted by mortality, YLLs and DALYs. Negative values indicates underfunded, and positive values indicates overfunded.

spectrum in China in recent 20 years. These trends may have influenced the allocation of research resources, because some disease may become more, while others less prevalent. We, therefore, evaluated the impacts of changes of mortality, YLLs, DALYs between 1990 and 2010 on disease funding. Data of disease burden, mortality, YLLs and DALYs for China in 1990, were also retrieved from GBD Study [9].

Some diseases are more prevalent, and pose an extra burden in China compared to the world average level. These diseases deserve extra research resource to accelerate improvements in prevention and management. Therefore, we evaluated the differences of mortality, YLLs and DALYs of each disease between China and the world average level. Data of mortality, YLLs and DALYs for the world average level in 2010 were retrieved from GBD Study [11–13].

Statistic Analysis

Univariate linear regression was performed to assess the relationship between funding levels and disease burden metrics. For each measure that had a significant association with funding, regression-derived estimates were used to calculate the expected NSFC funding for each disease. The expected and the actual funding magnitudes were then compared. In univaritate regression analyses, we also evaluated the association of funding levels with changes of disease burden during 1990 and 2010, and with differences of disease burden between China and the worldwide average. The SPSS statistical package (Version 16, Chicago, Ill) was used for all statistic analyses.

Results

The total NSFC budget of 2012 fiscal year was 16.93 billion RMB (US $2.69 billion), with 4.12 billion RMB allocated to health research (disease targeted), of which 2.57 billion RMB (62.4%) was devoted to the 53 diseases included in this study. Disease funding ranged from about 2 million RMB for multiple myeloma, to 328 million for leukemia, with a median of 31 million RMB (4.8±5.5 million RMB, **Table 1**).

In the univariate regression analysis, NSFC health funding was associated with burden of disease measured in mortality ($R = 0.33$, $P = 0.02$), YLLs ($R = 0.39$, $P = 0.004$), and DALYs ($R = 0.40$, $P = 0.003$, **Table 1**).

Since 1990, the burdens decreased in some diseases, while increased in others in large extents (**Table 1**). The mortality of chronic obstructive pulmonary disorder (COPD) decreased from 1427 thousand in 1990 to 934 thousand in 2010, with a decrement of 493 thousand which ranked top among diseases. The mortality of neonatal disorders decreased from 343 thousand to 83 thousand, with a decrement of 260 thousand which ranked second among diseases. Progress in neonatal disorders contributed the largest reduction of DALYs (a decrement of 22534), followed by pneumonia (a decrement of 20166). On the other hand, ischemic heart disease induced the largest increment of mortality (499 thousand) during 1990 to 2010, followed by stroke (387 thousand). Ischemic heart disease also induced the largest increment of DALYs (7759 thousand), followed by stroke (5262 thousand). Because these transitional trends of disease burden may be a reflection of past research strength, and could have been used as indicators for allocating research resources, we analyzed the changes of disease burdens during 1990 to 2010. But none of the changes of mortality ($R = 0.22$, $P = 0.12$), YLLs ($R = -0.04$, $P = 0.79$) and DALYs ($R = -0.003$, $P = 0.98$) was associated with NSFC funding magnitudes (**Table 1**).

Some diseases pose extra burden in China compare to the world averages, while others pose less burden. Of note, stroke demonstrated the largest extra mortality (126.1/100000 higher), YLLs (614/100000 higher) and DALYs (618/100000 higher) than the world averages. Ischemic heart disease induced the least extra mortality than the world average (35.6/100000 lower), and neonatal disorders induced the least extra YLLs (1985/100000 lower) and DALYs (2004/100000 lower) than the world averages. We analyzed differences of disease burden metrics in 2010 between China and world averages. But none of the differences of mortality ($R = -0.11$, $P = 0.45$), YLLs ($R = -0.11$, $P = 0.43$) and DALYs ($R = -0.12$, $P = 0.38$) to the world averages were associated with NFSC funding magnitudes (**Table 2**).

In standard multivariable analysis, DALYs became the only significant predictor for NSFC funding. The amount of predicted and actual NSFC funding as a function of DALYs is shown in **Figure 1**. The line represents the predicted funding levels if DALYs were the sole criterion for funding.

The difference between actual and predicted funding for each disease, with mortality, YLLs and DALYs as explanatory variables, is shown in **Figure 2**. Stroke, and COPD received the least funding compared to expected, while the leukemia and diabetes received the most funding compared to expected.

Discussion

In this study we analyzed the relationship between NSFC funding and burden of disease measured in mortality, YLLs and DALYs. Although the NSFC health funding was associated with disease burden, measured in mortality ($R = 0.33$, $P = 0.02$), YLLs ($R = 0.39$, $P = 0.004$), and DALYs ($R = 0.40$, $P = 0.003$), there exist significant differences between the actual and expected funding in some diseases according to these measures.

The relationship between disease research funding and burden of disease has been investigated in US National Institute of Health (NIH) system in several studies [6,7,14]. Disease incidence and prevalence were unrelated to funding, while mortality and YLLs weakly correlated with funding. DALYs were more strongly predictive [6,7]. In this study, mortality also weakly correlated with funding. Both YLLs and DALYs correlated significantly with NSFC funding. Although NSFC has a smaller total funding budget for health research, and is more inclusive and involves several subjects other than health, its organization is roughly similar to those of NIH. So it is not surprise that the overall profiles of NSFC funding distribution among diseases are similar to that of NIH.

The funding programs in NSFC can be classified as three types: free-applying, predetermined and investigator-targeted programs, which accounts for about 93%, 5% and 2% of the total budget respectively. For free-applying programs, there is no preset research scope, so applicants can choose any health research topics. For predetermined programs, every year one or two research topics were preset in each institute according to expertise and scientific needs. For the investigator-targeted programs, prominent investigators younger than 45 years were selected base on their previous academic achievements, and 1.5–3.0 million RMB was arranged to each awarder. With the money, they can choose any health research topics in five years. These arrange-

Table 2. Funding levels of NSFC and disease burden of world.

Condition or disease	NSFC research fund	Measure of disease burden in 2010					
		Age-standardized rate per 100000 (rank)					
	thousands in RMB (% of total)	Mortality,	Mortality,	YLLs,	YLLs,	DALYs,	DALYs,
		World	China-World	World	China-World	World	China-World
Leukaemia	327854 (12.8)	4.2(27)	0.0 (12)	137(23)	45 (7)	139(31)	46 (7)
Diabetes	176635 (6.9)	19.5(9)	−8.0 (46)	378(13)	−160 (43)	680(11)	−148 (41)
Ischemic heart disease	169185 (6.6)	105.7(1)	−35.6 (53)	1757(3)	−636 (48)	1884(3)	−642 (48)
Dementia	115785 (4.5)	7.1(18)	−3.2 (39)	66(34)	−20 (27)	165(28)	−46 (33)
Liver cancer	114225 (4.5)	11.5(14)	13.5 (4)	275(14)	379 (2)	277(17)	382 (2)
Injury	103560 (4.0)	74.3(3)	−17.6 (49)	3347(1)	−1024 (50)	4058(1)	−1118 (50)
Breast cancer	95360 (3.7)	6.6(19)	−3.1 (38)	161(21)	−62 (36)	174(27)	−67 (35)
Asthma	80060 (3.1)	5.2(23)	−3.7 (42)	125(27)	−100 (41)	326(15)	−242 (44)
Colorectal cancer	75990 (3.0)	10.8(17)	−0.2 (18)	201(19)	22 (9)	209(25)	21 (9)
Chronic kidney diseases	75389 (2.9)	11.1(16)	−5.3 (43)	249(15)	−108 (42)	307(16)	−116 (39)
Cirrhosis	68085 (2.7)	15.6(12)	−7.9 (45)	441(11)	−233 (45)	450(13)	−233 (43)
Neonatal disorders	63730 (2.5)	31.0(6)	−21.6 (51)	2794(2)	−1985 (53)	2931(2)	−2004 (53)
Lung cancer	63580 (2.5)	23.4(7)	12.4 (5)	465(10)	287 (3)	470(12)	290 (3)
Hypertensive heart disease	61463 (2.4)	13.1(13)	−0.3 (19)	216(17)	−23 (29)	222(23)	−28 (27)
Stroke	55330 (2.2)	88.4(2)	38.5 (1)	1421(5)	614 (1)	1484(5)	618 (1)
Stomach cancer	53610 (2.1)	11.5(15)	17.3 (3)	235(16)	204 (5)	238(20)	207 (4)
Hepatitis	53245 (2.1)	4.6(26)	−1.6 (33)	185(20)	−97 (40)	192(26)	−95 (37)
Brain cancers	52610 (2.1)	3(33)	0.3 (9)	87(32)	14 (10)	88(37)	14 (10)
Depression	51335 (2.0)	0(53)	0.0 (14)	0(53)	0 (16)	1078(9)	−260 (45)
Pneumonia	46600 (1.8)	41(5)	−25.1 (52)	1639(4)	−1204 (52)	1672(4)	−1208 (52)
Schizophrenia	43260 (1.7)	0.3(50)	0.3 (10)	9(49)	10 (12)	218(24)	8 (11)
HIV-AIDS	40075 (1.6)	21.4(8)	−19.0 (50)	1121(7)	−1010 (49)	1184(7)	−1065 (49)
Peptic ulcer	39870 (1.6)	3.7(29)	−2.3 (36)	93(28)	−67 (37)	98(33)	−67 (34)
Atrial fibrillation and flutter	39150 (1.5)	1.7(40)	−0.7 (25)	17(46)	−6 (21)	52(41)	−10 (21)
Prostate cancer	34530 (1.3)	3.8(28)	−2.9 (37)	48(38)	−36 (31)	55(39)	−42 (30)
Nasopharynx cancer	31250 (1.2)	1(46)	1.3 (7)	29(43)	39 (8)	29(47)	40 (8)
Epilepsy	31240 (1.2)	2.6(34)	−1.7 (35)	126(26)	−84 (39)	253(19)	−141 (40)
Maternal disorders	30260 (1.2)	3.7(30)	−3.4 (40)	208(18)	−189 (44)	234(21)	−196 (42)
COPD	29450 (1.2)	43.8(4)	26.8 (2)	687(8)	250 (4)	1114(8)	77 (6)
Parkinson disease	29160 (1.1)	1.7(41)	−1.2 (30)	19(45)	−11 (23)	28(48)	−9 (20)
Tuberculosis	26710 (1.0)	18(10)	−14.9 (47)	619(9)	−538 (47)	717(10)	−599 (47)

Table 2. Cont.

Condition or disease		NSFC research fund	Measure of disease burden in 2010					
			Age-standardized rate per 100000 (rank)					
		thousands in RMB (% of total)	Mortality,	Mortality,	YLLs,	YLLs,	DALYs,	DALYs,
			World	China-World	World	China-World	World	China-World
Cervical cancer		26245 (1.0)	3.4(32)	−1.7 (34)	92(30)	−45 (34)	94(35)	−46 (31)
Pancreatic cancer		24051 (0.9)	4.7(25)	−0.7 (24)	89(31)	−1 (18)	89(36)	−1 (15)
Ovarian cancer		22270 (0.9)	2.4(37)	−1.0 (28)	59(35)	−20 (26)	60(38)	−21 (25)
Mouth cancer		19970 (0.8)	1.9(39)	−0.9 (27)	45(39)	−22 (28)	47(43)	−23 (26)
Oesophageal cancer		19480 (0.8)	6.1(20)	6.2 (6)	129(24)	128 (6)	130(32)	129 (5)
Multiple sclerosis		18085 (0.7)	0.3(51)	−0.2 (17)	8(50)	−5 (20)	16(51)	−6 (18)
Lymphoma		16400 (0.6)	3.5(31)	−1.4 (31)	93(29)	−33 (30)	94(34)	−34 (29)
Malaria		15050 (0.6)	16.7(11)	−16.7 (48)	1141(6)	−1141 (51)	1200(6)	−1199 (51)
Schistosomiasis		14650 (0.6)	0.2(52)	0.4 (8)	5(52)	10 (11)	48(42)	−31 (28)
Bladder cancer		13280 (0.5)	2.6(35)	−0.9 (26)	42(41)	−14 (24)	44(45)	−15 (22)
Pancreatitis		13110 (0.5)	1.2(44)	−0.6 (23)	31(42)	−19 (25)	34(46)	−20 (24)
Anaemias		12860 (0.5)	1.7(42)	−0.5 (22)	79(33)	−46 (35)	227(22)	−105 (38)
Cardiomyopathy/myocarditis		12710 (0.5)	6.1(21)	−3.6 (41)	156(22)	−84 (38)	162(29)	−87 (36)
Alcohole Chinae disorders		10720 (0.4)	1.7(43)	−1.4 (32)	55(36)	−45 (33)	256(18)	−20 (23)
Kidney cancer		10020 (0.4)	2.5(36)	−0.3 (20)	52(37)	5 (13)	53(40)	4 (12)
Melanoma		8330 (0.3)	0.7(47)	−0.2 (16)	16(47)	−6 (22)	17(50)	−6 (19)
Gallbladder cancer		7560 (0.3)	2.3(38)	−0.2 (15)	44(40)	0 (17)	44(44)	0 (14)
Peripheral vascular disease		6990 (0.3)	0.7(48)	0.0 (13)	8(51)	0 (15)	14(52)	−1 (16)
Thyroid cancer		6660 (0.3)	0.5(49)	0.1 (11)	11(48)	2 (14)	12(53)	2 (13)
Meningitis		5350 (0.2)	6.1(22)	−5.5 (44)	389(12)	−357 (46)	426(14)	−372 (46)
Rheumatic heart disease		4470 (0.2)	5.2(24)	−1.2 (29)	127(25)	−41 (32)	147(30)	−46 (32)
Multiple myeloma		1710 (0.1)	1.1(45)	−0.4 (21)	21(44)	−4 (19)	21(49)	−4 (17)
Association with NSFC research fund	R		0.33	−0.11	0.24	−0.11	0.25	−0.12
	P		0.02	0.45	0.09	0.43	0.07	0.38

ments made the distribution of NSFC health research fund among diseases largely determined by numbers of applications and applicants' interests in individual disease, which may be further influenced by international research trends, governmental policies and public opinions.

Based on the limited data of the present study, it is unlikely to determine why some diseases were underfunded, while others overfunded relative to disease burden. The over-funding of leukemia in China may be explained by the governmental reinforce of children health after the implementation of One-Child Policy in 1978. Successes in treating some types of leukemia in resent years, arsenic trioxide for acute promyelocytic leukemia as an example, which was originally discovered by Chinese researchers and they also contributed remarkably in the subsequent studies [15,16], may have further incited the enthusiasm for leukemia research in China. On the other hand, stroke and COPD remained as the most underfunded diseases. The limited data suggested that incidence, prevalence of stroke, COPD and several other chronic diseases are increasing rapidly in China in recent year due to population ageing, lifestyle transition and environment pollution [17,18]. These rapid changes in disease burdens have not reflected in the current NSFC funding assignment, possibly due to the unawareness of impact of these changes to public health or delayed responses to these changes. Furthermore, lack of major progress in managing stroke and COPD in recent years probably have depressed the interests for studying these chronic diseases.

Given the limited resource for health research, developing countries like China should allocate more research fund to their country-specific diseases–those with extra burden than other countries [19]. But in analyzing NCSF allocation, we failed to find this association. Measured by mortality, YLLs or DALYs, stroke poses the heaviest disease burden in China. The mortality, YLLs and DALYs of stroke in China is 38.5/100000, 614/100000 and 618/100000 higher than the world average level respectively, and all of these differences rank first among diseases. On the other hand, mortality, YLLs and DALYs of ischemic heart disease is 35.6/100000, 636/100000 and 642/100000 lower than the world average level respectively, which make it one of the least country-specific diseases in China. Although DALYs caused by stroke in 2010 (30139 thousand) is about two times of DALYs caused by ischemic heart disease (17886 thousand), the NSFC fund allocated for stroke is only one third of that for ischemic heart disease (55 vs 169 million RMB). This phenomenon of disproportionally underfunding of stroke and overfunding of ischemic heart disease in reference to disease burden was not observed in the recent NIH fund allocation [7].

The disease spectrum in China has changed significant in recent 20 years. Measured by DALYs, the disease burden of neonatal disorders and pneumonia decreased with the largest extent (22534/100000 and 20166/100000) during 1990 to 2010; while DALYs due to ischemic heart disease and stroke increased with the largest extent (7759/100000 and 5262/100000) [9]. Theoretically, those with disease burden increased rapidly deserve more research resources to find approach for counteracting the trends. But we failed to find this association in NCSF allocation.

There are several limitations in this study which should be addressed when interpreting the results. First, we did not evaluate other sources, such as health research funds from government agencies other than NSFC. Other national funds, such as 863 projects, 973 projects, and National Supporting Programs administrated by Ministry of Science and Technology (MOST), account for about 10% of all governmental funds dedicated to health research in 2012 [20]. Funds from provincial government account for about 20% of all governmental funds dedicated to health research. Thus, contribution of resources other than NSFC for health research is unremarkable. Second, we did not include prevalence and incidence as measures for disease burden due to lack of recent data. In the previous studies, prevalence and incidence were not associated with NIH funding levels. We presume this is also the case in NSFC funding. Third, there may be fluctuation of funding magnitudes for a given diseases over years. The annual fluctuation of funding may be more predominant in less common diseases, for which the number of applicants is relatively small.

In conclusion, although the funding levels of NSFC were roughly associated with diseases burden as measured with mortality, YLLs and DALYs, some major diseases such as stroke were underfunded; with others such as leukemia were overfunded. Changes of disease burden during the past 20 years, and differences of disease burden from the world average have not been considered in allocating the current NSFC health funds.

Acknowledgments

This study was sponsored by Nature Science Foundation of Jiangsu (BE2013713) to GX. Authors thank Dr. Heqin Cao from NSFC for providing the annual funding data of NSFC, and for his suggestions in the study design and manuscript revision.

Author Contributions

Conceived and designed the experiments: GX ZZ QL YL RY YX YJ XL. Performed the experiments: GX ZZ QL YL. Analyzed the data: GX ZZ. Contributed reagents/materials/analysis tools: GX ZZ QL YJ XL. Wrote the paper: GX ZZ XL.

References

1. Van Noorden R (2014) China tops Europe in R&D intensity. Nature 505:144–145.
2. Qiu J (2014) China goes back to basics on research funding. Nature 507:148–149.
3. Morello L, Morrison J, Reardon S, Tollefson J, Witze A (2014) Obama's budget request falls flat. Nature 507:147–148.
4. Shi Y, Rao Y (2010) China's research culture. Science 329:1128.
5. Cao C, Li N, Li X, Liu L (2013) Science and Government. Reforming China's S&T system. Science 341:460–462.
6. Gross CP, Anderson GF, Powe NR (1999) The relation between funding by the National Institutes of Health and the burden of disease. N Engl J Med 340:1881–1887.
7. Gillum LA, Gouveia C, Dorsey ER, Pletcher M, Mathers CD, et al. (2011) NIH disease funding levels and burden of disease. PLoS One 6:e16837.
8. McCarthy M, Harvey G, Conceição C, la Torre G, Gulis G (2009) Comparing public-health research priorities in Europe. Health Res Policy Syst 7:17.
9. Yang G, Wang Y, Zeng Y, Gao GF, Liang X, et al. (2013) Rapid health transition in China, 1990–2010: findings from the Global Burden of Disease Study 2010. Lancet 381:1987–2015.
10. Murray CJ, Ezzati M, Flaxman AD, Lim S, Lozano R, et al. (2012) GBD 2010: design, definitions, and metrics. Lancet 380:2063–2066.
11. Lozano R, Naghavi M, Foreman K, Lim S, Shibuya K, et al. (2012) Global and regional mortality from 235 causes of death for 20 age groups in 1990 and 2010: a systematic analysis for the Global Burden of Disease Study 2010. Lancet 380:2095–2128.
12. Murray CJ, Vos T, Lozano R, Naghavi M, Flaxman AD, et al. (2012) Disability-adjusted life years (DALYs) for 291 diseases and injuries in 21 regions, 1990–2010: a systematic analysis for the Global Burden of Disease Study 2010. Lancet 380:2197–2223.
13. Vos T, Flaxman AD, Naghavi M, Lozano R, Michaud C, et al. (2012) Years lived with disability (YLDs) for 1160 sequelae of 289 diseases and injuries 1990–2010: a systematic analysis for the Global Burden of Disease Study 2010. Lancet 380:2163–2196.

14. Sampat BN, Buterbaugh K, Perl M (2013) New evidence on the allocation of NIH funds across diseases. Milbank Q 91:163–185.
15. Rao Y, Li R, Zhang D (2013) A drug from poison: how the therapeutic effect of arsenic trioxide on acute promyelocytic leukemia was discovered. Sci China Life Sci 56:495–502.
16. Wang ZY, Chen Z (2008) Acute promyelocytic leukemia: from highly fatal to highly curable. Blood 111:2505–2515.
17. Liu M, Wu B, Wang WZ, Lee LM, Zhang SH, et al. (2007) Stroke in China: epidemiology, prevention, and management strategies. Lancet Neurol 6:456–464.
18. Fang X, Wang X, Bai C (2011) COPD in China: the burden and importance of proper management. Chest 139:920–929.
19. Viergever RF, Olifson S, Ghaffar A, Terry RF (2010) A checklist for health research priority setting: nine common themes of good practice. Health Res Policy Syst 8:36.
20. National Bureau of Statistics Ministry of Science and Technology (2013) China Statistical Yearbook on Science and Technology. China Statistics Press. Beijing.

19

Cellular Intrinsic Mechanism Affecting the Outcome of AML Treated with Ara-C in a Syngeneic Mouse Model

Wenjun Zhao[1], Lirong Wei[1], Dongming Tan[1], Guangsong Su[1], Yanwen Zheng[1], Chao He[1], Zhengwei J. Mao[2], Timothy P. Singleton[3], Bin Yin[1,4,5]*

1 Cyrus Tang Hematology Center, Jiangsu Institute of Hematology, the First Affiliated Hospital, Soochow University, Suzhou, Jiangsu Province, PR China, **2** Division of Hematopathology, Department of Laboratory Medicine and Pathology, University of Minnesota Medical Center-Fairview, Minneapolis, Minnesota, United States of America, **3** Department of Laboratory of Medicine and Pathology, University of Minnesota, Minneapolis, Minnesota, United States of America, **4** Thrombosis and Hemostasis Key Lab of the Ministry of Health, Soochow University, Suzhou, Jiangsu Province, PR China, **5** Collaborative Innovation Center of Hematology, Soochow University, Suzhou, Jiangsu Province, PR China

Abstract

The mechanisms underlying acute myeloid leukemia (AML) treatment failure are not clear. Here, we established a mouse model of AML by syngeneic transplantation of BXH-2 derived myeloid leukemic cells and developed an efficacious Ara-C-based regimen for treatment of these mice. We proved that leukemic cell load was correlated with survival. We also demonstrated that the susceptibility of leukemia cells to Ara-C could significantly affect the survival. To examine the molecular alterations in cells with different sensitivity, genome-wide expression of the leukemic cells was profiled, revealing that overall 366 and 212 genes became upregulated or downregulated, respectively, in the resistant cells. Many of these genes are involved in the regulation of cell cycle, cellular proliferation, and apoptosis. Some of them were further validated by quantitative PCR. Interestingly, the Ara-C resistant cells retained the sensitivity to ABT-737, an inhibitor of anti-apoptosis proteins, and treatment with ABT-737 prolonged the life span of mice engrafted with resistant cells. These results suggest that leukemic load and intrinsic cellular resistance can affect the outcome of AML treated with Ara-C. Incorporation of apoptosis inhibitors, such as ABT-737, into traditional cytotoxic regimens merits consideration for the treatment of AML in a subset of patients with resistance to Ara-C. This work provided direct in vivo evidence that leukemic load and intrinsic cellular resistance can affect the outcome of AML treated with Ara-C, suggesting that incorporation of apoptosis inhibitors into traditional cytotoxic regimens merits consideration for the treatment of AML in a subset of patients with resistance to Ara-C.

Editor: Linda Bendall, University of Sydney, Australia

Funding: This study is supported by the National Key Scientific Project of China ("973 Program", No. 2011CB933501), the NSFC Project (No. 81070417), and the Priority Academic Program Development of Jiangsu Higher Education Institutions (PAPD program). The funders had no role in study design, data collection and analysis, decision to publish, or preparation of the manuscript.

Competing Interests: The authors have declared that no competing interests exist.

* Email: yinbin@hotmail.com

These authors contributed equally to this work.

Introduction

Acute myeloid leukemia (AML) is an aggressive hematologic malignancy characterized by a clonal expansion of myeloid blasts in the marrow and other sites. Despite the progresses made in AML therapy, such as hematopoietic stem cell transplantation, all-trans retinoic acid [1] and arsenic trioxide [2], the outcomes of most AML patients remain poor. In fact, the 5-year survival for patients with AML diagnosed from 2006 to 2010 was reported to be around 20% [3]. Failures in treatment of AML can be largely attributed to the refractoriness of leukemic cells to current therapies. However, the biological mechanisms underlying leukemic resistance to treatment are unclear.

Mouse models of leukemia have been attractive because of their close mimicking of human diseases in many aspects [4]. The past few years have witnessed a large amount of effort in the search for and the assessment of novel anti-leukemia treatment strategies in these mouse models. Recently, Mulloy's group evaluated standard cytosine-arabinoside (Ara-C) and doxorubicin regimens in AML xenografts using an immunodeficient mouse model, and showed that this system is useful for evaluation of novel chemotherapy in combination with standard induction treatment [5]. Because the microenvironment plays an important role in leukemic progression and response to therapy [6] and because immune cells are part of the tumor microenvironment [6], we investigated the effects of chemotherapy in immunocompetent mice and attempted to explore the mechanisms for differential drug responses.

Although enormous effort has been put into the exploration of targeted treatment of AML in the recent years, Ara-C remains one of the most effective drugs in the treatment of myeloid malignancies and demands more attentions [7,8]. It is specific to the S-phase of the cell cycle and therefore exhibits more toxicity to neoplastic cells that are in active synthesis of DNA. However, the outcomes of Ara-C-based treatment vary among patients. Genetic factors of leukemic cells have been associated with their response to treatment. MLL translocations predict poor outcome, whereas other chromosomal abnormalities such as AML1-ETO and inv(16), are associated with better prognosis [9,10]. Our earlier work demonstrated that Nf1 deficiency conferred Ara-C resistance to AML cells and that leukemic cells with loss-of-function mutation in p53 were selected for and grew out during the acquirement of resistance to Ara-C, indicating these genetic changes affected chemotherapeutic responses of leukemia [11,12]. Recently, p53 status has also been reported to significantly affect tumor response to targeted therapy [13]. Other factors contributing to the chemotherapeutic response need to be investigated.

To investigate the cellular mechanisms responsible for poor treatment response, we established a syngeneic mouse model of AML by transplanting BXH-2 derived myeloid leukemic cells to immunocompetent mice. The BXH-2 strain of mice spontaneously develops AML at a high incidence, mainly through retrovirally insertional mutagenesis arising from infection by a murine leukemia virus (MuLV) [14] Using this AML mouse model treated with an efficacious Ara-C-based regimen that we developed, we found that leukemic cell load, and the sensitivity of leukemic cells to Ara-C determined the survival. Gene expression profiling was performed to reveal the molecular changes in Ara-C resistant leukemic cells. Of interest, we demonstrated that the Ara-C resistant leukemic cells could be suppressed in vitro and in vivo by inhibition of anti-apoptosis proteins.

Materials and Methods

1. Ethics Statement

The cell line used in this study, B117, was originally established from primary AML cells developed in BXH-2 strain of mice, and published in independent studies thereafter [15]. This cell line is available upon request. All animal work was done in accordance with protocols approved by the Soochow University Institutional Animal Care and Use Committee.

2. Cell culture, drug and chemical

B117P and its derived cells were grown as described previously [15]. All culture media and supplements, except noted individually, were obtained from Invitrogen (Carlsbad, CA, USA). Ara-C was purchased from Pfizer Italia S.R.L (Neriviano, Italy). ABT-737 was obtained from Biochempartner Co. (Shanghai, China).

3. Animals

C57BL/6J and C3H/HeJ strains of mouse were obtained from Model Animal Research Center of Nanjing, and maintained in a Special Pathogen Free environment in our university animal facility. Six- to eight-week-old B6C3F1 mice generated by mating C57BL/6 and C3H/HeJ were used for leukemia transplantation and drug treatment. Moribund animals were euthanized as the end point in the survival experiments. Since this is an acute leukemia mouse model, these animals did not show obviously detectable sickness until a few hours prior to being moribund. To minimize suffering and difficulty of the mice, the husbandry conditions and health status of mice were monitored on a daily basis for any signs of sickness and maintained from fighting or tail clipping. During the late stage of the experiments, wet food was put on the floor of the cages. Moribund mice were euthanized using a CO_2 chamber. The criteria for humane euthanasia of mice involved in this study were determined by observation of signs of illness including lethargy, hunched posture, rough coat, and significant body weight loss. For collection of peripheral blood to count cells, mice were bled quickly followed by an immediate application of antibiotic analgesics.

4. Cytotoxicity assays

The MTS (3-(4,5-dimethylthiazol-2-yl)-5-(3-carboxymethoxyphenyl)-2-(4-sulfophenyl)- 2H-tetrazolium, Amresco, USA) tetrazolium assay was used to determine cytotoxic response of AML cell lines, as described before [12]. 1×10^5 cells were plated into flat-bottom 96-well plates (Corning Inc., Corning, NY, USA) in 200 μL of ASM media with various concentrations of Ara-C. After three days of incubation, 20 μL of MTS solution was added to each well and incubated at 37°C for 2 hours. The optical density at 650 nm was recorded as a reference, and subtracted from OD490 readings to eliminate nonspecific absorbance. Data from individual experiments are presented as the mean percentage of corrected OD490 of triplicate cultures ± SD.

5. Histopathology

The various mouse organ specimens were processed for histological analysis according to standard procedure [16]. Briefly, tissues were fixed in 4% paraformaldehyde, paraffin embedded, sectioned, and stained with hematoxylin and eosin. Morphological examination of leukemic cells and peripheral blood from leukemic recipient mice or normal mice used Wright-Giemsa staining method. Images were captured using an Olympus FSX100 at 20X for hematoxylin and eosin stained tissue sections, and 200X for hematoxylin and eosin or 600X for slides stained by Wright-Giemsa, respectively.

6. Flow cytometry

B117 cells and bone marrow cells flushed from mouse femurs and tibias were blocked prior to incubation with antibodies staining for Mac-1 and Gr-1 (BD Pharmingen, New Jersey, USA). To detect apoptosis, cells were stained with Annexin V-FITC apoptosis detection kit (Biouniquer, Nanjing, China) following the manufacturer's protocol. After staining, cells were washed and analyzed on a FACScan (BD Biosciences, Franklin Lakes, USA) using FlowJo software (Tree-Star Inc, Ashland, USA).

7. Measurement of B117P cell load using a specific proviral insertion tag

Genomic DNA was extracted from B117P and mouse white blood cells using the TIANamp Genomic DNA Kit (TianGen Co., China), according to the manufacturer's instructions. B117P specific proviral insertion tags were isolated using APE-PCR, as recently reported [17]. One of the tags was chosen as a molecular marker for B117P cells whose abundance can be reflected by measuring this tag using quantitative real-time polymerase chain reaction (See the following description of qPCR for details). The primers used for amplification of B117 tag were 5′ CTGAGATGAGGCGCAACAT 3′ (forward) and 5′ CCTGTGGTTCAAGTGAAGC 3′ (reverse), and β-actin gene as the internal reference 5′ GATCATTGCTCCTCCTGAGC 3′ (forward) and 5′ GACTCATCGTACTCCTGCTTG 3′ (reverse).

8. Gene expression profiling

Total RNA was extracted with TRIzol reagent according to the protocol (Molecular Research Center, Cincinnati, OH, USA), followed by DNase I treatment to eliminate potential genomic DNA contamination. Three samples of B117P and B117HS were analyzed by Super Biotek Co. Briefly, RNA was amplified and labeled using the OneArray Amino Allyl aRNA Amplification Kit

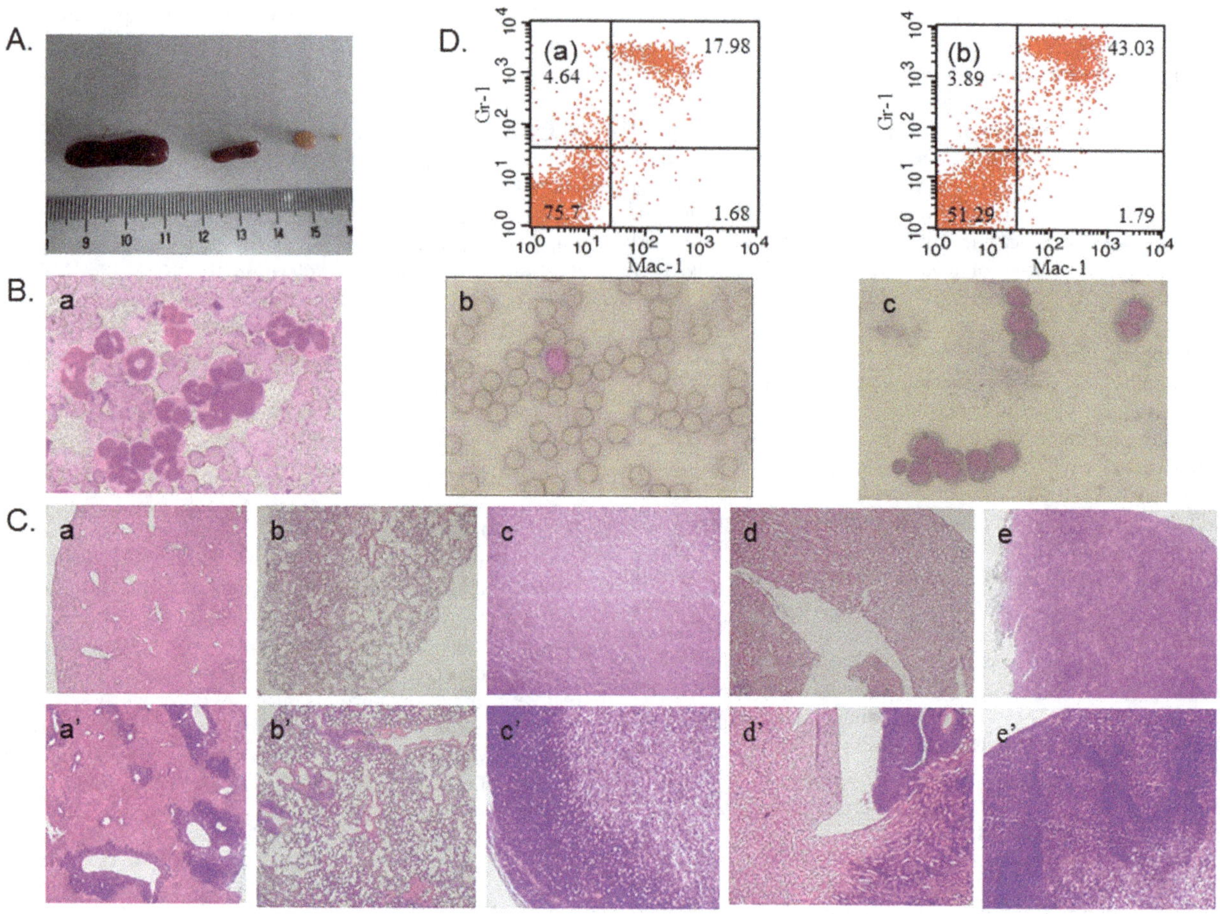

Figure 1. Establishment and characterization of an AML mouse model for evaluating treatment response by transplanting of BXH-2 derived myeloid leukemic cells into syngeneic mice (B6C3F1). Fig. 1A) Gross anatomic examination of spleen and lymph node collected from leukemic (left) or normal (right) mice. Fig. 1B) Morphological examination of peripheral blood smears from (a) recipient mice, (b) normal mice and (c) of B117 cells (Wright-Giemsa staining). Representative fields are shown here. Fig. 1C) Pathologic examination of organ sections, including liver (a & a'), lung (b & b'), lymph node (c & c'), kidney (d & d'), and spleen (e & e'), obtained from normal (a~e) versus leukemic (a'~e') mice (H & E staining). Fig. 1D) Immunophenotypic analysis of bone marrow cells recovered from normal (a) or leukemic (b) mice.

(Phalanx Biotech Group, Taiwan) and Cy5 dyes (Amersham Pharmacia, Piscataway, NJ, USA) and hybridized to Mouse Whole Genome OneArray with Phalanx hybridization buffer using Phalanx Hybridization System. Data was normalized using Rosetta Resolver System (Rosetta Biosoftware). A heat map of genes with $\log_2$ ratio ≥ 1 or $\log_2$ ratio ≤ -1 and p-value<0.05 was generated using Cluster 3.0 and TreeView and Gene set enrichment analysis was performed using ArrayTrack software (http://edkb.fda.gov/webstart/arraytrack/).

9. Quantitative real-time polymerase chain reaction (qPCR)

0.1 μg of total RNA was reverse transcribed with oligo(dT)n, using the SuperScript II First Strand cDNA Synthesis system (Invitrogen) according to the manual. qPCR was performed using SYBR Green method (Applied Biosystems, Foster city, CA, USA). Individual reaction contains diluted cDNA, 400 nM forward and reverse primers each, and 12.5 μL 2x PCR master mixes. PCR reaction was denatured at 95°C for 10 minutes, followed by 40 cycles of 95°C for 15 seconds and 60°C for 1 minute. The fold changes were calculated by the $2^{-\Delta\Delta Ct}$ method using ABI Prism 7500 SDS Software. The specific primers used for amplification of Dnmt3L were 5′ CTCTGGAAGAGCAATGGCTG 3′ (forward) and 5′ GACTTCGTACCTGATCATCTC 3′ (reverse), Plau 5′ GTGGCAGTGTACTTGGAGCT 3′ (forward) and 5′ GCATC-TATCTCACAGTGCTC 3′ (reverse), CD72 5′ GAACAGCG-CATCTAACCATCT 3′ (forward) and 5′ GTCGCAGTTGGTTGCTCTG 3′ (reverse), Uba7 5′ GAGT-TATACTCCAGGCAGCT 3′ (forward) and 5′ CACTGAG-CAGCCAAGTCAG 3′ (reverse), Pdrg1 5′ GAGTGTCTCT-GAAGATGTGAT 3′ (forward) and 5′ GTTGACTCCGCAGCCTTTCT 3′ (reverse), and β-actin transcript levels for normalization 5′ CAAGCAGGAGTACGAT-GAGT 3′ (forward) and 5′ GCCATGCCAATGTTGTCTCT 3′ (reverse), respectively.

10. Statistical analysis

Two-tailed Student's t-tests were performed using Microsoft Excel. A p-value of <0.05 was considered statistically significant. Kaplan-Meier estimates were used to calculate survival, and log-rank was used to calculate the p-value. Survival was defined as from the day of injection of tumor cells.

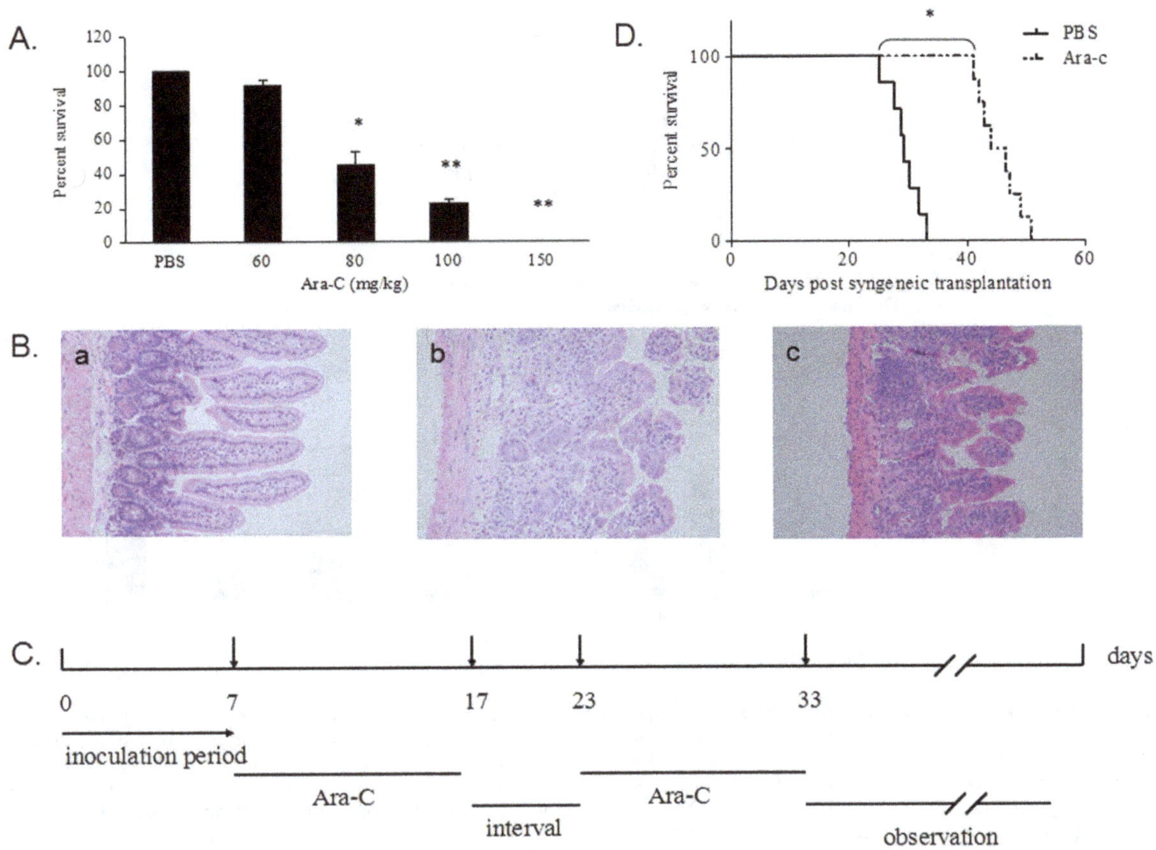

Figure 2. Development of an efficacious Ara-C-based regimen for the treatment of AML in mice. Fig. 2A) The survival rate of mice treated with Ara-C at various doses or with 100 μL of PBS control, in accordance with the treatment scheme described in the text. The mice were watched for a period of 50 days. The results shown here are representative of data obtained from 3 separate experiments. Fig. 2B) Histopathological examination of intestine affects Ara-C treatment. Fig. 2C) Treatment protocol for AML mice. The day of infusion of leukemic cells was considered as day 0. Fig. 2D) Suppression of leukemia using the treatment protocol. B6C3F1 mice transplanted with 2×10^5 B117P cells via tail vein were treated with either Ara-C (n = 12) or PBS (n = 12) as the control. *$p<0.05$.

Results

1. Establishment and characterization of a syngeneically transplanted AML mouse model for evaluation of treatment response

To establish an AML mouse model that is suitable for evaluation of chemotherapeutic response, we intravenously infused 2×10^5 B117 cells into a syngeneic B6C3F1 mouse. All recipient B6C3F1 mice (n = 12) reproducibly developed a hematologic disease resembling AML around a month following the transplantation, manifested by body weight loss, increased white blood cell counts, and being moribund. The necropsy showed enlarged spleen, lymph nodes and liver (Fig. 1A). Wright-Giemsa stained peripheral blood smears from diseased mice highlighted aggregates of heterogeneous blast cells with prominent nucleoli and nuclear indentations (Fig. 1B). Histopathological studies of liver, lung, lymph node, kidney and spleen revealed diffuse infiltration of the tissues with blast cells (Fig. 1C). Immunophenotypic staining of the bone marrow cells harvested from sick recipient mice showed an increased percentage of Mac-1^+Gr-1^+ cells (43%), compared with that for normal mice (18%) (Fig. 1D). These results indicated that an AML mouse model had been successfully created through a syngeneic transplantation of BXH-2 derived leukemia cells.

2. Development of an efficacious Ara-C based regimen for the treatment of AML in mice

One adverse effect of Ara-C treatment lies in its cause of damage to normal tissues. For the development of a protocol for Ara-C treatment of the mouse AML, it was important to determine the maximum tolerable dose (MTD) of Ara-C that could not only kill the tumor cells in vivo but also spare mice from the damage. To do so, we tested a range of doses of Ara-C on B6C3F1 mice that were intraperitoneally administered once a day for two courses of consecutive ten-day treatments with a five-day interval. We found that injection of 60 mg/kg of Ara-C gave rise to 5%~10% moribund animals which was further increased as the dose went up, till 100% reaching the end point mostly within the first course at 150 mg/kg (Fig. 2A). During the treatment, a significant body weight loss, a decrease in white blood cell counts, and frequent diarrhea were observed. Histopathological examination of intestine tissues of treated mice was indicative of a damage that became more severe with the increasing doses of Ara-C (Fig. 2B). These symptoms were consistent with the cytotoxicity of Ara-C. Therefore, the dose of 50 mg/kg of Ara-C was chosen for further studies.

Following several rounds of testings, we optimized the treatment scheme as illustrated in Fig. 2C. In order to examine its efficacy, AML mice created by intravenous infusion of 2×10^5 B117 cells were then treated with the protocol. Compared with the control

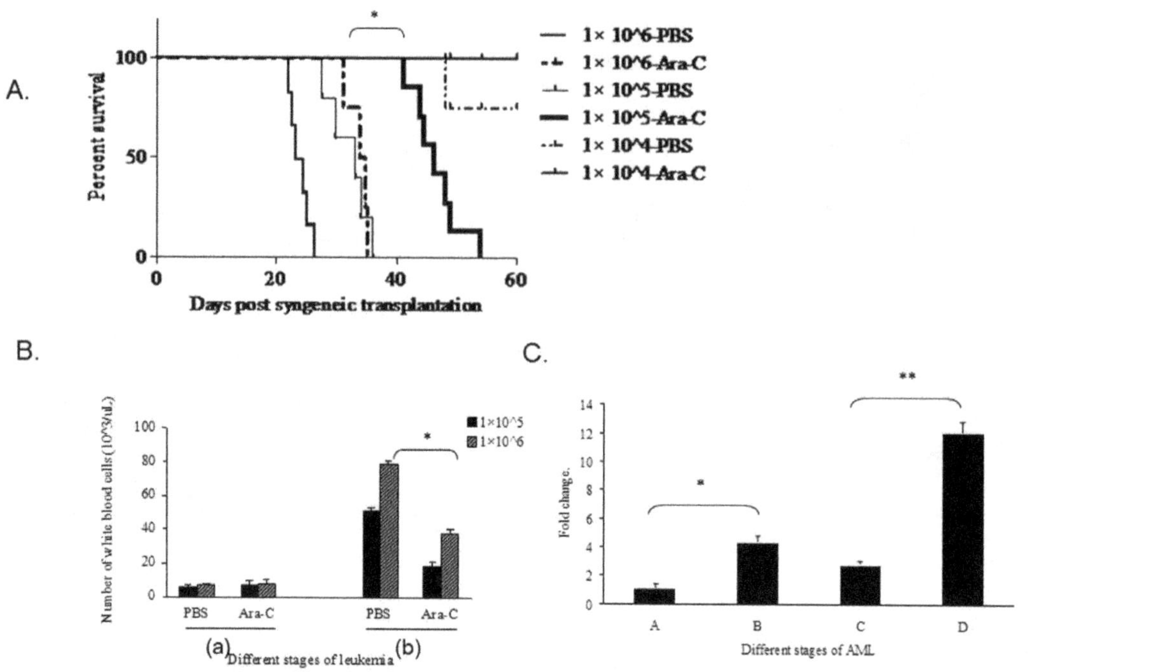

Figure 3. The effect of leukemic load on the survival of recipient mice. Fig. 3A) The survival of B6C3F1 mice receiving different dose of B117P cells and treated with either Ara-C or PBS. Each group included 12 mice. The mice were watched for 60 days. Fig. 3B) The white blood cell counts at different stages of transplanted leukemia in the mouse model. (a) before transplant, (b) after the first course of treatment. Fig. 3C) The abundance of B117 tag in the peripheral blood of recipient mice detected by q-PCR, taking β-actin as the reference, at different time points, (A) 2 days following the transplantation, (B) right before the treatment, (C) following the first course of treatment, (D) following the second course of treatment. $^*p<0.05$, $^{**}p<0.01$. The data were presented as mean +/− SD of triplicate.

(PBS) group, Ara-C treatment significantly prolonged the survival of mice for 12~14 days (Fig. 2D), suggesting that this Ara-C treatment protocol did not kill B6C3F1 mice but effectively suppressed leukemic cell growth in vivo.

3. The effect of leukemic load on the outcome of Ara-C treatment

To examine whether AML load had an impact on the treatment outcome, three different numbers of B117P cells were transplanted into B6C3F1 mice, followed by treatment either with PBS as control groups, or with Ara-C according to the above described protocol. As can be seen in Fig. 3A, infusion of 1×10^4 of B117P cells followed by Ara-C treatment did not cause moribund animal within the period of observation, whereas only 3 (25%) mice died in the PBS control group, indicative of an insufficient induction of reproducible leukemia at this cell dose. When the number of cells increased up to 1×10^5 and 1×10^6, the survival of recipient mice became shorter. Consistent with our previous observations, Ara-C treatment delayed the onset of disease, relative to the control groups. Notably, Ara-C treated mice infused with 1×10^5 B117P cells survived significantly longer than those with 1×10^6 cells, indicating that a higher level of blast cell load was associated with poor survival of Ara-C treated mice.

The recipient mice, when they became moribund, showed typical leukemic manifestations, with regard to their changed appearance and enlarged hematopoietic organs. The peripheral white blood cells of mice obtained at different stages of transplanted leukemia were counted, and the B117P tag quantified by qPCR. Following the first course of treatment, all four groups of mice displayed high counts of white blood cells, compared to normal B6C3F1 mice (Fig. 3B), consistent with moribund mice from transplanted leukemia and not from Ara-C toxicity. In PBS control groups, mice initially receiving 1×10^6 B117P cells died gradually, and had a greater increase in the numbers of white blood cells than mice injected with 1×10^5 cells which were still normal (Fig. 3C). Interestingly, Ara-C treated mice transplanted with either 1×10^5 or 1×10^6 cells had decreased cell counts in comparison with respective PBS control mice (Fig. 3B). This is consistent with our observation of the prolonged survival of Ara-C treated recipient mice, indicating, again, that this Ara-C treatment protocol could effectively reduce the number of blast cells. In addition, Ara-C treated mice infused with 1×10^6 cells exhibited an increased cell counts relative to mice receiving 1×10^5 cells (Fig. 3B). When they became sick after surviving the second course of treatment, mice showed markedly increased white blood cells (data not shown).

The abundance of B117P cells present in peripheral blood was also monitored by measuring the B117P-specific proviral insertion tag that has previously been identified by APE-PCR [17]. As shown in Fig. 3C, the B117P tag was detected as early as 2 days following the transplantation, and found to be increased later. The levels of B117P tag were decreased following the first course of Ara-C treatment, but became high again when animals were moribund after the second course of treatment. This indicated that changes of the number of B117P cells in the peripheral blood of mice followed a pattern similar to those of white blood cell counts.

The differential survival of mice receiving between 1×10^5 and 1×10^6 leukemic cells shown here suggested that leukemic load affected the survival of untreated recipient mice and the outcome of Ara-C therapy for AML.

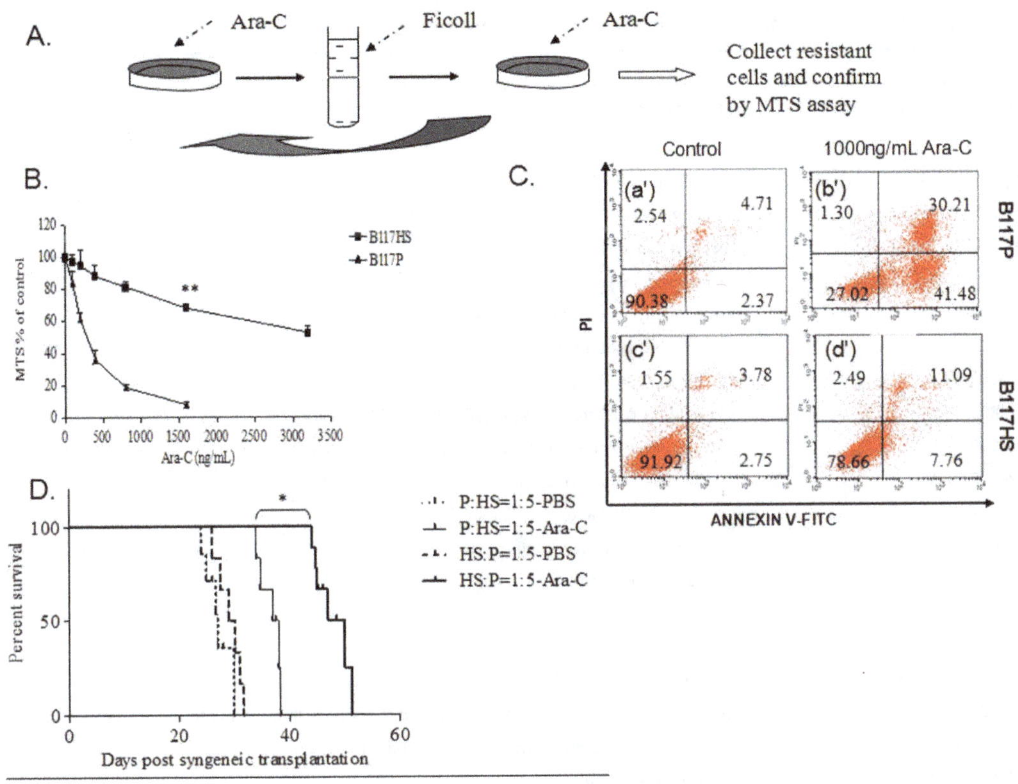

Figure 4. Sensitivity of leukemic cells to Ara-C determined the survival of treated AML mice. Fig. 4A) Selection scheme for generation of Ara-C resistant AML cells (B117HS). Fig. 4B) Comparision of B117P with B117HS in their sensitivities to Ara-C by MTS assay. **$p<0.01$. Fig. 4C) B117P or B117HS treated either with cell culture medium (a' and c') as control or with 1000 ng/mL Ara-C for 48 hours (b' and d') were subjected to flow cytometry analysis, according to the Methods. Fig. 4D) Survival of B6C3F1 mice transplanted with 2×10^5 leukemic cells containing different proportions of B117P and B117HS cells, followed by the treatment with Ara-C or PBS control. Each group included 12 B6C3F1 mice. *$p<0.05$.

4. Sensitivity of leukemia cells to Ara-C determined the survival of treated AML mice

We next asked whether the presence of drug-resistant cells in the leukemic population could impact the outcome of chemotherapy. Firstly, to generate isogenic leukemic cells with different drug sensitivity, we put B117P cells under selection against Ara-C at an initial concentration of 160 ng/mL. This concentration was chosen based on our previous observation that it could give rise to marked cytotoxicity but was no higher than the IC50 of B117P [12]. Thus, over 50% of treated cells could survive this initial treatment (data not shown). As depicted in Fig. 4A, a highly Ara-C resistant cell line, designated as B117HS, was derived from B117P by consecutive exposure to increasing concentrations of Ara-C, as described before [12]. It took about 10 weeks to produce B117HS. To verify the drug resistance of B117HS cells, we then performed MTS assay to determine their sensitivity to Ara-C. As shown in Fig. 4B, the IC50 of B117HS to Ara-C was about ten times higher than that of B117P. Flow cytometry analysis showed that treatment with 1000 ng/mL Ara-C induced apparent apoptosis of B117P and B117HS cells (Fig. 4C).

With the Ara-C resistant cells obtained, we next evaluated the effects of drug sensitivity of leukemic cells on the survival of transplanted animals. To better mimic the clinical context, we mixed B117P and B117HS at the ratio of 1:5 or 5:1, and transplanted the mixtures into B6C3F1 mice, prior to the drug treatment. All mice displayed similar signs of illness including lethargy, hunched posture, rough coat, and body weight loss, and eventually being moribund from AML. As shown in Fig. 4D, no obvious difference in the survival of mice between control groups B117P:B117HS (1:5) and B117P:B117HS (5:1) was detected. However, Kaplan-Meier analysis showed that, among Ara-C treated mice, B117P:B117HS (5:1) group survived significantly ($p<0.05$) longer than B117P:B117HS (1:5) group, indicating that an increased proportion of B117HS cells resulted in a poor outcome of chemotherapy. These data suggested that the existence of drug-resistant cells in leukemic population could affect the outcome of Ara-C treatment in vivo.

5. Gene expression profiling of leukemic cells sensitive or resistant to Ara-C

In order to further explore the intrinsic mechanism determining response to chemotherapy at a molecular level, a comparison of gene expression profiles between Ara-C resistant B117HS cells and their parental B117P-derived passage control cells was performed by Super Biotek using Mouse OneArray Microarray. Fluorescent aRNA targets were prepared from 1 or 2.5 µg total RNA samples using OneArray Amino Allyl aRNA Amplification Kit (Phalanx Biotech Group, Taiwan) and Cy5 dyes (Amersham Pharmacia, Piscataway, NJ, USA). Fluorescent targets were hybridized to the Mouse Whole Genome OneArray with Phalanx hybridization buffer using Phalanx Hybridization System. After 16 hrs hybridization at 50°C, non-specific binding targets were washed away by three different washing steps (Wash I 42°C 5 min; Wash II 42°C 5 min, 25°C 5 min; Wash III rinse 20 times), and the slides were dried by centrifugation and scanned by Axon 4000B scanner (Molecular Devices, Sunnyvale, CA, USA). The intensities of each probe were obtained by GenePix 4.1 software (Molecular Devices). Genechip hybridization data were collected,

Table 1. Genes upregulated or downregulated in B117HS compared with B117P.

Gene name	Super biotek probe set ID	Gene description	n-fold
Upregulated			
Thbs1	PH_mM_0014241	thrombospondin 1	99.99
CD63	PH_mM_0009050	CD63 antigen	99.99
Dnmt3L	PH_mM_0000812	DNA (cytosine-5-)-methyltransferase 3-like	70.09
Plau	mMC007080	plasminogen activator, urokinase	47.5
Tgfb3	mMC024423	transforming growth factor, beta 3	33.15
Rbpms	mMC016216	RNA binding protein gene with multiple splicing	19.03
Zmat3	mMC026312	zinc finger matrin type 3	18.95
ABCB9	mMR028795	ATP-binding cassette, sub-family B (MDR/TAP), member 9	16.46
Vopp1	mMC008041	vesicular, overexpressed in cancer, prosurvival protein 1	12.89
Gdf5	mMC004863	growth differentiation factor 5	11.9
Vegfa	PH_mM_0001624	vascular endothelial growth factor A	10.43
Kdr	PH_mM_0001297	kinase insert domain protein receptor	9.51
Stim1	PH_mM_0014218	stromal interaction molecule 1	8.05
Bcl2	mMR026887	B cell leukemia/lymphoma 2	5.26
Downregulated			
CD72	PH_mM_0008460	CD72 antigen	68.63
Psmb9	mMC008677	proteasome (prosome, macropain) subunit, beta type 9 (large multifunc- tional peptidase 2)	46.48
Parp8	mMC009866	poly (ADP-ribose) polymerase famil- y, member 8	33.08
Ripk3	PH_mM_0001581	receptor-interacting serine-threonine kinase 3	23.91
Traf3ip2	mMC006086	TRAF3 interacting protein 2	17.8
SOX4	mMR027907	SRY-box containing gene 4	16.22
Uba7	mMC023220	ubiquitin-like modifier activating enzyme 7	15.13
Pdrg1	mMC022475	p53 and DNA damage regulated 1	14.69
Cmpk2	mMC005508	cytidine monophosphate (UMP-CMP) kinase 2, mitochondrial	9.9
Lgals1	mMC003871	lectin, galactose binding, soluble 1	9.85
Ttc3	mMR026668	tetratricopeptide repeat domain 3	9.04

corrected, normalized, and statistically analyzed using programs including statistical Analysis of Microarray, GeneData Analyst, Principal Components Analysis and Cluster. As shown in Fig. 5A, a list of 578 genes with t-test ($p<0.01$) and fold-change (≥ 5.5) analysis was obtained, including 366 up-regulated and 266 down-regulated known genes in B117HS cells. Many of these genes were involved in resistance to chemotherapy or tumor formation and metastasis (Table 1). Expression changes for Dnmt3L, Plau, Bcl2, CD72, Uba7 and Pdrgl genes were confirmed by quantitative real-time PCR analysis using the ABI7500 (Fig. 5B). Our microarray study revealed extensive changes in gene expression levels of Ara-C resistant cells, and some of these may influence chemotherapy response and warrant further exploration.

6. Sensitivity of Ara-C resistant leukemic cells to an inhibitor of anti-apoptosis proteins (ABT-737)

Because of the result of gene expression profiling including up-regulated Bcl-2, we were curious whether Ara-C resistant cells were responsive to inhibition of anti-apoptotic proteins. Previous studies have shown that ABT-737, a BH3 mimetic, inhibited the pro-survival function of Bcl-2, Bcl-xL and Bcl-w, and induced apoptosis in a variety of cancer cell types [18–21]. We first examined the response of B117HS to ABT-737 in vitro. As shown in Fig. 6A, ABT-737 treated B117HS cells exhibited considerable apoptosis and/or necrosis compared to the control. To examine if B117P cells can be effectively treated by ABT-737, we performed MTS assay to measure the sensitivity of B117P to ABT-737. We found that B117P cells were sensitive to ABT-737 treatment, with an estimated IC50 of 2 μM (figure 6B(a)). Interestingly, B117HS exhibited a significantly lower IC50 compared with B117P ($p< 0.05$; figure 6B(a)), indicating that B117HS became even more sensitive to ABT-737 than B117P cells. Then, we determined the sensitivity of cultured B117HS to the combined treatment with Ara-C plus ABT-737 by MTS assay, and found that combined use of 0.4 μM of ABT-737 and an escalation of concentrations of Ara-C ranging from 200 ng/mL to 3200 ng/mL significantly reduced the viability of B117HS cells relative to the treatment with Ara-C alone (Fig. 6B(b)). These data indicated that ABT-737 had a suppressive effect on Ara-C resistant cells, and encouraged us to further examine the in vivo activity of ABT-737. As we observed previously, single agent Ara-C was effective in delaying the progression of leukemia in recipient mice. Excitingly, the combined treatment with Ara-C and ABT-737 suppressed leukemia and prolonged the survival to an even greater extent than the group treated with Ara-C alone (Fig. 6C(a)). However, mice transplanted with B117P-dervied leukaemia had no significantly different survival following the treatment with ABT-737 plus Ara-C compared with Ara-C treatment alone (Fig. 6C(b)).

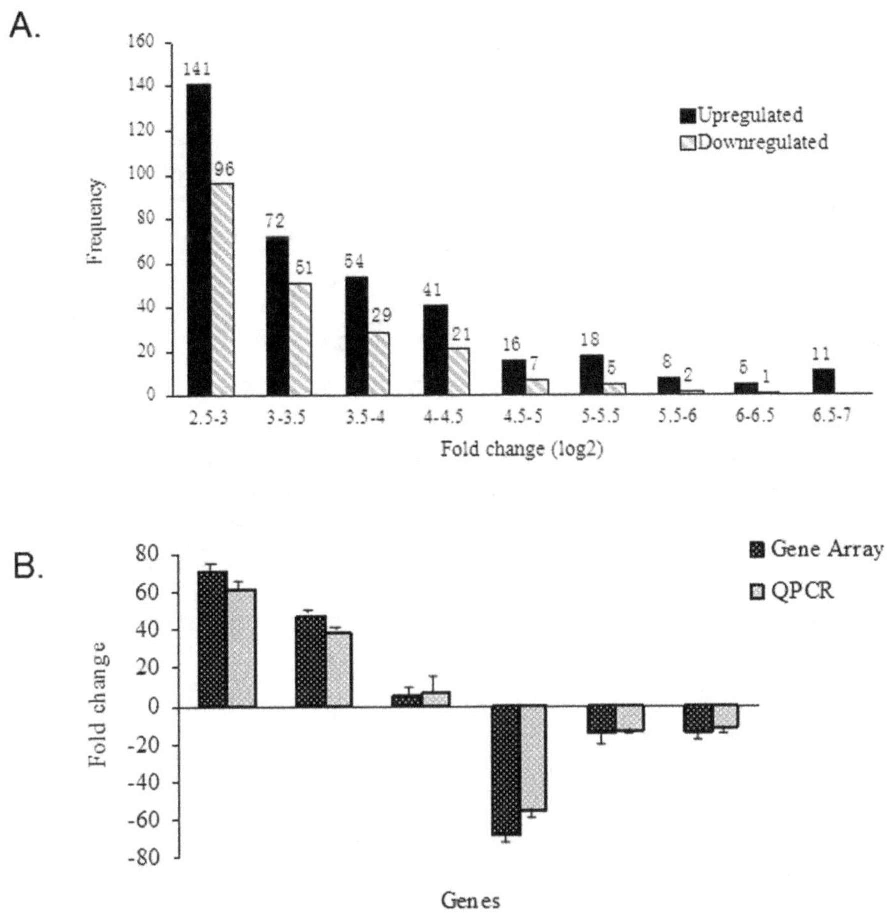

Figure 5. Gene expression profiling of leukemic cells sensitive or resistant to Ara-C. Fig. 5A) Histogram plot shows the distribution of genes with a fold change (log_2) over 2.5. Fold changes were calculated by Rosetta Resolver 7.2 with error model adjusted by Amersham Pairwise Ration Builder for signal comparison of samples. Fig. 5B) Validation of the differences in expression of Dnmt3L, Plau, Bcl-2, CD72, Uba7 and Pdrg1 genes by quantitative PCR. In order to verify the direction and magnitude of the changes in gene expression induced by resistance of Ara-C in the gene microarrays, q-PCR was performed using primers to the selected genes whose expression levels were significantly altered in the array analysis.

Ara-C resistance of AML cells could be partially reversed by the treatment with ABT-737. These results suggest that inhibition of anti-apoptosis may improve the outcome of Ara-C treatment of AML with intrinsic resistance.

Discussion

The cure of AML represents a clinical challenge. Although a large body of work has focused on the responses of leukemic cells to a variety of chemotherapeutics, most patients die from relapse. In this report, we investigated the cellular factors contributing to poor prognosis. We found that leukemic cell load within a certain range and intrinsic cellular chemosensitivity are important factors determining the outcome of in vivo treatment of AML.

Targeted therapy of AML with small molecules has been intensely pursued over the past decade. The small compounds act on certain genes or their encoded products that are specifically or preferentially critical to malignant cell survival or proliferation, and can effectively kill tumor cells while having minor side effects. However, the array of molecules that have been developed so far have not proven efficacious in patients, in general [22]. On the other hand, since the standard first line of chemotherapy includes Ara-C we focused on the investigation of AML response to this classic drug.

A variety of mouse models have been developed to study the initiation, progression, and maintenance of AML including chromosome translocation-associated leukemia [23,24], and mutant gene-induced myeloid malignancy [25]. Recently, by crossing PML-RARA transgenic mice with BXH-2 mice, Kogan's group has identified a new cooperating pathway to leukemogenesis: Sox4 overexpression accelerated PML-RARα initiated acute promyelocytic leukemia with increased penetrance and reduced latency of disease [26]. Most of the AML mouse models that have been reported are xenografts of human leukemic cells. In contrast to ALL, AML xenotransplantation models are hampered by the problems of inadequate engraftment and a short life span of the animals [27]. Importantly, these systems are usually immunocompromised to facilitate successful engraftment. In this study, we developed an immunocompetent AML mouse model to complement xenotransplant models and mirror the pathology and response to chemotherapy in patients because it is known that the microenvironment can significantly affect tumor response to therapeutics. Based on this mouse model, we developed an Ara-C treatment protocol that has a minimum toxicity but this confirms that suppressed the growth of transplanted AML cells and prolonged the survival of recipient mice. In our study, we found that the two courses of 10-day consecutive treatment scheme with 50 mg/kg of Ara-C worked well.

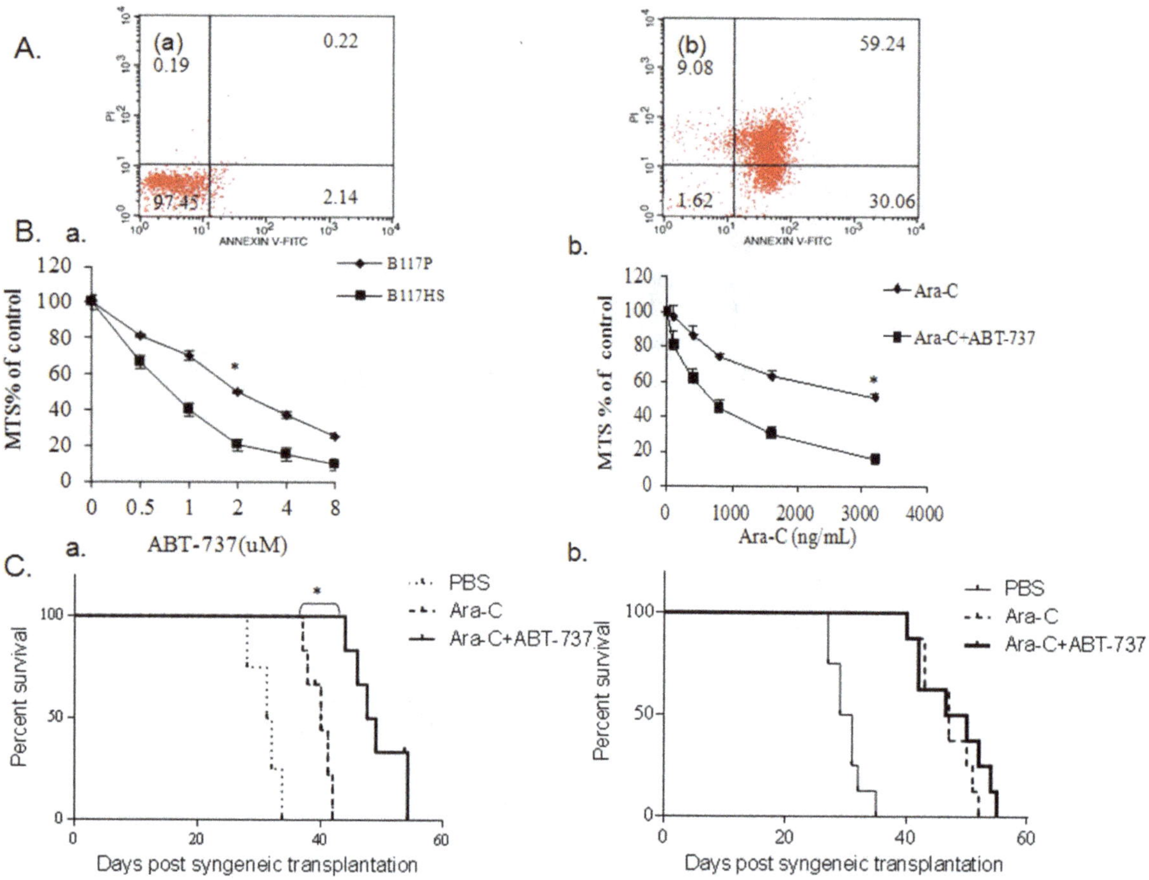

Figure 6. Sensitivity of Ara-C resistant leukemic cells to an inhibitor of anti-apoptosis proteins (ABT-737). Fig. 6A) In vitro induced apoptosis of B117HS cells by ABT-737. B117HS cells were treated with either DMEM medium as control (a) or with 2.0 μM of ABT-737 (b) for two days, followed by apoptosis analysis according to the Methods. Fig. 6B) Sensitivity of B117P and B117HS cells to ABT-737 (a). Cells were treated with 0.5 μM~8 μM of ABT-737 for three days prior to the MTS assay as described in the Methods. *$p<0.05$. Sensitivity of B117HS cells to Ara-C alone or in combination with ABT-737. (b). B117HS cells were treated with Ara-C alone or Ara-C combined with 0.4 μM of ABT-737 for three days prior to the MTS assay as described in the Methods. *$p<0.05$. Fig. 6C) Kaplan-Meier curves of recipient mice treated with Ara-C alone or in combination with ABT-737. B6C3F1 mice were infused with 2×10^5 B117HS cells (a) or B117P cells (b), followed by the treatment with PBS, Ara-C (50 mg/kg), or Ara-C (50 mg/kg) and ABT-737 (25 mg/kg), respectively. Each group contained 8 mice. *$p<0.05$.

In clinical practice, the number of leukemic blast cells is associated with the outcome of treatment. Measurement of leukemic load can be a useful tool in order to predict risk of relapse in patients [28]. Tumor load is also an important index for AML treatment by allogeneic bone marrow transplantation (BMT), and intermediate dose of Ara-C is suggested to be used to reduce leukemic load prior to allogeneic BMT [29]. In addition, it is helpful to monitor changes in tumor load following transplantation, since immunotherapy is known to be effective for low tumor burden. Some investigators have found an association between persistence of minimum residual disease and risk of relapse. Nevertheless, data from the literature remain contradictory and further correlations should be established [30]. Using a syngeneic transplantation mouse model, we showed that AML cell load of $1\times10^{5\sim6}$ were correlated with the survival of Ara-C treated recipient mice. In agreement, Mulloy observed that early treatment of transplanted AML cells before they expanded out could result in some cures, whereas mice with significant leukemic grafts were not cured using treatment by Ara-C plus doxorubicin [5]. Furthermore, Esteve et al. recently reported that patients with AML harboring a low burden of FLT3-ITD mutation and concomitant NPM1 mutation have a favorable outcome [31]. It appears that heavy leukemic load disrupts normal hematopoiesis more severely or more frequently results in leukemic infiltration of extramedullary organs which is commonly seen in patients with AML. Indeed, we noticed the marked infiltration of transplanted leukemia cells into organs, such as liver, lung, kidney, gastrointestinal tract (data not shown).

It is well established that tumor microenvironment and chronic inflammation play an important role in malignant transformation and progression [6]. Furthermore, it has been found that microenvironment can provide protection from cell death induced by treatment with chemotherapeutics or targeted small molecules for various types of tumors, including solid tumors, multiple myeloma, CLL, CML, AML as well [32–34]. Paradoxically, chemotherapy induced damage to tumor niches promote the development of tumor therapy resistance in some instances [35,36]. Therefore, to evaluate the intrinsic cellular effect on treatment outcome, it would be more appropriate to have a model with a normal microenvironment. Instead of immunodeficient mice, we have established a mouse model with syngeneic transplantation of AML. By following an optimized Ara-C treatment protocol, we demonstrated that the portion of leukemic cells ($>1\times10^5$) with intrinsic drug resistance affected the survival of treated mice. The intrinsic sensitivity of AML cells affected the outcome of AML treatment with Ara-C. This may help explain the observations that AML cells from different patients showed differential sensitivity to chemotherapy in a xenograft model [5]. Furthermore, heavy tumor load may also give rise to an increased probability of having resistant cell clones or of deriving them during chemotherapy, and influencing leukemia treatment response. Interestingly, our molecular study found extensive changes between sensitive and resistant cells in the expression levels of many genes that are involved in the regulation of several important cellular properties, such as proliferation, survival, metabolism, etc. These results reinforce the idea of intrinsic cellular mechanisms contributing to the treatment outcome of AML. Whether the differentially expressed genes are directly involved in the regulation of leukemic drug response awaits further exploration.

When they become resistant to chemotherapeutics, leukemic cells may retain or even upregulate their intrinsic anti-apoptotic mechanisms. We found that the growth of both Ara-C sensitive and resistant leukemic cells could be inhibited by a Bcl-2-specific BH3 mimetic, called ABT-737. Interestingly, resistant B117HS cells were even more effectively treated by ABT-737 than B117P cells in vitro and in vivo, which may be at least in part explained by the so-called onco-addiction hypothesis. This was a surprise to us, initially, even it was within our conceptual assumptions beforehand, because, although the onco-addiction is an interesting concept which can be translated into efficacious therapy for tumors in some cases, this concept may not equally well suit into every cases. Therefore, based on these analyses, and given the fact that the Ara-C sensitive and resistant B117 cells have similar expression levels of BCL-XL but are different for BCL-2, it seems that the Ara-C resistant B117HS cells are now reliant on BCL-2 function, and that Ara-C resistant leukemic cells with increased BCL-2 expression can become more sensitive to BCL-2 inhibition. ABT-737 has previously been demonstrated to be effective against AML and other forms of hematologic malignancies [18,19,21,37–39]. The inhibition of resistant cells by ABT-737 suggests that AML cells with intrinsic resistance to Ara-C remain sensitive to the suppression of anti-apoptotic pathway. There may be potential benefit from using this novel therapy in combination with standard induction Ara-C. In consistence, Jordan and collaborators found that BCL-2 was upregulated in leukemia stem cells enriched primary AML populations, and that BCL-2 inhibitors (ABT-263 or ABT-737) induced cell death by targeting leukemia stem cell mitochondrial energy generation and showed in vivo therapeutic effects against engrafted primary human AML cells [40]. Recently, Abbott Laboratories developed a new Bcl-2-specific BH3 mimetic, ABT-199, which was shown to be efficacious against aggressive Myc-driven murine lymphomas with significantly reduced adverse side effects [41]. Although it seems to be an improved version, whether the new Bcl-2 inhibitory compound can also have in vivo activities against AML cells, especially those with intrinsic chemoresistance, merits further investigations using animal models such as the one that we developed and described in this study.

We have described a syngeneic engraftment mouse model for AML, and showed that this immunocompetent mouse system is valuable for investigating the therapeutic response. The leukemic cell load above certain range and cellular intrinsic chemosensitivity are important factors contributing to the outcome of therapy for AML.

Acknowledgments

We would like to thank Dr. David A. Largaespada for his critical review.

Author Contributions

Conceived and designed the experiments: BY ZJM. Performed the experiments: WZ LW DT. Analyzed the data: BY ZJM GS. Contributed reagents/materials/analysis tools: BY TPS. Assisted with the experiments: YZ CH.

References

1. Ipek Y, Hulya D, Melih A (2012) Disseminated exfoliative dermatitis associated with all-transretinoic Acid in the treatment of acute promyelocytic leukemia. Case Rep Med 2012: 236174.
2. Liu P, Han ZC (2003) Treatment of acute promyelocytic leukemia and other hematologic malignancies with arsenic trioxide: review of clinical and basic studies. Int J Hematol 78: 32–39.
3. Pulte D, Gondos A, Brenner H (2010) Expected long-term survival of patients diagnosed with acute myeloblastic leukemia during 2006–2010. Ann Oncol 21: 335–341.
4. Bin Yin, Largaespada DA (2006) Models of acute myeloid leukemia: Prospects for drug development and testing. Drug Discovery Today 3: 137–142.
5. Wunderlich M, Mizukawa B, Chou FS, Sexton C, Shrestha M, et al. (2013) AML cells are differentially sensitive to chemotherapy treatment in a human xenograft model. Blood 121: e90–97.
6. Coussens LM, Zitvogel L, Palucka AK (2013) Neutralizing tumor-promoting chronic inflammation: a magic bullet? Science 339: 286–291.
7. Connelly P, Quinn BP (2011) Manufacturing decline yields drug shortages. Science 333: 156–157.
8. Kaiser J (2011) Shortages of cancer drugs put patients, trials at risk. Science 332: 523–523.
9. Coenen EA, Raimondi SC, Harbott J, Zimmermann M, Alonzo TA, et al. (2011) Prognostic significance of additional cytogenetic aberrations in 733 de novo pediatric 11q23/MLL-rearranged AML patients: results of an international study. Blood 117: 7102–7111.
10. Marcucci G, Mrozek K, Ruppert AS, Maharry K, Kolitz JE, et al. (2005) Prognostic factors and outcome of core binding factor acute myeloid leukemia patients with t(8;21) differ from those of patients with inv(16): a Cancer and Leukemia Group B study. J Clin Oncol 23: 5705–5717.
11. Yin B, Morgan K, Hasz DE, Mao Z, Largaespada DA (2006) Nfl gene inactivation in acute myeloid leukemia cells confers cytarabine resistance through MAPK and mTOR pathways. Leukemia 20: 151–154.
12. Yin B, Kogan SC, Dickins RA, Lowe SW, Largaespada DA (2006) Trp53 loss during in vitro selection contributes to acquired Ara-C resistance in acute myeloid leukemia. Experimental hematology 34: 631–641.
13. Yu JL, Rak JW, Coomber BL, Hicklin DJ, Kerbel RS (2002) Effect of p53 status on tumor response to antiangiogenic therapy. Science 295: 1526–1528.
14. Jenkins NA, Copeland NG, Taylor BA, Bedigian HG, Lee BK (1982) Ecotropic murine leukemia virus DNA content of normal and lymphomatous tissues of BXH-2 recombinant inbred mice. Journal of virology 42: 379–388.
15. Largaespada DA, Shaughnessy JD Jr, Jenkins NA, Copeland NG (1995) Retroviral integration at the Evi-2 locus in BXH-2 myeloid leukemia cell lines disrupts Nf1 expression without changes in steady-state Ras-GTP levels. Journal of virology 69: 5095–5102.
16. Konoplev S, Huang X, Drabkin HA, Koeppen H, Jones D, et al. (2009) Cytoplasmic localization of nucleophosmin in bone marrow blasts of acute myeloid leukemia patients is not completely concordant with NPM1 mutation and is not predictive of prognosis. Cancer 115: 4737–4744.
17. Xu Z, Li Y, Mao ZJ, Yin B (2013) The development of APE-PCR for the cloning of genomic insertion sites of DNA elements. Biologia 68: 766–772.
18. Del Gaizo Moore V, Schlis KD, Sallan SE, Armstrong SA, Letai A (2008) BCL-2 dependence and ABT-737 sensitivity in acute lymphoblastic leukemia. Blood 111: 2300–2309.
19. Deng J, Carlson N, Takeyama K, Dal Cin P, Shipp M, et al. (2007) BH3 profiling identifies three distinct classes of apoptotic blocks to predict response to ABT-737 and conventional chemotherapeutic agents. Cancer cell 12: 171–185.
20. Kang MH, Kang YH, Szymanska B, Wilczynska-Kalak U, Sheard MA, et al. (2007) Activity of vincristine, L-ASP, and dexamethasone against acute lymphoblastic leukemia is enhanced by the BH3-mimetic ABT-737 in vitro and in vivo. Blood 110: 2057–2066.
21. High LM, Szymanska B, Wilczynska-Kalak U, Barber N, O'Brien R, et al. (2010) The Bcl-2 homology domain 3 mimetic ABT-737 targets the apoptotic machinery in acute lymphoblastic leukemia resulting in synergistic in vitro and in vivo interactions with established drugs. Molecular pharmacology 77: 483–494.
22. Gillies RJ, Verduzco D, Gatenby RA (2012) Evolutionary dynamics of carcinogenesis and why targeted therapy does not work. Nature reviews 12: 487–493.
23. Barabe F, Kennedy JA, Hope KJ, Dick JE (2007) Modeling the initiation and progression of human acute leukemia in mice. Science 316: 600–604.

24. Kumar AR, Sarver AL, Wu B, Kersey JH (2010) Meis1 maintains stemness signature in MLL-AF9 leukemia. Blood 115: 3642–3643.
25. Nardi V, Naveiras O, Azam M, Daley GQ (2009) ICSBP-mediated immune protection against BCR-ABL-induced leukemia requires the CCL6 and CCL9 chemokines. Blood 113: 3813–3820.
26. Omidvar N, Maunakea ML, Jones L, Sevcikova S, Yin B, et al. (2013) PML-RARalpha co-operates with Sox4 in acute myeloid leukemia development in mice. Haematologica 98: 424–427.
27. Malaise M, Neumeier M, Botteron C, Dohner K, Reinhardt D, et al. (2011) Stable and reproducible engraftment of primary adult and pediatric acute myeloid leukemia in NSG mice. Leukemia 25: 1635–1639.
28. Zhu H-H, Zhang X-H, Qin Y-Z, Liu D-H, Jiang H, et al. (2013) MRD-directed risk stratification treatment may improve outcomes of t (8; 21) AML in the first complete remission: results from the AML05 multicenter trial. Blood 121: 4056–4062.
29. Beran M (2000) Intensive chemotherapy for patients with high-risk myelodysplastic syndrome. Int J Hematol 72: 139–150.
30. Perez-Simon JA, Caballero D, Diez-Campelo M, Lopez-Perez R, Mateos G, et al. (2002) Chimerism and minimal residual disease monitoring after reduced intensity conditioning (RIC) allogeneic transplantation. Leukemia 16: 1423–1431.
31. Pratcorona M, Brunet S, Nomdedeu J, Ribera JM, Tormo M, et al. (2013) Favorable outcome of patients with acute myeloid leukemia harboring a low-allelic burden FLT3-ITD mutation and concomitant NPM1 mutation: relevance to post-remission therapy. Blood 121: 2734–2738.
32. Zhang B, Li M, McDonald T, Holyoake TL, Moon RT, et al. (2013) Microenvironmental protection of CML stem and progenitor cells from tyrosine kinase inhibitors through N-cadherin and Wnt-beta-catenin signaling. Blood 121: 1824–1838.
33. Straussman R, Morikawa T, Shee K, Barzily-Rokni M, Qian ZR, et al. (2012) Tumour micro-environment elicits innate resistance to RAF inhibitors through HGF secretion. Nature 487: 500–504.
34. Uy GL, Rettig MP, Motabi IH, McFarland K, Trinkaus KM, et al. (2012) A phase 1/2 study of chemosensitization with the CXCR4 antagonist plerixafor in relapsed or refractory acute myeloid leukemia. Blood 119: 3917–3924.
35. Sun Y, Campisi J, Higano C, Beer TM, Porter P, et al. (2012) Treatment-induced damage to the tumor microenvironment promotes prostate cancer therapy resistance through WNT16B. Nature medicine 18: 1359–1368.
36. Kessenbrock K, Plaks V, Werb Z (2010) Matrix metalloproteinases: regulators of the tumor microenvironment. Cell 141: 52–67.
37. Oltersdorf T, Elmore SW, Shoemaker AR, Armstrong RC, Augeri DJ, et al. (2005) An inhibitor of Bcl-2 family proteins induces regression of solid tumours. Nature 435: 677–681.
38. Szymanska B, Wilczynska-Kalak U, Kang MH, Liem NL, Carol H, et al. (2012) Pharmacokinetic modeling of an induction regimen for in vivo combined testing of novel drugs against pediatric acute lymphoblastic leukemia xenografts. PloS one 7: e33894.
39. Beurlet S, Omidvar N, Gorombei P, Krief P, Le Pogam C, et al. (2013) BCL-2 inhibition with ABT-737 prolongs survival in an NRAS/BCL-2 mouse model of AML by targeting primitive LSK and progenitor cells. Blood 122: 2864–2876.
40. Lagadinou ED, Sach A, Callahan K, Rossi RM, Neering SJ, et al. (2013) BCL-2 inhibition targets oxidative phosphorylation and selectively eradicates quiescent human leukemia stem cells. Cell stem cell 12: 329–341.
41. Vandenberg CJ, Cory S (2013) ABT-199, a new Bcl-2-specific BH3 mimetic, has in vivo efficacy against aggressive Myc-driven mouse lymphomas without provoking thrombocytopenia. Blood 121: 2285–2288.

20

The *NPM1* Mutation Type has no Impact on Survival in Cytogenetically Normal AML

Friederike Pastore[1,2,3,4]*, Philipp A. Greif[1,2,3,4], Stephanie Schneider[1], Bianka Ksienzyk[1], Gudrun Mellert[1], Evelyn Zellmeier[1], Jan Braess[5], Cristina M. Sauerland[6], Achim Heinecke[6], Utz Krug[7], Wolfgang E. Berdel[7], Thomas Buechner[7], Bernhard Woermann[8], Wolfgang Hiddemann[1,2,3,4], Karsten Spiekermann[1,2,3,4]

1 Laboratory for Leukemia Diagnostics, Dept. of Internal Medicine III, University Hospital Munich Großhadern, Ludwig-Maximilian-University (LMU), Munich, Germany, **2** Clinical Cooperative Group Pathogenesis of Acute Myeloid Leukemia, Helmholtz Zentrum München, German Research Center for Environmental Health, Munich, Germany, **3** German Cancer Consortium (DKTK), Heidelberg, Germany, **4** German Cancer Research Center (DKFZ), Heidelberg, Germany, **5** Dept. of Oncology and Hematology, Krankenhaus Barmherzige Brüder, Regensburg, Germany, **6** Institute of Biostatistics and Clinical Research, University of Muenster, Muenster, Germany, **7** Dept. of Internal Medicine A, Hematology and Oncology, University of Muenster, Muenster, Germany, **8** German Society of Hematology and Oncology, Berlin, Germany

Abstract

NPM1 mutations represent frequent genetic alterations in patients with acute myeloid leukemia (AML) associated with a favorable prognosis. Different types of *NPM1* mutations have been described. The purpose of our study was to evaluate the relevance of different *NPM1* mutation types with regard to clinical outcome. Our analyses were based on 349 *NPM1*-mutated AML patients treated in the AMLCG99 trial. Complete remission rates, overall survival and relapse-free survival were not significantly different between patients with *NPM1* type A or rare type mutations. The *NPM1* mutation type does not seem to play a role in risk stratification of cytogenetically normal AML.

Editor: Ralf Krahe, University of Texas MD Anderson Cancer Center, United States of America

Funding: The authors have no support or funding to report.

Competing Interests: The authors have declared that no competing interests exist.

* Email: Friederike.Pastore@med.uni-muenchen.de

Introduction

The gene encoding nucleophosmin (*NPM1*), a nucleo-cytoplasmatic shuttling protein with prominent nucleolar localization is located on 5q35.1 and contains 12 exons. *NPM1* is involved in epigenetic control (binding of nucleic acids, centrosome duplication), ribosomal protein assembly as molecular chaperon and regulation of the ARF-p53-tumor suppressor pathway [1,2].

NPM1 mutations can be found in 35% of patients with cytogenetically normal acute myeloid leukemia (AML). They are associated with a favorable prognosis in the absence of an additional internal tandem duplication in the fms-related tyrosine 3 gene (*FLT3-ITD*), female gender, high white blood count (WBC), high amount of bone marrow blasts as well as a high platelet count [1].

In the vast majority of cases *NPM1* mutations result in a frameshift due to an insertion of four bases, which cluster in exon 12. Different types of *NPM1* mutations have been described according to the inserted tetranucleotide, the most common being type A mutations (TCTG) in 80%, followed by type B (CATG) and type D (CCTG) mutations in about 10%, and a spectrum of other mutations accounting for 10% of cases. In rare cases, insertions from 2 to 9 bases can occur (e.g. types E, F) [1].

The altered *NPM1* protein (*NPM1*c+) contains an additional C terminal nuclear export signal (NES) motif and loses at least one tryptophan residue, causing an aberrant cytoplasmatic localization of the protein [3].

Little is known about the prognostic relevance of the variable *NPM1* mutation types. In *FLT3-ITD* negative patients, a Korean study found an adverse impact on overall survival (OS) and duration of complete remission (CR) in *NPM1* mutations other than type A [4]. In *FLT3-ITD* positive patients, another recent study reported an adverse OS in *NPM1* type A mutations [5] whereas - in contrast to Koh et al. - they did not observe an effect of *NPM1* mutation type in *FLT3-ITD* negative patients.

We aimed at studying the clinical relevance of *NPM1* mutation types on prognosis in a large homogeneously treated cohort of cytogenetically normal AML patients.

Patients and Methods

Patients

Our analyses were based on a total of 783 patients with newly diagnosed cytogenetically normal AML treated within the randomized multicenter German AML Cooperative Group 99 (AMLCG99) trial comparing a double induction therapy with thioguanine, cytarabine and daunorubicin (TAD) and high dose mitoxantrone (HAM) versus HAM-HAM [6].

The AMLCG99 trial is registered at ClinicalTrials.gov (NCT00266136) and was approved by the local institutional review boards of all participating centers. Informed consent was obtained from all patients in accordance with the Declaration of Helsinki.

Cytogenetic and molecular analyses

All cytogenetic and molecular analyses were performed on bone marrow aspirates. Cytogenetic analyses were based on the assessment of at least 20 metaphases and performed according to the international system of cytogenetic nomenclature (ISCN) guidelines [7]. Mutations of *NPM1* [1], *FLT3-ITD* [8], the *FLT3-ITD* mRNA level [9,10], *CEBPA* [11,12], were analyzed as previously described. The nomenclature of the *NPM1* mutation type was performed according to the literature [1,13,14]. *NPM1* mutations other than type A mutations were grouped together as rare type mutations (*NPM1*-rare), *NPM1* mutations other than type A, B or D were grouped together as other mutations (*NPM1*-other).

Outcome Parameters

OS was calculated from the date of randomization until death from any cause. Surviving patients were censored at the date of last follow-up. Relapse-free survival (RFS) was determined for responders from the first day of CR until relapse or death from any cause. Patients in CR that did not experience a relapse were censored at the last disease assessment.

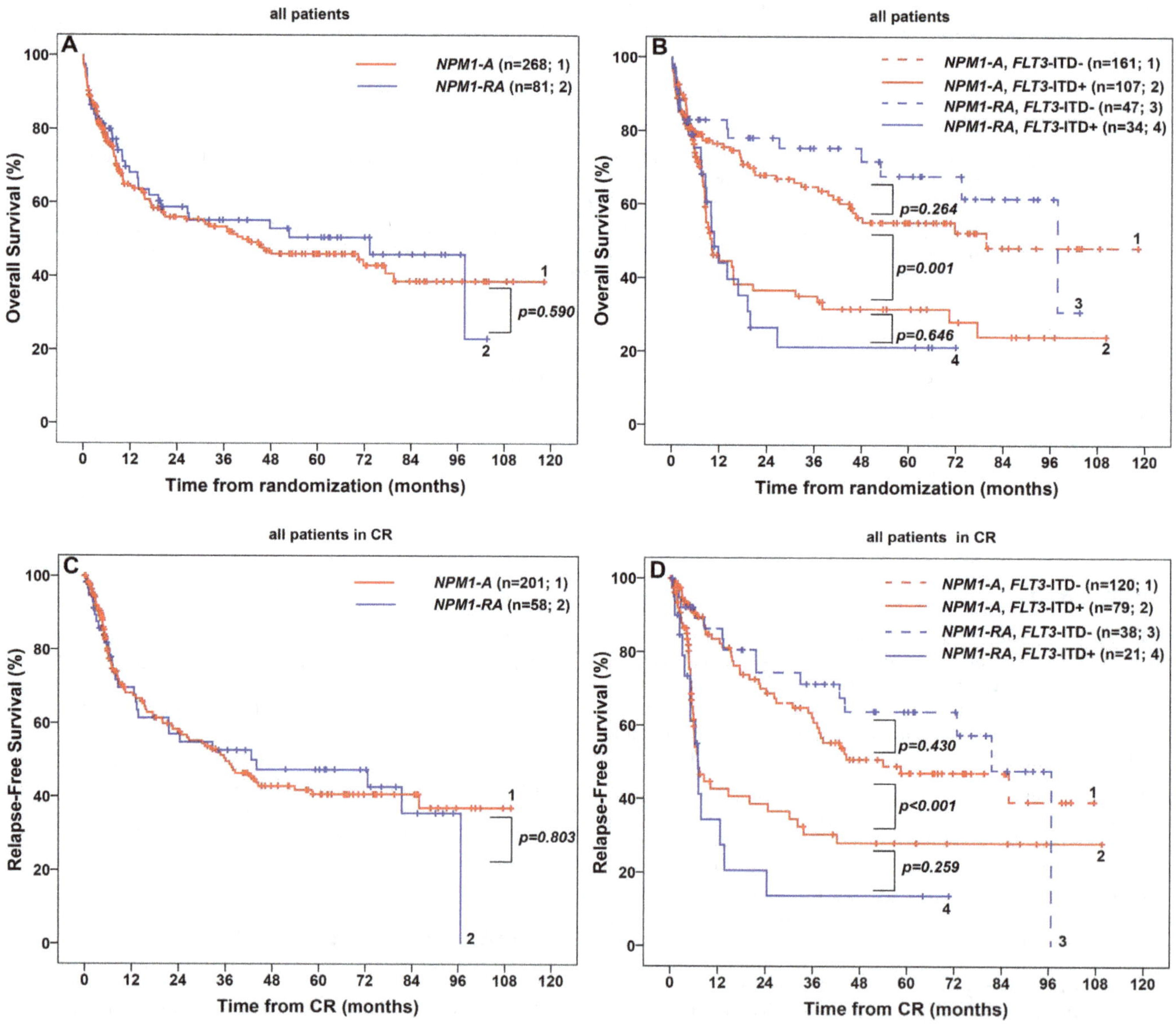

Figure 1. Overall Survival (OS) and Relapse-Free Survival (RFS) in 349 patients with cytogenetically normal acute myeloid leukemia and *NPM1* mutation treated in the AMLCG99 study. (A) OS in patients with *NPM1* type A mutation versus *NPM1* rare type mutation. (B) OS in patients with *NPM1* type A mutation versus *NPM1* rare type mutation with or without an additional *FLT3-ITD.* (C) RFS in patients with *NPM1* type A mutation versus *NPM1* rare type mutation. (D) RFS in patients with *NPM1* type A mutation versus *NPM1* rare type mutation with or without an additional *FLT3-ITD*. **Abbreviations**: CR, complete remission; *FLT3-ITD+*, presence of an internal tandem duplication in the fms-related tyrosine 3 gene; *FLT3-ITD-*, absence of an internal tandem duplication in the fms-related tyrosine 3 gene; *NPM1-A*, mutation in the nucleophosmin gene consisting of an insertion of the tetranucleotide TCTG; *NPM1-RA*, mutation in the nucleophosmin gene other than type A.

For patients who had undergone allogeneic transplantation according to the study protocol, OS and RFS times were censored at the time of transplantation.

Statistical Analysis

Continuous characteristics between patient groups were compared using the Mann-Whitney U test for 2 groups and the Kruskal-Wallis test for 3 groups. The x^2-test for was applied for categorical variables. Kaplan-Meier estimation for OS and RFS was performed comparing *NPM1*-mutated patients with a type A mutation (*NPM1-A*) versus *NPM1*-mutated patients with another type of *NPM1* mutation (rare type: *NPM1-RA*) as well as both groups combined with either *FLT3-ITD* or without *FLT3-ITD*. In a second analysis, patients with *NPM1* mutations types A, B and D were analyzed independently and compared to patients carrying other mutations than A, B and D who were grouped together as "*NPM1*- other".

Hazard ratios and 95% confidence intervals between the different groups were estimated by Cox regression analyses.

Independent prognostic parameters for OS and RFS were identified by univariable Cox regression analyses and a multivariable Cox regression model using backward elimination with an exclusion significance level of 5%. For all analyses, a p-value<0.05 was considered significant. For the estimation of the median follow-up time, the reversed Kaplan-Meier method was applied [15].

Results

Patient characteristics

Analyses were performed in 349 *NPM1*-mutated patients of 667 patients with CN-AML treated within the AMLCG99 trial, after exclusion of 106 patients without information of the *NPM1* mutation status. For an overview of patient selection, please refer to **Figure S1 in File S1**.

Out of 349 patients, 16% underwent allogeneic stem cell transplantation in first CR. Median follow-up for OS was 45.3 months. Median OS was 45.6 months with 151 events. In 74% of patients who achieved a CR, median RFS was 37.1 months with 115 events.

Patient characteristics are summarized in **Table S1 in File S1**. The selected 677 patients from whom the 349 *NPM1*-mutated patients were analyzed displayed similar patient characteristics and outcome (OS and RFS, not significantly different) as the unselected patients.

The majority of patients (77%) carried *NPM1* type A mutations, followed by 9% with *NPM1* type D, 5% with *NPM1* type B mutations and 2% with *NPM1* type I mutations. All other mutations occurred in ≤1% of patients (**Table S2 in File S1**).

NPM1 mutation type does not influence outcome

A) *NPM1* mutation type A versus rare type mutations. We did not observe any significant difference between patients with *NPM1 type* A and rare mutations in clinical or molecular parameters, in particular, there was no difference regarding OS and RFS (**Figures 1A and 1C, Table S1 in File S1**).

In patients with *NPM1* mutation (*NPM1+*), the presence of an *FLT3-ITD* (*FLT3-ITD+*) caused significant changes in WBC, LDH level, amount of bone marrow blasts and a decrease in OS and RFS compared to patients without *FLT3-ITD* (*FLT3-ITD-*) (**Figure S2 in File S1**).

Table 1. Multivariable Cox regression models for OS and RFS in 349 *NPM1*-mutated patients.

independent prognostic factors	comparison	OS HR	OS 95% CI	OS p	RFS HR	RFS 95% CI	RFS p
Age	per 10 years	1.71	1.44–2.03	<0.001	1.55	1.28–1.87	<0.001
WBC	10^9/L, per 10-fold increase	1.63	1.16–2.30	0.005	1.71	1.15–2.56	0.009
FLT3-ITD	positive versus negative	2.04	1.40–2.96	<0.001	2.45	1.60–3.75	<0.001
NPM1 mutation type	*NPM1-A* versus *NPM1-RA*	1.06	0.71–1.59	0.764	0.89	0.57–1.38	0.590

White blood cell count, platelet count, hemoglobin level, lactase dehydrogenase level, bone marrow blasts, de novo AML versus non de novo AML, performance status, sex, age, type A versus rare type *NPM1* mutation, *FLT3-ITD*, monoallelic *CEBPA* mutations, biallelic *CEBPA* mutations were included in the Cox regression models for OS and RFS with backward elimination. The analyses were performed using 313 patients for OS and 227 RFS who had data for all these variables. A p-value of <0.05 was considered as indicating significant differences. All parameters that did not have a significant impact on OS or RFS are not shown in the table, except for the *NPM1* mutation type.

Abbreviations: *CEBPA*, CCAAT/enhancer-binding protein alpha gene; CI, confidence interval; *FLT3-ITD*, internal tandem duplication of the *FLT3* gene; HR, hazard ratio; negative, absence of *FLT3-ITD*; *NPM1*, nucleophosmin gene; *NPM1-A*, mutation in the nucleophosmin gene leading to the insertion of the tetranucleotide TCTG; *NPM1-RA*, mutation in the nucleophosmin gene other than type A; OS, Overall survival; p, p value; positive, presence of *FLT3-ITD*; RFS, Relapse-free survival; WBC, white blood cell count.

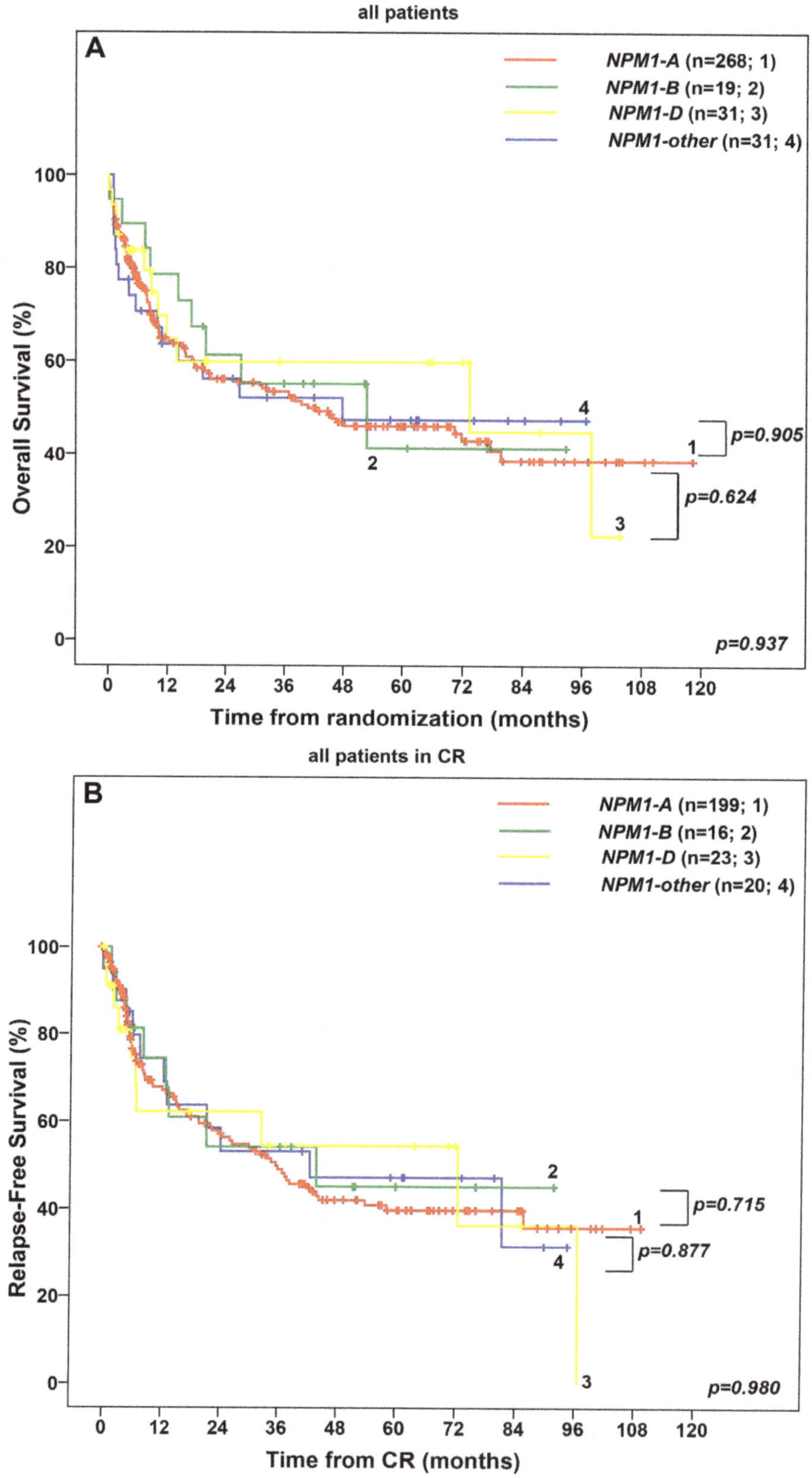

Figure 2. Overall Survival (OS) and Relapse-Free Survival (RFS) in 349 patients with cytogenetically normal acute myeloid leukemia and *NPM1* mutation treated in the AMLCG99 study. (A) OS in patients with *NPM1* type A mutation versus *NPM1* type B mutation versus *NPM1* type D mutation versus *NPM1* type other mutation. (B) RFS in patients with *NPM1* type A mutation versus *NPM1* type B mutation versus *NPM1* type D mutation versus *NPM1* type other mutation. **Abbreviations**: CR, complete remission; *FLT3-ITD+*, presence of an internal tandem duplication in the fms-related tyrosine 3 gene; *FLT3-ITD-*, absence of an internal tandem duplication in the fms-related tyrosine 3 gene; *NPM1-A*, mutation in the nucleophosmin gene consisting of an insertion of the tetranucleotide TCTG; *NPM1-B*, mutation in the nucleophosmin gene consisting of an insertion of the tetranucleotide CATG, *NPM1-D*, mutation in the nucleophosmin gene consisting of an insertion of the tetranucleotide CCTG, *NPM1-other*, mutation in the nucleophosmin gene other than *NPM1* mutation types A, B, D.

We did not observe any difference in patient characteristics, OS or RFS between *NPM1-A/FLT3-ITD-* versus *NPM1-RA/FLT3-ITD-* patients (**Figure 1B and 1D, Table S1 in File S1**). Similar results were obtained for *NPM1-A/FLT3-ITD+* versus *NPM1-RA/FLT3-ITD+* patients, except for WBC which was higher in the rare type group ($p = 0.005$).

In multivariable Cox regression analysis, parameters with independent adverse impact on OS and RFS were older age, a high WBC and the presence of an *FLT3-ITD*. Importantly, the *NPM1* mutation type (*NPM1-A* versus *NPM1-RA*) was not significantly correlated with OS or RFS, neither in univariable, (**Table S3 in File S1**) nor in multivariable Cox regression models (**Table 1**).

Similar results were obtained for the effect of *NPM1-A* versus *NPM1-RA* on OS and RFS in patients receiving chemotherapy only (without allogeneic transplantation in first CR), patients with de novo AML and patients <60 or ≥60 years (**text and Figures S3, S4 and S5 in File S1**).

B) *NPM1* mutation types A versus B versus D versus other mutations. We did not find a statistical difference with regard to OS and RFS in patients with *NPM1* type A, B, D and other mutations ($p = 0.937$, $p = 0.980$) (**Figures 2A and 2B**). Furthermore, OS and RFS were similar between patients with type A, B, D and other mutations without an additional *FLT3-ITD* (data not shown). *NPM1-A/FLT3-ITD+* patients showed similar OS and RFS as patients with *NPM1-B/FLT3-ITD+*, *NPM1-D/FLT3-ITD+* and *NPM1-other/FLT3-ITD+* patiens (data not shown). In multivariable Cox regression analysis, older age, a high WBC and presence of a *FLT3-ITD* were associated with an adverse prognosis, whereas the type of *NPM1* mutation (A versus B versus D versus other) was not significantly associated with OS or RFS (**Table S4 in File S1**). Similar results were obtained for patients not receiving allogeneic transplantation (**text in File S1**).

Conclusions and Discussion

The aim of this study was to assess the relevance of different *NPM1* mutation types with regard to clinical and molecular patient characteristics and outcome.

In the literature only few published studies have addressed this topic revealing controversial results. Koh et al who investigated only patients without an additional *FLT3-ITD*, found a negative prognostic impact of rare type mutations on OS and duration of CR [4]. Their analyses were based on 18 *NPM1*-mutated de novo AML patients, 13 of which had a type A mutation versus 5 with a rare type mutation. Thus, conclusions are limited due to small sample size and, furthermore, patients were not treated homogeneously within a clinical trial.

In contrast, another study recently presented at the ASH meeting involving 603 *NPM1*-mutated patients with intermediate risk karyotype showed a trend towards a longer OS in rare type versus type A *NPM1* mutations [5]. In the presence of an *FLT3-ITD*, type A patients had a worse OS compared to rare type mutations, whereas there was no difference between these groups in the absence of a *FLT3-ITD*.

Our study of a homogenous cohort with respect to treatment (all patients are treated within one clinical trial) and cytogenetics (all patients had a normal karyotype) did not reveal any difference in molecular and clinical parameters including CR rates, OS and RFS between type A and rare type *NPM1* mutations. Even when our patients were stratified according to *FLT3-ITD* status the type of *NPM1* mutation was not relevant for clinical outcome. This was also true comparing *NPM1* mutation types A, B, D versus other. Moreover, the type of *NPM1* mutation was not an independent prognostic factor in a multivariable analysis.

Except for the addition of a NES causing an aberrant cytoplasmatic localization of the mutated *NPM1* protein, other biochemical consequences of different *NPM1* mutation types on a protein level which might alter the binding of *NPM1* targets have not been fully explored and warrant further investigation.

In light of the low frequency and diversity of rare *NPM1* mutations, however, it is very challenging to assess their individual clinical relevance.

We conclude that the type of *NPM1* mutation does not seem to play a role in risk stratification of cytogenetically normal AML.

Supporting Information

File S1 Data supplement. Text, *NPM1* mutation type does not influence outcome - Subgroup analyses. A) *NPM1* mutation type A versus rare type mutationsin 292 patients receiving chemotherapy only in 292 patients receiving chemotherapy only; in 330 patients with de novo AML; in patients <60 and ≥60 years of age. B) *NPM1* mutation types A versus B versus D versus other mutations in 292 patients receiving chemotherapy only. Table S1, Characteristics of *NPM1*-mutated patients and comparison between those with type A and rare type with or without a *FLT3-ITD*. Table S2, Frequency of different types of *NPM1* mutations. Table S3, Univariable Cox regression for overall survival (OS) and relapse-free survival (RFS). Table S4, Multivariable Cox regression models for OS and RFS in 349 *NPM1*-mutated patients. Figure S1, Overview of patient Selection. Figure S2, Influence of a *FLT3-ITD* in 349 *NPM1*-mutated patients on outcome. (A) OS in 349 *NPM1*-mutated patients. (B) RFS in *NPM1*-mutated patients in CR. Figure S3, Overall Survival (OS) and Relapse-Free Survival (RFS) in 292 patients with cytogenetically normal acute myeloid leukemia and *NPM1* mutation treated in the AMLCG99 study, not receiving allogeneic transplantation. (A) OS in patients with *NPM1* type A mutation versus *NPM1* rare type mutation. (B) OS in patients with *NPM1* type A mutation versus *NPM1* rare type mutation with or without an additional *FLT3-ITD*. (C) RFS in patients with *NPM1* type A mutation versus *NPM1* rare type mutation. (D) RFS in patients with *NPM1* type A mutation versus *NPM1* rare type mutation with or without an additional *FLT3-ITD*. Figure S4, Overall Survival (OS) and Relapse-Free Survival (RFS) in 330 patients with de novo cytogenetically normal acute myeloid leukemia and *NPM1* mutation treated in the AMLCG99 study. (A) OS in patients with *NPM1* type A mutation versus *NPM1* rare type mutation. (B) OS in patients with *NPM1* type A mutation versus *NPM1* rare type mutation with or without an additional *FLT3-ITD*. (C) RFS in patients with *NPM1* type A mutation versus *NPM1* rare type mutation. (D) RFS in patients with *NPM1* type A mutation versus *NPM1* rare type mutation with or without an additional *FLT3-ITD*. Figure S5, Overall Survival (OS) and Relapse-Free Survival (RFS) in 197 patients <60 years and 152 patients ≥60 years with cytogenetically normal acute myeloid leukemia and *NPM1* mutation treated in the AMLCG99 study. (A) OS in patients <60 years with *NPM1* type A mutation versus *NPM1* rare type mutation. (B) OS in patients ≥60 years with *NPM1* type A mutation versus *NPM1* rare type mutation. (C) RFS in patients <60 with *NPM1* type A mutation versus *NPM1* rare type mutation. (D) RFS in patients ≥60 with *NPM1* type A mutation versus *NPM1* rare type mutation.

Acknowledgments

We would like to thank all centers and patients that participated in the AMLCG99 trial.

Author Contributions

Conceived and designed the experiments: FP KS PAG WH. Wrote the paper: FP PAG SS BK GM EZ JB CMS AH UK WEB TB BW WH KS. Collection and assembly of data: FP SS BK GM EZ JB CMS AH UK WEB TB BW WH KS. Data analysis and interpretation: FP KS PAG WH. Final approval of manuscript: FP PAG SS BK GM EZ JB CMS AH UK WEB TB BW WH KS.

References

1. Falini B, Mecucci C, Tiacci E, Alcalay M, Rosati R, et al. (2005) Cytoplasmic nucleophosmin in acute myelogenous leukemia with a normal karyotype. N Engl J Med 352: 254–266. doi:10.1056/NEJMoa041974.
2. Federici L, Falini B (2013) Nucleophosmin mutations in acute myeloid leukemia: a tale of protein unfolding and mislocalization. Protein Sci 22: 545–556. doi:10.1002/pro.2240.
3. Falini B, Bolli N, Shan J, Martelli MP, Liso A, et al. (2006) Both carboxy-terminus NES motif and mutated tryptophan(s) are crucial for aberrant nuclear export of nucleophosmin leukemic mutants in NPMc+ AML. Blood 107: 4514–4523. doi:10.1182/blood-2005-11-4745.
4. Koh Y, Park J, Bae EK, Ahn KS, Kim I, et al. (2009) Non-A type nucleophosmin 1 gene mutation predicts poor clinical outcome in de novo adult acute myeloid leukemia: differential clinical importance of *NPM1* mutation according to subtype. Int J Hematol 90: 1–5.
5. Alpermann T, Haferlach C, Dicker F, Eder C, Kohlmann A, et al. (2013) Evaluation Of Different *NPM1* Mutations In AML Patients According To Clinical, Cytogenetic and Molecular Features and Impact On Outcome. Blood 122: 51–51. Available: http://bloodjournal.hematologylibrary.org/content/122/21/51.abstract.
6. Büchner T, Berdel WE, Haferlach C, Haferlach T, Schnittger S, et al. (2009) Age-related risk profile and chemotherapy dose response in acute myeloid leukemia: a study by the German Acute Myeloid Leukemia Cooperative Group. J Clin Oncol 27: 61–69. doi:10.1200/JCO.2007.15.4245.
7. Shaffer LG, McGowan-Jordan J, Schmid M (2013) ISCN 2013: An International System for Human Cytogenetic Nomenclature (2013) - International Standing Committee on Human Cytogenetic Nomenclature. Karger publishers.
8. Thiede C, Steudel C, Mohr B, Schaich M, Schäkel U, et al. (2002) Analysis of *FLT3*-activating mutations in 979 patients with acute myelogenous leukemia: association with FAB subtypes and identification of subgroups with poor prognosis. Blood 99: 4326–4335.
9. Schnittger S, Schoch C, Dugas M, Kern W, Staib P, et al. (2002) Analysis of *FLT3* length mutations in 1003 patients with acute myeloid leukemia: correlation to cytogenetics, FAB subtype, and prognosis in the AMLCG study and usefulness as a marker for the detection of minimal residual disease. Blood 100: 59–66.
10. Schneider F, Hoster E, Unterhalt M, Schneider S, Dufour A, et al. (2012) The *FLT3*ITD mRNA level has a high prognostic impact in *NPM1* mutated, but not in *NPM1* unmutated, AML with a normal karyotype. Blood 119: 4383–4386. doi:10.1182/blood-2010-12-327072.
11. Dufour A, Schneider F, Metzeler KH, Hoster E, Schneider S, et al. (2010) Acute myeloid leukemia with biallelic CEBPA gene mutations and normal karyotype represents a distinct genetic entity associated with a favorable clinical outcome. J Clin Oncol 28: 570–577. doi:10.1200/JCO.2008.21.6010.
12. Benthaus T, Schneider F, Mellert G, Zellmeier E, Schneider S, et al. (2008) Rapid and sensitive screening for CEBPA mutations in acute myeloid leukaemia. Br J Haematol 143: 230–239. doi:10.1111/j.1365-2141.2008.07328.x.
13. Schnittger S, Schoch C, Kern W, Mecucci C, Tschulik C, et al. (2005) Nucleophosmin gene mutations are predictors of favorable prognosis in acute myelogenous leukemia with a normal karyotype. Blood 106: 3733–3739. doi:10.1182/blood-2005-06-2248.
14. Dohner K, Schlenk RF, Habdank M, Scholl C, Rücker FG, et al. (2005) Mutant nucleophosmin (*NPM1*) predicts favorable prognosis in younger adults with acute myeloid leukemia and normal cytogenetics: interaction with other gene mutations. Blood 106: 3740–3746. doi:10.1182/blood-2005-05-2164.
15. Schemper M, Smith TL (1996) A note on quantifying follow-up in studies of failure time. Control Clin Trials 17: 343–346.

21

Establishment of a Humanized APL Model via the Transplantation of *PML-RARA*-Transduced Human Common Myeloid Progenitors into Immunodeficient Mice

Hiromichi Matsushita[1,2,3]*, Takashi Yahata[1,2,4], Yin Sheng[1], Yoshihiko Nakamura[1], Yukari Muguruma[1], Hideyuki Matsuzawa[1,5], Masayuki Tanaka[5], Hideki Hayashi[5], Tadayuki Sato[5], Anar Damdinsuren[3], Makoto Onizuka[6], Mamoru Ito[7], Hayato Miyachi[3], Pier Paolo Pandolfi[8], Kiyoshi Ando[1,2,6]*

1 Research Center for Cancer Stem Cell, Tokai University School of Medicine, Isehara, Kanagawa, Japan, **2** Medical Research Institute, Tokai University, Isehara, Kanagawa, Japan, **3** Department of Laboratory Medicine, Tokai University School of Medicine, Isehara, Kanagawa, Japan, **4** Department of Cell Transplantation, Tokai University School of Medicine, Isehara, Kanagawa, Japan, **5** Support Center for Medical Research and Education, Tokai University, Isehara, Kanagawa, Japan, **6** Division of Hematology and Oncology, Department of Internal Medicine, Tokai University School of Medicine, Isehara, Kanagawa, Japan, **7** Central Institute for Experimental Animals, Kawasaki, Kanagawa, Japan, **8** Cancer Research Institute, Beth Israel Deaconess Cancer Center, Departments of Medicine and Pathology, Beth Israel Deaconess Medical Center, Harvard Medical School, Boston, Massachusetts, United States of America

Abstract

Recent advances in cancer biology have revealed that many malignancies possess a hierarchal system, and leukemic stem cells (LSC) or leukemia-initiating cells (LIC) appear to be obligatory for disease progression. Acute promyelocytic leukemia (APL), a subtype of acute myeloid leukemia characterized by the formation of a PML-RARα fusion protein, leads to the accumulation of abnormal promyelocytes. In order to understand the precise mechanisms involved in human APL leukemogenesis, we established a humanized *in vivo* APL model involving retroviral transduction of *PML-RARA* into CD34$^+$ hematopoietic cells from human cord blood and transplantation of these cells into immunodeficient mice. The leukemia well recapitulated human APL, consisting of leukemic cells with abundant azurophilic abnormal granules in the cytoplasm, which expressed CD13, CD33 and CD117, but not HLA-DR and CD34, were clustered in the same category as human APL samples in the gene expression analysis, and demonstrated sensitivity to ATRA. As seen in human APL, the induced APL cells showed a low transplantation efficiency in the secondary recipients, which was also exhibited in the transplantations that were carried out using the sorted CD34$^-$ fraction. In order to analyze the mechanisms underlying APL initiation and development, fractionated human cord blood was transduced with *PML-RARA*. Common myeloid progenitors (CMP) from CD34$^+$/CD38$^+$ cells developed APL. These findings demonstrate that CMP are a target fraction for *PML-RARA* in APL, whereas the resultant CD34$^-$ APL cells may share the ability to maintain the tumor.

Editor: Marina Konopleva, University of Texas M.D. Anderson Cancer Center, United States of America

Funding: Hiromichi Matsushita received funding from a Grant-in-Aid for Scientific Research from The Ministry of Education, Culture, Sports, Science and Technology of Japan (#24591411, URL http://www.jsps.go.jp/english/e-grants/), Tokai University School of Medicine Project Research (http://www.med.u-tokai.ac.jp/web/international/about_us/message_from_the_dean.html), and the Takeda Science Foundation (http://www.takeda-sci.or.jp/index.html). Kiyoshi Ando received support from a Grant-in-Aid for Scientific Research from The Ministry of Education, Culture, Sports, Science and Technology of Japan (#24390248). The funders had no role in study design, data collection and analysis, decision to publish, or preparation of the manuscript.

Competing Interests: The authors have declared that no competing interests exist.

* Email: hmatsu@is.ic.cc.u-tokai.ac.jp (H. Matsushita); andok@keyaki.cc.u-tokai.ac.jp (KA)

Introduction

Acute myeloid leukemia (AML) constitutes a heterogeneous group of tumors in myeloid lineage cells characterized by the proliferation and accumulation of immature myeloblasts [1]. Recent advances in cancer biology have revealed that various genetic events result in the blockage of differentiation with subsequent uncontrolled cellular proliferation. In addition, *in vivo* analyses using a xenograft model with immunodeficient mice have shown that a very immature subset of AML cells called leukemic stem cells (LSC), which are typically characterized as CD34$^+$/CD38$^-$ cells, as observed in normal hematopoietic stem cells (HSCs), have been shown to slowly undergo cell division to both yield progenitor cells and sustain the LSC population, thus resulting in the maintenance of the tumor [2–6]. More recently, several reports have shown that CD34$^+$/CD38$^+$ hematopoietic progenitors are able to acquire the ability to maintain populations of LSC or leukemia-initiating cells (LIC) [7]. It is therefore possible that the phenotypes of LIC differ among the subtypes of AML.

Acute promyelocytic leukemia (APL) is a subset of AML defined by the formation of a chimeric gene, promyelocytic leukemia-retinoic acid receptor α (*PML-RARA*) [8]. It is characterized by the accumulation of abnormal promyelocytes with abundant large azurophilic granules, suggesting that APL cells undergo maturation arrest in the later steps of myeloid differentiation. The typical pattern of cellular surface markers of APL is positive for CD13,

CD33 and CD117, and negative for CD34, which is usually presumed to indicate cellular immaturity, and HLA-DR [9]. It is very difficult to engraft primary APL samples in immunodeficient mice. They did not become engrafted into the NOD/SCID mice to any degree [3]. In NOD/Shi-SCID/IL-2Rγ^{null} (NOG) mice, which are more profoundly immunocompromised than NOD/SCID mice [10,11], six out of eight APL samples were not engrafted or only very little engrafted [12]. It is therefore possible that the mechanisms underlying the development of APL differ from those involved in the pathogenesis of AML uncovered to date. Elucidating the pathogenesis of APL is important for improving the treatment of APL patients, and will provide clues to understand the development of other subtypes of AML.

In vivo analyses using transgenic APL mice models with *PML-RARA* have revealed that a population of committed myeloid progenitor cells (CD34$^+$, c-kit$^+$, FcγRIII/II$^+$, Gr1^{int}) was identified as the APL-LIC [13,14]. However, the cellular surface antigens and the gene expression pattern in humans are different from those in mice. In particularly, in transgenic systems, murine APL developed after a long latent period through a myelodysplastic/proliferative phase, which does not usually precede human APL [15–18]. There have been no *in vivo* models for exploring leukemogenesis of human APL to date; largely because human primary APL cells are difficult to engraft as a xenograft [3,12]. *PML-RARA*-retrovirally transduced human CD34$^+$ cells from cord blood have therefore only been evaluated *in vitro* [19].

Therefore, the aim of this study was to establish a humanized xenograft APL model using the retroviral transduction of *PML-RARA* into human CD34$^+$ cells and NOG mice in order to investigate the mechanisms of APL leukemogenesis, such as that involving disease initiation and maintenance in the model.

Materials and Methods

Fractionation of human hematopoietic cells from cord blood

Cord blood (CB) and patients' APL samples were obtained after written informed consent was provided in accordance with the Declaration of Helsinki and with approval from the Tokai University Committee on Clinical Investigation (Permit number: #12I-46 and #12I-49). CD34 positive and negative specimens were primarily prepared using the CD34 Progenitor Cell Isolation Kit (Miltenyi Biotec, Bergisch Gladbach, Germany). CD34$^+$ cells were then purified again using anti-human CD34 mAbs (Beckman Coulter, Brea, CA), in combination with or without an anti-CD38 antibody (BD, Franklin Lakes, NJ), with a FACS vantage instrument (BD). CD34$^-$/CD33$^+$ cells were also purified again using anti-human CD34 and CD33 mAbs (Beckman Coulter) and the FACS vantage instrument. The preparation of common myeloid progenitors (CMP), granulocyte-monocytic progenitors (GMP) and megakaryocyte-erythrocyte progenitors (MEP) was performed using an anti-CD123 antibody (BD) and anti-CD45RA (Biolegend, San Diego, CA) antibody, according to a previous report [20].

Retrovirus transduction of *PML-RARA* into human hematopoietic cells

The MIGR1 retroviral vector [21] or MIGR1-*PML-RARA* (bcr3/short form) [22] in combination with the vesicular stomatitis virus-G protein (VSV-G) envelope vector (pCMV-VSV-G) was transiently transfected into PLAT-gp cells using the Fugene 6 transfection reagent (Roche Diagnostics, Basel, Switzerland). The culture supernatant was concentrated 100 to 200 times by ultracentrifugation. After overnight culture of the fractionated cells in StemPro-34 (Life Technologies, Carlsbad, CA) with TPO, SCF, and FLT3 ligand (50 ng/ml each), they were incubated with the concentrated supernatant on retronectin-coated plates (Takara-Bio, Otsu, Japan). Retroviral transduction was performed twice, and then transplantation was performed the next day.

Colony-forming unit-cells assay

PML-RARA transduced cells were sorted by their EGFP, CD34 and CD38 expression by FACS vantage 48 h after infection. The colony-forming unit-cells (CFU-C) assay was performed as described previously [23]. The fluorescent images were captured using a HS All-in-One Fluorescence Microscope Biorevo 9000 (Keyence Corporation, Osaka, Japan) and were analyzed by the BZ II software program (Keyence Corporation).

RNA extraction and RT-PCR

Total RNA was isolated using the RNeasy micro kit (Qiagen, Hilden, Germany) or Isogen (Nippon gene, Tokyo, Japan), and the reverse-transcribed cDNA was amplified by qualitative PCR. The qualitative-PCR analysis was performed by SRL Inc. (Hachioji, Tokyo, Japan). The sequences of PCR primers and probes were shown in **Table S1**.

Transplantation, serial transplantation and ATRA treatment

Nine- to 20-week-old NOD/Shi-scid, IL-2Rγc^{null} (NOG) mice [10,11] were irradiated with 220 cGy of X-rays. On the following day, the whole infected cells or primary AML cells were intravenously injected. The EGFP-positive cells in the peripheral blood were monitored. The mice with induced APL were defined as those bearing more than 0.1% EGFP$^+$ cells which dominantly expressed CD33 (more than 70%) in their bone marrow at four months after transplantation. In the initial analysis, the occurrence of APL was confirmed by the morphological observations using cytospin slides after EGFP sorting. For serial transplantation, bone marrow cells were obtained from recipient mice, and the sorted EGFP-positive cells were injected intravenously or intramedullary into the irradiated mice [24]. The engrafted mice were treated intraperitoneally with 1.5 µg/g of body weight/day of all-*trans* retinoic acid (ATRA, Sigma) for 21 days [25], and were then sacrificed to collect the EGFP-positive cells in the bone marrow by sorting. All the experiments using animals were approved by the animal care committee of Tokai University (Permit number: #132028).

Flow cytometric analysis

The cells were stained with APC-conjugated anti-human CD45, CD33, CD34, HLA-DR (Beckman Coulter), CD13, and CD117 (BD) mAbs. They were subjected to flow cytometry using a FACSCalibur instrument (BD) and the CellQuest software program (BD).

Cell preparation, Wright-Giemsa staining and immunofluorescence microscopy

Cytospin slides were prepared using a Cytospin 4 Cytocentrifuge (Thermo Scientific, Waltham, MA) at 500 rounds per minute for 5 min. To observe the cellular morphology, Wright-Giemsa staining was performed. For the immunofluorescent study, cells were seeded onto poly-L-lysine coated slides and fixed with ice cold 70% ethanol for 15 min. After permeabilization with 0.2% Triton X-100 for 20 min, the slides were treated with PBS containing 5% normal goat serum for 1 hour to block the nonspecific binding of antibodies. The anti-PML antibody (Merck

Millipore, Billerica, MA) was applied overnight at 4°C. Cells were counterstained with DAPI. Images were captured with an LSM510 META confocal microscope (Carl Zeiss, Oberkochen, Germany) and processed using Adobe Photoshop 7.0 (Adobe Systems, San Jose, CA).

Southern blot analysis

Genomic DNA was extracted from the cells using a DNeasy kit (Qiagen). Ten micrograms of the DNA were electrophoresed and transferred to nylon membranes (Hybond-N+, GE Healthcare, Fairfield, CT). The DNA was then crosslinked to the membrane by ultraviolet light. The EGFP probe was prepared from MIGR1 vector by cutting it using NcoI and SalI, and was labeled with ^{32}P-dCTP using the Rediprime II DNA Labelling System (GE Healthcare). The membrane was hybridized with the probe in Rapid-hyb buffer (GE Healthcare), and was analyzed by a Phosphoimager (LAS1000, Fuji Film, Tokyo, Japan).

Microarray

Total RNA was labeled and hybridized to Affymetrix Human Genome U133 Plus 2.0 Array GeneChip microarrays (Affymetrix, Santa Clara, CA) using the manufacturer's protocols. The results were deposited in the Gene Expression Omnibus (GEO; http://www.ncbi.nlm.nih.gov/geo/; accession no. GSE49344). The microarray data from normal human promyelocytes and clinical samples bearing AML, including APL, were obtained from the deposited data on the GEO (GSE12662). The APL-specific expressed genes have been described in detail in a previous study [26]. The probe set data were generated using standard normalization algorithms included in the Affymetrix Microarray Suite software program, v.5 (MAS5.0). The clustering analysis was performed by the Gene spring GX software program, version 11 (Agilent technology, Santa Clara, CA).

To identify the genes that are differentially expressed in a specific cellular subset, all probe sets with fewer than 10% present calls in both groups and a coefficient of variation <0.5 across all samples were eliminated prior to the subsequent analysis; (i) The genes differently expressed in the induced APL cases among the AML cases were defined as genes whose expression change (upregulation or downregulation) was ≥2.0 fold in comparison to those in AML other than APL, (ii) The genes associated with immaturity in the induced APL cases were expressed at significantly higher levels in CD34$^+$ cells than the other normal cells (FDR <0.05, fold-change >2.0 upregulated), and were also expressed in the induced APL cells at similar levels (induced APL: CD34$^+$ ≥1:1), and moreover, these genes were expressed at higher levels in promyelocytes (induced APL: Pros ≥2:1). (iii) The genes upregulated during promyelocyte differentiation were expressed at significantly higher levels in promyelocytes than in the other normal cells (FDR <0.05, fold-change >2.0 upregulated), and were expressed at lower levels in the induced APL (induced APL: Pros ≤1:2), (iv) The genes induced by *PML-RARA* were expressed at higher levels in the induced APL than in all the normal cells (induced APL: normal ≥2:1), and were not expressed in any normal cells (more than 75% absent calls, as summarized by the MAS5.0). Statistical significance was assessed by the unpaired unequal variance Welch test (P<0.05), and correction for multiple testing was performed by the Benjamini and Hochberg False Discovery Rate (FDR), using a cutoff of 0.05.

The gene set specific for induced APL was defined to fulfill one or more of the above criteria (ii) to (iv) in the gene set identified in (i).

The integration site analysis of *PML-RARA* using linear amplification-mediated PCR

To identify the genomic-proviral junction sequence, linear amplification-mediated polymerase chain reaction (LAM-PCR) was performed as described previously, with minor modifications [27,28]. In brief, genomic DNA from bone marrow cells was first digested with Tsp509I. A linear amplification of target DNA in the digested genome was performed by repeated primer extension using a vector-specific 5′-biotinylated primer, LTR1.5, and Taq polymerase. After selection with Dynabeads MyOne Streptavidin C1 (Life Technologies), a double-stranded asymmetrical linker cassette was ligated to the Tsp509I-digested site using T4 DNA Ligase. The DNA products were then amplified by PCR using a vector-specific primer, LTR3, and linker cassette primer, LC1. The nested PCR was performed using internal primers LTR5 and LC2. The final products were sequenced after cloning them into the TOPO TA cloning vector (Life Technologies). The primer sequences are shown in **Table S1**.

Statistical analyses

The Kaplan-Meier method was used to estimate the leukemia-free survival (LFS) of mice. Log-rank p values were used for comparisons of the LFS among three subgroups. The analyses were conducted using the GraphPad Prism software package (GraphPad Software, La Jolla, CA). The other statistical analyses were performed using the Mann-Whitney U Test with the IBM SPSS Statistics software program (New York, NY). Values of $p<0.05$ were considered to be statistically significant.

Results

Functions of PML-RARα in human CD34 cells *in vitro*

To examine the functions of PML-RARα *in vitro*, a MIGR1-*PML-RARA* or MIGR1 control vector was retrovirally infected into human CD34$^+$ cells from cord blood. The transduction efficiency evaluated by EGFP positivity was 0.5% to 18.6% (n = 10, median: 5.7%) and 2.1% to 19.7% (n = 25, median: 6.8%), respectively. The expression of *PML-RARA* in these cells was confirmed by RT-PCR (**Figure S1**). The induction of *PML-RARA* in CD34$^+$ cells disrupted PML nuclear bodies by interacting with wild-type PML via the PML portion of the chimeric transcript, and the distribution of PML in the nucleus was altered to show a microspeckled pattern in these cells [29–31] (**Figure 1A**). Additionally, the induction of *PML-RARA* reduced all the colony formation capacity (**Figure 1B**). The *PML-RARA* expression was confirmed in these colonies by EGFP fluorescence (**Figure S1 and S2**) and RT-PCR, although the expression levels were 37 times lower compared to those in the CD34$^+$ cells 48 hours after *PML-RARA* transduction (**Figure S3**). Regarding the content of colonies, MIGR1-infected CD34$^+$ cells mainly generated the erythroid lineage-containing colonies, such as CFU-mix and BFU-E, whereas more than half of the colonies from the CD34$^+$ cells with *PML-RARA* were of the myeloid lineage, like CFU-GM (**Figures 1C**). These data demonstrate that *PML-RARA* induces the myeloid commitment of human CD34$^+$ cells.

Establishment of a humanized *in vivo* APL model

The cells transduced with *PML-RARA* or the MIGR1 control vector were then transplanted into NOG mice. The EGFP$^+$ cells survived and proliferated three to four months after transplantation only in the NOG mice transplanted with *PML-RARA*-, not control vector at all, infected human CD34$^+$ cells. The median proportion of EGFP$^+$/CD45$^+$ cells in the bone marrow obtained from the transplanted mice was 23.7% (0.95% to 96.5%, n = 24)

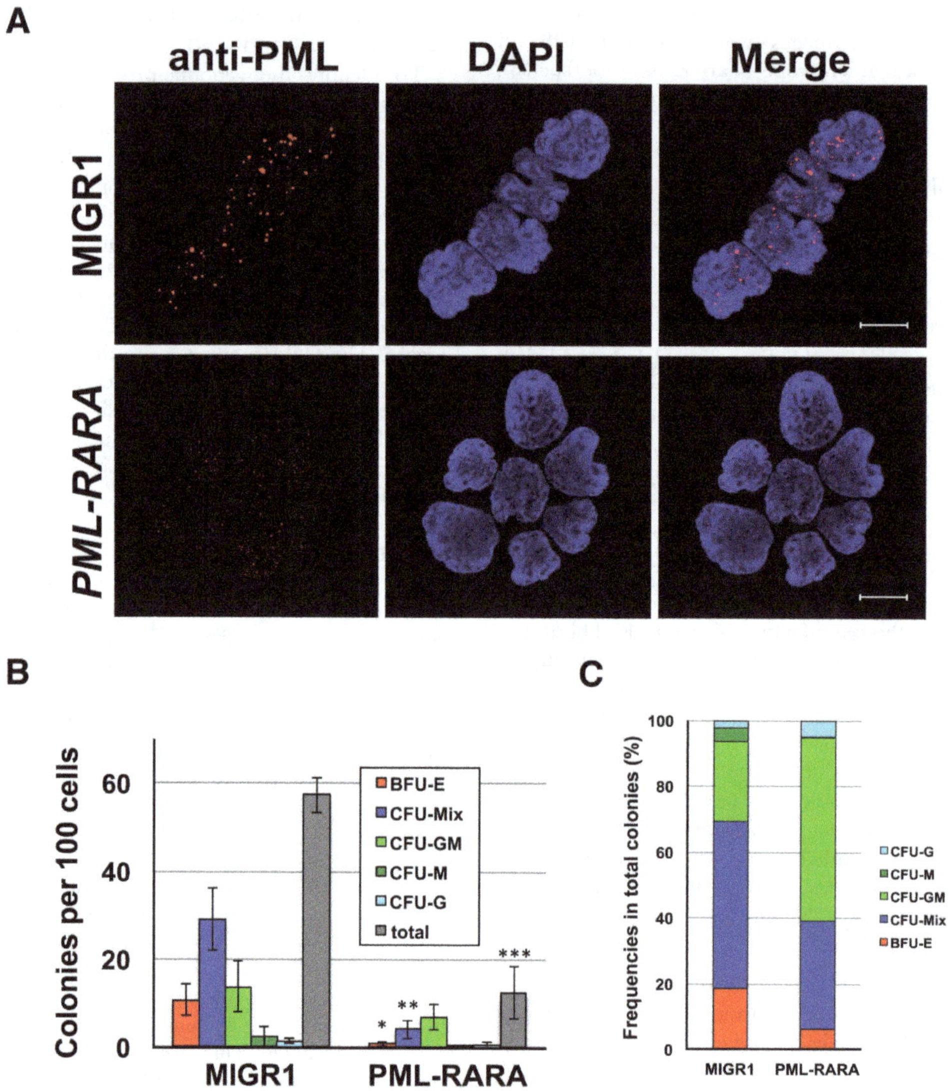

Figure 1. The function of *PML-RARA* in human CD34$^+$ cells *in vitro*. (**A**) The results of an immunofluorescent analysis of PML distribution in human CD34$^+$ cells transduced with *PML-RARA*. The images were captured with an LSM510 META confocal microscope (Carl Zeiss). The bars indicate 10 μm. (**B**) The colony-forming assay using *PML-RARA*-transduced CD34$^+$ cells. The cells were sorted by EGFP expression 48 h after infection. Colony formation was evaluated on days 10 to 12 after plating the cells. The average numbers of colonies from three independent experiments are shown. Data represent the means ± SD. The asterisks (*) indicate $p<0.05$. (**C**) The proportion of each kind of colony was calculated from the results of the colony-forming assay shown in (B). The percentages of CFU-GM are higher in *PML-RARA*-infected cells than in control (MIGR1) cells ($p=0.013$).

(**Figure 2A**). The majority of the engrafted EGFP$^+$/human CD45$^+$ cells expressed human CD33 (70.2% to 100%, median 90.6%, n = 24) (**Figure 2B**), thus suggesting that they were of the myeloid lineage. The *PML-RARA* expression was detected only in the EGFP$^+$ fraction and not in the EGFP$^-$ fraction of the sorted human CD45$^+$/CD33$^+$ cells from the NOG mice (**Figure 2C**). The expression levels of *PML-RARA* were decreased about 17-fold in comparison to those in the CD34$^+$ cells 48 hours after *PML-RARA* transduction (**Figure S3**), but the presence of *PML-RARA* in the human myeloid cells, recognized as EGFP$^+$ cells, caused marked accumulation of promyelocytes, in comparison to the control EGFP$^-$ human myeloid cells (52.8% in EGFP$^+$ cells vs 19.4% EGFP$^-$ cells in the 13 paired samples, $p<0.0001$). On the other hand, the proportions of myeloblasts, mature neutrophils and monocytes were decreased (5.2% vs 14.4%, $p=0.010$; 2.5% vs 12.7%, $p=0.005$; 4.0% vs 10.1%, $p=0.016$) (**Figure 2D**). These findings confirmed that the expression of *PML-RARA* induced the myeloid differentiation of human CD34$^+$ cells and blocked them at the promyelocytic stage. Morphologically, the promyelocytes had abundant large azurophilic granules and round nuclei with a high nucleocytoplasmic ratio. Some of them had a number of Auer bodies and looked like Faggot cells, which are the typical morphological features of APL cells, and were not seen in the previous murine models (**Figure 2E**). A Southern blot analysis using an EGFP probe revealed that the EGFP$^+$/CD45$^+$/CD33$^+$ cells oligoclonally proliferated *in vivo* (**Figure 2F**).

The induced APL cells were detected in 24 out of the 34 mice (71%) transplanted with *PML-RARA*-transduced CD34 cells ($p=0.0184$ in comparison to the control). They were detected in all 16 mice when the calculated number of the transplanted EGFP$^+$/CD34$^+$ cells per mouse was more than 3,000 (4,655 to 29,728 cells, median: 11,085 cells) ($p=0.0006$ in comparison to the control). On the other hand, they were only detected in eight out of 18 mice (44%) transplanted with EGFP$^+$/CD34$^+$ cells at a

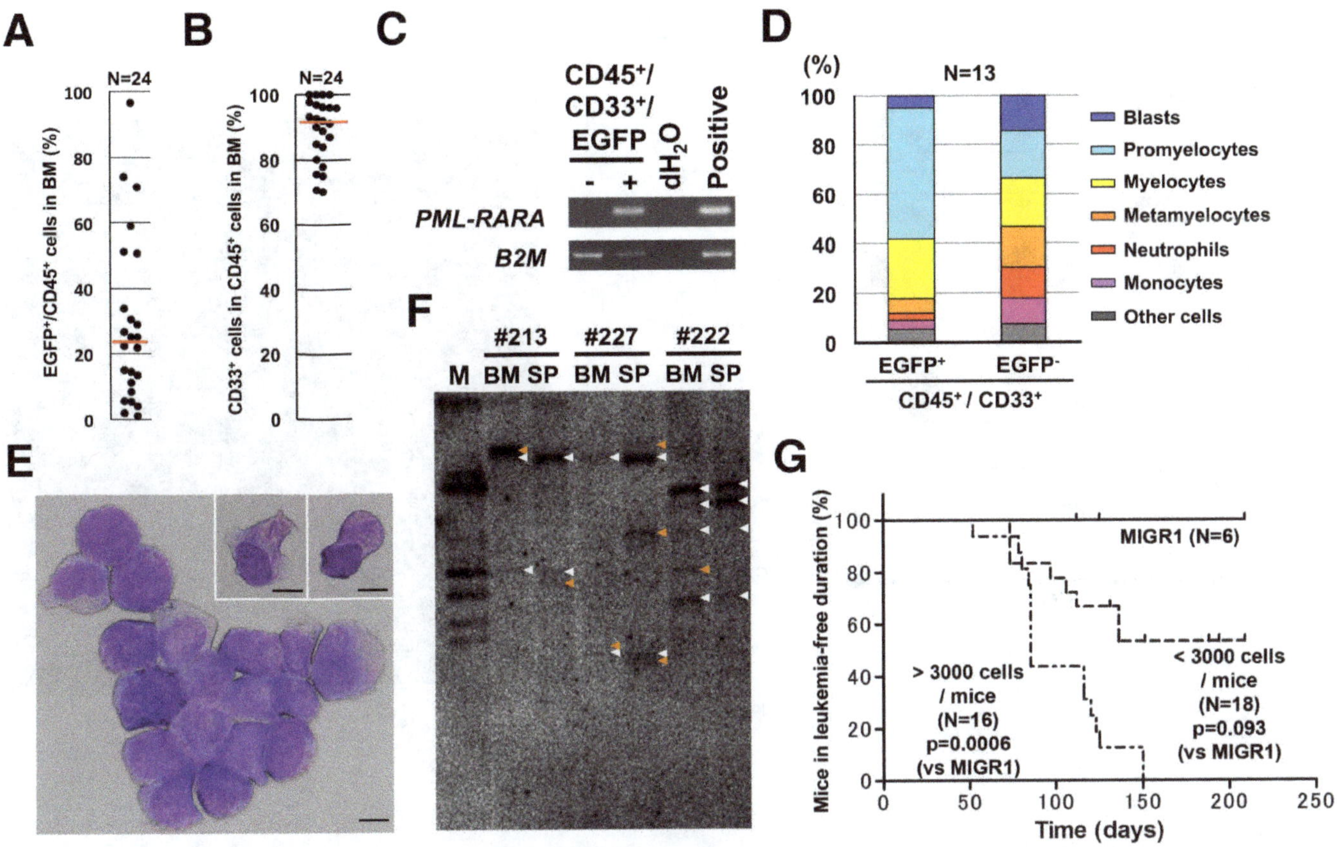

Figure 2. Establishment of humanized APL *in vivo*. (**A**) The proportion of EGFP$^+$/human CD45$^+$ cells in the bone marrow of leukemic NOG mice. Each dot represents a single mouse. The horizontal line represents the median value. (**B**) The proportion of CD33$^+$ cells among the EGFP$^+$/human CD45$^+$ cells in the bone marrow of the leukemic NOG mice. Each dot represents a single mouse. The horizontal line represents the median value. (**C**) The expression of *PML-RARA* in RT-PCR was detected only in the EGFP$^+$ fraction obtained from the engrafted human CD45$^+$/CD33$^+$ cells. The cells were obtained from bone marrow 16 weeks after transplantation. *B2M, beta 2 microglobulin.* The *PML-RARA* expression vector and human CD34$^+$ cells were used as a positive control for the *PML-RARA* and *B2M* analysis, respectively. (**D**) The differential counts of the engrafted CD45$^+$/CD33$^+$/EGFP$^+$ and EGFP$^-$ cells from the mice transplanted with *PML-RARA*-induced human CD34$^+$ cells. They were obtained from bone marrow 16 to 20 weeks after transplantation. The data represent the means. (**E**) A representative photograph of the resulting leukemic cells which morphologically recapitulated APL. Faggot cells were recognized, as seen in the right top corner. The images were captured with a BX41 microscope (Olympus). The bar indicates 10 μm. (**F**) The results of a Southern blot analysis of the genomic DNA from induced APL cells with an EGFP probe. Clonal bands are shown by arrow heads: white, seen in both BM and SP; orange, seen only in BM or SP. BM, bone marrow; SP, spleen. (**G**) The leukemia-free duration in NOG mice transplanted with *PML-RARA*-transduced CD34$^+$ cells.

density of less than 3,000 (480 to 2,660 cells, median: 1,861 cells) (p = 0.093 in comparison to the control) (**Figure 2G**). This proportion was not dependent on the number of transplanted EGFP$^+$/CD34$^+$ cells.

These findings demonstrate that a humanized APL model can be successfully established by the transplantation of *PML-RARA*–transduced human CD34 cells into NOG mice.

Characteristics of the induced APL cells obtained from the humanized *in vivo* model

The induced APL cells were positive for human myeloid markers such as CD13, CD33 and CD117, and were negative for CD34 and HLA-DR, as seen in typical human APL [32]. *PML-RARA* did not contribute to the development of lymphocytes. Human CD19$^+$ B-cells in the spleen and human CD4$^+$/CD8$^+$ T-cells in the thymus were negative for EGFP (**Figure 3A**).

To evaluate the gene expression of the induced APL cells, a microarray analysis was performed, and the expression of the 510 APL-specific genes identified in a previous study was compared with that observed in the clinical AML samples [26]. Two clinical APL samples from our patients were simultaneously evaluated and were aligned in the APL category defined in the study, suggesting that our microarray results were comparable with those in the previous study. The induced APL cells from our models were also classified into the APL category when compared to normal promyelocytes and AML samples other than APL (**Figure 3B**).

In common with this previous study [26], the 3,439 probes (3278 genes) differentially expressed in the induced APL and the AML other than APL ((i) in the Materials and Methods) grouped the induced APL and human primary APL together, separately from the other types of AML (**Figure S4**). The gene sets whose expression in the induced APL cases was not dependent on the myeloid differentiation were also filtered by comparison with the data for normal myeloid cells. They included the genes for immaturity expressed in the induced APL (1,782 probes, including 1,720 genes), the genes upregulated in promyelocyte differentiation not in the induced APL (447 probes, including 427 genes) and the genes specifically induced by *PML-RARA* (466 probes, including 429 genes) ((ii), (iii) and (iv) in the Materials and Methods). Each gene set was analyzed using the DAVID website

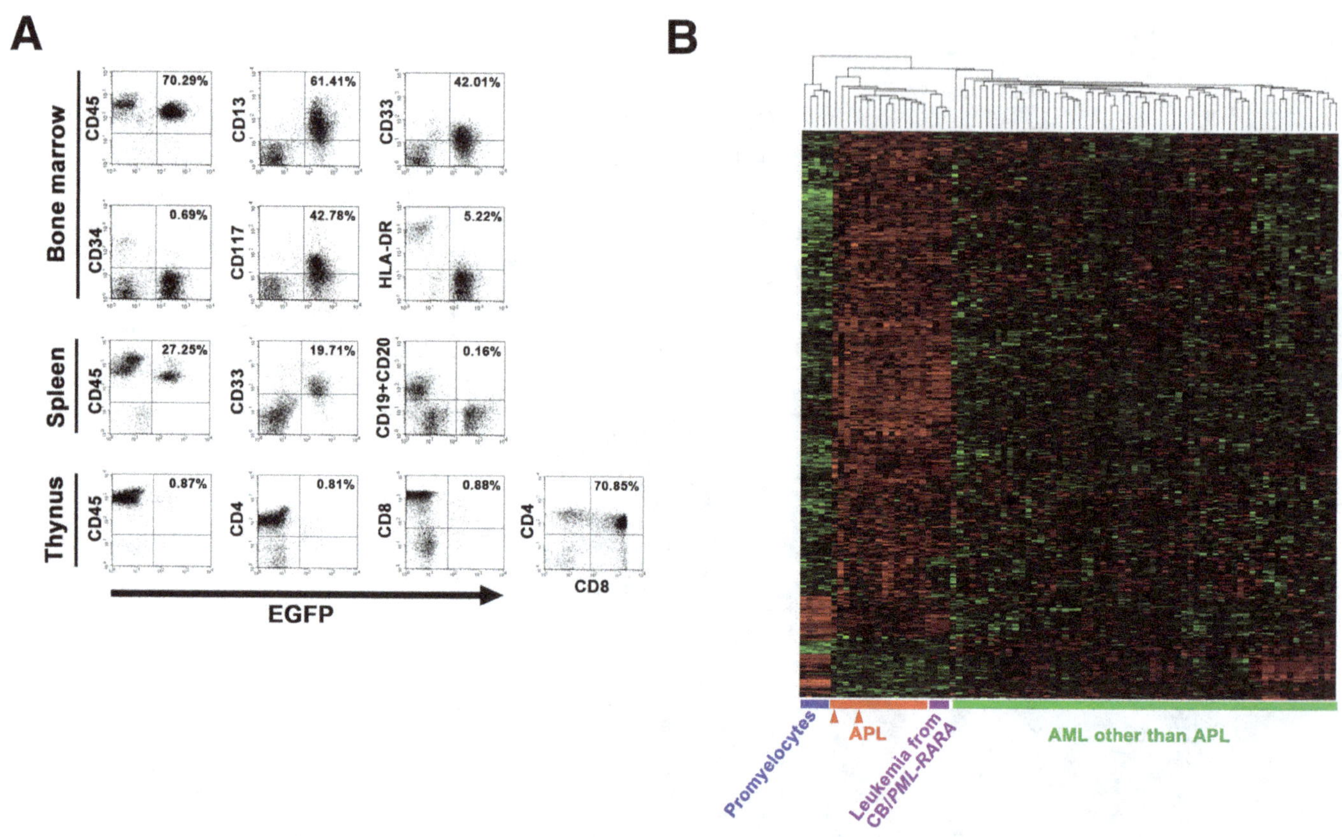

Figure 3. Characteristics of the induced APL *in vivo*. (**A**) The representative expression pattern of cell surface markers in the induced APL cells determined by a flow cytometric analysis. All the scatter plots show the relationships between the EGFP positivity and cell surface marker expression. The whole living cells gated as a propidium iodide-negative fraction in the bone marrow were analyzed. The induced APL cells were recognized as EGFP$^+$ cells. A few murine hematopoietic cells, recognized as a human CD45$^-$ fraction, were detected in this mouse. (**B**) The heat map of the microarray analysis using the 510 APL-specific genes for the comparison of the induced APL cells (purple, n = 3) with APL (red, n = 16), other types of AML (M0, 1, 2 and 4 in FAB classification, green, n = 62) and normal promyelocytes (blue, n = 5) in a previous study [26]. The red triangles (n = 2) for a total 16 APL cases show the clinical APL samples whose microarray data were obtained in this study.

(david.abcc.ncifcrf.gov/). In the induced APL cases, the genes related to N-Glycan, steroid and heparan sulfate biosynthesis, the spliceosome and pyrimidine metabolism were expressed similar to the levels in normal CD34$^+$ cells, and those related to the MAPK signaling pathway were exclusively expressed in comparison to normal myeloid cells, including normal CD34$^+$ cells. On the other hand, the genes related to neurotrophin signaling and the cell cycle, as well as those associated with metabolic processes, such as glycolysis/gluconeogenesis, the pentose phosphate pathway and sphingolipid metabolism were downregulated (**Table S2**), thus suggesting that the induced APL exhibited dysregulated signaling and metabolism as differentiated myeloid cells. Additionally, the gene set composed of 573 probes including 547 genes, which fulfilled one or more above criteria (ii) to (iv) in the gene set identified in (i), clearly separated the normal and malignant promyelocytes, such as those of induced and human primary APL (**Figure S5 and Table S3**), as described in the previous study using primary APL cases [26].

To evaluate the additional genetic events that accompanied the integration of *PML-RARA* in the genome, the insertion sites of *PML-RARA* were analyzed. Some of the integration sites of *PML-RARA* were in the introns or exons of genes (**Table S4**). However, they were neither recurrent nor found in the previous whole genome sequence analysis of the APL patients [33]. These findings suggest that *PML-RARA* was a common key event, but that there were various additional genetic events in these induced APL cells, and this finding was compatible with the previous analysis using human primary APL [33].

The induced APL cells differentiated into mature neutrophils following treatment with all-*trans* retinoic acid (ATRA) *in vitro* (**Figures 4A and 4B**), which was accompanied by alterations in the PML distribution in the nucleus, from a microspeckled to a speckled pattern (**Figure 4C**). Similarly, ATRA induced transient myeloid differentiation *in vivo* (n = 4), as has been seen in APL patients (**Figures 4D and 4E**).

These findings demonstrate that our induced APL cells recapitulate human APL both phenotypically and functionally.

Re-transplantable cellular fraction in the induced APL cells

It is necessary to prove that the resultant induced APL cells possess the reproducibility of APL in the secondary recipients in order to demonstrate their capacity for leukemogenesis. However, previous studies have revealed that primary APL cells exhibit difficultly in engrafting in immunodeficient mice [3,12]. When the induced APL cells were transplanted into the second recipients, they were proven to be re-transplantable intravenously; 500,000 to 1,000,000 leukemic cells, but not 50,000 cells, were required, and the frequency of APL cells in the secondary recipients was low (0.04% to 1.41%, n = 6). The frequency was still low, even though

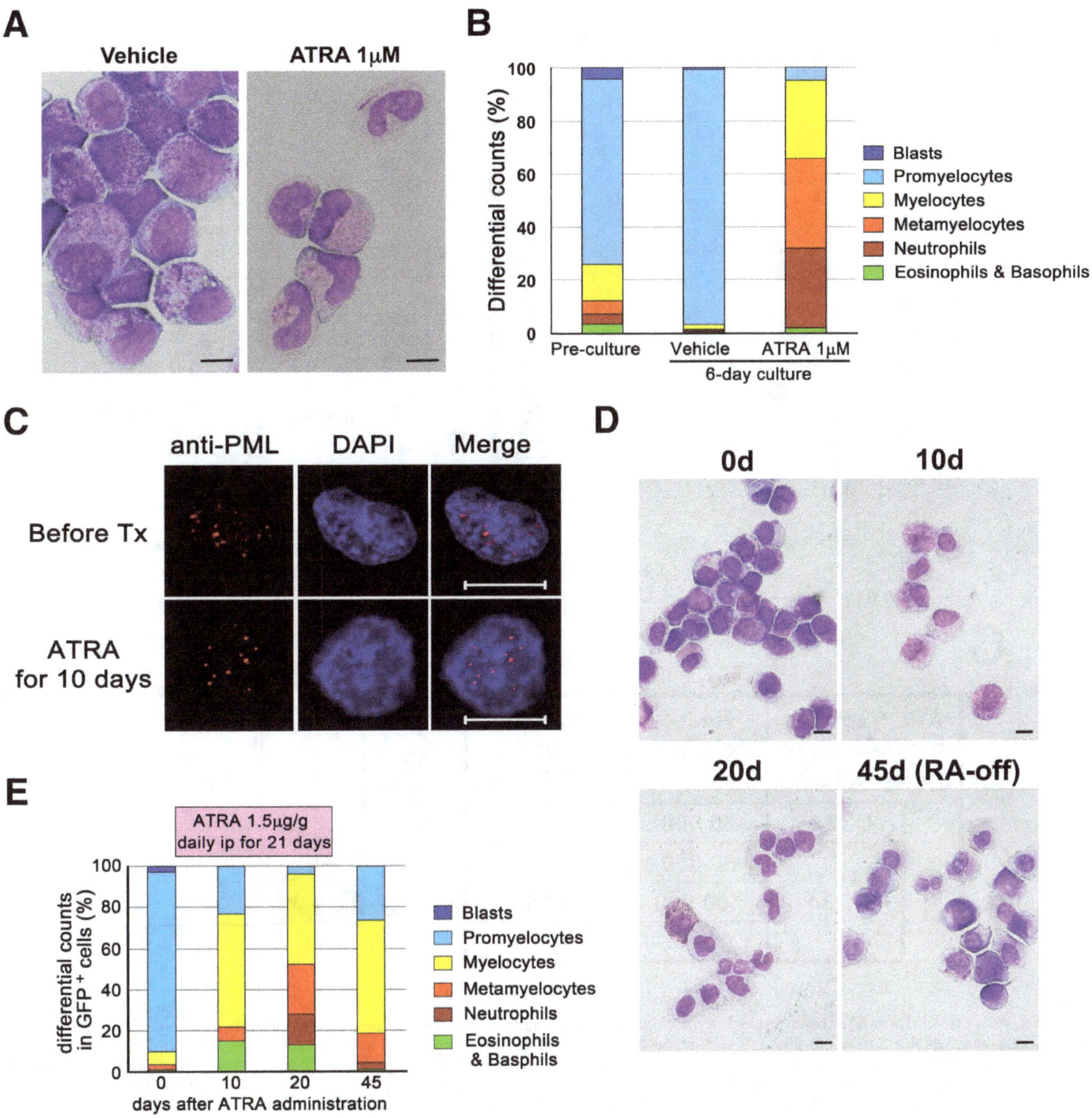

Figure 4. The induction of myeloid differentiation in the APL cells induced by ATRA treatment *in vitro* and *in vivo*. (**A**) Cytospin slides of the induced APL cells cultured with or without 1 μM ATRA for 6 days. The mature neutrophils with Auer rods are seen in the ATRA-treated group. The images were captured with a BX41 microscope (Olympus). The bar indicates 10 μm. (**B**) The differential cellular counts of the induced APL cells cultured with or without ATRA. The average leukocyte differentiation in three independent experiments is shown. (**C**) The results of an immunofluorescent analysis of the PML distribution in the induced APL cells before and after treatment with ATRA. The images were captured with an LSM510 META confocal microscope (Carl Zeiss). All the bars indicate 10 μm. (**D, E**) The induction of myeloid differentiation in the induced APL cells by ATRA *in vivo*. The secondary recipients transplanted with the induced APL cells were then intraperitoneally treated with ATRA for 21 days. Cytospin slides of EGFP$^+$/hCD45$^+$/hCD33$^+$ cells from the secondary recipients transplanted with the induced APL cells are shown (**D**). The images were captured with a BX41 microscope (Olympus). The bar indicates 10 μm. Their differentiated cellular counts were evaluated, and the representative series data are indicated (**E**).

they were transplanted intramedullary (iBM, 2.00% to 5.98%, n = 2) (**Figure 5A**). The immunophenotype of the engrafted cells was the same as that seen in the primary induced APL cells: they were positive for CD13 and CD33, without the expression of CD34 or HLA-DR (**Figure 5B**), demonstrating that the induced APL retains self-renewal capacity with a low level of transplan-

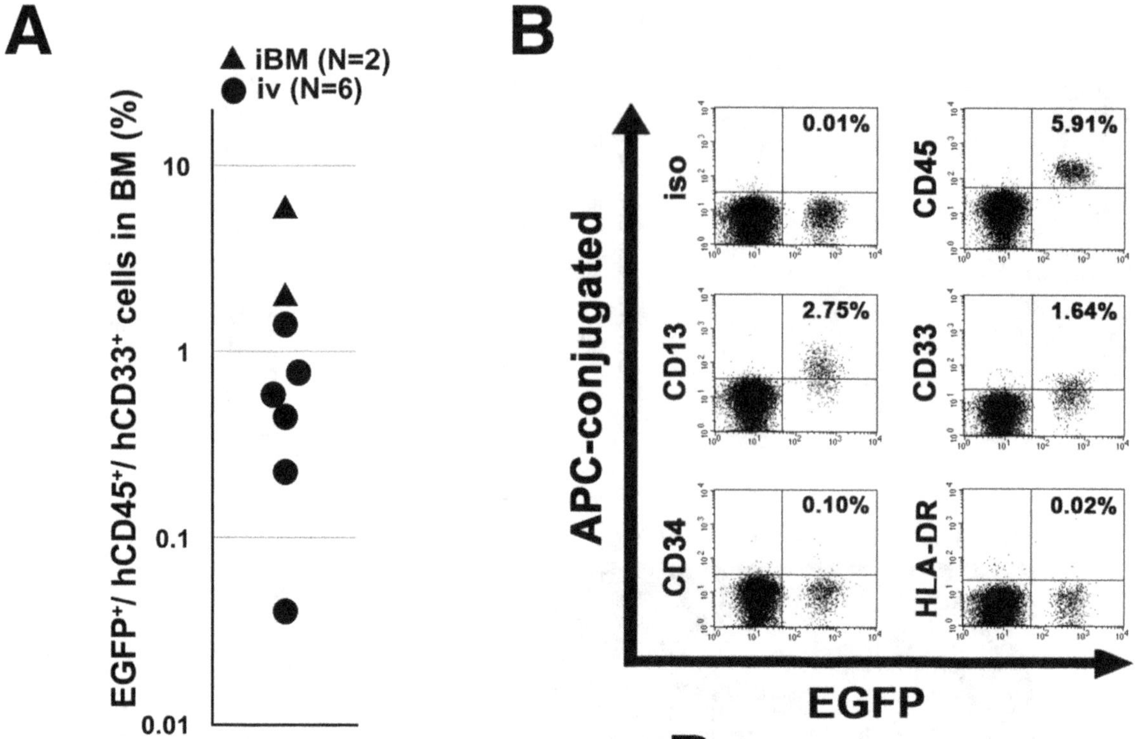

C

APL fractions for secondary transplantation		No. of cells per mouse	Detection of engraftment
EGFP+	CD34+	50 000	0 / 4
	CD34-	50 000	0 / 4
		500 000	0 / 1
		1 000 000	4 / 4

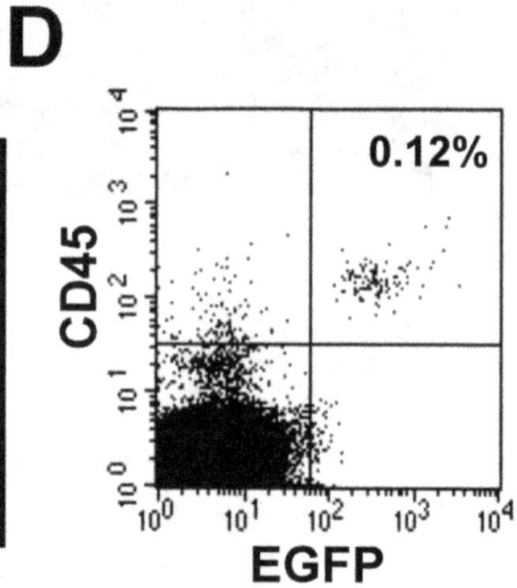

Figure 5. APL-LIC in the humanized APL *in vivo* model. (**A**) The engraftment of the induced APL cells in the secondary recipients. The bone marrow cells were obtained 16 weeks after transplantation and evaluated. Each dot represents a single mouse. (**B**) The immunophenotype of the induced APL cells in the secondary recipients. The representative pattern is shown. (**C**) The engraftment capacity in each fraction from the induced APL cells in the secondary recipients. The bone marrow cells were obtained 16 weeks after transplantation and evaluated. (**D**) The engraftment of the $CD34^-$ fraction in the secondary recipients. The engrafted cells are shown as $EGFP^+/CD45^+$ cells.

tation efficiency. In addition, the results suggested that the capacity for engraftment in this xenograft model differed between the $CD34^+$ cells transduced with *PML-RARA* and the APL cells mostly composed of the $CD34^-$ fraction.

To identify a fraction responsible for the APL maintenance in the induced APL cases, $CD34^+$ and $CD34^-$ APL fractions were separately collected and transplanted intravenously. The $CD34^+$ fraction was pooled because there were very few $CD34^+$ cells in each induced APL case (**Figures 3A and 5B**). The $CD34^-$ fraction was sorted twice to exclude the $CD34^+$ fraction completely. Fifty thousand APL cells in both the $CD34^+$ and $CD34^-$ fractions failed to engraft in the secondary recipients (0 out of 4 mice in each fraction). Similar to the unsorted cells, one million $CD34^-$ fraction cells were able to engraft in recipient mice (4 out of 4 mice) (**Figures 5C and 5D**).

These findings revealed that $CD34^-$ induced APL cells exhibit the ability to function as APL-LIC *in vivo*, although the LIC function was not excluded in the $CD34^+$ APL fraction.

The $CD34^+/CD38^+$ progenitors trigger APL by *PML-RARA* induction *in vivo*

The findings that the *PML-RARA* transduced-$CD34^+$ cells developed APL while the resultant $CD34^-$ APL cells exhibited transplantability indicate the possibility that the initiation and maintenance of APL arise at different steps of differentiation, which are not likely to involve the $CD34^+/CD38^-$ fraction, as originally reported in human AML. Therefore, in order to identify a cellular target for *PML-RARA* that effectively develops APL, *PML-RARA* was transduced into fractionated cells: CD34$^+$/CD38$^-$, CD34$^+$/CD38$^+$ and CD34$^-$/CD33$^+$ cells from the cord blood (**Figures 6A and 6B**). The transduction efficiency, as evaluated by EGFP expression, ranged from 1.9% to 5.0% (median: 3.53%, n = 6) in CD34$^+$/CD38$^-$ cells, 4.5% to 10.6% (median: 10.07%, n = 6) in CD34$^+$/CD38$^+$ cells and 19.1% to 22.1% (median: 20.63%, n = 4) in CD34$^-$/CD33$^+$ cells. Because the CD34$^+$ fraction from human cord blood possessed a higher proportion of CD34$^+$/CD38$^+$ (74.5% to 94.2%) than that of CD34$^+$/CD38$^-$ cells, the presumed absolute number of *PML-RARA* transplanted cells was higher in CD34$^+$/CD38$^+$ cells than in CD34$^+$/CD38$^-$ cells (3,430 to 31,800 cells vs 140 to 450 cells per mouse; 22,900 to 27,700 CD34$^-$/CD33$^+$ cells). One hundred unfractionated human CD34$^+$ cells, including both CD34$^+$/CD38$^-$ and CD34$^+$/CD38$^+$ cells, were engrafted with multilineage differentiation in our previous study [10], thus suggesting that the transplanted cell numbers were adequate for engraftment in the NOG mice. The induction of *PML-RARA* in CD34$^+$/CD38$^+$ cells reduced the colony formation capacity and favored the formation of myeloid colonies, as seen in CD34$^+$ cells (**Figures 1B and 1C**). On the other hand, the induction of *PML-RARA* in CD34$^+$/CD38$^-$ cells generated very few colonies in comparison to the MIGR1 control vector-infected CD34$^+$/CD38$^-$ cells (**Figures 6C and 6D**). Consistent with the results, the induced APL cells were detected mostly in the mice transplanted with CD34$^+$/CD38$^+$ cells (median, 16.4% in the whole bone marrow cells) (**Figure 6E**). These findings suggest that CD34$^+$/CD38$^+$ progenitors proliferate and survive more efficiently than CD34$^+$/CD38$^-$ cells *in vitro* and trigger APL *in vivo* by inducing *PML-RARA*.

Human common myeloid progenitors develop into APL by inducing *PML-RARA* among CD34$^+$/CD38$^+$ progenitors

In order to identify the detailed target fraction in CD34$^+$/CD38$^+$ cells that generates APL with *PML-RARA*, the CD34$^+$/CD38$^+$ cells were then divided into three fractions based on their expression of CD123 and CD45RA; CMP, GMP and MEP (**Figure 6F**). The retroviral transduction efficiencies of *PML-RARA* into CMP, GMP and MEP were 6.0% to 15.2% (median: 6.6%, n = 9), 3.3% to 8.8% (median: 7.1%, n = 8), and 7.8% to 24.6% (median: 8.5%, n = 7) (**Figure 6G**), and the presumed absolute numbers of *PML-RARA* transduced cells in CMP, GMP and MEP utilized for the transplantation were 5,850 to 15,200, 830 to 4,250, and 1,150 to 2,550 cells per mouse, respectively, which were deduced to directly reflect their proportion in the human cord blood. The frequency of induced APL cells in whole bone marrow cells from transplanted NOG mice was higher when using CMP (median, 25.2%) than GMP and MEP (median, 0.15% and 0.01%, respectively) (**Figure 6H**).

Taken together, these findings obtained using our humanized *in vivo* APL model demonstrate that CMP are a target fraction for *PML-RARA* in the development of APL.

Discussion

Our present study revealed that a humanized APL model was successfully established by transplantation of human CD34$^+$ cord blood transduced with *PML-RARA* into immunodeficient mice. Using this model, we demonstrated that the CMP develop into APL by transducing *PML-RARA* whereas the resultant CD34$^-$ APL cells had the ability to maintain the tumor. Our system improves in the following points: The induced APL cells were detected in all of the mice within 150 days if more than 3,000 human CD34$^+$ cells infected with *PML-RARA* were transplanted into NOG mice. The resultant leukemia well recapitulated the human disease phenotypically, genetically and functionally, including the presence of Auer rods and Faggot cells, and the expression pattern of cellular surface markers and transcripts, as well as ATRA sensitivity and low leukemia transplantability. These findings demonstrated that this humanized *in vivo* model is suitable for prospectively analyzing the process of APL development in humans.

The cellular subset from which the APL originates is still controversial. Several lines of evidence using *in vivo* experiments have suggested that APL arises in the committed myeloid progenitors, whereas several clinical observations using FISH and RT-PCR analyses suggest that APL arises in earlier progenitors [4]. A recent report using conditional knock-in mice showed that the induction of *PML-RARA* led to dominant proliferation in a stem cell compartment with multilineage potential, but did not result in myeloproliferation, as if the stem cell compartment would not support leukemogenesis in this model [34,35]. Our *in vitro* and *in vivo* findings are compatible with the previous findings which showed that the generation of *PML-RARA* transgenic mice was only possible by expressing *PML-RARA* in early myeloid cells using the human cathepsin G (hCG) and MRP8 promoters, not the promoters of β-actin, a housekeeping gene, and CD11b which is expressed at a later stage of myeloid differentiation [36].

The leukemogenic function of PML-RARα may require subtle myeloid differentiation, as seen in CMP in the present study; PML-RARα has been reported to possess the inhibitory or toxic effects on the cellular survival, senescence or apoptosis [18,37,38]. CMP are still immature enough to easily acquire stemness and are already committed to the myeloid lineage, which may allow *PML-RARA* to dysregulate RARα-dependent myelopoiesis, rather than hematopoietic stem cells, in agreement with the fact that *RARA* is implicated in the regulation of myelopoiesis, including both early stage and terminal differentiation. In this scenario, the expression of *PML-RARA* would induce differentiation of CMP to promyelocytes, but inhibit their terminal differentiation at the same time [19,39,40]. Therefore, if the CMP expressing *PML-RARA* acquires stemness, this can result in the development of APL. Our findings showed no engraftment of CD34$^+$/CD38$^-$ cells with *PML-RARA* transduction *in vivo*, although their leukemogenic activity cannot be denied, as fewer cells were transplanted in comparison to the CD34$^+$/CD38$^+$ cells. Further analyses are required to evaluate whether CD34$^+$/CD38$^-$ cells possess the ability to cause APL.

Xenograft models using immunodeficient mice are at present the only method for evaluating the maintenance of human leukemia as LIC. The induced APL generated in the NOG mice had a low engraftment efficiency; however, this biological feature well-reproduced the properties of APL cells found in human patients [3,12]. It is possible that the difficulty associated with engrafting APL cells, both primary samples and induced APL cells obtained from cord blood, into NOG mice may depend on the different preferences of human hematopoietic cells between humans and mice. The reconstitution of the human hematopoietic system in NOG mice is achieved with the dominant engraftment of B-cells, in comparison to the myeloid lineage cells [10]. This technical feature may affect the engraftment of each of the transplanted cellular subsets in our study. The slow progressive myeloid tumor cells, such as those involved in myelodysplastic syndromes and chronic myeloid leukemia in the chronic phase, were shown to be difficult to engraft in NOD/SCID-β2-

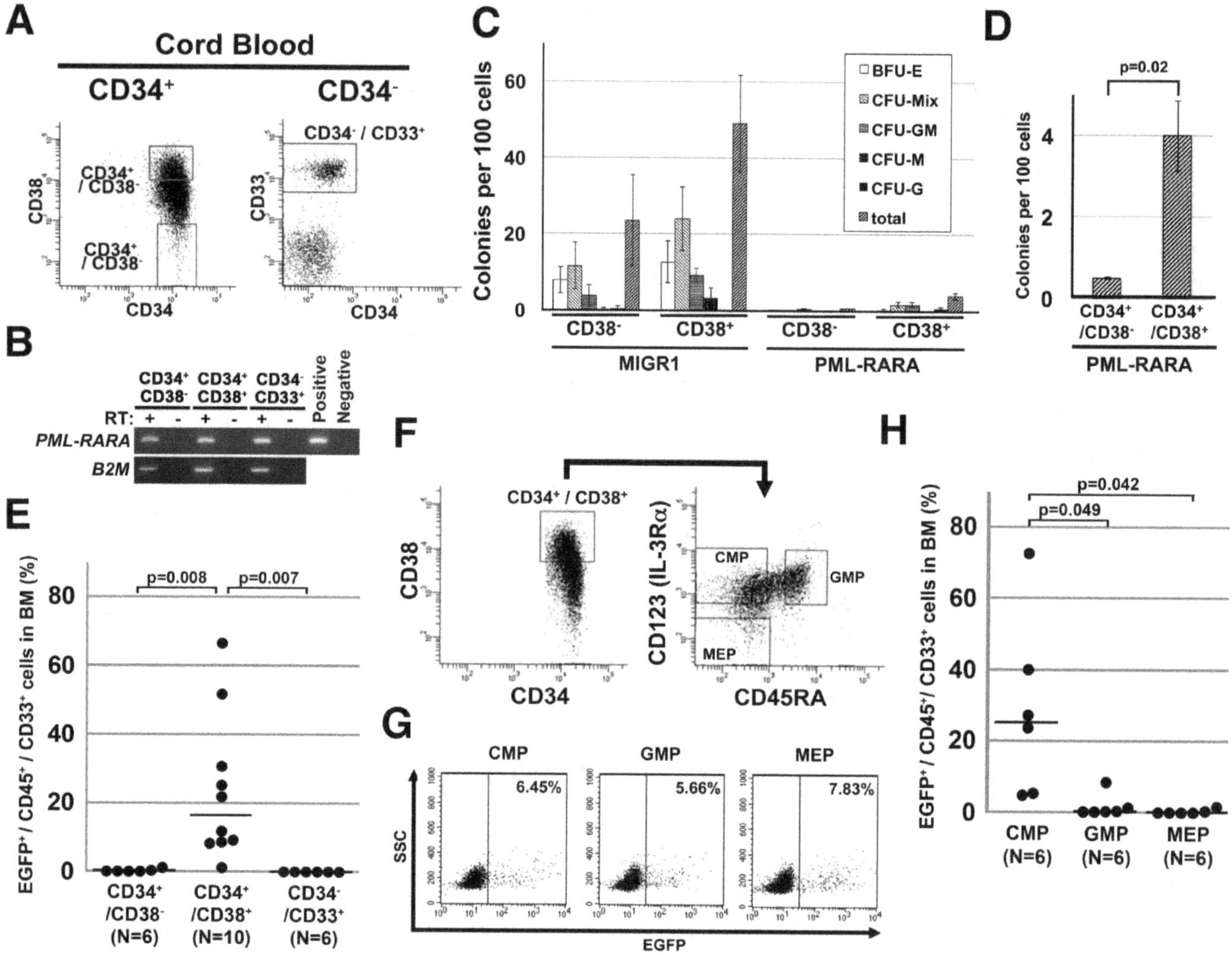

Figure 6. ***PML-RARA*** **targeted human common myeloid progenitors for APL leukemogenesis.** (**A**) The sorting strategy for CD34$^+$/CD38$^-$, CD34$^+$/CD38$^+$ and CD34$^-$/CD33$^+$ cells. Human cord blood was first separated into CD34$^+$ and CD34$^-$ cells by magnetic beads, and then sorted into three fractions by a FACS vantage instrument. (**B**) The expression of *PML-RARA* mRNA in each of the fractions after retroviral transfection. *B2M, beta 2 microglobulin.* The *PML-RARA* expression vector was used as a positive control for the *PML-RARA* analysis. (**C**) A colony-forming assay using *PML-RARA*-transduced CD34$^+$/CD38$^+$ and CD34$^+$/CD38$^-$ cells. The average of three independent experiments is shown. The data represent the means ± SD. (**D**) The total numbers of colonies of *PML-RARA*-transduced CD34$^+$/CD38$^+$ and CD34$^+$/CD38$^-$ cells shown in (C) are highlighted. The data represent the means ± SD (n = 3). (**E**) The development of the induced APL from CD34$^+$/CD38$^+$ cells in NOG mice. Each sorted fraction from human cord blood, as seen in (A), was retrovirally transduced with *PML-RARA* and transplanted into irradiated NOG mice. The percentages were determined by the frequency of EGFP$^+$/CD45$^+$/CD33$^+$ cells at 16 to 20 weeks after transplantation. Each dot represents a single mouse. The horizontal line represents the median value. (**F**) The sorting strategy for common myeloid progenitors (CMP), granulocyte-monocytic progenitors (GMP), and megakaryocyte-erythrocyte progenitors (MEP). Human cord blood was separated into CD34$^+$ cells by magnetic beads, CD34$^+$/CD38$^+$ cells were sorted out, and were finally divided into CMP, GMP and MEP by the FACS vantage instrument. (**G**) The transduction efficiency of *PML-RARA* in CMP, GMP and MEP. Representative data are shown. (**H**) The development of the induced APL from the human hematopoietic progenitors in NOG mice. Each sorted progenitor fraction from human cord blood, as seen in (F), was retrovirally transduced with *PML-RARA* and transplanted into irradiated NOG mice. The percentages were determined by the frequency of EGFP$^+$/CD45$^+$/CD33$^+$ cells at 16 to 20 weeks after transplantation. Each dot represents a single mouse. The horizontal line represents the median value.

microglobulin-deficient or NOG mice (the previous reports [41–43] and our unpublished data), suggesting that the engraftment failure did not always indicate a lack of leukemogenecity of the transplanted cells. Therefore, our study confirmed the leukemogenic activity of the CD34$^-$ induced APL fraction, although it was not strong. These results are consistent with the previous *in vivo* reports which described the some primary CD34$^+$/CD38$^+$ and CD34$^-$ AML cells could function as LIC *in vivo* [44,45].

In conclusion, we demonstrated that the induction of *PML-RARA* targeted human CD34$^+$ cells, including CMP, and led to their ability to cause APL, and that CD34$^-$ APL cells have the capability of maintaining the disease. These findings suggest that it is not necessary that LIC are always consistent with a cellular fraction where leukemia-inducing events occur. Tumor-specific oncogenes, such as *PML-RARA*, effectively function to form tumors with specific characteristics in specific hierarchal stages of myelopoiesis. This model differs from the conventional hierarchal system of AML, in which LIC possess an immature phenotype as seen in hematopoietic stem cells. Since AML is a group of heterogeneous diseases with various causal genetic abnormalities, the present findings will be helpful for the analysis of leukemogenesis in other types of AML which display differentiated leukemic blasts.

Supporting Information

Figure S1 The detection of *PML-RARA* expression in $CD34^+$ cells transduced with *PML-RARA* and their descendent colonies by qualitative RT-PCR. RT, reverse transcription.

Figure S2 Fluorescent images of the colonies derived from the $EGFP^+$ and $EGFP^-$ fractions of the $CD34^+$ cells transduced with *PML-RARA*.

Figure S3 The results of a quantitative analysis of the *PML-RARA* expression in the $CD34^+$ cells 48 hours after *PML-RARA* transduction, the differentiated cells from the resultant colonies and the induced APL cells. There were significant differences in the comparison of the expression level of *PML-RARA*. * indicates p values <0.05.

Figure S4 The heat map of the microarray analysis using the 3,439 probes (3,278 genes) that were differentially expressed in the induced APL (n = 3) and the AML other than APL (n = 62). The gene set separated the induced and human primary APL from the cases of AML other than APL. Red triangles (n = 2 from the total of 16 APL cases) show the clinical APL samples whose microarray data were obtained in this study.

Figure S5 The heat map of the microarray analysis performed using the gene set composed of 573 probes (547 genes), which were specifically expressed in the induced APL in comparison to cases of AML other than APL and normal promyelocytes. The gene set clearly clustered the malignant promyelocytes, such as the induced and human primary APL, apart from the normal promyelocytes. Red triangles (n = 2 of a total 16 APL cases) show the clinical APL samples whose microarray data were obtained in this study.

Table S1 The sequences of the PCR primers and probes.

Table S2 KEGG pathway analysis with the gene sets aberrantly expressed in the induced APL.

Table S3 The gene set apllied in Figure S5 (573 probes).

Table S4 The integration sites of PML-RARA in the induced APL cells.

Acknowledgments

We thank Dr. Warren S. Pear (University of Pennsylvania) for providing the MIGR1 retroviral vector, Dr. Toshio Kitamura (The University of Tokyo) for providing the PLAT-gp packaging cells, Dr. Guilherme Santos (Beth Israel Deaconess Medical Center, Harvard Medical School) for his valuable suggestions and comments, and Tomoko Uno and Tomomi Takanashi (Tokai University School of Medicine) for their expert technical assistance.

Author Contributions

Conceived and designed the experiments: H. Matsushita KA. Performed the experiments: H. Matsushita TY YS YN YM H. Matsuzawa TS AD H. Miyachi. Analyzed the data: H. Matsushita TY MT HH. Contributed reagents/materials/analysis tools: MO MI PPP. Wrote the paper: H. Matsushita TY KA.

References

1. Lowenberg B (2008) Acute myeloid leukemia: the challenge of capturing disease variety. Hematology Am Soc Hematol Educ Program: 1–11.
2. Lapidot T, Sirard C, Vormoor J, Murdoch B, Hoang T, et al. (1994) A cell initiating human acute myeloid leukaemia after transplantation into SCID mice. Nature 367: 645–648.
3. Bonnet D, Dick JE (1997) Human acute myeloid leukemia is organized as a hierarchy that originates from a primitive hematopoietic cell. Nat Med 3: 730–737.
4. Grimwade D, Enver T (2004) Acute promyelocytic leukemia: where does it stem from? Leukemia 18: 375–384.
5. Hope KJ, Jin L, Dick JE (2004) Acute myeloid leukemia originates from a hierarchy of leukemic stem cell classes that differ in self-renewal capacity. Nat Immunol 5: 738–743.
6. Dick JE (2008) Stem cell concepts renew cancer research. Blood 112: 4793–4807.
7. Becker MW, Jordan CT (2011) Leukemia stem cells in 2010: current understanding and future directions. Blood Rev 25: 75–81.
8. de The H, Chen Z (2010) Acute promyelocytic leukaemia: novel insights into the mechanisms of cure. Nat Rev Cancer 10: 775–783.
9. Paietta E (2003) Expression of cell-surface antigens in acute promyelocytic leukaemia. Best Pract Res Clin Haematol 16: 369–385.
10. Ito M, Hiramatsu H, Kobayashi K, Suzue K, Kawahata M, et al. (2002) NOD/SCID/gamma(c)(null) mouse: an excellent recipient mouse model for engraftment of human cells. Blood 100: 3175–3182.
11. Yahata T, Ando K, Nakamura Y, Ueyama Y, Shimamura K, et al. (2002) Functional human T lymphocyte development from cord blood CD34+ cells in nonobese diabetic/Shi-scid, IL-2 receptor gamma null mice. J Immunol 169: 204–209.
12. Patel S, Zhang Y, Cassinat B, Zassadowski F, Ferre N, et al. (2012) Successful xenografts of AML3 samples in immunodeficient NOD/shi-SCID IL2R-gamma(-/-) mice. Leukemia 26: 2432–2435.
13. Guibal FC, Alberich-Jorda M, Hirai H, Ebralidze A, Levantini E, et al. (2009) Identification of a myeloid committed progenitor as the cancer-initiating cell in acute promyelocytic leukemia. Blood 114: 5415–5425.
14. Wojiski S, Guibal FC, Kindler T, Lee BH, Jesneck JL, et al. (2009) PML-RARalpha initiates leukemia by conferring properties of self-renewal to committed promyelocytic progenitors. Leukemia 23: 1462–1471.
15. Brown D, Kogan S, Lagasse E, Weissman I, Alcalay M, et al. (1997) A PMLRARalpha transgene initiates murine acute promyelocytic leukemia. Proc Natl Acad Sci U S A 94: 2551–2556.
16. Grisolano JL, Wesselschmidt RL, Pelicci PG, Ley TJ (1997) Altered myeloid development and acute leukemia in transgenic mice expressing PML-RAR alpha under control of cathepsin G regulatory sequences. Blood 89: 376–387.
17. He LZ, Tribioli C, Rivi R, Peruzzi D, Pelicci PG, et al. (1997) Acute leukemia with promyelocytic features in PML/RARalpha transgenic mice. Proc Natl Acad Sci U S A 94: 5302–5307.
18. Westervelt P, Lane AA, Pollock JL, Oldfather K, Holt MS, et al. (2003) High-penetrance mouse model of acute promyelocytic leukemia with very low levels of PML-RARalpha expression. Blood 102: 1857–1865.
19. Grignani F, Valtieri M, Gabbianelli M, Gelmetti V, Botta R, et al. (2000) PML/RAR alpha fusion protein expression in normal human hematopoietic progenitors dictates myeloid commitment and the promyelocytic phenotype. Blood 96: 1531–1537.
20. Manz MG, Miyamoto T, Akashi K, Weissman IL (2002) Prospective isolation of human clonogenic common myeloid progenitors. Proc Natl Acad Sci U S A 99: 11872–11877.
21. Pear WS, Miller JP, Xu L, Pui JC, Soffer B, et al. (1998) Efficient and rapid induction of a chronic myelogenous leukemia-like myeloproliferative disease in mice receiving P210 bcr/abl-transduced bone marrow. Blood 92: 3780–3792.
22. Matsushita H, Scaglioni PP, Bhaumik M, Rego EM, Cai LF, et al. (2006) In vivo analysis of the role of aberrant histone deacetylase recruitment and RAR alpha blockade in the pathogenesis of acute promyelocytic leukemia. J Exp Med 203: 821–828.
23. Kawada H, Ando K, Tsuji T, Shimakura Y, Nakamura Y, et al. (1999) Rapid ex vivo expansion of human umbilical cord hematopoietic progenitors using a novel culture system. Exp Hematol 27: 904–915.
24. Yahata T, Takanashi T, Muguruma Y, Ibrahim AA, Matsuzawa H, et al. (2011) Accumulation of oxidative DNA damage restricts the self-renewal capacity of human hematopoietic stem cells. Blood 118: 2941–2950.

25. Rego EM, He LZ, Warrell RP Jr, Wang ZG, Pandolfi PP (2000) Retinoic acid (RA) and As2O3 treatment in transgenic models of acute promyelocytic leukemia (APL) unravel the distinct nature of the leukemogenic process induced by the PML-RARalpha and PLZF-RARalpha oncoproteins. Proc Natl Acad Sci U S A 97: 10173–10178.
26. Payton JE, Grieselhuber NR, Chang LW, Murakami M, Geiss GK, et al. (2009) High throughput digital quantification of mRNA abundance in primary human acute myeloid leukemia samples. J Clin Invest 119: 1714–1726.
27. Ando K, Yahata T, Sato T, Miyatake H, Matsuzawa H, et al. (2006) Direct evidence for ex vivo expansion of human hematopoietic stem cells. Blood 107: 3371–3377.
28. Schmidt M, Hoffmann G, Wissler M, Lemke N, Mussig A, et al. (2001) Detection and direct genomic sequencing of multiple rare unknown flanking DNA in highly complex samples. Hum Gene Ther 12: 743–749.
29. Dyck JA, Maul GG, Miller WH Jr, Chen JD, Kakizuka A, et al. (1994) A novel macromolecular structure is a target of the promyelocyte-retinoic acid receptor oncoprotein. Cell 76: 333–343.
30. Weis K, Rambaud S, Lavau C, Jansen J, Carvalho T, et al. (1994) Retinoic acid regulates aberrant nuclear localization of PML-RAR alpha in acute promyelocytic leukemia cells. Cell 76: 345–356.
31. Grignani F, Testa U, Rogaia D, Ferrucci PF, Samoggia P, et al. (1996) Effects on differentiation by the promyelocytic leukemia PML/RARalpha protein depend on the fusion of the PML protein dimerization and RARalpha DNA binding domains. EMBO J 15: 4949–4958.
32. Paietta E, Goloubeva O, Neuberg D, Bennett JM, Gallagher R, et al. (2004) A surrogate marker profile for PML/RAR alpha expressing acute promyelocytic leukemia and the association of immunophenotypic markers with morphologic and molecular subtypes. Cytometry B Clin Cytom 59: 1–9.
33. Welch JS, Ley TJ, Link DC, Miller CA, Larson DE, et al. (2012) The origin and evolution of mutations in acute myeloid leukemia. Cell 150: 264–278.
34. Welch JS, Yuan W, Ley TJ (2011) PML-RARA can increase hematopoietic self-renewal without causing a myeloproliferative disease in mice. J Clin Invest 121: 1636–1645.
35. Wartman LD, Welch JS, Uy GL, Klco JM, Lamprecht T, et al. (2012) Expression and function of PML-RARA in the hematopoietic progenitor cells of Ctsg-PML-RARA mice. PLoS One 7: e46529.
36. Puccetti E, Ruthardt M (2004) Acute promyelocytic leukemia: PML/RARalpha and the leukemic stem cell. Leukemia 18: 1169–1175.
37. Ferrucci PF, Grignani F, Pearson M, Fagioli M, Nicoletti I, et al. (1997) Cell death induction by the acute promyelocytic leukemia-specific PML/RARalpha fusion protein. Proc Natl Acad Sci U S A 94: 10901–10906.
38. Grignani F, Ferrucci PF, Testa U, Talamo G, Fagioli M, et al. (1993) The acute promyelocytic leukemia-specific PML-RAR alpha fusion protein inhibits differentiation and promotes survival of myeloid precursor cells. Cell 74: 423–431.
39. Collins SJ (2002) The role of retinoids and retinoic acid receptors in normal hematopoiesis. Leukemia 16: 1896–1905.
40. Du C, Redner RL, Cooke MP, Lavau C (1999) Overexpression of wild-type retinoic acid receptor alpha (RARalpha) recapitulates retinoic acid-sensitive transformation of primary myeloid progenitors by acute promyelocytic leukemia RARalpha-fusion genes. Blood 94: 793–802.
41. Thanopoulou E, Cashman J, Kakagianne T, Eaves A, Zoumbos N, et al. (2004) Engraftment of NOD/SCID-beta2 microglobulin null mice with multilineage neoplastic cells from patients with myelodysplastic syndrome. Blood 103: 4285–4293.
42. Kerbauy DM, Lesnikov V, Torok-Storb B, Bryant E, Deeg HJ (2004) Engraftment of distinct clonal MDS-derived hematopoietic precursors in NOD/SCID-beta2-microglobulin-deficient mice after intramedullary transplantation of hematopoietic and stromal cells. Blood 104: 2202–2203.
43. Muguruma Y, Matsushita H, Yahata T, Yumino S, Tanaka Y, et al. (2011) Establishment of a xenograft model of human myelodysplastic syndromes. Haematologica 96: 543–551.
44. Taussig DC, Vargaftig J, Miraki-Moud F, Griessinger E, Sharrock K, et al. (2010) Leukemia-initiating cells from some acute myeloid leukemia patients with mutated nucleophosmin reside in the CD34(-) fraction. Blood 115: 1976–1984.
45. Eppert K, Takenaka K, Lechman ER, Waldron L, Nilsson B, et al. (2011) Stem cell gene expression programs influence clinical outcome in human leukemia. Nat Med 17: 1086–1093.

Permissions

All chapters in this book were first published in PLOS ONE, by The Public Library of Science; hereby published with permission under the Creative Commons Attribution License or equivalent. Every chapter published in this book has been scrutinized by our experts. Their significance has been extensively debated. The topics covered herein carry significant findings which will fuel the growth of the discipline. They may even be implemented as practical applications or may be referred to as a beginning point for another development.

The contributors of this book come from diverse backgrounds, making this book a truly international effort. This book will bring forth new frontiers with its revolutionizing research information and detailed analysis of the nascent developments around the world.

We would like to thank all the contributing authors for lending their expertise to make the book truly unique. They have played a crucial role in the development of this book. Without their invaluable contributions this book wouldn't have been possible. They have made vital efforts to compile up to date information on the varied aspects of this subject to make this book a valuable addition to the collection of many professionals and students.

This book was conceptualized with the vision of imparting up-to-date information and advanced data in this field. To ensure the same, a matchless editorial board was set up. Every individual on the board went through rigorous rounds of assessment to prove their worth. After which they invested a large part of their time researching and compiling the most relevant data for our readers.

The editorial board has been involved in producing this book since its inception. They have spent rigorous hours researching and exploring the diverse topics which have resulted in the successful publishing of this book. They have passed on their knowledge of decades through this book. To expedite this challenging task, the publisher supported the team at every step. A small team of assistant editors was also appointed to further simplify the editing procedure and attain best results for the readers.

Apart from the editorial board, the designing team has also invested a significant amount of their time in understanding the subject and creating the most relevant covers. They scrutinized every image to scout for the most suitable representation of the subject and create an appropriate cover for the book.

The publishing team has been an ardent support to the editorial, designing and production team. Their endless efforts to recruit the best for this project, has resulted in the accomplishment of this book. They are a veteran in the field of academics and their pool of knowledge is as vast as their experience in printing. Their expertise and guidance has proved useful at every step. Their uncompromising quality standards have made this book an exceptional effort. Their encouragement from time to time has been an inspiration for everyone.

The publisher and the editorial board hope that this book will prove to be a valuable piece of knowledge for researchers, students, practitioners and scholars across the globe.

List of Contributors

Hailong Zhang, Lubing Gu, Tao Liu, Kuang-Yueh Chiang and Muxiang Zhou
Department of Pediatrics and Aflac C ancer and Blood Disorders Center, Emory University School of Medicine, Atlanta, Georgia, United States of America

Sheila Xinxuan Soh and John W. J. Huang
Cancer and Stem Cell Biology Program, Duke-NUS Graduate Medical School, Singapore, Singapore

S. Tiong Ong
Cancer and Stem Cell Biology Program, Duke-NUS Graduate Medical School, Singapore, Singapore
Department of Haematology, Singapore General Hospital, Singapore, Singapore
Department of Medical Oncology, National Cancer Centre, Singapore, Singapore
Division of Medical Oncology, Duke University Medical Center, Durham, North Carolina, United States of America

Joshua Yew Suang Lim and Nan Jiang
Department of Paediatrics, Yong Loo Lin School of Medicine, National University of Singapore, Singapore, Singapore

Allen Eng Juh Yeoh
Department of Paediatrics, Yong Loo Lin School of Medicine, National University of Singapore, Singapore, Singapore
National University Cancer Institute, National University Health System, Singapore, Singapore,
Viva-University Children's Cancer Centre, University Children's Medical Institute, National University Health System, Singapore, Singapore
Cancer Science Institute, National University of Singapore, Singapore, Singapore

Martijn E. T. Dollé, Bhawani Nagarajah, Marianne Roodbergen and Piet de With
National Institute for Public Health and the Environment, Bilthoven, The Netherlands

Erwin Reiling
National Institute for Public Health and the Environment, Bilthoven, The Netherlands
Department of Cell Biology and Genetics, Center for Biomedical Genetics, Erasmus MC, Rotterdam, The Netherlands

Harry van Steeg
National Institute for Public Health and the Environment, Bilthoven, The Netherlands
Department of Toxicogenetics, Leiden University Medical Center, Leiden, The Netherlands

Jan H. Hoeijmakers
Department of Cell Biology and Genetics, Center for Biomedical Genetics, Erasmus MC, Rotterdam, The Netherlands

Sameh A. Youssef and Alain de Bruin
Faculty of Veterinary Medicine, Department of Pathobiology, Utrecht University, Utrecht, The Netherlands

Moonsook Lee and Jan Vijg
Department of Genetics, Albert Einstein College of Medicine, Bronx, New York, United States of America

Paul Hasty
Department of Molecular Medicine and Institute of Biotechnology, Barshop Institute for Longevity and Aging Studies, Cancer Therapy and Research Center, University of Texas Health Science Center at San Antonio, San Antonio, Texas, United States of America

Ioannis Panagopoulos and Ludmila Gorunova
Section for Cancer Cytogenetics, Institute for Cancer Genetics and Informatics, The Norwegian Radium Hospital, Oslo University Hospital, Oslo, Norway
Centre for Cancer Biomedicine, Faculty of Medicine, University of Oslo, Oslo, Norway

Synne Torkildsen
Section for Cancer Cytogenetics, Institute for Cancer Genetics and Informatics, The Norwegian Radium Hospital, Oslo University Hospital, Oslo, Norway
Centre for Cancer Biomedicine, Faculty of Medicine, University of Oslo, Oslo, Norway
Department of Hematology, Oslo University Hospital, Oslo, Norway

Sverre Heim
Section for Cancer Cytogenetics, Institute for Cancer Genetics and Informatics, The Norwegian Radium Hospital, Oslo University Hospital, Oslo, Norway
Centre for Cancer Biomedicine, Faculty of Medicine, University of Oslo, Oslo, Norway
Faculty of Medicine, University of Oslo, Oslo, Norway

Geir E. Tjønnfjord
Department of Hematology, Oslo University Hospital, Oslo, Norway
Faculty of Medicine, University of Oslo, Oslo, Norway

Anne Tierens
Department of Pathology, The Norwegian Radium Hospital, Oslo University Hospital, Oslo, Norway

Dongmin Gu, Isere Kuiatse, Hua Wang, Jin He, Richard J. Jones, Chad C. Bjorklund and Jing Yang
Department of Lymphoma/Myeloma, The University of Texas MD Anderson Cancer Center, Houston, Texas, United States of America

Robert Z. Orlowski
Department of Lymphoma/Myeloma, The University of Texas MD Anderson Cancer Center, Houston, Texas, United States of America
Department of Experimental Therapeutics, The University of Texas MD Anderson Cancer Center, Houston, Texas, United States of America

Shuhong Wang
Department of Hematology, Chinese PLA General Hospital, Beijing, China

Yun Dai and Steven Grant
Department of Medicine, Virginia Commonwealth University, Richmond, Virginia, United States of America

Kaini Shen, Daobin Zhou and Jian Li
Department of Hematology, Peking Union Medical College Hospital, Chinese Academy of Medical Sciences and Peking Union Medical College, Beijing, People's Republic of China

Gufeng Xu
Zhejiang University, School of Medicine, Hangzhou, Zhejiang, People's Republic of China

Qing Wu
Division of Health Sciences Research, Mayo Clinic, Scottsdale, Arizona, United States of America

Li-Xu Yan, Yan-Hui Liu, Dong-Lan Luo, Fen Zhang, Yu Cheng, Xin-Lan Luo, Jie Xu, Jie Cheng and Heng-Guo Zhuang
Department of Pathology, Guangdong General Hospital, Guangdong Academy of Medical Science, Guangzhou, China

Leila Dardaei, Livia Modica, Giorgio Iotti and Francesco Blasi
Fondazione Istituto FIRC di Oncologia Molecolare (IFOM), Milan, Italy

Nicole Bethge, Vera Hilden and Erlend B. Smeland
Department of Immunology, Institute for Cancer Research, Oslo University Hospital, Oslo, Norway
Centre for Cancer Biomedicine, University of Oslo, Oslo, Norway

Hilde Honne, Kim Andresen and Guro E. Lind
Centre for Cancer Biomedicine, University of Oslo, Oslo, Norway
Department of Cancer Prevention, Institute for Cancer Research, Oslo University Hospital, Oslo, Norway

Knut Liestøl
Centre for Cancer Biomedicine, University of Oslo, Oslo, Norway
Department of Informatics, University of Oslo, Oslo, Norway

Harald Holte
Centre for Cancer Biomedicine, University of Oslo, Oslo, Norway
Department of Oncology, The Norwegian Radium Hospital, Oslo University Hospital, Oslo, Norway

Gunhild Trøen and Jan Delabie
Department of Pathology, Oslo University Hospital, Oslo, Norway

Wei-da Wang, Qi-rong Geng, Liang Wang, Xiao-qin Chen, Cheng-cheng Liu and Yue Lv
Department of Hematologic Oncology, Sun Yat-Sen University Cancer Center, Guangzhou, Guangdong, P.R.China
State Key Laboratory of Oncology in South China, Guangzhou, Guangdong, P. R. China

Jing Zhang
Department of Hematologic Oncology, Sun Yat-Sen University Cancer Center, Guangzhou, Guangdong, P.R.China
State Key Laboratory of Oncology in South China, Guangzhou, Guangdong, P. R. China
Department of Medical Oncology, Hubei Cancer Hospital, Wuhan, Hubei, P. R. China

Adil D. Duru, Johan Liwing and Gösta Gahrton
Department of Medicine, Karolinska Institutet Huddinge, Stockholm, Sweden

Katarina Uttervall, Johan Lund, Evren Alici and Hareth Nahi
Department of Medicine, Karolinska Institutet Huddinge, Stockholm, Sweden
Hematology Center, Karolinska University Hospital Huddinge, Stockholm, Sweden

Erik Holmberg
Department of Oncology, Institute of Clinical Sciences, Sahlgrenska Academy at University of Gothenburg, Sweden

Johan Aschan
Janssen-Cilag AB, Sollentuna, Sweden

Michael M. Weil, F. Andrew Ray, Paula C. Genik and Christina M. Fallgren
Colorado State University, Fort Collins, Colorado, United States of America

Yongjia Yu, Maureen McCarthy and Robert L. Ullrich
University of Texas Medical Branch, Galveston, Texas, United States of America

Serena De Vita, Michael Garcia, Jenna Wood, Mathilde Gavillet and David A. Williams
Division of Hematology/Oncology, Boston Children's Hospital, Harvard Medical School, Boston, Massachusetts, United States of America

Rebekka K. Schneider, Benjamin L. Ebert and Ann Mullally
Division of Hematology, Department of Medicine, Brigham and Women's Hospital, Harvard Medical School, Boston, Massachusetts, United States of America

Alexander Gerbaulet and Axel Roers
Institute for Immunology, Medical Faculty Carl Gustav Carus, Dresden University of Technology, Dresden, Germany

Ross L. Levine
Human Oncology and Pathogenesis Program, and Leukemia Service, Department of Medicine, Memorial Sloan-Kettering Cancer Center, New York, New York, United States of America

Eszter Szánthó, Harjit Pal Bhattoa, Mária Csobán, Péter Antal-Szalmás, Anikó Újfalusi, János Kappelmayer and Zsuzsanna Hevessy
Department of Laboratory Medicine, Medical and Health Science Center, University of Debrecen, Debrecen, Hungary

Liu-Fei Luo,Yuan-Fang Liu, Sai-Juan Chen and Keqin Kathy Li
State Key Laboratory of Medical Genomics, Shanghai Institute of Hematology, Rui Jin Hospital Affiliated to Shanghai Jiao Tong University School of Medicine, Shanghai, China

Limin Chen
State Key Laboratory of Medical Genomics, Shanghai Institute of Hematology, Rui Jin Hospital Affiliated to Shanghai Jiao Tong University School of Medicine, Shanghai, China
Drug Discovery and Design Center, State Key Laboratory of Drug Research, Shanghai Institute of Materia Medica, Chinese Academy of Sciences, Shanghai, China

Junyan Lu, Lianchun Li, Jiang Wang, Hong Liu, Hualiang Jiang and Cheng Luo
Drug Discovery and Design Center, State Key Laboratory of Drug Research, Shanghai Institute of Materia Medica, Chinese Academy of Sciences, Shanghai, China

Heng Song
Department of Chemistry, East China University of Science and Technology, Shanghai, China

Enrique M. Ocio
Centro de Investigación del Cáncer, Instituto de Biología Molecular y Celular del Cáncer/Consejo Superior de Investigaciones Científicas-Universidad de Salamanca, Salamanca, Spain
Hospital Universitario de Salamanca, Salamanca, Spain
Instituto de Investigación Biomédica de Salamanca (IBSAL), Salamanca, Spain

Teresa Paíno, Patryk Krzeminski, Laura San-Segundo and Mercedes Garayoa
Centro de Investigación del Cáncer, Instituto de Biología Molecular y Celular del Cáncer/Consejo Superior de Investigaciones Científicas-Universidad de Salamanca, Salamanca, Spain
Instituto de Investigación Biomédica de Salamanca (IBSAL), Salamanca, Spain

Luis A. Corchete and Alba Redondo
Hospital Universitario de Salamanca, Salamanca, Spain

María E. Sarasquete, Ramón García-Sanz and Norma C. Gutiérrez
Hospital Universitario de Salamanca, Salamanca, Spain
Instituto de Investigación Biomédica de Salamanca (IBSAL), Salamanca, Spain

Bruno Paiva and Jesús F. San-Miguel
Clínica Universidad de Navarra; Centro de Investigaciones Me´dicas Aplicadas (CIMA), Pamplona, Spain

Dammy Pinheiro, Hannah Bryant and Tim Dalessandri
Department of Clinical Sciences and Services, Immune Regulation Laboratory, The Royal Veterinary College, London, United Kingdom

Oliver A. Garden
Department of Clinical Sciences and Services, Immune Regulation Laboratory, The Royal Veterinary College, London, United Kingdom
Department of Clinical Sciences and Services, Queen Mother Hospital for Animals, The Royal Veterinary College, Hatfield, Hertfordshire, United Kingdom

Yu-Mei Chang
Research Office, The Royal Veterinary College, London, United Kingdom

Balazs Szladovits
Department of Pathology and Pathogen Biology, The Royal Veterinary College, Hatfield, Hertfordshire, United Kingdom

Lucy J. Davison
Henry Wellcome Building, Centre for Cellular and Molecular Physiology, University of Oxford, Oxford, United Kingdom
Department of Veterinary Medicine, University of Cambridge, Cambridge, United Kingdom

Elizabeth Yallop and Emily Mills
Clinical Investigation Centre, The Royal Veterinary College, Hatfield, Hertfordshire, United Kingdom

Chiara Leo, Ana Lara and Anneliese Stell
Department of Clinical Sciences and Services, Queen Mother Hospital for Animals, The Royal Veterinary College, Hatfield, Hertfordshire, United Kingdom

Gerry Polton
Oncology Service, North Downs Specialist Referrals, Bletchingley, Surrey, United Kingdom

Gelin Xu, Zhizhong Zhang, Qiushi Lv, Yun Li, Ruidong Ye, Yunyun Xiong, Yongjun Jiang and Xinfeng Liu
Department of Neurology, Jinling Hospital, Nanjing University School of Medicine, Nanjing, Jiangsu Province, China

Wenjun Zhao, Lirong Wei, Dongming Tan, Guangsong Su, Yanwen Zheng and Chao He
Cyrus Tang Hematology Center, Jiangsu Institute of Hematology, the First Affiliated Hospital, Soochow University, Suzhou, Jiangsu Province, PR China

Bin Yin
Cyrus Tang Hematology Center, Jiangsu Institute of Hematology, the First Affiliated Hospital, Soochow University, Suzhou, Jiangsu Province, PR China
Thrombosis and Hemostasis Key Lab of the Ministry of Health, Soochow University, Suzhou, Jiangsu Province, PR China
Collaborative Innovation Center of Hematology, Soochow University, Suzhou, Jiangsu Province, PR China

Zhengwei J. Mao
Division of Hematopathology, Department of Laboratory Medicine and Pathology, University of Minnesota Medical Center-Fairview, Minneapolis, Minnesota, United States of America

Timothy P. Singleton
Department of Laboratory of Medicine and Pathology, University of Minnesota, Minneapolis, Minnesota, United States of America

Stephanie Schneider, Bianka Ksienzyk, Gudrun Mellert and Evelyn Zellmeier
Laboratory for Leukemia Diagnostics, Dept. of Internal Medicine III, University Hospital Munich Großhadern, Ludwig-Maximilian-University (LMU), Munich, Germany

Friederike Pastore, Philipp A. Greif, Wolfgang Hiddemann and Karsten Spiekermann
Laboratory for Leukemia Diagnostics, Dept. of Internal Medicine III, University Hospital Munich Großhadern, Ludwig-Maximilian-University (LMU), Munich, Germany
Clinical Cooperative Group Pathogenesis of Acute Myeloid Leukemia, Helmholtz Zentrum München, German Research Center for Environmental Health, Munich, Germany
German Cancer Consortium (DKTK), Heidelberg, Germany
German Cancer Research Center (DKFZ), Heidelberg, Germany

Jan Braess
Dept. of Oncology and Hematology, Krankenhaus Barmherzige Brüder, Regensburg, Germany

Cristina M. Sauerland and Achim Heinecke
Institute of Biostatistics and Clinical Research, University of Muenster, Muenster, Germany

Utz Krug, Wolfgang E. Berdel and Thomas Buechner
Dept. of Internal Medicine A, Hematology and Oncology, University of Muenster, Muenster, Germany

Bernhard Woermann
German Society of Hematology and Oncology, Berlin, Germany

Yin Sheng, Yoshihiko Nakamura and Yukari Muguruma
Research Center for Cancer Stem Cell, Tokai University School of Medicine, Isehara, Kanagawa, Japan

Hideyuki Matsuzawa
Research Center for Cancer Stem Cell, Tokai University School of Medicine, Isehara, Kanagawa, Japan
Support Center for Medical Research and Education, Tokai University, Isehara, Kanagawa, Japan

Hiromichi Matsushita
Research Center for Cancer Stem Cell, Tokai University School of Medicine, Isehara, Kanagawa, Japan
Medical Research Institute, Tokai University, Isehara, Kanagawa,Japan
Department of Laboratory Medicine, Tokai University School of Medicine, Isehara, Kanagawa, Japan

Takashi Yahata
Research Center for Cancer Stem Cell, Tokai University School of Medicine, Isehara, Kanagawa, Japan
Medical Research Institute, Tokai University, Isehara, Kanagawa,Japan
Department of Cell Transplantation, Tokai University School of Medicine, Isehara, Kanagawa, Japan

Kiyoshi Ando
Research Center for Cancer Stem Cell, Tokai University School of Medicine, Isehara, Kanagawa, Japan
Medical Research Institute, Tokai University, Isehara, Kanagawa,Japan
Division of Hematology and Oncology, Department of Internal Medicine, Tokai University School of Medicine, Isehara, Kanagawa, Japan

Anar Damdinsuren and Hayato Miyachi
Department of Laboratory Medicine, Tokai University School of Medicine, Isehara, Kanagawa, Japan

Masayuki Tanaka, Hideki Hayashi and Tadayuki Sato
Support Center for Medical Research and Education, Tokai University, Isehara, Kanagawa, Japan

Makoto Onizuka
Division of Hematology and Oncology, Department of Internal Medicine, Tokai University School of Medicine, Isehara, Kanagawa, Japan

Mamoru Ito
Central Institute for Experimental Animals, Kawasaki, Kanagawa, Japan

Pier Paolo Pandolfi
Cancer Research Institute, Beth Israel Deaconess Cancer Center, Departments of Medicine and Pathology, Beth Israel Deaconess Medical Center, Harvard Medical School, Boston, Massachusetts, United States of America

Index

A

Active Kit, 116, 127

Acute Lymphoblastic Leukemia, 1, 8-10, 19-20, 120, 128, 139, 148, 195-196

Acute Myeloid Leukemia, 30-31, 35, 73, 79, 108, 110, 114, 128, 136, 139, 147-148, 159, 186, 195-198, 200-203, 213-214

Ara-c, 136-137, 139-140, 142, 145-146, 186-187, 189-195

Autoimmune Disease, 49, 55-56, 175

Autophagy, 37-39, 41-42, 44, 48, 148

B

Bcl2, 9, 19, 57-68, 70-72, 80-81, 148, 192

Bcl6, 57-68, 70-72, 158

Bim Deletion, 9-12, 14, 16-17, 19

Bortezomib, 37-38, 44, 47-48, 98-101, 103-107, 149, 151-152, 154, 157

Breast Cancer, 87, 130, 135, 159, 175, 177, 182

C

Cd138++, 149, 151-155, 157-158

Cd138low, 149, 151-155, 157-159

Cell Apoptosis, 1-2, 136-137, 141, 145

Cell Death, 8-10, 14, 28, 37, 39, 41, 44, 46-48, 88, 126, 136-137, 139, 141, 144-148, 194-195

Chromosomal Copy Number, 48

Chronic Lymphocytic Leukemia, 129, 135, 147

Chronic Myelogenous Leukemia, 1, 148, 213

Cirrhosis, 113, 177, 182

Clonogenic Cells, 149, 157, 159

Cyclophosphamide, 57, 72, 89, 99, 165, 168, 173-175

Cytosol, 39, 138

Cytotoxicity, 1, 4, 41, 48, 99, 106, 147, 187, 189, 191

D

D184v Mutation, 120

Dermatomyositis, 54-55

Diffuse Large B-cell Lymphoma, 57, 71-72, 80-81, 83-84, 86, 88, 91, 96, 174-175

Dna-pkcs, 21-24, 27-28

Dusp4, 80-86

E

E3 Ligase, 37, 48

Endogenous Ceramide, 136, 147

F

Flow Cytometry, 3-4, 7, 37-39, 41-42, 44, 47, 77-79, 130, 137, 139, 141-142, 144-145, 151-152, 157, 162, 174, 187, 191, 204

Flt3-itd, 194, 196-201

Fluorescence in Situ Hybridization, 30, 39, 57, 71, 130

Foxp3+ T Cells, 161, 166, 170-171, 175

Fty720, 136-148

G

G-banding, 30-32

Glucocorticoids, 9

H

Hematopoietic Cells, 2, 8, 73-75, 96, 122, 128, 203-204, 208, 211

Hepatocellular Carcinoma, 108, 111, 113-115, 134

Hodgkin's Lymphoma, 56, 71-72, 86, 88, 96, 129, 134-135, 173-174

Hypermethylated, 80, 86

I

Interleukin-9, 88, 96-97

K

Kat6a-crebbp, 30-33, 35

Ku80 Deficiency, 21, 28

L

Lenalidomide, 37-38, 44, 46-48, 98-99, 101, 103-106, 159

Leukemia-initiating Cells, 203, 214

Leukemic Cells, 7, 19, 30-31, 73, 75-77, 138-139, 148, 186-195, 203, 207-208

Lrp12, 80-86

Lymphomagenesis, 79, 88, 91, 127, 175

M

Malignant Plasma Cells, 55, 149, 159

Mast Cell Leukemia, 116-117

Mdm2, 1-8, 37-40, 42, 44, 46-48

Meis1, 73-79, 196

Mm-csc, 149, 157-158

Multi-agent Chemotherapy, 9-10

Multiple Myeloma, 37, 44, 46-56, 86, 98-99, 101-103, 106-107, 149, 151-152, 159-160, 178, 181, 183

Myeloid Progenitors, 79, 136, 203-204, 211-214
Myeloproliferative Neoplasms, 116, 148

N
Neutropenic, 218
Nilotinib, 1-8
Nk/t-cell Lymphoma, 88, 91
Non-hodgkin Lymphoma, 56, 161, 173-174
Npm1 Mutation, 194-201

P
Peripheral Blood Mononuclear Cells, 80-81, 127, 137
Philadelphia Positive, 1
Pml-rara, 193, 203-208, 210-214
Polymyositis, 54-55
Prep1, 73-76, 78-79
Primary Mediastinal B-cell Lymphoma, 80, 83-84

R
Renal Impairment, 98-107
Rheumatoid Arthritis, 49, 51-52, 56
Rna- Sequencing, 30
Rt-pcr, 2-3, 5-6, 12, 30-33, 35, 147-148, 204-205, 207, 211, 213

S
Schizophrenia, 177, 182
Serum Thymidine Kinase Activity, 129, 131-134
Sphingolipid Metabolism, 136-137, 140, 142-143, 146-148, 208
Systemic Mastocytosis, 116, 118, 122, 127-128

T
Thalidomide, 37, 98-99, 101, 103-106
Tyrosine Kinase Inhibitors, 1, 8-10, 19, 116

www.ingramcontent.com/pod-product-compliance
Lightning Source LLC
LaVergne TN
LVHW060559210926
848485LV00005B/1342